NURSING IN TODAY'S WORLD

Challenges

NURSING IN TODAY'S WORLD

Challenges, Issues, and Trends

7th Edition

Janice Rider Ellis, RN, PhD
Professor of Nursing
Director of Nursing Education
Shoreline Community College
Seattle, WA

Celia Love Hartley, RN, MN
Professor Emerita
Nursing and Health Sciences
College of the Desert
Palm Desert, CA

Illustrations by Kari Berger

Lippincott
Philadelphia · New York · Baltimore

Acquisitions Editor: Margaret Zuccarini
Editorial Assistant: Helen Kogut
Project Editor: Debra Schiff
Senior Production Manager: Helen Ewan
Senior Production Coordinator: Nannette Winski
Design Coordinator: Risa Clow
Indexer: Michael Ferreira
Manufacturing Manager: William Alberti
7th Edition

Library of Congress Cataloging-in-Publication Data

Ellis, Janice Rider.
 Nursing in today's world : challenges, issues, and trends / Janice Rider Ellis, Celia Love
Hartley; illustrations by Kari Berger.—7th ed.
  p. ; cm.
 Includes bibliographical references and index.
 ISBN 0-7817-2455-4 (alk. paper)
 1. Nursing. 2. Nursing—Practice—United States. I. Hartley, Celia Love. II. Title.
 [DNLM: 1. Nursing—trends—United States. 2. Delivery of Health Care—trends—United
States. 3. Education, Nursing—United States. 4. Ethics, Nursing—United States. 5
Legislation, Nursing—United States. 6. Licensure, Nursing—United States. WY 16 E47n 2000]
RT82 .E45 2000
610.73—dc21
                                                                              00-042402

Care has been taken to confirm the accuracy of the information presented and to describe generally accepted practices. However, the authors, editors, and publisher are not responsible for errors or omissions or for any consequences from application of the information in this book and make no warranty, express or implied, with respect to the contents of the publication.

The authors, editors, and publisher have exerted every effort to ensure that drug selection and dosage set forth in this text are in accordance with current recommendations and practice at the time of publication. However, in view of ongoing research, changes in government regulations, and the constant flow of information relating to drug therapy and drug reactions, the reader is urged to check the package insert for each drug for any change in indications and dosage and for added warnings and precautions. This is particularly important when the recommended agent is a new or infrequently employed drug.

Some drugs and medical devices presented in this publication have Food and Drug Administration (FDA) clearance for limited use in restricted research settings. It is the responsibility of the health care provider to ascertain the FDA status of each drug or device planned for use in his or her clinical practice.

Reviewers

Mary Ann Cosgarea, RN, BA, BSN
Nurse Administrator
Portage Lakes Career Center
W. Howard Nicol School of Practical Nursing
Green, Ohio

Mary Jane Hanson, RN, CRNP, CS, PhD
Assistant Professor, Director of Graduate Programs
University of Scranton
Scranton, Pennsylvania

Nancy Harms, RN, PhD
Chair of Nursing Division
Midland Lutheran College
Fremont, Nebraska

Mabel H. Smith, RN, JD, PhD
Associate Professor
Old Dominion University
College of Health Sciences, School of Nursing
Norfolk, Virginia

Russell Tranbarger, RN, EdD, CNAA
Associate Professor
East Carolina University
School of Nursing
Greenville, North Carolina

Robert H. Welton, RN, MSN
Professional Development Coordinator
Patient Care Services
University of Maryland Medical System
Baltimore, Maryland

Ruth Yanos, RN, BSN, MSN
Chair, Department of Nursing
Delaware Technical and Community College
Dover, Delaware

Preface

With this, the seventh edition, *Nursing in Today's World: Challenges, Issues, and Trends* celebrates its twenty-first birthday. There have been many changes in nursing since the first edition was published in 1980. Nursing care delivery has moved from one focused on primary care with a single individual planning care for a client from admission until discharge within an acute care facility, to one of managed care where a multidisciplinary team is involved in care through a variety of levels and institutions. Care was provided primarily in acute care facilities, many of which were non-profit organizations owned by communities or religious organizations. Today care occurs as much outside the acute care facility (which likely is owned by a health care conglomerate) as it occurs within it. The advent of diagnosis related groups (DRGs) revolutionized the payment for services, moving the United States from a fee-for-service method of charging for health services to a prospective payment system. The clientele we serve also has changed to represent an older, more diverse population that is looking forward to an increased life span. Consumers have become more involved in decisions that are to be reached about their health and carry more responsibility for acting and living responsibly. New technology and research have revolutionized what can be accomplished in treatment. Better diagnostic measures, more effective pharmaceutical agents, and treatment modalities that provide miraculous recovery for once fatal conditions have significantly influenced patient outcomes.

In a serious effort to bring the student the realities of the health care delivery system and nursing, this textbook also has changed throughout the metamorphosis of health care. This remains true in this seventh edition.

WHAT'S NEW?

- *Web site information provided two ways*—within each chapter you will find **references to Web sites** that will assist in locating information pertinent to the topics discussed; at the end of each chapter are separate lists of **relevant Web sites**. In an age of information and knowledge explosion, being able to access the most recent information is critical to informed decision making.
- *Critical Thinking Activity* (feature)—Another element that dominates the educational environment is that of greater learner interactivity and critical thinking. Interspersed throughout each chapter of *Nursing in Today's World* are activities that stimulate and perfect critical thinking abilities.

- *New and Update Chapter Content*—All content is updated. Examples include an exploration of issues related to multistate licensure, a discussion about maintaining professional boundaries, tables reflecting the distribution of NCLEX examinations content, expansion of workplace concerns, a new appendix on commonly used acronyms, and more.

TEXT ORGANIZATION

We begin the text with an overview of economic and political aspects of health care delivery, believing that students can better determine nursing's place in the health care delivery system if they have some introduction to that system, how it got to where it is today, how it operates, how it is financed, and how it is politically influenced. Some of you like this approach; others prefer a more traditional organizational approach. For those who opt for a chronological approach, we encourage you to adapt your use of the various chapters to match this preference. Each chapter is written to stand alone with regard to content and each chapter provides a reference to other areas in the text where a particular content area is addressed. Therefore, if you prefer to study the origins of nursing first, that section of this text (Chapter 4) can be read and deliberated before studying the first three chapters.

The content is arranged into four major units of study.

- Unit I includes three chapters that discuss the health care delivery system, its financing, and the politics that impact upon it.
- Unit II includes three chapters that focus on nursing itself and brings to the student an understanding of nursing through studying it as a profession, by exploring nursing origins, and the various paths providing preparation for a career in nursing.
- Unit III includes four chapters that focus on legal and ethical accountability and includes a discussion of the credentials found among health care providers, tracing the history of credentialing in the United States as well as an exploration of the legal issues facing today's nurse. The unit discusses ethics and lays a foundation for ethical decision making, including a broad discussion of various bioethical issues that impact nursing and nursing practice.
- The final unit, Unit IV, includes two chapters that focus on today's health care world of work. Students will learn about ways to seek and secure employment, gaining an understanding of the workplace environment.

PEDAGOGICAL FEATURES

- Objectives introduce each chapter to guide learning efforts
- Key terms used in the chapter discussion are listed
- Key concepts summarize each chapter

SPECIAL TEXT FEATURE

Each chapter is illustrated with cartoon-like characters that have been a hallmark of the text. Though it seemed revolutionary when the first edition was published, it has become something of a trend in nursing texts of this nature. Through them, we hope you gain a varied visual introduction to nursing issues that will provide some humor, as well as gratification, to your commitment to nursing.

INSTRUCTOR'S MANUAL AND TESTBANK

Available to faculty adopting this text is an Instructor's Manual and Testbank. This invaluable resource manual includes chapter overviews; Situations to Foster Critical Thinking, which are different from the Critical Thinking Activities feature included within the textbook; Discussion/Essay Questions; and a variety of testing items including Fill in the Blanks/Short Answer, True-False Questions, Matching Questions, and NCLEX-style multiple choice test items, each of which is tied to a chapter objective. An additional unique feature presented in the Instructor's Manual is instructions for using "Gaming in the Classroom" as a teaching strategy.

WE WELCOME AND APPRECIATE YOUR INVOLVEMENT

We continue to appreciate the comments and suggestions of colleagues, friends, and students. We encourage you to review this text critically and advise us of ways in which we can make it better meet classroom needs. We thank the many educators who continue to select *Nursing in Today's World: Challenges, Issues, and Trends* as the textbook for your class. In this competitive market, we know there are many texts from which to choose. We appreciate your support and strive to bring to you the book that will continue to meet your needs.

SPECIAL ACKNOWLEDGMENTS

We want to express our appreciation to our respective husbands, Ivan and Gordon, for their continued support and encouragement during the development of another edition of the text. Their willingness to let deadlines take precedence over home or social activities and their assistance with household duties and errands has allowed us to meet publication deadlines. And finally, we would like to thank the editors of Lippincott Williams & Wilkins for support of this text and their help and assistance in seeing it published.

Janice Rider Ellis
Celia Love Hartley

Contents

UNIT **II**   Appreciating the Development of Nursing as a
Profession   119

UNIT I

Economic and Political Aspects of Health Care Delivery

A significant part of the economic and political life of any nation relates to the health care available to its people. The percentage of a country's gross national product devoted to health care is a frequently quoted figure. It helps to reflect much of what is best about life but also serves to point out those areas in which a serious problem exists.

Because of the importance of this topic, the first unit in this text provides you with a basic overview of the health care delivery system in the United States. It is impossible within the limitations of a single chapter to discuss fully the complexity of the system.

Beginning with the part of the system with which you are probably most familiar—those settings that employ nurses—content is expanded to include some of those less commonly understood. The specific characteristics of these settings—their roles in health care, the roles of nurses in these settings, the colleagues with whom nurses work, and alternative health care resources—are the focus of the first chapter in the unit.

The second chapter in this unit discusses the financial aspects of the health care delivery system. Because this topic is much too complex to discuss in detail in a single chapter, an overview must suffice. You should gain an understanding of the various players in the system that will help you analyze specific financial issues as they arise: issues related to access to the system, and issues related to power and control.

The unit concludes with a discussion of the political process: how it affects nursing, and how nurses can affect it. An understanding of the various aspects of the health care delivery system can be relevant to your professional experience.

1

Understanding the Health Care Environment

Nurses are experts on reality. No one has roots that penetrate so deeply into our health care institutions. No one sees so much, nor understands so thoroughly.

(Joel, 1996)

OBJECTIVES

After completing this chapter, you should be able to:

1. Identify the various ways of classifying health care agencies and analyze how the classifications differ in their focus.

2. Describe major health care settings (hospitals, long-term care facilities, and community agencies) in terms of the usual length of stay, ownership, types of services offered, and the roles that registered nurses perform in each.

3. Differentiate the approach to the client/resident of acute care hospitals and long-term care facilities.

4. Discuss the roles and interrelationships of the various health care providers in the health care system.

5. Analyze the issues related to education, credentialing, and scope of practice of individual health care occupations.

6. Describe the various types of alternative health care and analyze their relationship to traditional medical care.

KEY TERMS

Accreditation

Acupuncture

Acute care facility

Alternative health care

Assisted-living facility

Community mental health centers

Complementary therapy

Continuing care retirement community (CCRC)

Herbal medicine

Homeopathy

Hospital

Long-term care facility

Naturopathy

Nonprofit

Nursing home

Osteopathy

Primary care provider

Proprietary agency

Skilled nursing facility (SNF)

Subacute care

Tertiary care hospital

Therapeutic touch

Transitional care

Health care is an exciting and challenging field that is also filled with controversy and uncertainty. The entire health care system reverberates with change. The roles of nurses in this system are expanding and changing. You can function more effectively within this system if you understand the various health care agencies and their services, the roles that nurses perform in those agencies, and the colleagues in other disciplines with whom you work.

As we discuss each type of health care agency, we point out the roles that nurses play in that agency and the type of services the agency provides. As alternative health care practices grow in popularity with the public and with providers, health care providers are challenged to understand alternative approaches to health care and also to work effectively with clients who choose those resources. To help you with this task, we discuss alternative and traditional health care options (Fig. 1-1).

CLASSIFICATION OF HEALTH CARE AGENCIES

The health care industry is so large, so diverse, and so complex, that it is sometimes difficult to understand. Generally, agencies providing care are classified according to one of three ways: length of stay, ownership, or type of service (Display 1-1). You need to understand that these classifications are somewhat arbitrary, and that any agency may be placed in more than one classification. With the systemic changes that are occurring, one

FIGURE 1–1   The many aspects of health care in the United States are not coordinated into a single system.

Display 1–1

CLASSIFICATIONS FOR HEALTH CARE AGENCIES

Length of Stay
Short-stay
Traditional acute care
Long-term care

Type of Ownership
Governmental
Proprietary/for-profit
Nonprofit

Type of Service
General vs. specialty
Community vs. tertiary
Subacute care/transitional care
In-home care
Ambulatory care

agency may now include multiple lengths of stay and different types of service, and may combine many segments with different ownership patterns under one large entity. Nevertheless, understanding these categories is useful because they are still used to describe institutions. Your understanding can also be used to guide clients and families through what sometimes seems a maze of confusion in the health care system (Fig. 1-2).

FIGURE 1–2 Clients often need assistance in finding their way through the modern health care system.

Classification According to Length of Stay

One way of classifying in-patient agencies is according to the average length of time patients remain in the facility; that is, the *length of stay*. Short-stay, traditional acute care, and long-term care are terms that reflect the average length of stay in a facility.

SHORT-STAY

Short-stay facilities provide services to patients who are suffering from acute conditions or who have treatment needs that usually require less than 24 hours of care. In some areas the average length of stay for a person having an appendectomy or cholecystectomy is now less than 24 hours. Short-stay may take place in separate units in a hospital, or in freestanding short-stay centers, or even in one section of an emergency department. Many types of short-stay procedures have been made possible by modern developments in minimally invasive surgery or the use of conscious sedation instead of traditional anesthesia.

ACUTE CARE

Traditional acute care takes place in hospitals. In general, acute care encompasses patients staying more than 24 hours but fewer than 30 days. However, the average length of stay for all acute care patients regardless of diagnosis has been declining steadily over the past few years. Stays have become significantly shorter since the implementation of diagnosis-related groups (DRGs) in 1983 and the spread of managed care in the 1990s. (DRGs are discussed in greater detail in Chapter 2.) In many hospitals the average length of stay after general surgery is 3 to 5 days.

LONG-TERM CARE

Long-term care facilities include those that offer services to patients with major rehabilitation needs, chronic disease, functional losses, or mental illness. The average length of stay extends from 30 days to years. State institutions for the mentally ill are usually considered long-term hospitals, although they may have units designated for shorter, acute care stays. Some hospitals have long-term rehabilitation as their only focus. Long-term rehabilitation also may be located on one unit of an acute care hospital. Nursing homes traditionally provide care for those who will be residents for the remainder of their lives, but many also serve people who need a period of convalescence and rehabilitation before returning to their homes or other living settings. Assisted-living facilities for the dependent elderly and group care homes for the developmentally disabled are designed to be permanent residences for clients. In long-term care settings, managing the living environment is as critical as managing health-related concerns.

Classification According to Ownership

The second method of classifying health care agencies is according to *ownership*. Agencies may be classified as governmental or public, proprietary, or nonprofit.

GOVERNMENT-OWNED FACILITIES

Public or government agencies, which receive some tax support for capital or operational costs, may be owned and operated by federal, state, or local governments. The federal facilities usually serve the needs of a special group of individuals, such as veterans, military personnel, Native Americans, or inmates in federal prisons. State mental facilities and hospitals operated by the state are also governmental institutions. Cities, counties, and hospital districts may operate acute care and long-term care agencies and public health departments.

PROPRIETARY AGENCIES

Proprietary agencies (also known as for-profit) are investor owned and operated. Proprietary agencies are commonly part of a corporation owned by stockholders. Some small nursing homes or group homes are owned by an individual. In proprietary agencies, the original capital costs were provided by the owners and investors. Profits from a proprietary institution provide a return on the money invested by the stockholders or individual owners. Historically, some proprietary hospitals were owned and operated by a small group of physicians, but over the years many of these have been sold to community groups or to corporations. In the past few years, there has been a significant trend toward the acquisition of health care enterprises by investor-owned corporations and the formation of multi-unit, for-profit systems. Examples include Columbia/HCA Healthcare Corporation, which is based in Nashville, and Humana Incorporated of Louisville. Each of these groups owns more than 80 hospitals and operates several others. In some areas of the country, most hospitals are proprietary; however, this is not true for the country as a whole. In the long-term care field, Beverly Enterprises and Hillhaven Corporation are examples of corporations that own and operate many nursing homes across the country.

NONPROFIT AGENCIES

Voluntary or nonprofit agencies are those operated by nonprofit groups such as universities, religious bodies, fraternal groups, and community boards. More than 50% of the nation's short-term hospitals and most of the large medical centers fall into this classification. Original capital costs are obtained in a variety of ways, but most often through donations. Community fund-raising campaigns often raise donations for building, capital start-up costs, and special projects. One current concern is the purchase of nonprofit agencies by profit-making corporations. Communities often believe their interests and contributions are discounted in these large business mergers.

The term *nonprofit* may be somewhat misleading. All facilities must make a sufficient income to meet the current costs of the care provided, to maintain facilities and services, and to plan for capital improvement and development. However, those facilities that are classified as nonprofit must put any profit to work in the facility rather than distribute it to stockholders.

Classification by Type of Care

Health care agencies may also be classified according to *type of care* provided. Many agencies provide more than one type of care.

ACUTE CARE

Acute care refers both to a type of care and a length of stay. Acuity refers to the seriousness and rate of change of the patient's condition. Individuals with major surgery, trauma, newly developing illness, and exacerbations of chronic disease may all need acute care because of the high acuity of their conditions. Their conditions are serious and subject to rapid deterioration. In acute care, the conditions require highly skilled patient care. Acute care has a high concentration of professional care providers from a variety of disciplines. The physician is expected to visit daily to manage the rapid changes that may occur. In large hospitals, resident physicians may be available 24 hours a day to respond to problems and emergencies. Registered nurses are always in charge of patient care and present 24 hours a day in the acute care environment.

SUBACUTE CARE

Subacute care is a growing type of service that may be offered in a special unit of a hospital (where it is sometimes termed *transitional care*) or in a long-term care setting. This care is seen as a "middle ground" between the high level of care provided to those in the acute care hospital and the care provided to more traditional long-term care clients. The typical length of stay in short-term subacute units is up to 30 days. Some units focus on intermediate lengths of stay, usually ranging from 31 to 90 days, when clients may recover enough to be discharged to home or stabilize their conditions so that their needs can be met in a nursing home. Still other subacute units offer care that can extend for up to 2 years. The units that offer primarily medical services, where discharge is rapid, are most commonly located in hospitals; those that provide rehabilitative services are usually located in long-term care facilities (Taylor, 1994).

SKILLED NURSING CARE

Skilled nursing care provides specific health care related to skilled rehabilitation services, observation and assessment of the patient's condition, patient teaching and training, direct skilled nursing services (such as tube feedings), and management and evaluation of the patient's care plan (Hawryluk, 1999). A registered nurse must be in charge of the care. The designation of skilled care originated in Medicare and Medicaid legislation and has been adopted by insurers and managed care. The assumption is that all hospital care requires skilled nursing care, but that only some long-term care requires skilled nursing. Skilled nursing care also may take place in skilled nursing facilities, often referred to as SNFs (pronounced "sniffs") and in the home. People who need close monitoring during and after hospitalization and those progressing toward independent care are recognized as having skilled nursing needs. Skilled care includes care of individuals with continuing high-intensity needs, such as those who remain permanently dependent on a ventilator or individuals with the multiple problems of advanced acquired immunodeficiency syndrome (AIDS). Reimbursement for skilled nursing care provided outside the hospital depends on careful documentation of the specific skilled nursing tasks required by the patient.

CUSTODIAL CARE

Custodial care refers to care focused on meeting deficits in multiple areas of daily living. Although the individual may have some routine health care needs, the reason that in-patient care is required is the need for assistance with activities of daily living (ADLs). Unfortunately, people often associate this term with a low level of care that does not require special educational preparation to plan or deliver. Even though maintaining function and preventing decline in the person with multiple deficits requires a broad background of nursing knowledge and careful attention to details of care, there is limited recognition of the difference that skilled nurses can make to individual well-being. Custodial care may take place in private homes, group homes, large institutions, and nursing homes. Understanding the difference between custodial care and skilled care is important when funding is considered. Medicare and health insurance plans do not cover custodial care. These costs must be borne by the individual unless that individual is eligible for public assistance of some type.

HOSPICE CARE

Hospice care is considered still another type of service for both planning and reimbursement. Hospice care is by definition multidisciplinary, providing medical, nursing, social work, a variety of therapies, and spritual support to individuals who are dying and their families and friends. Hospice care may be provided either at home or in a hospice facility. The focus is symptom management, comfort, and individual autonomy in determining what care is needed. Additionally, hospices usually provide bereavement counseling and support to family and care providers.

REHABILITATION CARE

Rehabilitation is designed to support restoration of function, the ability to complete daily living activities, or to engage in an occupation (vocational rehabilitation). The multidisciplinary team may include physicians, nurses, therapists, psychologists, social workers, and vocational counselors, and creates the most effective approach to rehabilitation. Most rehabilitation clients also have skilled nursing care needs. Active rehabilitation is considered skilled care for reimbursement purposes.

AMBULATORY CARE

Ambulatory care also is referred to as *outpatient care*. Traditionally, ambulatory care focused on individuals who came for visits to clinics or primary care offices. This is still the major focus of ambulatory care. In fact, clinic locations are expanding into schools, workplaces, and senior communities. Today's ambulatory care, however, includes a wide variety of diagnostic and treatment services.

Day surgery centers provide an ever-increasing percentage of all surgical procedures. Presurgical care on a day prior to surgery also may be provided, and can include assessment, laboratory tests, and preoperative education. On the day of surgery, the patient arrives at a scheduled time, which may be as early as 6:00 AM, for preoperative care before surgery. The pace in these preoperative units is rapid, with patients being admitted, transferred to the operating room, and discharged in a continuing process throughout the day.

Medical treatment services originally established for those in the hospital gradually have expanded to include services for outpatients. Physical therapy, occupational therapy, respiratory therapy, and other treatments support health care for whole segments of the community. Special outpatient units provide chemotherapy, dialysis, parenteral nutrition, antibiotic therapy, intervention radiology, and other medical treatments.

Sophisticated *diagnostic services* are provided as ambulatory care. Where once individuals were admitted to hospitals to have major diagnostic procedures, this is rare today. Some diagnostic services occur in hospital departments, others occur in physician offices. Individuals may provide self-care for all preparation, including enemas, medications, and dietary restrictions. After brief periods of post-procedure monitoring, patients are sent home with instructions for self-care.

HOME CARE

Home care now encompasses nursing care, therapies, and personal and household assistance. Traditionally, home care agencies were independent organizations, but the number of hospitals offering *home care services* (including hospice home care) is growing as hospital stays have been shortened or eliminated for some conditions. Home services may operate as independent departments, in conjunction with other services, or through a contractual relationship with a home care agency. Examples include home infusion therapy that is connected to a medical treatment center, and home postpartum visits that are administered through a mother-baby unit. Just as with long-term care facilities, home care agencies often are restricted in the care for which they will be reimbursed by definitions of skilled care and by specific mandated limitations on number of visits.

UNDERSTANDING TODAY'S HOSPITAL

The modern hospital may be viewed as the hub or center of the health care delivery system and as central to the health care of a community. In addition to supplying health care to clients, hospitals also provide education to a wide variety of health care workers and to the community. In many cases, they also serve as centers for research and its dissemination. Hospitals are using their status and position in health care to enter into cooperative agreements and alliances with other types of providers, insurance companies, and even other hospitals. To better understand the hospitals of today, you will find it useful to look at their history and development in Chapter 4.

Inpatient versus Outpatient Care

Two terms used frequently to describe today's modern hospital services are *inpatient* and *outpatient*. Individuals are termed "inpatient" when they have been admitted for the purpose of staying 24 hours or longer. The outpatient comes to the hospital for services but is expected to stay less than 24 hours. A primary characteristic of hospital care, whether inpatient or outpatient, is its focus on the current problem, rapid assessment, stabilization or treatment, and then discharge to home care or to long-term care.

INPATIENT SERVICES

Hospitals provide inpatient care in a variety of departments that are commonly designed around the acuity or seriousness of the patient's condition. These units compose what most people think of when they use the designation "acute care hospital." See Display 1-2 for an overview of the services provided. Inpatients may be admitted for acute care but many hospitals also provide long-term inpatient services such as rehabilitation, transitional care, and hospice care. Nurses work in all of these service departments, coordinating the nursing care for individual clients, managing the care environment, delegating and supervising care provided by others, and providing direct skilled care.

Display 1–2
TYPES OF HOSPITAL SERVICES

- Acute care
  - Intensive care units
  - Coronary care units
  - Step-down units
  - Medical–surgical units
  - Mother–baby units
  - Surgery suites
  - Emergency rooms
- Diagnostic services
  - Diagnostic imaging
  - Endoscopic centers
  - Laboratory services
- Day surgery centers
  - Pre- and postoperative care
- Medical treatment (outpatient)
  - Physical and occupational therapy
  - Respiratory therapy
  - Dialysis
  - Chemotherapy
  - Parenteral nutrition
  - Antibiotic therapy

- Rehabilitation (inpatient and outpatient)
  - Nursing care
  - Physical and occupational therapy
  - Vocational and personal counseling
- Transitional care
- Hospice inpatient care
- Hospitality units
- Home care
  - Medical services
  - Hospice home care
  - Infusion therapy
  - Postpartum visits
- Health professional education
  - Schools of nursing
  - Respiratory therapy programs
  - Dietetics
  - Medical residency programs

The person admitted for surgery is an inpatient when he or she is expected to remain in the hospital for at least 24 hours postoperatively. The woman admitted in labor becomes an inpatient because the stay is expected to be at least 24 hours in total and may extend longer if needed. Lengths of stay for acute care are now short, averaging 3 to 5 days for many diagnoses.

Many hospitals have had empty beds because of shortened lengths of stay and the shift to outpatient procedures. In an effort to use costly resources effectively to generate income, hospitals have developed transitional care and rehabilitation units that provide long-term care services. A transitional care or rehabilitation unit allows a hospital to discharge an individual from acute, inpatient care in a timely fashion because the next level of services is guaranteed to be available. Reimbursement is based on long-term care guidelines and the care must meet long-term care standards for skilled nursing care. Even rehabilitation stays are becoming shorter. Inpatient rehabilitation services may be provided for only a brief period of time, followed by outpatient rehabilitation services.

OUTPATIENT SERVICES

Many diagnostic and treatment procedures, surgeries, and emergency health needs are treated as outpatient care. The outpatient goes through an admission process, has a procedure performed or care delivered, is determined to be ready for home care, and subsequently is discharged.

Sometimes an outpatient is retained for observation beyond the standard 24 hours. Although this individual may be moved to a conventional hospital room, admission as an inpatient may never occur and the person may be discharged as an outpatient with an extended stay. The distinction between the categories of inpatient and outpatient is important in regard to both billing and discharge to a nursing home. Both Medicare and Medicaid are billed differently for outpatient care than for inpatient care. Medicare payments for nursing home care after hospitalization require that the person be admitted as an inpatient with a minimum 3-day hospital stay. When these conditions are not met, Medicare payment is denied. Older patients and their families may not understand this distinction and how it affects the bills they receive and their eligibility for some types of reimbursement. Nurses must understand this difference as they help patients to plan for needed care after discharge.

Mix of Hospital Services

Hospitals are often referred to by the mix of traditional inpatient services that are offered. Not every hospital offers each of the services mentioned earlier, but more are becoming part of a corporate entity that provides all of these services (see Display 1-2). The terms most commonly used to describe the mix of services are the general or community hospital, the tertiary care hospital, and the specialty hospital.

GENERAL OR COMMUNITY HOSPITAL

The most common facility is the *general hospital* that offers medical, surgical, obstetric, emergency, and diagnostic and laboratory services. The term *community hospital* is interchangeable in many ways with the term general hospital. Community hospitals provide general hospital services for a specific community. The majority of hospitals in the United States fall into this category.

TERTIARY CARE HOSPITAL

Tertiary care hospitals serve as referral centers for clients with complex or unusual health problems. These hospitals have the facilities for specialized care such as level 1 trauma, major burns, bone marrow transplant, and research-based oncology, along with resources for general care. They serve a wide geographic area in addition to their own community. Tertiary care hospitals usually are associated with a university or are part of a large medical center.

SPECIALTY HOSPITAL

Specialty hospitals offer only a particular type of care, such as that provided by psychiatric hospitals, women's hospitals, or children's hospitals. Specialty hospitals tend to be less common than general hospitals. Many specialty hospitals have become part of larger health care systems in order to have a sufficient referral base and offer their patients wider options.

Other Services

Hospitals may offer a wide variety of other services that are not directed solely at client care, such as hospitality units and education for health professionals.

Day procedures and early discharge for inpatient care may present travel difficulties for individuals who live a long distance from a major care center. To facilitate care for these patients and their families, some hospitals have developed hotel-like services, often termed *hospitality units*. The patient scheduled for day surgery may plan to arrive the day before and stay overnight at a hospitality unit to be present for the morning surgery appointment. A family member can stay in the unit during the individual's hospitalization. After discharge, both the patient and the family member may stay one or more days before traveling home. Although the cost of staying in a hospitality unit usually is not covered by insurance, staying at a nearby hotel or motel might not be as convenient. Additionally, if an emergency occurs, the patient in a hospitality unit has care immediately available.

The *education of health care providers* is an important function of many hospitals. Although the number of hospital-based schools of nursing offering diplomas has been decreasing steadily, some are well supported and expect to continue operation. There are also hospital-based programs for respiratory therapy, dietetics, and other health-related occupations. Many hospitals serve as clinical laboratory sites for individuals enrolled in colleges and universities that provide education for health care professionals.

A physician in a residency program is considered to be in an educational program. Residents receive a salary from the hospital, and are responsible for providing services in return. In addition to augmenting the services of primary physicians, residents often provide medical services for individuals who are part of the medically underserved in a community.

As pressure mounts to reduce the number of specialists and increase the number of primary care physicians, there is speculation about what will happen to some medical residency programs. At this time, part of the funding for these programs comes from Medicare reimbursement policies. These policies allow hospitals to identify educational costs and receive "pass-through" money (that is, money not related to specific individual patient care needs) from Medicare to support educational programs. If these funds were withdrawn, diminished, or designated to be used for primary care preparation (such as family practice), many residency programs would not be sustained at their current size. This would also have profound effects on the function of hospitals that rely on resident physicians for day-to-day, 24-hour services. Some hospitals are already moving to augment services by interns and residents with the use of acute care nurse practitioners.

THE LONG-TERM CARE FACILITY

Long-term care provides assistance with activities of daily living and health care for people of any age who are physically or mentally unable to provide adequate self-care. These conditions may extend over a limited period of time (such as during recovery from a major surgery) or may last a lifetime (as with a developmental disability). Care involves coordination of the entire multidisciplinary team to provide counseling, nursing care, rehabilitation, nutritional support, social services, and sometimes special education programs. Managing a positive living environment is as important as managing health problems for long-term care residents. Long-term care facilities include nursing homes, chronic disease hospitals, psychiatric hospitals, tuberculosis hospitals, and psychiatric and mental retardation facilities. The majority of long-term care facilities are nursing homes that care primarily for the elderly.

The Nursing Home Today

The nursing home is the care facility most often associated with long-term care. Although nursing homes suffer from negative images of the past, they offer a far different environment than they did even 10 years ago. Nursing homes in the United States provide care and a positive living environment for individuals who have the greatest number of deficits in activities of daily living and who need ongoing skilled nursing care. Just as in the acute care hospital, the nursing home is expanding services beyond those traditionally associated with nursing home care.

WHO ARE THE RESIDENTS?

Although most of the elderly live in community settings, many will spend their last years in a nursing home. Approximately two thirds of the residents are women, reflecting the longer life span of women and the greater likelihood that a woman's spouse will precede her in death (Lipowski & Bigelow, 1996). Nursing home residents range in age from 65 to older than 100, with an average age of about 84.

HEALTH SERVICES IN NURSING HOMES

The majority of residents in nursing homes remain there because of major deficits in self-care abilities and the need for ongoing care that is custodial in focus rather than treatment oriented. Maintenance of function, independence, autonomy, and rehabilitation are all goals for nursing home residents. Residents are concerned with the living environment and the health care environment.

Units designed for the cognitively impaired provide facilities constructed without barriers to mobility and without the need for restraints. Facility design and alarm systems prevent residents from wandering out. A unit for the cognitively impaired has special approaches to care delivery that decrease stress and reduce the potential for catastrophic reactions such as hostile, angry outbursts. Reality orientation is used for those who might benefit from this therapy. Validation therapy and reminiscence also are planned to provide a supportive and rich environment. Staff development assists caregivers in responding appropriately to the special challenges of working with the cognitively impaired.

Some nursing homes have entire wings for individuals receiving posthospital convalescent care in subacute units. These individuals are admitted with a specific planned stay of 14 to 30 days. During this time the individual is aided in restoring functional abilities and planning for self or family care. Rehabilitation is a major focus of some subacute units. This might include physical therapy for the person with a hip replacement or speech therapy after a stroke. The goal is to enable residents to return to independent living in the community.

The level of autonomy expected of nurses in nursing homes where physicians visit monthly is often surprising to those who have always worked in acute care hospitals where physicians visit patients daily and resident physicians are available when needed. In nursing homes the individual may be a permanent resident and the nurse may be charged with managing both quality of life and quality of care. Additionally, nurses in these settings must manage care conducted by a variety of assistive personnel and work effectively with an interdisciplinary team.

FUNDING NURSING HOME CARE

The cost of nursing home care is a concern for many because it often exceeds $3,500 per month, depending on the care needs of the individual and the geographic location of the nursing home. Medicare pays for only a limited number of days for individuals who meet specific criteria regarding hospitalization and who need skilled care or rehabilitation rather than custodial care. A few individuals have long-term care insurance that will pay some of their costs. Because this type of insurance is fairly new and quite expensive, few residents have purchased policies. The personal financial resources of most individuals will be exhausted by a prolonged nursing home stay. State-administered public assistance in the form of programs such as Medicaid and Medi-Cal pays for nursing home care when an individual's personal financial resources have fallen below a certain state-determined level. As the number of elderly individuals requiring nursing home care has risen, these costs are becoming a serious budget concern in most states.

REGULATION OF NURSING HOME CARE

Nursing homes have become the most regulated of all health care settings. In fact, only industries such as nuclear power face more regulations. Because the federal government pays for some of the care, there are federal regulations affecting nursing homes across the country. These have resulted in specific mandated assessment tools, planning processes, standards of care, and evaluation tools. Data collected according to specific standards must be transmitted electronically to state centers for reimbursement to occur. The regulations contained in the Federal Budget Act of 1987 (OBRA 87) created sweeping changes in everything from the use of restraints and psychoactive medications to the documentation systems used. State regulations may place additional constrait on nursing homes. Nursing homes are visited by a survey team that is responsible for assuring adherence to regulatory standards. The results of nursing home surveys are public documents and must be displayed in each facility in a place accessible to the public and to residents who wish to review it.

Critical Thinking Activity

Investigate a hospital or nursing home in your community. Find out its average length of stay, the types of services it offers, and its type of ownership. Analyze its overall contribution to health care in your community.

Assisted-Living Facilities

A more recent development is the *assisted-living facility*, which provides care for those needing help with up to three activities of daily living. In an assisted-living arrangement, the resident can maintain maximum independence and use a shared decision-making model to decide when additional help or support is needed (DeYoung, Just, & VanDyk, 1994). Husbands and wives reside together and may often bring their own furniture and belongings to create a homelike atmosphere. As the costs of nursing home care have risen, those who are able to perform any activities of daily living are seeking the less costly and more flexible living found in assisted living. Assisted-living facilities have been much less regulated than nursing homes. As these facilities admit more impaired individuals or as individuals living in them want to "age in place," concerns are being raised about the quality of care provided. Increasing regulation is expected. The Joint Commission on Accreditation of Healthcare Organizations has announced the development of a voluntary accrediting process for assisted-living centers.

CARE IN ASSISTED-LIVING FACILITIES

In an assisted-living facility, all instrumental activities of daily living such as shopping, cleaning, meal preparation, and laundry are provided. A resident is expected to have some mobility (even though it may require a walker or a cane) and to eat in a dining room. Residents also are expected to manage their own medication and health needs, although they may be assisted with remembering to take medications. Assistance is provided with bathing, dressing, and other personal care as needed. Most care is provided by unlicensed assistive personnel. One area of controversy is the level of assistance with medications and health needs that can be provided by unlicensed, unregulated personnel. Nurses may be employed in a supervisory capacity and may plan for care.

When the ability to perform activities of daily living is lost, transfer to a nursing home is required by regulation. For some individuals, the transitions from independent living to assisted living and from assisted living to nursing home care are smooth ones. This is particularly true when multiple levels of care are available in the same retirement living setting. (See discussion of continuing care communities below.) When the older individual must move from one living situation to another, transition or relocation stress impacts well-being.

FUNDING ASSISTED LIVING

Assisted living is not supported with Medicare funds and therefore does not have to meet the stringent regulatory standards of federal legislation (Hawryluk, 1995). Public assistance, in the form of Medicaid, Medi-Cal, or other programs, may provide some support for assisted living when the alternative would be expensive nursing home care for which the state would be responsible. However, this is not true in all jurisdictions. Most assisted living is paid for by the individual or family.

Retirement Communities

Recent years have witnessed the development of several forms of retirement communities. These communities may be self-contained towns, retirement villages, retirement subdivisions, retirement residences, or continuing-care retirement communities. The basic retirement complex is designed to provide self-care and may support independence longer than would a regular house or apartment. Home care services are provided to those in retirement communities in the same way that they are provided to those in regular homes or apartments.

Continuing care retirement communities (CCRC) provide a variety of levels of independent living and care to residents based on each resident's need. Most residents enter the community to reside in a retirement apartment. The community also maintains an assisted living section and a convalescent or nursing home center. Services such as occupational therapy, physical therapy, and dental care also may be available as home care or for those in the convalescent center. The aim is for people to reside in the setting that provides maximum autonomy and independence while assuring that needs are met. There is data to suggest that residents of continuing care retirement communities maintain better health and require less nursing home care than the general population (Sloan, Shayne, & Conover, 1995). A major limiting factor is the cost of such communities to the individual residents. There is no governmental financial assistance available in these residences.

Rehabilitation Centers

Rehabilitation centers typically focus on a specific health care problem just as rehabilitation units in acute care hospitals do. For example, there are centers for those with spinal cord injuries and other centers focusing on head injuries or cerebral vascular accidents. Although many of these agencies prefer nurses who have taken advanced courses in rehabilitation nursing, many employ nurses with different backgrounds such as those who have worked in a nursing home focused on rehabilitation principles.

AMBULATORY CARE SETTINGS

Ambulatory care has long been provided in offices, clinics, and the day procedure units of hospitals. Some ambulatory care is provided in settings where people work and go to school. Providing care where people routinely spend their days rather than requiring them to go to a different site for health care often results in more effective use of health care services. All ambulatory care settings rely heavily on the skills of registered nurses.

Primary Care Offices

The health care provider contacted initially by clients who seek health care is considered a primary care provider. Today the federal government considers general practitioners, family practice specialists, pediatricians, internal medicine specialists, and obstetricians as primary care physicians. Physician's assistants and nurse practitioners also are recognized as primary care providers. The primary care provider is the mainstay of basic care for most individuals.

One of the major changes in health care has been the decrease in the number of solo practice offices and the growth of group and organizational practices. In 1996, for the first time, more physicians were employed in group practice settings than in solo practice offices. Advanced practice nurses and physician's assistants also are working in many of these group practice settings. Other registered nurses in these settings may have responsibility for answering questions on the telephone as well as teaching and providing care for patients in the office. Nursing roles in ambulatory care are expanding as the need for cost-effective use of physician time is modifying practice patterns.

Walk-in Clinics

Walk-in clinics treat clients with emergent conditions that do not require the high-technology resources of the emergency room. Walk-in clinics may be referred to as immediate care facilities, urgent care centers, or emergent care centers and are usually open during extended hours that include evenings and weekends in addition to the traditional Monday through Friday office hours. Walk-in clinics have grown in popularity as people have found it increasingly difficult to gain access to traditional health care settings because of time constraints in their personal lives. Many walk-in clinics have gradually added services such as sports physical examinations for school-age children, pelvic examinations and Pap tests for women, and routine immunizations. As these clinics mature, some are beginning to act as primary care settings, advertising the willingness of staff doctors to become "family doctors." Walk-in clinics have relatively small nursing staffs, often employing only one registered nurse during a shift; therefore, each nurse must have a wide variety of skills and be able to function with a high degree of autonomy. Some settings do not use registered nurses in direct care; they are hired in these settings only to supervise other clinic staff members. Licensed practical nurses may be employed in ambulatory care to collect data, carry out specific treatments, and give medications.

COMMUNITY AGENCIES

Agencies providing care in the community include public health agencies, traditional home care agencies, and home hospice care (Display 1-3).

Public Health Agencies

Public health departments are operated as agencies of the government. In general, the focus of health departments has been on broad community issues, communicable diseases, and infant and child health. Although public health nurses originally did a great deal of individual family visiting, today fewer funds are available for visits. As a result, public health nurses now focus on individuals who are high risk and whose health affects the entire community. Public health nurses responsible for community health issues are required to have a baccalaureate degree in nursing; however, some agencies operate a variety of clinics (such as immunization clinics) in which registered nurses with an associate degree or diploma provide teaching and direct care services.

Traditional Home Care Agencies

Home care agencies, such as the traditional visiting nurse services and the proprietary home health care companies, provide a broad spectrum of care that may include nursing care, personal care assistance, minor housekeeping, physical therapy, and respiratory therapy for individuals in their homes. Teaching family and caregivers is a large part of the home care professional's responsibility. Some home care agencies focus on providing short-term visits for clients who need assistance after a hospital stay or acute illness. Others focus on clients who will need ongoing home care for years, such those requiring dialysis or ventilator support in the home. Some agencies provide nursing care for 8- to 12-hour shifts in the home in an effort to provide support and respite for family caregivers. Others provide episodic visits that last from 15 to 60 minutes.

Display 1–3
COMMUNITY AGENCIES

- Public health departments
- Home care agencies
- Hospice home care
- Community mental health centers
- Day care centers for older adults
- Ambulatory care dialysis centers

Hospice Home Care

Hospice care has gained momentum as a way to provide maximum quality of life to terminally ill people. Multidisciplinary teams may include physicians, nurses, clergy, occupational and physical therapists, home health aides, social workers, and volunteers. The goal of hospice care is to assist the individual in living as he or she wishes until death. The members of multidisciplinary teams work with both the hospice patient and the family. Nurses provide special skills in symptom management for physical problems such as pain, nausea, anorexia, and constipation and psychosocial support for end-of-life events and issues.

Community Mental Health Centers

Community mental health centers were established to allow individuals with psychiatric problems to remain in their communities. Evidence supports the belief that psychiatric clients who remain in their communities on an outpatient basis, with family and community ties intact, have more successful treatment outcomes. For those who must be hospitalized, the community mental health center provides follow-up care that facilitates early discharge. Another advantage of community mental health centers is that people seek help more readily when it is available within the community. These centers usually employ a variety of mental health workers including psychiatrists, clinical psychologists, social workers, marriage and family counselors, psychiatric nurses, and community workers. Services may include individual counseling and therapy, group or family counseling, evaluation, and referral.

In actual practice, community mental health centers have not been funded adequately to meet the many and varied needs of individuals with mental health problems. Mentally ill clients often are not eligible for care that can maintain their health, but are eligible for care only when they become acutely ill. Some people are not eligible for help because of the complex rules and regulations governing funding. Some do not continue with prescribed treatment and thus relapse; legal constraints do not allow involuntary treatment. Although recognition of the rights of the mentally ill has been important, there also is concern that society expects mentally ill people to make rational decisions about their own best interests when they are not mentally capable of understanding the consequences of their actions. The entire area of community mental health has many problems and challenges.

Critical Thinking Activity

Identify an agency in your community that offers home health care. Investigate the services offered by this agency. Compare these with the list of possible services offered by home care agencies mentioned in this chapter. If the lists do not match, analyze the factors in your community that may be responsible for the difference.

Day Care Centers for the Elderly

Day care centers have been established for elderly people who cannot safely be alone throughout the day. Clients are transported to the center each day by family or by a van operated by the center. While at the center, clients receive a variety of social and health services that enable them to continue to live in their own home or a family member's home. Various maintenance and rehabilitative services usually are available, including exercise classes, medication education and supervision, recreational activities, mental health care, and an opportunity to interact with other people. Some centers provide "drop in" or intermittent services for clients who need only one aspect of the program. Other centers provide care each day for clients who need continuing supervision while family members are at work or school. The nursing role in these settings may vary considerably. Some settings have advanced practice nurses who plan care and work with families. Others have registered nurses who provide medication supervision, assessment for ongoing health problems, and who may lead groups in reminiscence, reality orientation, or validation therapy. They may have LPNs who give medications and carry out specific treatments.

Ambulatory Care Dialysis Centers

Individuals with chronic renal failure who need ongoing renal dialysis may be managed by home dialysis or by dialysis performed in a dialysis center. A dialysis center provides an environment where the individual who does not have a family care provider or a home dialysis assistant can go two to three times a week for dialysis. Nurses in dialysis centers must have high-level skills because clients with renal failure who need in-center dialysis usually have the most complex problems and coexisting illnesses. Both LPNs and RNs may be employed in these centers.

COLLEAGUES IN HEALTH CARE

Many different groups deliver health care. Various providers exist because they meet the needs of our society in some way. Some groups are believed to provide a valuable service; the services of others are of questionable benefit. There is a short supply of qualified individuals in some areas. In other areas there are enough qualified providers, but the providers tend to be of a single gender or ethnic background. This may pose difficulties for both the client and the care provider when the two are unable to communicate effectively. Many programs are in place that strive to increase diversity among health care providers to better meet the needs of all clients. As the health care workforce changes, some clients must alter their perspectives to adapt to a wider diversity in health care providers (Fig. 1-3).

Hundreds of different types of health care workers have been identified in the United States. It is not within the scope of this book to discuss each of these occupations individually, but we do attempt to outline the general categories of health care providers with whom you may be working. Table 1-1 provides an overview of the education and licensure for some of the more common health care providers.

FIGURE 1–3 As the health care workforce changes, some clients must adapt their perceptions.

Primary Health Care Providers

The primary health care provider furnishes entry into the health care system. This person is consulted by the client for routine health maintenance and for care of episodic illnesses. This health care provider traditionally has been a medical doctor, osteopathic physician, or dentist. These professionals are licensed in all states and are authorized to treat illness and prescribe drugs.

The planned cornerstone of health care reform is an increased emphasis on the primary health care provider as the "gatekeeper" for the system. The primary provider implements health maintenance activities that prevent the need for more expensive care. This individual provides referral to more specialized care when it is needed. Lack of access to primary care has been one of the health care problems for individuals residing in rural areas, economically disadvantaged areas in large cities, and those on welfare programs. The lack of access often has resulted in delaying care until the problem is more complex and requires greater resources to resolve. In urban areas the lack of access to primary care has often resulted in the inappropriate use of emergency room services for routine illnesses. To meet the needs of society, there is pressure to increase the number of professionals who are authorized to deliver primary care.

TABLE 1–1. Allied Health Occupations With Accredited Education Programs*

Occupational Group	Number of Accredited Programs	Education Required — Certificate (1 Year)	Associate Degree (2 Year)	Baccalaureate Degree	Graduate Program	Credential — Professional Certification	Legal License
Anesthesiology assistant	2				X	X	
Athletic trainer	17			X		X	
Cardiovascular technologist	7		X			X	
Clinical lab scientist	383			X		X	
Clinical lab technician	216	|—	—X			X	
Cytotechnologist	38	|—	—|	—X—	⊤	X	
Diagnostic medical sonographer	65	|—	—X—	—|	⊤	X	
Electroneurodiagnostic technologist	67	|—	—X—			X	
Emergency medical technician-paramedic	14	|—	—X—	—|		X	X
Health information administrator	88			—X—	⊤	X	
Health information technician	54	|—X	—|			X	
Histologic technician	137	X—|				X	
Histologic technologist	32	|—	⊤	X—|	⊤	X	
Medical assistant	221	X—|	⊤			X	
Medical illustrator	25			—|	X	X	
Nuclear medicine technologist	17121	X—|		|X	⊤	X	
Occupational therapist	785			|X	⊤	X	X
Occupational therapy assistant	38394	|—	—X—			X	
Ophthalmic medical technician/technologist	21611	X—|	—⊤			X	
Perfusionist	35	|—		—X—	—X	X	X
Physician's assistant (surgeon's assistant was consolidated with PA in 1994)	61	|—		—X—	⊤	X	X
Radiation therapist	125	X—|	—|	⊤		X	X
Radiographer	693	|—	—X—	⊤		X	X
Respiratory therapist	275	|—	—X—	⊤		X	X
Respiratory therapy technician	179	X—|	⊤			X	
Specialist in blood bank technology	28				X	X	
Surgical technologist	140	X—|	⊤			X	X

*When more than one educational level is available, a line is shown between the highest and lowest levels. A large X is placed in the column where the largest number of programs lies.

PHYSICIANS

The term *physician* refers to the doctor of medicine or the doctor of osteopathic medicine. The differences between traditional (allopathic) medicine and osteopathic medicine are becoming less distinct. Historically, the philosophy of care and remedial techniques of osteopathic physicians included treatments such as back manipulation and nutritional counseling, whereas allopathic physicians prescribed more drugs and performed more surgery. Osteopathic physicians and allopathic physicians practiced entirely independently of each other and used separate hospitals; a visible antagonism between the two groups was often apparent. The current environment is one of greater cooperation, with physicians from both backgrounds practicing side by side in clinics and hospitals. The osteopathic group is considerably smaller and less well known, and has far fewer specialists and fewer resources for research. However, the educational patterns for both groups are similar.

Undergraduate medical education may vary in focus, but a strong biological science background is required. This is followed by 4 years of medical school. During these 4 years, formal education is stressed, with client contact occurring most often during the latter part of the program. Some medical schools are beginning to provide client contact earlier in the educational process. After completion of medical school, licensing examinations are taken.

Once individuals are licensed as physicians, they must participate in a residency program to prepare for autonomous practice. Although licensed to practice, a physician is not accepted into any group practice or awarded privileges at a hospital without first completing a residency. Residency programs are developed by hospitals or health care delivery systems and primarily focus on extensive experiences in providing medical care. The length of these programs varies depending on the specialty. The resident is paid a salary by the sponsoring health care agency. In state, county, and city hospitals, the resident physician may serve as the primary physician for some patients, with senior staff physicians or medical school professors providing oversight. For patients who are responsible for their own medical bills (either directly or through insurance), the admitting personal physician usually remains in charge and the resident serves a supporting role in the patient's medical care. At the end of the residency, the resident physician can practice independently, in a group practice, or as an employee of a health care agency.

After residency training is completed, the physician also is prepared to take written examinations for certification in a specialty. The person who successfully passes the specialty examination is termed *board certified*, although it is not legally required that a physician be board certified to practice in a specialty area. Certification in family practice increasingly is being considered the preferred credential for general practice.

Subspecialty training occurs after specialty training is completed and may add another 3 to 4 years. Given this pattern of education and training, a physician may have a total of 10 or more years of postsecondary education and training before beginning to work independently.

PODIATRISTS

Podiatrists (formerly called chiropodists) are educated in the care and surgery of the foot. They care for corns, bunions, and toenails; prescribe and fit corrective shoes and arch supports; and perform surgery on the feet, such as correcting deformities and removing bunions and small tumors. Podiatrists may become expert in treating wounds of the feet because of the high incidence of these as health problems for an aging population. A podiatrist does not prescribe systemic medication or care for generalized diseases. With an aging society and an increase in sports-related foot problems, the work of podiatrists is receiving more recognition.

NURSE PRACTITIONERS

As demands on the system have increased, additional categories of professionals have been added to the group of primary care providers. Nurses working in specialized roles as primary care nurses and nurse practitioners (NP) are examples. These nurses have obtained education in addition to that required for basic licensure (most commonly in a master's degree program) and have earned certification in a particular specialty. They may have a state-issued license allowing expanded practice. Nurse practitioners may work with a physician in an office or clinic, or they may function independently in nursing clinics. Most states grant nurse practitioners who meet special guidelines the authority to write prescriptions. This prescriptive authority is the subject of heated debate in states not providing this option. In some areas, acute care nurse practitioners are being educated to provide medical support in hospitals that historically has been provided only by resident physicians. Acute care nurse practitioners are found most commonly in critical care units.

Supporters suggest the increased use of the nurse practitioner as a primary care provider is a major aspect of health care reform. They point to geographic availability and cost savings as critical elements. In keeping with this approach, most of the federal money for nursing education has been allocated to advanced preparation.

PHYSICIAN'S ASSISTANTS

Another primary caregiver is the physician's assistant (PA), sometimes called the *medex*. This person often has medical and emergency training, perhaps from military service or other health care occupations, and has completed a university program. Physician's assistant programs vary from 1-year certificate programs to 4-year baccalaureate programs. Physician's assistants must work under the direction of a physician at all times.

Physician's assistants usually see clients with commonly recurring health problems such as colds, flu, fractures, and cuts needing suturing. Physician's assistants also may provide some primary health care, such as routine physical examinations. If the client needs referral to a specialist or hospital admission, the physician's assistant first refers the client to the physician with whom he or she works. In some settings the roles of the nurse practitioner and physician's assistant are similar. Some physician's assistants work with a specialty physician, such as an orthopedic surgeon, and have responsibilities related to that specialty: applying and removing casts, for example. Some physician's assistants work with surgeons in the role of surgical first assistant.

The use of physician's assistants is sometimes controversial. Some clients believe that they are receiving less than quality care if they are treated by a physician's assistant instead of seeing the physician. The appropriateness of physician's assistants writing prescriptions and orders on the charts of hospitalized clients has been questioned among health care workers. Nurses have been concerned because their own licensure laws sometimes state that they can administer medications only on the order of a licensed physician, osteopath, or dentist, yet, in some instances, nurses are asked to give medications on the order of a physician's assistant.

Another area of concern has been whether nurses working in expanded roles should be classified as physician's assistants and be governed by the Board of Medicine rather than the Board of Nursing. Some nurses have enrolled in and completed the regular physician's assistant programs and are working in this capacity. Other nurses strongly believe that the nurse in primary care should be considered an independent nurse rather than a physician's assistant. The American Nurses Association (ANA) has supported the position that the nurse in primary care is better prepared to address the whole person's health needs than a physician's assistant.

OTHER PRIMARY CARE PROVIDERS

Social workers and clinical psychologists historically have performed a primary care role by providing client entry into the mental health care system, serving as counselors and supervisors of care, and furnishing referrals as needed. Because social workers and psychologists are not able to treat physical problems, they often work in cooperation with psychiatrists or psychiatric-mental health nurse practitioners who are able to manage this aspect of care. Within most health plans, clients can see these mental health workers only on referral from a primary physician.

Social problems, including lack of a social support network and the financial resources for care, create major barriers to accessing health care for many people. Clinical social workers are prepared at the master's degree level and are employed in health care agencies to provide services upon referral. Social workers work with family and significant friends to arrange the support that permits early discharge and facilitates home care. Social workers sometimes face a difficult task in obtaining financial support for their services. Some institutional providers and third-party payers are recognizing that social supports may play a large role in an individual's movement from expensive acute care environments to home care, and therefore are increasing their willingness to reimburse social workers for care.

Clinical psychologists have completed doctoral programs followed by a 1-year internship in a mental health setting, typically a hospital or large clinic. They may practice privately after successful completion of either a licensing or a certification examination, depending on specific state laws. Clinical psychologists diagnose various forms of mental illness, provide psychotherapy, administer and interpret psychological tests, and engage in research. In addition to independent practice, they are found in many settings, including hospitals, clinics, schools, and institutions for the mentally ill.

Optometrists provide vision testing and prescribe glasses, contact lenses, and corrective exercises for eye problems. They have a general background in the assessment of eye diseases and can screen clients and refer them to an ophthalmologist (a physician who specializes in eye diseases) when diagnosis and treatment are needed. The scope of practice of optometrists is being expanded in some states to enable them to provide more comprehensive eye care. Because ophthalmologists and optometrists offer some of the same services, there is some disagreement between them as to the proper scope of practice for each group. Whether eye examinations and corrective lenses for vision should be part of basic health care is another area of debate in health care reform legislation.

Dentists provide primary care of the teeth and mouth. Many dentists are beginning to provide general health screening, such as examining the mouth and throat for tumors or disease and taking blood pressure during their basic examination. A client is referred to a physician if an abnormality is noted. Dentists have an educational background similar in length to that of the physician—4 years of baccalaureate education followed by dental school. There is no residency period, and dentists begin independent practice after passing state licensing examinations. Dentists are empowered to prescribe medications in addition to providing care for the mouth and teeth. There are specialty areas in dentistry, such as orthodontics (the application of devices to change the occlusion of the teeth), just as there are in medicine. Education for specialties occurs in universities that have dental schools. After the student has graduated, the diploma indicates competence in the specialty. There is no legal requirement for advanced education to practice a dental specialty, although strong professional constraints exist.

Dental care is one of the basic health care concerns being debated. Certainly dental health is a part of overall health. Some, however, suggest that for health care to be economically viable, we must limit demands and not try to cover every aspect of health for all individuals. The expanded use of the dental hygienist has been suggested as one avenue to broadening the availability of preventive dental services while limiting costs.

Allied Health Care Workers

The Allied Health Education Directory (1999) lists 29 different allied health occupations. Most allied health care professionals (eg, the clinical laboratory technician) provide diagnostic and treatment services related to a medical plan for care. Some professionals, such as those who work with records, serve to support the system but do not have direct care responsibilities. Many allied health professions evolved in response to demand for individuals trained to manage complex technology; an example is the perfusionist who manages the cardiopulmonary bypass machine used in cardiac surgery.

Table 1-1 (p 22) outlines the educational background required of some of these professions. You will notice that some professions require education ranging in length from 1 year (certificate programs) to 4 years (baccalaureate programs). This reveals that education is not standardized in many health professions. The five organizations listed in Display 1-4 provide accreditation for programs preparing these providers.

In addition to the allied health programs listed in Table 1-1, new allied health occupations are being added by health care facilities. Over 240 different titles for allied health personnel are found in health-related literature. The stated goals of developing new occupations are to provide technical expertise for clients, decrease costs, and offer the expertise of professionals to more clients. Many health professional groups are joining nurses in expressing concern about the trend toward adding assistive personnel who function without education or credentials. For example, the American Speech

Display 1–4
ORGANIZATIONS PROVIDING ALLIED HEALTH ACCREDITATION

1. Accreditation Council for Occupational Therapy Education
2. Commission on Accreditation of Allied Health Education Programs (CAAHEP has 17 separate committees on accreditation; each focuses on a different allied health area.)
3. Joint Review Committee on Educational Programs in Nuclear Medicine Technology
4. Joint Review Committee on Education in Radiologic Technology
5. National Accrediting Agency for Clinical Laboratory Sciences

Language and Hearing Association established a task force on support personnel (Task Force, 1996). The task force developed guidelines related to training, credentialing, use, and supervision of assistive personnel in the field of speech pathology. The Association has adopted these guidelines.

The following sections provide information about some of the major allied health professionals with whom you may work on an interdisciplinary team (Fig. 1-4).

FIGURE 1–4   Overlapping roles and unclear boundaries between health care occupations can lead to conflict.

LABORATORY AND DIAGNOSTIC SERVICES

Included in the category of laboratory and diagnostic technologists and technicians are those who work in the clinical laboratory, such as the medical technologist (MT) and medical laboratory technician (MLT), as well as those who work in specialized diagnostic fields, such as the nuclear medicine technician, the electroencephalograph (EEG) technician, and the radiologic technician (RT). These people assist with the tests now used to diagnose and monitor the progression of illnesses. As new sophisticated diagnostic technology is introduced, new technical fields are created to operate and monitor the equipment. Some occupations, such as medical technologist, require a baccalaureate degree. Others, such as radiology technician (RT) and medical laboratory technician, usually have 2-year associate degrees. Still other occupations, such as electrocardiographic (ECG) technician, may be learned on the job.

ADMINISTRATIVE AND BUSINESS PERSONNEL

As health care facilities become more complex, the administrative and business aspects of health care grow more demanding. Many people are needed to maintain and retrieve information from medical records. These workers include health information administrators, health information technicians, and medical secretaries. The positions of hospital administrator and assistant administrator are changing. In the past, these appointments might have been filled by a physician, an attorney, or a nurse. Because the health care system now has such specialized demands, the administrative positions increasingly are being filled by those with a baccalaureate or master's degree in health care administration. A special certification is required for those who administer nursing homes.

COMMUNITY HEALTH CARE WORKERS

Community health is a growing field that requires an increasing number of workers. The major focus of community health care is the promotion of health rather than care of illness. Some workers, such as the health educator and community health visitor, work directly with individual clients. Others, such as the sanitarian, assist the community as a whole toward better health through maintenance of standards for cleanliness and infectious disease control.

Other community health care workers help individuals with health and personal care after discharge from the hospital. Although some workers are registered nurses who provide skilled care, many more are home health aides who assist with nontechnical aspects of care and may even help with household tasks and shopping. Education for home health aides in the past consisted of on-the-job training; now it also takes place in courses leading to certification.

MAKERS OF PROSTHETIC AND ASSISTIVE DEVICES

With technologic advances, the number of different prostheses and assistive devices increases. Those who make and fit devices such as eyeglasses, braces, and artificial limbs need specialized education. They do not usually have licenses, but may be certified by a professional organization. Most are employed by health care institutions, although some (eg, dispensing opticians who make eyeglasses) may be in private business.

DIETARY SERVICES

The nutritionist or dietitian spends a large percentage of time planning for the special dietary needs of clients as a group—that is, determining the menu for those on a diabetic diet, a low-salt diet, or any other special diet ordered by the physician and provided by the facility. In addition, dietitians work with individual clients in planning appropriate diets and teaching nutrition. Nutritionists long have advocated healthy diets for health promotion and maintenance. Increasing numbers of third-party payers now will support nutrition counseling for those whose health clearly would be improved by sound nutrition. Registered dietitians have 4 years of college plus an internship. Dietetic technicians have a 2-year associate degree education.

RESPIRATORY CARE

Those who provide direct care related to respiratory treatments and the use of respiratory devices are called respiratory therapists (RT). Recent changes in educational requirements now specify a minimum of an associate degree for certification. A baccalaureate degree in respiratory therapy is also available. Respiratory care professionals are employed by hospitals, long-term care facilities, and home health care agencies. They may provide client teaching as well as administer specific treatments and inhaled medications for respiratory care.

PHARMACY SERVICES

Pharmacists are altering their practice focus from dispensing drugs to managing drug therapy. Baccalaureate pharmacy programs are gradually closing, and pharmacy is moving into graduate programs (the Master of Pharmacy program and the Pharmacy doctorate, or PharmD, program) designed to prepare clinical pharmacists who will consult with physicians, recommend therapy, assist with monitoring therapy, provide consultation for nurses, and teach clients. In most universities, a pharmacy program involves clinical work in a hospital or other patient care setting. As drug therapy becomes more complex and drug interactions a greater concern, the presence of this specialist enhances the interdisciplinary team. Although pharmacists are involved with dispensing medications, they increasingly provide drug therapy consultation to physicians and nurses and directly teach clients how to comply with their drug regimens. Many pharmacies also employ pharmacy technicians trained on the job or in community colleges to conduct many dispensing activities.

PHYSICAL THERAPY

The physical therapist (PT) is educated in a master's degree program or in a 5-year baccalaureate program. There is a strong movement within the profession toward requiring physical therapists to obtain the master's degree to practice. The focus of physical therapy is the restoration of normal function of large muscle groups, bones, and joints.

Treatment includes exercise, heat and cold therapy, electrical stimulation, and the use of other physical agents. The physical therapist also teaches the client to use crutches, prostheses, and other assistive devices. As emphasis on rehabilitation and the maintenance and restoration of functional abilities increases, the physical therapist may assume the role of leader of an interdisciplinary team. Physical therapists are moving into areas of health promotion and maintenance through teaching individuals about safe exercise, providing direction for exercise fitness, and helping individuals with health problems to gain maximum function. Physical therapy assistants (PTA) are educated in 2-year associate degree programs and work with registered physical therapists to carry out planned therapeutic regimens.

OCCUPATIONAL THERAPY

The occupational therapist (OT) assists the client in restoring fine motor skills and performing activities of daily living. Treatment includes exercise, the making of splints and assistive devices, and identifying ways to modify the environment to make the performance of daily living activities possible. The need for analyzing work environments to determine ergonomic hazards and identify ergonomically sound conditions and practices has generated new opportunities for the occupational therapist. Meaningful activities such as crafts and games often are used to provide clients with needed exercise. Occupational therapists also provide diversional activities appropriate to the client's strength, ability, and interest that are designed to help the client achieve physical or psychosocial goals. The occupational therapist has a baccalaureate degree and a 1-year internship. Occupational therapy assistants (OTA) have associate degrees and carry out plans for therapy that have been established by the registered occupational therapist.

SPEECH THERAPY

The speech therapist usually completes a graduate program in speech pathology. In addition to working with those with rehabilitation needs in speech and language function, the speech therapist works with clients who have swallowing difficulties. Often the speech therapist serves as a consultant to nursing staff as they plan for care of individuals with stroke or head injury.

OTHER SPECIFIC THERAPIES

Many health professionals provide specific types of therapy. The radiation therapy technician is one example. Also included in this group, but more rarely seen, are the massage therapist, the music therapist, the bibliotherapist, and the art therapist.

Critical Thinking Activity

Choose an allied health profession other than nursing. Investigate the current education requirements for that health profession in your state. Identify the usual responsibilities associated with this profession. Provide a carefully supported argument for or against legal licensure for this health profession.

ISSUES RELATED TO INDIVIDUAL HEALTH PROFESSIONS

The many changes in the health care delivery system as it struggles with cost and providing care demand corresponding changes in the education of health professionals and their function within the system.

Issues Related to Primary Health Care

One of the problems in U.S. health care is the maldistribution of primary care providers. Urban areas have proportionately more health care workers of every kind than do rural areas. In large cities, care providers are concentrated in the more affluent areas. Many programs have attempted to provide incentives to establish practices in insufficiently served areas. In some programs, educational loans are forgiven or canceled if a person works in an underserved area after completing a course of study. In other instances, schools have tried to recruit students from underserved areas, hoping that after graduation the students would return home to practice. Some schools incorporate into their programs learning experiences in rural or poorly served areas with the hope that graduates will be attracted to these areas and return later to work. In 1999, the University of Iowa announced that its efforts to prepare physicians for rural practice were showing success: 86 new physicians entering rural practice in Iowa exceeded the 48 who either were retiring or moving away ("College dean," 1999).

However, insufficiently served areas still exist for several reasons. Physicians prefer to practice where there is access to specialized medical centers and where opportunities for consultation are readily available. The tremendous physical strain involved in being the only care provider is another factor that deters physicians from practicing in rural areas. The rural physician often receives little respite from 24-hours-a-day, 7-days-a-week availability to the community. The income of a rural physician also tends to be lower than that of a physician in an urban area. Nurse practitioners increasingly are providing health care to underserved populations and have been more willing to relocate to rural or impoverished areas.

Another concern is the number of physicians prepared as specialists relative to the number who act as primary care providers. In the United States, approximately 60% of physicians practice in specialties and 40% practice in some area of primary care such as general practice, family practice, pediatrics, and obstetrics/gynecology. This has resulted in too few primary care providers and an excess of specialists in some areas. Part of the health care reform legislation being introduced provides for incentives and support for those entering primary care practice.

The trend in private medical practice is toward group practices. Several specialties may be represented within a group. Although each client may have a private physician, group practice clients also may receive care from other members of the group. Group practice assures the individual physician more time for personal and family life.

Care in private practice usually is based on fee for service. Although some physicians attempt to make adjustments for clients with less ability to pay, the cost of health care for even middle-class individuals is a serious problem today. Insurance may pay for some outpatient care, and it funds most of the care given during hospitalization, but increasing numbers of people are underinsured or uninsured.

Accreditation of Health Professional Education Programs

Specialized accreditation of programs providing education for health professionals has created nationwide standards when individual state licensing laws differ greatly. State laws, in most instances, do not require that schools have national accreditation; in some states, however, national accreditation has been accepted in place of individual state monitoring of programs. The accrediting organizations seek to remain abreast of current practice and to be nondiscriminatory in their decision making.

The U.S. Department of Education now includes an office that reviews accrediting agencies and associations and publishes a list of those that the Department of Education recognizes as reliable authorities on educational quality. Although the Department of Education does not control the organizations offering accreditation and cannot create or eliminate them, the Department's approval confers recognition of standards being met. This federal office began operation in the 1990s, and gradually is reviewing organizations against their criteria for accreditation. Because application of the Department of Education's standards is new, some organizations are finding that they must make changes in their accreditation systems. A serious concern is that federal requirements are moving away from a system based on the overall professional judgment of colleagues about the quality of programs toward one that uses specific checklists of measurable data that may or may not measure actual excellence.

The Pew Reports

The Pew Health Professions Commission supported a series of studies and reports regarding the ability of the health professions to meet public needs for health care (Pew Health Professions Commission, 1995; O'Neill, 1993; Shugars et al., 1991). Much of what was reported supported trends others had identified. However, these three reports generated discussion and controversy among health professionals, educators, and regulators. The final report (Pew Health Professions Commission, 1995) identified four major concerns regarding the future of health professional education and licensure (Display 1-5).

SKILLS NEEDED IN THE FUTURE

The first issue that the Pew Commission addressed was redesign of the health care workforce. The Pew Commission suggested that the development of excellent generalists rather than narrow specialists urgently is needed. The trend of much health care has been toward developing more highly specialized individuals with extraordinary skills in a narrow field. Although this may provide excellence in certain areas, it does not provide for the overall health support of the nation. Demand will increase for generalists who look at the whole person and focus on prevention and health maintenance.

Display 1–5
PEW COMMISSION RECOMMENDATIONS

1. Redesign the health care workforce
2. Develop an interdisciplinary focus in health professional education
3. Examine and alter health professional regulations to make them more standardized, accountable, flexible, effective, and efficient
4. Right-size the health professions, which will include closing some nursing and medical schools

THE NEED FOR AN INTERDISCIPLINARY FOCUS

The Pew Commission also examined the consumer's need for interdisciplinary care and the need for a more organized system perspective. The Commission strongly recommended that educational programs emphasize these needs in the education of all health care professionals.

CHANGES IN REGULATION OF HEALTH CARE PROVIDERS

The regulatory system for both health professional education and for practice settings represents another barrier to effective delivery of care, according to the Commission (1995). They set goals that all regulation be standardized, accountable, flexible, effective, and efficient. These regulations affect issues such as entry into practice, the need for demonstrating continued competence by practitioners, and the need for effective systems to handle complaints and discipline. With regard to nursing, the Commission identified the multiple entry and exit points as a strength, but recommended clear differentiation of competencies at each level to guide both educators and employers and to establish clear avenues of articulation among levels.

THE SUPPLY OF HEALTH PROFESSIONALS

For many years, the federal government has supported a variety of efforts to increase the supply of many health professionals. In the 1990s, changes in the delivery of health care have raised questions about whether we need to increase the supply of health professionals or whether we might already have an oversupply in some areas. As hospitals restructured in the early 1990s, nurses were laid off and had difficulty finding positions outside the acute care setting that offered comparable salaries and benefits. The Pew Commission made recommendations about reducing the supply of nurses and some other health professionals.

As the 21st century begins, a nursing shortage is emerging with special concerns about highly technical areas such as critical care, the operating room, and emergency departments in hospitals. Long-term care facilities often have serious recruitment problems when jobs in acute care are abundant. There are also concerns that the numbers of nurses being prepared to fill positions requiring baccalaureate and higher degrees is inadequate. The shortage is also geographical with some areas of the country affected more than others. The nursing workforce is aging, with the average age being over 40 and the prospect of retirements increasingly affecting the adequacy of the supply of nurses (Fig. 1-5). Thus, the Pew recommendations about reducing the supply of nurses are no longer as relevant to health care needs.

The Pew Commission also recommended ensuring that foreign nationals who train in the United States return to their own countries after graduation. This was primarily focused on physicians who come to the United States for specialty residencies and then prefer to stay rather than return to the less sophisticated medical systems that exist in their own countries. Many large urban hospitals have met their needs for residents through recruiting foreign-educated physicians. Decreasing this supply of resident physicians has been another factor in the rapid emergence of the acute care nurse practitioner.

ALTERNATIVE HEALTH CARE

Professionals in health care often ignore the many alternative avenues of health care that people use, such as health foods, vitamins, chiropractors, and faith healers. When professionals consider these alternatives at all, they often dismiss them as quackery, with little understanding of why people turn to these resources. Increasingly, people are

FIGURE 1–5 The aging of the nursing workforce will affect the supply of nurses.

using what formerly were termed *alternative therapies* in addition to traditional medical care. In these situations, alternative therapies are often referred to as *complementary therapies*. According to an article in the *British Medical Journal* (1996), the increase in the use of complementary therapies is a worldwide phenomenon.

The Center for Alternative and Complementary Medicine (CACM) has defined this field as "those treatments and healthcare practices not taught widely in medical schools, not generally used in hospitals, and not usually reimbursed by medical insurance companies" (nccam.nih.gov, 1999). This definition focuses on what alternative care is *not* more than what it is. Part of that definition occurs because of the broad range of health care practices included in this category.

Major Types of Alternative Care

The CACM has categorized complementary and alternative medicine (CAM) into five types of treatment for the purpose of discussion and study. These are listed in Display 1-6.

Specific alternative care providers may use more than one type of treatment in their practice. Additionally, there are many areas of overlap between conventional medical practice and CAM. The major types of alternative care available are described briefly in the following sections and summarized in Display 1-6.

BIOELECTROMAGNETIC APPLICATIONS

The use of bioelectromagnetic (BEM) therapies is based on the understanding that electrical phenomena are found in all living organisms. There are magnetic fields that extend outside of the body that can be measured. Those magnetic fields that extend outside the body may be affected by external forces. The mechanisms by which the electromagnetic fields occur in the body, how these can be changed, and the effects of such changes are under study. Many modalities have been used for years without clear studies of their effectiveness. Some believe that bioelectromagnetics may be a unifying theory explaining why such widely diverse therapies as acupuncture and homeopathy produce results.

There are thermal applications of BEM therapy in the form of radio frequency hyperthermia and radio frequency diathermy. Nonthermal applications include magnets and nerve stimulation. One common application is the use of magnets to relieve musculoskeletal problems. Magnetic insoles for shoes and magnets to be worn on the

Display 1–6
ALTERNATIVE HEALTH CARE RESOURCES

- Bioelectromagnetic applications
- Diet, nutrition, lifestyle changes
- Herbal medicine
- Manual healing
- Mind–body control
- Pharmacologic and biologic treatment

body are widely sold. Research is progressing in the more sophisticated applications of this therapy for tissue regeneration and immune system stimulation (Alternative Medicine, 1992).

DIET, NUTRITION, LIFESTYLE CHANGES

The use of specific foods, overall diet plans, and changes in lifestyle are so widely used and accepted that many people do not consider them an alternative approach to health care. Ample evidence exists for the efficacy of a generally sound diet, exercise, and moderate lifestyle in enhancing health and longevity. There is less support, however, for the use of nutritional products as specific therapy for disease in the absence of a deficiency.

The health food movement in the United States is extraordinarily popular. Countless books are written and innumerable products are produced for this market. One of the appeals of this approach to health care is that it focuses on everyday, natural resources as opposed to science and technology. Poor dietary practices are common in the United States, with many individuals eating far more fat than is recommended and neglecting fruits, vegetables, and whole grains. Many people achieve better health by paying attention to good nutrition.

Medical research is beginning to identify some benefits of using food and vitamins in therapeutic ways. We have long known that many individuals who develop type 2 diabetes later in life may be able to manage their blood sugar through dietary control. The role of antioxidants in decreasing cell damage and the effect of certain phytochemicals contained in cruciferous vegetables in preventing bowel cancer are just two examples of the therapeutic benefits of nutrients.

There are hazards in this approach to health care, however. Megadoses of vitamins may prove toxic. Some nutrients interact with medications, decreasing their effectiveness. Individuals who choose to avoid all traditional medical care and rely on unsubstantiated claims about the therapeutic effects of nutrients may suffer a deterioration in health.

All health care professionals need to support and encourage healthy dietary practices. Often it is possible to assist clients who rely on the use of nutrients for health care by becoming knowledgeable about the research base regarding nutrition, accepting what clients believe helps them (as long as it is not detrimental to their well-being), and maintaining an open attitude. When you are willing to acknowledge the validity of some aspects of their preferred approach to health care, these clients may be willing to combine more conventional medical care along with their nutritional approaches.

HERBAL MEDICINES

Herbal medicines are plant products that are used to treat almost all illnesses. We know that plants often have active ingredients that affect the human body. Digitalis, for example, was originally a dried leaf of the foxglove plant. (Digitalis drugs are now synthesized in the laboratory.) It was indeed a potent and effective medication when used as an herb, but dosage was not accurate and little scientific information existed regarding its effects. As research into plant products continues, our understanding of the efficacy of herbs is increasing. Many herbalists in the United States are Asian Americans who received their training in herbs during an apprenticeship with an experienced herbalist. Some naturopathic physicians also use herbs.

It is wise to recognize the potential problems and the potential benefits of the use of herbal medicines. Individual plants may vary in their concentration of active chemicals. This makes accurate and stable dosage of herbs difficult. Sometimes the active ingredient may have potent side effects. For example, many individuals have used herbs that contain ephedra. Ephedra acts as a stimulant, dilates bronchioles, and decreases appetite. Therefore, it has been used for the herbal treatment of fatigue, asthma, and obesity. It also raises blood pressure, increases pulse rate, and creates feelings of tension and anxiety. These side effects have been severe enough to precipitate stroke and cardiac problems in some individuals.

Many herbs are imported from around the world. Rules and regulations regarding labeling and content purity may not be as strict in some countries as they are in the United States. This means that some herbs that are sold may contain contaminants. Serious illnesses and even deaths have been traced to contaminants in herbal medicines. At present, there are no laws regulating the potency or purity of herbs sold in the United States.

Clients taking herbal medicines should be encouraged to share this information with their health care provider. They also should be encouraged to question carefully the sources of the herbs that they take. These actions might help clients avoid potentially harmful interactions with prescribed medications, or other adverse effects.

MANUAL HEALING

Manual healing is the physical manipulation of the body to achieve health goals. Perhaps the most commonly known type of manual healing is chiropractic. Manual healing also is found in massage therapy and reflexology. Massage therapy uses both fixed and movable pressure and holding by the hands and sometimes the forearms, elbows, and feet. There is evidence that these techniques affect the musculoskeletal, circulatory-lymphatic, and nervous systems. Reflexology is massage of the feet.

Chiropractic care is based on the theory that disease is caused by interference with nerve function. It uses manipulation of the body joints, especially the spinal vertebrae, in seeking to restore normal function. The chiropractor also may use other treatments commonly associated with physical therapy, such as massage and exercise. There are definite differences among chiropractors. Some state that there are illnesses that cannot be treated through manual healing and do recommend that certain clients seek medical care. Others believe that all illnesses may be treated by chiropractic methods and do not refer clients for medical care. A major concern is that some clients may have more serious illnesses that may be missed altogether or not recognized in time to be given optimal medical attention. Another problem with chiropractic care is the use of chiropractic treatments on infants and young children in place of immunizations and other well child services.

Many people with joint and muscle strain and tension find that chiropractic treatments relieve discomfort and support effective functioning. The Agency for Health

Care Policy and Research recommends chiropractic treatment as a useful option in specific circumstances for relieving pain discomfort in acute back pain (ACHPR, 1994, www.ahrq.gov).

MIND-BODY CONTROL

Mind-body therapies seek to control physical processes through the mind's capacities. In addition, mind-body therapies treat emotional concerns. Traditional psychotherapy is a mind-body approach to health and wellness. Support groups, yoga, meditation, relaxation, biofeedback, and visualization are all mind-body therapies.

Relaxation exercises, hypnosis, and meditation are examples of controlling physiologic stress responses through mental processes. Relaxation exercises, breathing techniques, meditation, and visualization are used to reduce anxiety, reduce blood pressure, and lessen the body's response to stressors. These techniques also are designed to prevent stress-related problems from developing; for many people, they are part of a plan to increase health and well-being. These techniques also are suggested for the management of specific health problems. Such approaches may be used in conjunction with traditional medical treatment.

Visualization may be used to help children manage painful medical procedures. Suggestions regarding healing and postoperative recovery now are used in the operating room by some anesthesiologists and surgeons. The anesthesiologist may talk to the patient who is still anesthetized, suggesting that pain will be minimal, nausea will not occur, and recovery will be rapid. This is similar to posthypnotic suggestion. Hypnosis has been used in other illnesses for symptom relief (Fig. 1-6).

Biofeedback is a specific mechanism to assist individuals to alter physiologic responses through mental processes. The machines used for biofeedback provide visual

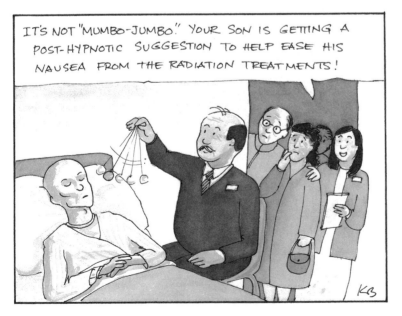

FIGURE 1–6 Alternative health care is moving more and more into mainstream practice.

or auditory feedback of physiological parameters such as blood pressure or galvanic skin response. By observing these parameters, the individual learns to change the underlying physiologic process. Some individuals with migraine headaches use biofeedback control over circulation to abort migraine attacks rather than taking medications.

Mind-body control therapies in general allow people to participate actively in their own care. People are often changed emotionally and psychologically in the process of treating illness or disease. A big advantage of the mind-body therapies is that they are safe and economical and can be used easily in conjunction with other therapies.

PHARMACOLOGIC AND BIOLOGIC TREATMENT

Pharmacologic and biologic treatments include a variety of substances not approved as medical treatment by the Food and Drug Administration. These products have been developed by individuals and organizations and are often sold as food supplements rather than as medicines. Cartilage products from sharks, cattle, sheep, and chickens are being used to treat both cancer and arthritis. Peptide fractions derived from human blood and urine, called antineoplastons, are being used to treat cancer. Coley's toxins are killed cultures of bacteria that have been used for treating cancer. Apitherapy is the use of honeybee venom to treat rheumatic diseases, dermatologic conditions, chronic pain, and cancer. Research on the efficacy of these treatments is costly, and sponsors willing to bear that cost are hard to find. Some small studies are being funded with federal grants.

Alternative Medical Systems

Alternative medical systems represent complete systems of theory and practice that approach health care differently from the traditional Western biomedical approach. Four subcategories are identified: acupuncture and Asian medicine; traditional indigenous systems; unconventional Western systems of medicine; and naturopathy (Display 1-7). Each of these systems uses a variety of specific therapies.

ACUPUNCTURE AND ASIAN MEDICINE

In acupuncture and Asian medicine, there are complete systems of explanation for health and illness. The therapies chosen are based on these theoretical systems of belief. Acupuncture and Asian medicine practitioners use a variety of approaches to

Display 1–7
ALTERNATIVE SYSTEMS OF HEALTH CARE

Acupuncture and Asian Medicine	Unconventional Western Systems of Medicine
Traditional Indigenous Systems	Naturopathy

health care. They often combine acupuncture with herbal medicines and diet. Some use traditional Chinese manual techniques such as Tui Na, a form of massage and manipulation.

TRADITIONAL INDIGENOUS SYSTEMS

Native Americans, Hispanic Americans, Asian Americans, and many other ethnic groups have traditional health care resources that are still used by many people. Often termed *folk medicine*, these traditions usually are handed down by word of mouth and are used to treat common health problems. Treatment often involves the use of herbs, foods, and traditional ceremonies. Little is understood about many of the herbs used, but some have demonstrated therapeutic effects. In a given ethnic group, certain people may be designated as healers or as having special knowledge and ability in regard to illness. The advice of such a person may be sought instead of the advice of a physician. To work most effectively with a client who uses folk medicine, you need to investigate the specific beliefs and resources that he or she is using.

Ayurvedic medicine from India is included in this category. Ayurvedic care has existed for more than 5,000 years and has a specific theoretical and therapeutic focus on imbalance in the individual's consciousness. Lifestyle interventions are the major form of Ayurvedic preventive and therapeutic treatment. There is one Ayurvedic hospital in North America.

Every major religion of the world responds in particular ways to those who are ill. A well-established way for supporting an ill person is through the prayers of others who care. Nurses recognize that spiritual distress has a significant impact on a client's ability to move toward wellness. Supporting the individual's quest for spiritual solace and healing has been a part of the mission of many health care agencies that were established by religious bodies. The separation of prayer and spiritual care from other health care is a modern phenomenon.

UNCONVENTIONAL WESTERN SYSTEMS OF MEDICINE

Unconventional Western systems of medicine originated in Western society but did not find general support. Some individuals continue to practice in the theoretical precepts of these systems.

Perhaps the most common of these unconventional systems is homeopathy. Homeopathy is based on the belief that exposure to extremely small quantities of either the substance causing an illness or a related substance will stimulate a cure. Of course, this principle is also the basis for immunization and allergy desensitization. The application of this principle to other diseases, however, has not been accepted by the medical community. The dilutions used in many homeopathic remedies are so great that a dosage may contain only a few molecules of a substance. Homeopathy was popular in the early 20th century, but fell into disrepute as standard medical research advanced. There is currently a resurgence of interest in this approach to therapy, and some new research is being done. Homeopathic practitioners once again are offering an alternative to standard medical care.

NATUROPATHY

Naturopathy gets its name from the natural agents used in treating disease, such as food, exercise, air, water, and sunshine. Because naturopathy has a different focus than systems that use chemical interventions, it was categorized separately from the other Western alternative systems. The naturopathic physician treats people by recommending changes in lifestyle, diet, and exercise, and the use of vitamins and herbs. For many, this is a successful form of treatment. Naturopathic physicians follow a prescribed course of study that includes clinical experiences with clients and results in the doctor of naturopathy (ND) degree. Naturopathy is licensed in some states.

Understanding the Use of Alternative Health Care

For many clients with chronic conditions, mainstream medical care offers few options. Long-term treatments with medications often produce their own iatrogenic (treatment-caused) health problems, some of which are as troubling to the individual as the original disease process. A common response to these problems has been to add more medications and more treatments, each with its own potential adverse effects. Mainstream health care providers often give little attention to the problems of daily living that are of greatest concern to the individual. Stress and anxiety also add to the burden of these clients. For clients with acute health conditions, certain treatments or medications may produce unpleasant or harmful side effects. Clients often are looking for alternative treatment methods that do not appear to have the same potential for harm.

Some alternative therapies have been available for many years, and there are people who believe that they have been significantly helped by these approaches. Unfortunately, traditional health care providers often have dismissed these therapies without investigating them thoroughly. On the other hand, few alternative therapies have been formally researched, and proponents rely on undocumented reports of effectiveness.

Research into alternative therapies now is supported by the federal government, but only in a small way compared to other research. The federal government now has an office of alternative health care and a Web page of references, the National Center for Complementary and Alternative Medicine. (See list of Web sites.) More attention is being paid to the responses of individuals. Concern about the role of stress in illness has prompted an increased openness to nonmedical methods of managing stress. The possibility of alternative care practices working in a complementary fashion with traditional medical care is gaining wider acceptance. Often these complementary therapies are used to address the whole person and not simply the disease.

Part of the appeal of alternative health care is the caring and personalized response that clients often receive. People who have been intimidated by businesslike clinics, and made to feel unimportant by impersonal professionals, may find that the warm, concerned, accepting atmosphere of the nonconventional setting meets many personal needs. The fact that stress and anxiety play a major role in any health problem may help explain why many people are helped by therapies that may not be based on sound scientific knowledge.

To learn more about any specific therapy, or to research alternative and complementary therapies for any condition, you can use the CAM Citation Index found on the Web site of the National Center for Complementary and Alternative Medicine (see references). You may also use MEDLINE at the National Library of Medicine to research various therapies.

Assisting Clients Who Choose Alternative Health Care

Many people who support conventional methods of health care have long ignored or repudiated the value of unorthodox health care traditions. We must recognize that alternative health care practices have persisted because people have found them to be valuable. Acknowledging health care alternatives and working cooperatively with them is usually much more productive than trying to oppose them.

One problem that clients face in seeking complementary or alternative health care is the lack of assurance that a practitioner they consult is well trained and ethical, because there are usually no universally accepted alternative health care standards (Lynn, 1996). Traditional health care providers have an obligation to assist their clients in formulating questions that reveal a practitioner's background, education, and training. We must help our clients to identify and avoid those alternative care providers who engage in unethical or harmful practices.

Many health care providers now support the use of various complementary therapies. According to Norton (1995), such issues as client choice, informed consent, and the ethical principles of beneficence and nonmaleficence (see Chapter 9) all must be considered in relation to alternative therapies. As alternative and complementary therapies move into the mainstream, greater accountability to the public is essential.

Critical Thinking Activity

Identify a specific form of alternative and complementary therapy. Do a literature search regarding this therapy. Review the information available in other sources. Analyze the information to determine whether the data supporting the use of this therapy are weak, moderate, or strong. Provide a rationale for your determination.

KEY CONCEPTS

- The various types of health care services are differentiated by the needs of the client being served, and range from specific specialized services to skilled care to custodial care.
- Many different types of agencies provide health care services; examples include long-term care settings, acute care hospitals, ambulatory care centers, home care agencies, and health care businesses, among others. There are a wide variety of nursing roles in these different settings. Health care agencies are classified according to length of stay, type of service provided, and ownership of the agency.

- Acute care facilities center around the work of the traditional hospital, which has become a hub for health care in most communities.
- Long-term care facilities provide many types of care. Nursing homes provide care for those without the ability to manage activities of daily living and who need ongoing care. Assisted-living centers provide fewer services. Rehabilitation centers assist the individual in returning to a maximum level of independence.
- Ambulatory care settings provide care on an outpatient basis. This care may range from simple office calls for common illnesses and health promotion activities such as immunizations to the performance of ambulatory surgery.
- Home health agencies offer a wide variety of care services that may include traditional public health services, high-intensity skilled care in the home, and rehabilitation services. Home care agencies offer services within the home that assist individuals in avoiding institutional care settings when they are unable to complete their own activities of daily living.
- Changes in the health care delivery system are creating many problems that affect health care workers. Among these, as presented by the Pew Commission, are issues related to primary care, accreditation of health professional education programs, and the future of health professional education and licensure.
- Alternative health care is growing in popularity. Some types of alternative care are being used along with traditional medical care as complementary therapies. Understanding the different types of alternative health care services, why people choose alternative health care, and how you may assist people who seek this care will form a foundation for more effective relationships with clients.

REFERENCES

Alternative Medicine: Expanding Medical Horizons. A report prepared under the auspices of the Workshop on Alternative Medicine, held in Chantilly, VA, September 14–16, 1992

College dean: "So close" to solving rural doctor shortage. (1999, Aug. 30). Sioux City Journal, p. A4.

Complementary medicine is booming worldwide. British Medical Journal 313(7050):131–133, 1996

DeYoung S, Just G, VanDyk R. Assisted living: Policy implications for nursing. Nurs Health Care 15(10):510–513, 1994

Hawryluk, M. Final rule clarifies coverage issue. Provider 25(10):33–34, 1999

Hawryluk M. Regulations in the assisted living community. Provider 21(10):71–72, 74, 1995

Joel LA. Hungry for the truth. Am J Nurs 96(3):7, 1996

Lanigan JM, Dodds L, Mechanic J. The ambulatory treatment unit: An innovative model. J Nurs Admin 24(4):41–44, 1994

Lipowski EE, Bigelow WE. Linkages for research on outcomes of long term care. The Gerontologist 36(4):441–447, 1996

Lynn J. The rising popularity of complementary therapies. Prof Nurse 11(4):266–269, 1996

Norton L. Complementary therapies in practice: The ethical issues. J Clin Nurs 4(6):343–348, 1995

O'Neil EH. Health Professions Education for the Future: Schools in Service to the Nation. San Francisco: Pew Health Professions Commission, 1993

Pew Health Professions Commission, Critical Challenges: Revitalizing the Health Professions for the Twenty-First Century. San Francisco: UCSF Center for the Health Professions, 1995

Shugars DA, O'Neill EH, Bader JD, eds. Healthy America: Practitioners for 2005, An Agenda for Action for U.S. Health Professional Schools. Durham, NC: The Pew Health Professions Commission, 1991

Task Force on Support Personnel (1996, Spring). Guidelines for the training, credentialing, use, and supervision of speech–language pathology assistants. ASHA Supplement, 38(2 Suppl. 16):21–34.

Taylor KS. Clamor over subacute care creates adversaries/new partners. Hospitals and Health Care Networks 68(6):102, March 20, 1994

FURTHER READING

Alexander CJ, Steefel L. Biofeedback: Listen to the body. RN 58(8):51–52, 1995

American Nurses Association. Standards for Clinical Nursing Practice. Washington, DC: American Nurses Publishing Co., 1991

Cassileth BR, Chapman CC. Alternative cancer medicine: A ten-year update. Cancer Investigation 14(4):396–404, 1996

Cleveland MJ, Biester DJ. Alternative and complementary therapies: Considerations for nursing practice. J Pediatr Nurs 10(2):121–123, 1995

Enskar K. Ethical aspects of judging the alternative treatment of children with cancer. Nursing Ethics 2(2):51–62, 1995

Lynn J. Using complementary therapies: Reflexology. Professional Nurse 11(5):321–322, 1996

Mackay RB. Complementary modalities: Part 1. Discover the healing of therapeutic touch. Am J Nurs 95(4):26–32, 1995

Mornhinweg GC, Voignier RR. Holistic nursing interventions. Orthopedic Nursing 14(4): 20–24, 1995

Nokes KM, Kendrew J, Longo M. Alternative/complementary therapies used by persons with HIV disease. Journal of the Association of Nurses in AIDS Care 6(4):19–24, 1995

Segal-Isaacson AE. Healing patients: Therapeutic touch in nursing practice. Np News 3(3):4, 9–10, 1995

Slater VE. Toward an understanding of energetic healing, Part 1: Energetic structure. J Holistic Nurs 13(3):209–224, 1995

Slater VE. Toward an understanding of energetic healing, Part 2: Energetic processes. J Holistic Nurs 13(3):225–238, 1995

Swackhamer AH. Complementary therapies: It's time to broaden our practice. RN 58(1):49–51, 1995

Talton CW. Touch—of all kinds—is therapeutic. RN 58(2):61–64, 1995

Relevant web sites

Agency for Healthcare Research and Quality (AHRQ—formerly Agency for Health Care Policy and Research: Practice Guidelines [AHCPR]) *www.ahrq.gov*

American Pain Society: Policies and Recommendations on Pain Management *www.ampainsoc.org*

Joint Commission for the Accreditation of Healthcare Organizations (JCAHO) *www.jcaho.org*

National Center for Complementary and Alternative Medicine: Federal Government database of scientific articles and abstracts *nccam.nih.gov*

National Guideline Clearinghouse *www.guideline.gov/index.asp*

National League for Nursing Accrediting Commission: Nursing Education Accreditation Standards and Criteria *www.nlnac.org*

National Library of Medicine, MEDLINE data base search through PubMed *ncbi.nlm.nih.gov/PubMed*

2

Health Care Finance and Control

How do we decide who will be cared for and who will not? Who will pay and how much?

(Moccia, 1988)

O B J E C T I V E S

After completing this chapter, you should be able to

1. Describe different mechanisms for financing health care.

2. Explain how the role of the federal government in health care financing has affected the system.

3. Discuss the various approaches to managing costs in the health care delivery system, including changing patterns of payment and controlling providers.

4. Analyze the issues related to access to health care, including types of barriers and indicators of access.

5. Discuss the mechanisms being used to measure and assure quality in organizations and agencies that are delivering health care.

6. Analyze the use of power by regulatory agencies, payers, providers, and consumers in the health care system.

7. Explain continuing concerns regarding the effective use of health care and concerns about changing the system.

K E Y   T E R M S

Acuity

Capitation

Case management

Comorbidity

Cost containment

Diagnosis–related groups (DRGs)

Fee-for-service

Health maintenance organization (HMO)

Insurance

Joint Commission for the Accreditation of Healthcare Organizations (JCAHO)

Key indicators

Long-term care

Managed care	Power	Quality indicators (QI)
Medicaid	Preferred provider organiza-	Restructuring
Medicare	tion (PPO)	Resource utilization groups
Medicare intermediary	Primary care provider	(RUGs)
Outcome measures	Prospective payment	Third-party payer
Point-of-service plan	Prospective payment system	Vertically integrated systems
	(PPS)	

Throughout the world, the concern over health care has everyone's attention. In most of what we call the industrialized world, health care is seen as a right of every citizen. Based on this right, health care is operated by governmental systems that provide universal health care coverage. In some countries, such as Sweden and the Netherlands, there is strong centralization of financing and control. In other countries, such as Canada and Germany, systems are controlled regionally through provincial authority. These governmental systems are successful in accomplishing overall health outcomes such as low maternal-infant mortality, high immunization rates, and reduction of preventable deaths. The problems found in these systems are related to the high cost of providing health care throughout the world and subsequent attempts to control those costs. Waits for care may be long and some care, especially care that is very costly such as dialysis, may be rationed. Because of these situations, private medical care that is paid for by individuals also may be available to those with sufficient income.

In developing nations, health care may be limited. Some care may be paid for by the government and some by private means, but there are not the individual or institutional providers to meet the needs of the population. The available resources may not meet the standards that those in more affluent countries have come to expect. Hospitals may lack adequate safe water and sanitation. Ordinary supplies such as dressing materials and sterile needles may be unavailable. Drugs may be in short supply, and diagnostic and laboratory testing may be nonexistent. Health care outcomes in these countries tend to be poor, especially regarding infant and child mortality. It is in these countries that the World Health Organization is most active in trying to improve health outcomes through immunization, sanitation, and other public health programs.

In the United States, health care has not been accepted as a right for the whole society. Therefore, no mechanism exists to build a coordinated health care system. Much of the complexity found in the U.S. health care system relates to the variety of mechanisms for funding and controlling health care. Although the United States has ready availability of the most sophisticated medical technology and expertise, at the same time there are deficiencies seen in some of the key measures of population health. Some individuals have access to the most effective health care in the world; others have no health care access except in cases of emergency when hospitals are required by law to provide care.

This chapter explains the various organizations and agencies responsible for health care financing and control in the United States, and how that affects the availability of health care and access to it. Understanding this aspect of the health care system can enable you to be a more effective participant in it.

FINANCING HEALTH CARE FOR INDIVIDUALS

Currently, there are many different approaches to financing health care for individuals. Personal payment, charitable care, insurance plans, health maintenance organizations, and a variety of government programs are all forms of health care financing. Agencies that pay caregivers for health services provided to individuals are termed *third-party payers*. These payers include insurance companies, health maintenance organizations, Medicare, Medicaid, and other governmental agencies (Display 2-1). Increasingly, individual health care decisions are made by the a combination of the patient-consumer, the provider, and the payer rather than by any one of them alone.

Personal Payment

Originally, health care was paid for each time it was provided. Although the payment was usually in cash, in a more rural society payment sometimes extended to barter, with garden produce, chickens, and eggs traded for medical care. Individuals who did not have the means to pay for a doctor or hospital visit did not receive needed care.

Today most individuals still pay for health care, but often in indirect ways that make them less aware of the specific costs. Health insurance premiums may be deducted from a paycheck, or an employer may pay premiums directly while considering them part of employee compensation. Federal and state taxes provide for some health services. Most health insurance plans require the subscriber to pay a deductible (a portion of the bill), which may be computed for each service or may be an aggregate for the year. The size of the deductible that is the individual's responsibility has been increasing in many insurance plans, giving people greater incentive to use services wisely.

Charitable Care

Charitable care has played a significant role in the history of health care. The earliest hospitals were religious institutions that provided health care as a form of ministry and as a charitable service. Some large charitable groups still provide a great deal of care

Display 2-1
APPROACHES TO FINANCING HEALTH CARE

- Personal payment
- Charitable care
- Health insurance plans
- Health maintenance organizations
- State-administered health plans
- Federal government programs

for people who are unable to pay, such as the Shriner's Children's Hospitals. Although these hospitals do collect insurance and payment from those who can afford care, they also raise money for the purpose of providing high-level care to children in need.

During the 1970s and 1980s, federal funds were made available through the Hill-Burton Act for hospital construction. Hospitals constructed with these funds accepted an obligation to provide some charitable care in their communities. As these obligations expired, concern about what was happening in emergency care led to legislation that requires hospitals to provide emergency care regardless of an individual's ability to pay.

Historically, some money for charitable care was raised through donations. As insurance became more widespread, hospitals often supported charitable care by charging paying clients more than the cost of their care and using the excess income to offset the costs of charitable care. However, as negotiations for lower health care costs for managed care continue and regulations have limited Medicare reimbursement, hospitals are experiencing a decreased ability to provide charitable care without severe financial difficulties.

Individual physicians also have provided forms of charitable care. Only rarely did people directly ask physicians for charitable care; often a physician did not pursue the payment of a bill that could not be paid by a family. Physicians and other care providers also have provided charitable care by volunteering their time at "free" clinics. Many people who could not afford care simply did without because they did not want to ask for charity.

Health Insurance Plans

Starting in the 1930s, insurance companies gradually began to pay a greater share of medical fees. The basic framework of insurance coverage is that of shared risk. Individuals pay for coverage whether or not they have health care costs; when a covered individual requires health care, the insurance pays for that care. Historically, health insurance was for hospital care and related services only. Outpatient visits, immunizations, costs of drugs, and other such services were not covered by insurance policies. One disadvantage of this system was that consumers had no incentive to reduce their use of services: they paid the same regardless of their needs. People sought to have services delivered on an inpatient basis to obtain reimbursement. Another disadvantage was that individuals often neglected preventive health care that had to be paid for out-of-pocket. Health insurance policies now cover many preventive services, outpatient costs, and some prescription costs.

At the heart of the process of setting insurance rates and specifying coverage is the process of identifying what will be covered, determining risks for different groups of individuals, and projecting the costs of care. The more heterogeneous the group, the more broadly the risk is spread and the more insurance costs are kept reasonable for all. Limitations on coverage protect insurance companies from excessive risk. When high-risk individuals are excluded from insurance, it makes the cost less for low-risk subscribers, but leaves those who are most in need of assistance without the benefit of broadly shared risk.

Many insurance companies are private profit-making companies owned by stockholders. They provide service to policyholders and also create profit for stockholders. The

"Blues" (Blue Cross and Blue Shield companies) originally were established as not-for-profit organizations. Historically, this has provided them with certain benefits in the marketplace and enabled them to offer services at a lower cost than for-profit companies such as Aetna. However, nonprofit corporations face restrictions on their functioning that private profit-making companies do not encounter. Recent changes in the health care system have blurred the distinctions between nonprofit and private profit-making companies. In some areas of the country, Blue Cross and Blue Shield have asked regulatory authorities for permission to convert to standard profit-making companies and to sell stock (and have changed their names in the process). In some states, courts have required that these corporations provide remuneration to their communities. In other states, these changes have occurred without public input.

As the cost of health care has increased, insurance premiums also have increased greatly. One of the concerns of the public is that health insurance is unobtainable for individuals with existing health problems and often economically beyond the means of those who are not insured as part of an employee group. Legislation to require insurance companies to cover everyone has passed in some jurisdictions and is being considered in others. Federal legislation, the Health Coverage Portability Act, was passed in 1996 to allow people to maintain coverage when they change jobs; it requires that an individual previously covered by an employer's health insurance policy be covered by the new employer's insurance without waiting periods or exclusions for preexisting conditions. This legislation also has provided tax incentives for those purchasing long-term care insurance.

Another cause for concern is the process of reviewing and denying insurance claims. All insurance plans have written rules regarding notification, acceptable providers, and precisely when and how reimbursement will occur. Sometimes these rules result in a denial of payment, as illustrated by the following example.

A young woman who delivered a baby at her preferred provider hospital expected the standard coverage for delivery to apply. To her surprise, however, she was reimbursed as if the hospital were a nonpreferred provider because she had not notified the insurance company in advance that she would be using that facility. She had submitted claims for all prenatal care to the company, had attended prenatal classes at the hospital, and had filled out all insurance forms early in her pregnancy. The hospital was expected to take care of all insurance papers, but subsequently denied responsibility for advance notice. This cost the young couple $500. Similar situations occur often and cause all consumers to be concerned about their health insurance plans.

Although insurance companies originally focused on paying for health care, they now are involved in establishing standards for care, evaluating care, and negotiating charges. They are active participants in all areas of health care and, because of the economic power they wield, have great influence. Insurance companies determine whom they will pay and what procedures they will reimburse. Thus, insurance companies can limit health care choices.

Health Maintenance Organizations

Health maintenance organizations (HMOs) have been in existence in the United States for more than 50 years, but their growth in number was slow until federal legislation in 1972 and 1974 provided the impetus to start new HMOs. Health maintenance organizations originated as an alternative to traditional insurance plans. Although traditional insurance plans paid for care when subscribers were ill, health maintenance organizations were the first to provide payment for care aimed at preventing illness. Health maintenance organizations provided well child care, prenatal care, immunizations, pelvic examinations, and other preventive services when insurance companies did not. A flat charge per month covered routine preventive health care, care for illness, hospitalization and, in some instances, prescription costs, outpatient care, and other services. Currently, HMO-enrolled individuals are responsible for a copayment (meaning the client pays a part of the bill). Copayments support part of the cost of care and give the consumer an incentive to use services wisely.

HMOs are characterized by differing patterns of finance and governance. Some are operated by insurance companies; some are private profit-making organizations; some are nonprofit organizations; and still others are consumer owned and operated. Many newer HMOs operate as business entities that manage the financial aspects of health care and, through financial management, access to services. Consumer Reports magazine (1996) has reported that there is greater consumer satisfaction with nonprofit HMOs.

HMOs are also characterized by differing patterns of providing health services. Primary health care providers may be employed by an HMO and receive a fixed salary. In some cases, a group of primary health care providers, termed an *independent practice association* (IPA), may contract with an HMO to provide services for a preset fee per individual in the program. HMOs also may employ many other health care workers, including nurses. In some HMOs clients have a choice of care providers; in others they do not. HMO plans that allow an individual to choose to go outside of the plan for services that the plan does not or will not provide are called *point-of-service* plans. Usually the subscriber is eligible for some reimbursement of costs in these plans, but at a greatly reduced rate. Two examples of HMOs are described in Display 2-2.

Because the HMO receives the same income (except for modest copayments) whether a client requires extensive care or very little care, there is a built-in incentive to emphasize preventive care and avoid costly hospitalization. HMOs were the first type of health plan to manage care. The concept of managed care has broadened considerably and includes many types of health plans.

Because HMOs have lower health care costs than conventional fee-for-service systems, the federal government has subsidized the creation of new HMOs and has encouraged employers to offer HMOs as alternatives to traditional health insurance plans. This has speeded the development of new HMOs. Federal subsidizing of HMOs also helps to contain costs in all health plans as a result of competition. People on Medicare now have the option of joining HMOs. Under such circumstances, Medicare makes capitated payments directly to the HMO. This may limit the flexibility of the individual to seek care outside the HMO, although some HMOs are offering plans with higher copayments that allow the individual to seek care from any desired provider.

Beginning in 1998, a crisis occurred in Medicare HMOs. Many plans found that overall costs were greater than anticipated. These HMOs refused to renew their contracts to provide Medicare-HMO services. This left many elderly individuals with difficult choices to make as they returned to conventional Medicare Supplemental Insur-

Display 2-2
HEALTH MAINTENANCE ORGANIZATIONS

THE KAISER FOUNDATION HEALTH PLAN

This nonprofit organization, which began in California and Oregon, owns and operates its own hospitals. The physicians are members of a group that contracts with the organization to provide medical services. The fee for membership covers almost all health care costs, including both outpatient and inpatient costs. Kaiser Health Plans are now available in many states.

GROUP HEALTH COOPERATIVE OF PUGET SOUND

Located in Washington State, this HMO is a consumer-owned and -operated cooperative that owns and operates its own clinics and employs physicians and other health care providers. For most of its history, it also operated its own hospitals but is gradually closing down inpatient services, maintaining a birthing center and outpatient surgery services, and contracting for most other hospital care. People who join the cooperative as members pay a monthly fee for comprehensive health care, which includes both outpatient and inpatient services. The membership elects the governing board; members serve on policy-making committees; and a vote of the entire membership decides some issues. In addition, Group Health Cooperative contracts with employers to provide comprehensive, prepaid coverage for employee groups. Members of the employment groups may choose to become members of the cooperative. The employer may pay the monthly fee directly or the employee may pay the fee through payroll deduction.

These two organizations are currently cooperating to provide multistate health care coverage.

ance. These conventional plans often did not provide outpatient pharmacy coverage, thus greatly increasing the costs of health management for the individual.

State-Administered Health Plans

States may operate a variety of health care resources for residents. All states manage some type of insurance plan for workers injured on the job. These workers' compensation plans may be managed as a state monopoly or may be contracted to private insurance companies. Employers are required to pay premiums based upon statistical information about covered injuries and hazards in various job categories. An individual injured on the job is assured of receiving care paid for by the workers' compensation plan.

Some states administer health insurance plans on a wider basis. Hawaii assures universal health care coverage for its residents. Minnesota has been a leader in attempting to provide health services for all its residents. The state of Washington has developed an insurance plan called the Basic Health Plan for working individuals who earn too much money to be eligible for tax-supported health care, but who do not have incomes high enough to afford regular insurance. Unfortunately, this plan, which is subsidized by tax revenue, cannot accommodate all who are eligible.

The federal government also provides funds through the Medicaid programs that are administered by the states and matched with state funds. Included in this funding are the costs of health care for families on public assistance and support of nursing home care for those who have exhausted their personal financial resources. In 1999 the federal government provided a mechanism for states to enlarge their Medicaid programs to enroll children from low income families who did not qualify for Medicaid and who would otherwise be without health care coverage. This Children's Health Insurance Plan (CHIP) represents the first time that the United States has supported health care as a right for all children. Not all states have agreed to participate in the plan because it requires their financial contribution and provides for some federal control of the program.

Most states support state mental hospitals and public health services. Further public health services may be supplied through county and city governments. Hospitals designed to provide care for those who are indigent may be operated by the city (such as the New York City hospitals) or by the county (such as Cook County Hospital in Chicago) (Fig. 2-1).

Federal Government Programs

The federal government in the United States is deeply involved in health care financing. Federal programs cover the elderly, the poor, federal workers, the military, veterans, and Native Americans and Native Alaskans. Some individuals are concerned about governmental involvement in our health care system; when all of these programs and agencies are considered together, it is clear that, for good or ill, the federal government already controls many aspects of health care.

FIGURE 2–1   Health care insurance plans are complex and often confusing to the ordinary consumer.

MEDICARE AND MEDICAID

In 1965, after years of effort and testimony by many health-related groups (including the ANA), and with widespread public support, an amendment to the Social Security Act was passed. Title XVIII of the act, which was termed *Medicare*, provided payment for hospitalization (Part A), and insurance that could be purchased to meet physicians' fees and outpatient costs (Part B), for people over age 65 and certain others who were receiving Social Security payments. Participation in Medicare Part A is automatic for those on Social Security, whereas participation in Medicare Part B is optional. Medicare is administered through a federal agency called the Health Care Financing Administration (HCFA, sometimes pronounced "hik-fah") which uses contracted insurance companies termed *Medicare intermediaries* to process claims.

Title IX of the Social Security Act, which was termed Medicaid, provides funds for health care for those dependent on public assistance and certain other low income individuals. Costs are shared between the federal government and each state. Each state is responsible for administering Medicaid: the state determines eligibility and level of coverage. Payments from the federal government to the states are administered by HCFA. Benefits vary greatly among states. California's plan, called Medi-Cal, historically has been one of the most comprehensive. As health care costs have risen, there has been great pressure to cut this program. A few states have not participated in the Medicaid program to avoid federal control. Some states have requested waivers from HCFA's usual regulations governing Medicaid and Medicare to allow experimentation with different plans that might help to control costs.

The complexity of filing claims with Medicare and also with an insurance company designed to supplement Medicare coverage is confusing for many people. Even when claims are filed by the provider, they may be denied payment if they do not conform to specific rules and regulations. Often elderly people accept an initial denial of payment for the claim as the final decision and do not pursue the matter further. There is a high rate of reconsideration when denials are appealed; therefore, it is often wise to encourage clients to appeal a denial of payment.

Many HMOs and insurance companies are seeking the business of those on Medicare. The plans they provide supplement what Medicare pays and often cover all health care. This coverage usually comes with a loss of choice of providers for the consumer, a feature some individuals do not understand when they sign up for such plans.

Medicare and Medicaid are important health care resources, but they have not been without problems. Costs have been much greater and have been rising faster than anticipated. There has been a great deal of publicity about instances of abuse, and even fraud, associated with these two program. The goals of providing cost-effective health care to the elderly and the indigent through these programs have yet to be achieved.

Impact on Nursing. The Medicare bill contains many provisions that have made a significant impact on nursing. A definition of skilled nursing care in the original bill was narrow and excluded many important aspects of care necessary to maintaining the health of clients. Through later efforts and testimony, nursing organizations were instrumental in convincing legislators to recognize that the definition of skilled nursing was a critical matter; as a result, a Senate subcommittee asked the ANA to study skilled nursing care to provide background data for the Senate. Amendments to the Medicare/Medicaid Act of 1972 encouraged study of alternative ways of providing health care to contain costs. These alternatives included the use of nurses in expanded roles and the use of HMOs.

Cost-Containment Initiatives. Amendments to the Medicare/Medicaid Act were also responsible for mandating review and evaluation of health care. This was done in the interests of cost control or containment. Institutions must review records of Medicare/Medicaid clients and compare them with specific criteria for care.

In 1982, the 97th Congress revised Medicare to prevent the serious financial deficits in the system that escalating costs could potentially create. The revisions increased the premium for Part B of Medicare (the optional portion that provides for out-of-hospital and physician care) and also increased the deductible that the individual must pay for covered service. The system of payment was changed to prospective payment based on diagnosis-related groups (DRGs). (See the discussion on patterns of payment later in this chapter.) The planners who revised Medicare also included a new mechanism for reimbursing hospice care.

In 1993, more changes, restrictions, and controls were instituted in the Medicare system: the payroll deduction for Medicare (paid by all employed individuals regardless of income level or age) was increased; the length of stay was further shortened; and rehabilitation and convalescent services moved from acute care environments to newly created subacute units in long-term care facilities and in hospitals. Many procedures that previously required an inpatient stay became outpatient services.

In 1996, the news media again predicted serious financial problems for the Medicare system in the near future. The growing numbers of elderly, the rising costs of medications, supplies, and wages, and the widespread use of costly, highly technical therapies all have contributed to escalating health care costs. Despite these concerns, Medicare and Medicaid have provided health care dollars and services to many people who would otherwise have done without.

Critical Thinking Activity

What changes are occurring in the health care systems in your community? Analyze how these changes may affect nursing practice.

MILITARY HEALTH CARE

The military branches of the Defense Department operate hospitals and clinics for service members and their families, and also finance health care through civilian health providers in an extensive program known as CHAMPUS. The latter program allows individuals to select care providers in their community who are reimbursed in much the same way that insurance reimburses for care. This comprehensive federal program covers both active and retired military personnel and their dependents.

OTHER FEDERAL HEALTH CARE PROGRAMS

The Public Health Service historically has operated hospitals for merchant seamen and the Coast Guard. These facilities were also available to veterans and certain government employees. Many of these public health hospitals have been closed and the care transferred to community resources. Individuals are then covered by an insurance reimbursement plan.

Within the Department of the Interior, the Bureau of Indian Affairs has operated hospitals and clinics on Indian reservations and in native villages in Alaska. Care in these settings is sometimes minimal, limited by a low budget.

The Department of Veterans' Affairs operates many clinics, hospitals, and nursing homes for veterans. These are found across the country. For those who are eligible for care from the Veterans' Administration, benefits are comprehensive. Restrictions have increased, however, on who is eligible for VA care and under what circumstances.

MANAGING THE RISING COSTS OF HEALTH CARE

Two of the major problems facing the health care system are rising costs and accessibility for all individuals. These two issues are related in that cost is one of the factors that can limit access to health care.

Understanding Increasing Costs

Many factors contribute to the rising costs of health care (Display 2-3). One important factor in cost increase is the price of new technology. New, more sophisticated diagnostic and treatment devices are developed each year. The rising cost of technology affects every area of the health care field, from the cardiac care unit to the laboratory.

An increasing population needs a greater number of facilities, and the construction of new care facilities also contributes to rising costs. In addition, existing facilities often require modifications. More space is needed for new technologies both at the bedside and in many hospital departments. Computer systems are used more often for documentation of care. Bedside computers that enable documentation to be done at the point of

Display 2–3
CONTRIBUTING FACTORS IN RISING HEALTH
CARE COSTS

- Price of new technology
- Construction of new facilities
- Higher survival rates leading to greater need for costly intensive or long-term care
- Growing population of elderly adults requiring health care
- Rise in salaries for health care workers
- High costs of drugs and health-related equipment

care decrease the amount of time required for "paperwork." More offices and conference rooms are needed. The regulations governing hospital construction also have become more stringent, requiring more fire safety and infection control measures, and protection against environmental hazards. These factors combine to make the "per bed" cost of new hospital construction or remodeling increasingly expensive. Additionally, decreases in the length of hospital stay and the move to outpatient services have left many hospital beds unused. Unoccupied hospital beds create a major drain on organizations, because large sums of capital investment are tied up and not returning any income.

The average length of hospital stay for standard diagnoses has decreased steadily. The typical client in today's hospital is discharged rapidly to convalesce at home or in a long-term care facility, leaving behind only the acutely ill. Many clients who would have died quickly in earlier years live through a crisis but require long and intensive care. All of these factors make the acuity level of a client today much greater. This in turn requires more intensive observation and care and the use of more specialized equipment.

The population as a whole is growing older and, statistically, the elderly have an increased incidence of all chronic illnesses. A greater percentage of the population requires health care on a regular basis and may depend on medications, treatments, and therapies for continued functioning.

Until recently, the salaries of health care workers (except for physicians) were far below those of the general society. To remedy this, for a time salaries of health care workers rose more rapidly than the general inflation rate. Physicians also had an increase in income greater than the relative inflation rate until the mid-nineties, when changes in the system began to affect income levels for physicians.

Companies that manufacture health-related devices and drugs reportedly have some of the highest profits in any industry. These companies justify their profits as appropriate relative to the risk and cost involved in research and development; however, some critics believe these companies take advantage of the public's dependence on their products. For example, recent evidence indicates that drug companies spend more on advertising than they do on research. For those health insurance plans providing prescription coverage and for HMOs, the costs of prescription drugs is cited as a key reason for premium increases. The public has expressed concern that drug companies sell identical drugs in other countries for far less money than the drugs cost to consumers in the United States. One of the realities contributing to this situation is that other countries place price controls on drugs and the United States does not.

Lack of competition in the health care field is one factor that may contribute to higher costs. Although physicians continue to be primary gatekeepers in the system, the advent of other primary care providers, such as nurse practitioners and nurse midwives, has offered alternate and less costly care for many routine problems, and for normal life processes such as pregnancy and childbirth. However, there has been opposition to allowing these practitioners to operate in collaborative rather than dependent or subsidiary roles.

One attempt to increase the availability of nonphysician care has been the movement to obtain legislation requiring that government agencies and third-party payers (eg, insurance companies) pay the nonphysician (eg, the nurse practitioner) who provides primary care service. The traditional pattern required that payment always be made to a physician, who in turn paid the nonphysician provider. Progress has been made in regard to third-party reimbursement for nurses in primary care; however, this continues to be a problem and a major thrust of political pressure by nurses (American Medical Association, 1995).

As health care costs have continued to rise, third-party payers have used several methods to control costs, including changing patterns of payment, controlling the actions of providers, and other techniques (Fig. 2-2).

Critical Thinking Activity

> Choose a patient. Make a list of all the therapies, medications, diagnostic tests, and surgeries or procedures that this patient has received. Research the cost of these therapies and the daily rate for hospital care in your area for 1 day. Research the DRG reimbursement for that diagnostic group. Compare the reimbursement with the costs being incurred for this individual patient. Identify ways that nurses could reduce the costs involved in this patient's care.

FIGURE 2–2 Federal legislation is encouraging hospitals to stop the rapid rise of health care costs.

Changing Patterns of Payment

Understanding the various methods of paying for health care services can help you understand what is happening in the organizations and agencies involved in the health care system.

FEE-FOR-SERVICE PAYMENT

Fee-for-service payment means that each time a service is provided, a fee is generated and then billed to the recipient of care. The more services provided, the more fees charged. This can be compared to ordering each dish in a restaurant separately and having each appear as a separate charge on the bill. This was the traditional method of charging for health care in the United States. Initially, almost all fees were paid by private individuals. When insurance companies began assisting with payment, the individual's bill was sent to the insurance company and to the client. The insurance company then paid its share (for example, 80%) and the client was required to pay the rest.

As costs rose, insurance companies began setting a standard rate of reimbursement. Under this system, if a policy stated that a company reimbursed at 80%, this meant 80% of a fee that the insurance company determined was reasonable. If the provider charged more than the "reasonable" fee, the client was responsible for the excess, in addition to 20% of the "reasonable" fee. Insurance companies usually set these fees based on statistical analysis of prevailing fees in a geographic area. In a time of rapid inflation, providers complained that there was often a serious discrepancy between the fee used for calculating benefits and the actual fees being charged.

PROSPECTIVE PAYMENT

A *prospective payment* is a reimbursement amount for a procedure or illness that has been determined in advance of the provision of service. The predetermined amount is paid without regard to actual costs in individual situations. Unlike fee-for-service payment, which reimburses each individual item of service provided, prospective payment is based on a fixed reimbursement amount for an identified major illness, procedure, or acuity category.

Prospective payment is designed to provide an incentive for hospitals to control costs. Another advantage to payers in a prospective payment system is that costs are predictable. The system transfers the burden of risk (the chance that an individual may require extraordinary services) from the payer to the provider. It can be compared to a fixed price for a dinner at a restaurant that includes appetizer, salad, main dish, dessert, and beverage. If you choose not to have the dessert, you still are charged the same amount. For the person who wants all five items, the fixed price typically is cheaper than paying for each item separately.

DIAGNOSIS-RELATED GROUPS

The major change in the method of payment for health care services began on October 1, 1983, when the federal government stopped using a fee-for-service reimbursement system for Medicare, and introduced a prospective payment system using *diagnosis-related groups* (DRGs) to determine the payment for each person admitted to the hospital. This change was designed to stop the spiraling costs of Medicare and to correct inequities that made the costs of care in one facility very different from those in another facility.

Calculation of Costs. The method of determining the rates to be paid in the Medicare prospective payment system—the creation of DRGs—resulted from a computerized analysis of costs that had been billed for hospitalized individuals in the past. This analysis led to the formation of categories of medical diagnoses that require similar treatment, and for which costs are similar. Each category (or DRG) has a name and number; for example, DRG 236 is "fracture of the hip and pelvis." In addition, a decision was made to increase the payment for care when another illness or condition is present. This second condition is termed a *comorbidity*. Thus, a person with heart failure whose basic DRG is "fractured hip" is designated "fractured hip with congestive heart failure." A hospital receives greater reimbursement for providing service to this person because care is more complex and costs are higher. Hospitals also receive additional amounts for cases that are determined to be "outliers." An *outlier* is a case in which the client stay significantly exceeds the average. The number of days needed to qualify a case as an outlier is predetermined. For example, the average length of stay for DRG 236, "Fractured hip and pelvis," is 6.2 days, but the stay must reach 29 days for the case to be considered an outlier.

Most hospital costs are included in the DRG reimbursement. The actual DRG reimbursement amount is calculated each year by HCFA through a complex formula that considers the area of the country in which the care was provided (eg, Northwest, Southeast), the urbanization of the area (eg, rural, suburban), and the type of care required. Some hospital costs still are reimbursed separately. In the past, these included costs for medical education and research conducted by the hospital; however, pressure is mounting to stop this separate payment. The goal is to include all costs in one reimbursement figure. Physician costs also are paid separately, but some suggest that these eventually should be included in the single rate.

Most of the controversy surrounding the implementation of DRGs has not concerned the incentives for cost control, or the prospective reimbursement system itself, but rather how the payment amounts are determined and how the system is being administered. There are conflicting studies regarding whether the DRGs adequately reflect the intensity of nursing care required (Halloran & Halloran, 1985; McKibbin et al., 1985; Yasko & Fleck, 1995). Another concern is that clients reportedly are discharged after much shorter stays, when they are still in need of care (the "quicker and sicker" concern—clients are discharged quicker and feeling sicker). Alterations and modifications of the system will continue, but the basic prospective plan probably will remain in place.

Implications for Nurses. There are a variety of implications for nurses in the current DRG system. The availability of documents that reflect the acuity level and multiple problems of a client when records are audited for compliance is essential. The need for discharge planning is always present but is more critical as the length of stay becomes shorter. A longer length of stay significantly increases the costs to the hospital; therefore, nursing actions that prevent complications, avoid inappropriate scheduling, and facilitate early discharge are important. Nurses in home health agencies and long-term care facilities are caring for clients with complex nursing needs. A major concern is whether the DRG reimbursement system provides adequate funds for quality nursing care to be delivered, and whether hospitals, in their attempt to cut costs, will cut quality of care.

In addition to Medicare, many states are adopting systems similar to DRGs, and some private insurance carriers are now using these basic concepts in their cost-control efforts through prospective payment. Therefore, DRGs will continue to be an issue of concern to nurses.

RESOURCE UTILIZATION GROUPS

Resource utilization groups (RUGs) are the categories used to determine prospective payment for nursing home clients. The RUGs represent groups that require differing amounts of care and thus will differ in how much it costs to support that care each day. Unlike the hospital prospective payment, which is a flat amount for the entire hospital stay, the prospective payment for nursing home care is a fixed daily rate. This daily rate must include all the services, including medications and treatments that a resident needs.

The basis for determining to which RUG a nursing home resident will be assigned for reimbursement purposes is the comprehensive minimum data set (MDS) prepared by the registered nurse. This assessment must be transmitted electronically to the appropriate center for review and payment categorization. If the assessments are not completed accurately or are not submitted in a timely manner, the resident automatically is assigned to the lowest reimbursement RUG category. The facility is then unable to recover missed costs even if the resident really needs a much higher level of care. Reassessments are required at specified intervals. These reassessments are used to reassign the resident to a RUG.

The use of a prospective payment system (PPS) was phased in over two years beginning in 1997 with the first pilot groups. The PPS has created great consternation throughout the nursing home industry. The costs of compliance are high, the reimbursements are lower, and there are more restrictions on such items as the provision of therapy services. Many nursing homes have reduced staff, changed practice patterns, and made other adjustments to adapt to the decrease in reimbursement. The nursing home industry is lobbying for changes in the reimbursement plan because they believe that low reimbursement is undermining their ability to provide appropriate care. Payments to nursing homes have dropped precipitously.

One unintended result of the move to PPS for the nursing home has been the refusal of nursing homes to admit high-cost residents. For example, an individual with an extensive wound that requires intensive wound care with expensive products might cost more per day for care than the highest RUG category allows. In the past, it was possible to bill separately for the expensive dressings and topical agents used. When this is not possible, the facility simply may refuse to admit the patient. This actually may increase costs for the payer, because the patient remains in the high-cost hospital if no long-term care facility will admit him.

CAPITATION

Capitation is yet another way of determining payment within the health care system. In a capitated system a fee is paid to a provider organization for each person (each "head," thus the term) whether or not that person uses any health care services. This shifts an even greater share of the risk of providing health care from the payment organization to the provider organization. Providers in a capitated system have an incentive to guide individuals to low-cost outpatient services or other care environments rather than to the acute care hospital. A goal of this payment system is to encourage preventive services that may make high-cost interventions unnecessary. Thus, in a capitated system you may find that services such as mammograms, immunizations, stop-smoking clinics, and back-injury classes do not have any copayments attached, or the copayments may be quite low. Health maintenance organizations were the original capitated systems. A criticism of a capitated system is that when the provider is at risk for providing care, there may be an unconscious (or even deliberate) attempt to deny needed care to keep costs down. In some capitated systems, consumers have complained that they were unable to obtain services they believed were appropriate.

Controlling Health Care Providers

Third-party payers and government and public agencies all have used different approaches to restrain rising health care costs.

CERTIFICATES OF NEED

To add new high-cost equipment or additional client care facilities, a health care institution may be required to apply for a certificate of need from the state. This establishes that there will not be unnecessary duplication of services in an area and that a need for them exists. For example, if every hospital purchased magnetic resonance imaging (MRI) equipment that was used to only one fourth or one third of its capacity, the cost per use would have to be higher to cover the investment and maintenance costs than if the device were used to capacity.

In many states, nonprofit hospitals must make application for rate increases. In their applications, they must document all the factors contributing to the need for an increase. Hearings are held, and permission for rate increases is given only when the evidence indicates that all possible economies are being observed. Private, profit-making hospitals are not held to these rules.

PREFERRED PROVIDERS

In an attempt to contain costs, third-party payers such as insurance companies, HMOs, and managed care organizations sometimes negotiate with providers of health care to supply certain kinds of care at an agreed-upon, usually lower, price. The third-party payers then provide incentives for clients to use these "preferred providers." These incentives may include the waiver of all or part of copayments by the insured, or coverage of additional conditions or situations.

Preferred provider organizations (PPOs) may be hospitals, nursing homes, corporations employing care providers, or groups of care providers who have cooperated to negotiate more successfully with third-party payers for these special contracts. The advantage to the provider is the assured number of clients and the guaranteed income. In a time of competition in health care, this may be a significant advantage. Each PPO operates independently without government regulation; therefore, the exact structure and contractual arrangements are independently determined.

MANAGED CARE

Managed care refers to any system in which the use of health care services is controlled and monitored carefully to ensure that policies are followed, that neither too much nor too little care is provided, and that costs are minimized. Owens (1995, p. 5) identifies managed care more specifically as "a system to control the cost of health care by using a select group of providers who have agreed to a predetermined payment, with the clinical interventions being managed via utilization and/or a case management process." A managed care plan may be controlled by the payer (such as an insurance company), may include both payers and providers, or may be a business entity that serves only as a go-between. HMOs always have acted as managed care systems. Many of the current health plans referred to as HMOs are in reality managed care systems that do not focus on health maintenance at all.

In a managed care system there is always someone assigned to the role of "gatekeeper." This person monitors and restricts the use of services by the client. In most managed care plans the primary physician is expected to serve as the "gatekeeper." The physician sees the client first and then determines whether referral or diagnostic services are needed. In some managed care systems, the primary physician has decision-making authority. However, in many managed care systems, the actual gatekeeper is a plan manager who must be consulted regarding the use of services. A written request may be required before the client receives permission for a referral. This may delay or deny needed care and is one source of consumer dissatisfaction with some managed care plans.

Many managed care decisions about individual clients are made based on a set of predetermined protocols for treatment. The original protocols were developed by physicians, based on broad statistical patterns. Thus the protocol may not be responsive to individual differences. These protocols often are administered by plan employees who are not health care providers. Physicians express dismay over a mechanism that allows a nonphysician who has never seen a client to make critical decisions about the care needed and to deny any individualization of the plan.

Managed care usually requires that care be authorized or approved for payment before it is provided. Clients identify the required approval of any type of care as a major problem. A managed care plan may not approve or pay for care that it considers nonessential. If a health care provider and a plan consultant disagree about which type of treatment is appropriate, the client often feels caught in the middle. This situation frequently occurs in emergency care. Even when approval is granted, the process may have been long and frustrating for the client and physician involved.

In some managed care plans, a subscriber who needs emergency care and is outside the appropriate service area is subject to what is called the standard of the "prudent consumer." This means that if a prudent layperson would consider the symptoms an emergency, the plan will pay for care. Thus, if a person with chest pain goes to an emergency room, the plan pays even if the chest pain turns out to be esophageal reflux. Some plans created a standard related to the final medical diagnosis. A plan with this standard would pay an individual who visited the emergency room with chest pain only if the final diagnosis were myocardial infarction, but would not pay if the final diagnosis were esophageal reflux. This approach caused such public consternation that legislation was enacted in some areas that required any kind of health plan to cover emergency care based on the "prudent consumer" model.

Some plans require that an individual travel to a designated hospital when an emergency is not life-threatening. Thus, one consumer was denied payment for a fractured ankle sustained while skiing because it was not life-threatening and because the injury was treated in the skiing community rather than back home in the consumer's designated hospital.

Managed care controls extend to such matters as the medications that can be prescribed. A managed care company may have a specific formulary of drugs for which it has negotiated purchase at low prices. For many conditions, there are clear therapeutic equivalents and medication restrictions are not a concern. For the person with a chronic health condition who has been stabilized on specific medications, however, moving into a managed care plan can pose a real threat to health maintenance if the plan will not approve the client's current drugs.

All of these actions are designed to hold down costs. Managed care plans that originally focused on health maintenance and keeping relatively healthy people healthy showed great promise for controlling health care costs. However, as managed care has encompassed people with serious chronic illnesses, controlling costs has become more difficult.

CASE MANAGEMENT

Case management is a technique used in some managed care systems to efficiently move an individual requiring major health services through the system. According to the Case Management Society of America (CMSA), case management is "a collaborative process which assesses, plans, implements, coordinates, monitors, and evaluates options and services to meet an individual's health needs through communication and available resources to promote quality cost-effective outcomes" (CMSA, 1995). Case managers most commonly are assigned to high-risk clients, such as those with chronic illnesses or major traumas, who will require rehabilitation. In some settings, the case manager specializes in a particular group of high-risk clients, such as those with diabetes, and is referred to as a "disease manager."

The case manager is an experienced health professional with knowledge of available resources who oversees or monitors a case to ensure that necessary care is instituted promptly and is provided in the most cost-effective setting. Nurses have often assumed the role of case manager. In this role, the nurse monitors the care as it is provided, ensuring that appropriate referrals are made, that changes in the plan of care are instituted appropriately, and that the care follows established standards. Because of their understanding of the whole person, both physiologically and psychosocially, and their understanding of how the system works, nurses are particularly well suited to this role. The CMSA provides a system for certifying professional case managers.

Case managers may operate within only one part of the system: for example, managing cases from admission through discharge in a nursing home or hospital. These managers are often referred to as *internal case managers*. Some may manage cases across all phases of care from outpatient through hospitalization, rehabilitation, and back to outpatient. These individuals are termed *external case managers*. At their best, case management systems ensure that delays in patient transfer or breaks in communication do not occur, and that costs are minimized through efficiency. Case managers often act as advocates for clients in the system. Physicians sometimes object to what they see as the interference of the case manager in a decision-making process that used to include only the client and the physician.

VERTICALLY INTEGRATED HEALTH CARE SYSTEMS

Organizations contracting to provide managed care also are expanding their own control through the development of *vertically integrated systems*, that is, those that provide every level of health care service. A vertically integrated system may have contracted physicians, laboratories, a hospital, a subacute facility, a rehabilitation facility, and a home care agency. This allows the contracting organization to offer managed care corporations a package that provides care at all levels for each enrolled member of the managed care plan for a capitated fee. The contracting organization then has an incentive to control costs by decreasing the use of high-cost services and more effectively using low-cost alternatives. It is also in a better position to negotiate with the managed care system about reimbursement. As large systems develop in this manner, hospitals become a cost center rather than a revenue center. This merging of systems is resulting in the closure of hospitals in many communities.

A more recent development has been the splitting off of subsidiaries that were added to large health systems. For example, in late 1999 Columbia/HCA, one of the largest health systems in the United States, announced that they were going to divest the corporation of the physician practices that had been purchased in the last 10 years. Their announcement indicated that they had found the system lacked the expertise to manage physician practices and that they were unable to manage costs and create profits as they had originally expected.

USING ACUITY MEASURES TO DETERMINE COSTS

Health care providers who are negotiating contracts and planning care need very accurate data regarding the specific cost of each service. One way of trying to understand and control these costs is through the development of *acuity* measures. Acuity in this context refers to how acutely ill a person is and how much skilled care is required.

Various ways of measuring acuity in both acute and long-term care settings have been devised. Most systems use categories that reflect the different types of care needed. Each category is assigned a numerical value on a scale of 1 to 4 (or on a similar scale). All applicable category values are summed and compared with a standard. For example, an acuity measuring system might have one category reflecting the need for assistance in personal hygiene. As a person needs more assistance, more points are assigned. Another category might reflect the amount of time needed for monitoring vital signs: the more time required, the more points assigned. Each category is assigned an appropriate number of points, and the total is computed. The points identified for an individual client are then compared with a standard and the client is assigned an acuity level. Clients with the fewest points are level 1 and require the least care. Those with the most points are level 4 and require the most care. Each system in use has its own scale for determining acuity. Acuity values are sometimes called "intensity measures" because they reflect the intensity of care needed.

In some settings acuity levels or intensity measures are used as a mechanism for determining the staffing needs of a client care unit. Acuity levels also are used as a means of billing for the level of nursing care needed, and are reflected in a variable rather than flat charge for the nursing portion of a client's room charge. It also has been suggested that prospective reimbursement might be based on acuity level rather than on medical diagnosis because acuity levels reflect the real impact on resources more accurately than do medical diagnoses (DRGs reflect nursing resources, 1985; Biordi, 1995). The RUGs developed for prospective reimbursement in long-term care are essentially an acuity measure based on the nursing assessment.

Other Cost-Containment Measures

In many medical facilities, personnel now are asked to be cost conscious. Cost consciousness involves such ordinary measures as being conservative with telephone use, canceling meal trays when clients are discharged, and using expensive supplies with care. Nursing personnel also must be aware of the tremendous cost of any complication or additional length-of-stay. Preventing complications and getting clients ready for early discharge have become a major focus of care. Care pathways are specifying care and identifying outcomes for each day of hospitalization with the goal of assuring that resources are used wisely. Physicians are asked to judge carefully the necessity of diagnostic studies and costly procedures. Some diagnostic studies must be preapproved by the managed care organization. In some hospitals physicians are asked to consult with pharmacists before prescribing certain high-cost drugs to determine whether a low-cost therapeutic alternative exists. Although the latest aminoglycoside antibiotic might be effective, for example, an inexpensive first generation cephalosporin antibiotic also might be effective while costing 90% less. When all medication costs must be covered by a prospective payment, the hospital has a strong incentive to limit physicians' choices. Many physicians are upset about these cost-containment measures because they may interfere with the physician's independent decision making about what care is needed and when.

Hospitals with a large population of extra-high-risk clients (eg, the very elderly or poor) have expressed concern that discharging a client for convalescence in a home with a caring family, good food, and a clean environment is much different from discharging a client to an impoverished environment. Many believe the individual situation should be considered when determining regulations for length of stay. The proponents of shortened stays point out that shortened stays are effective cost-containment measures. They argue further that a client's lack of a support system is a social problem and that hospitalization cannot be used to solve social problems.

The federal government has sought to control costs for Medicare and Medicaid by establishing higher deductibles (the portions that individual clients must pay) and by limiting the fees that the government will pay. Because the elderly and the poor are often unable to pay these deductible amounts, they become liabilities for health care providers, who cover these costs by collecting higher fees from those who do pay their bills. Hospitals and physicians argue that as more limits have been imposed, the limited reimbursement no longer covers the actual costs of care. This jeopardizes the entire system. Medicaid costs also have been contained by tightening eligibility requirements, which shuts more people out of the health care system.

As Medicare and Medicaid have become a larger and larger part of the financing of the health care system, fraud also has become a larger problem. The Health Insurance Portability and Accountability Act of 1996 (HIPAA) created a federal Health Care Fraud and Abuse Control Program. This program coordinates federal, state, and local law enforcement activities in fighting health care fraud and abuse. In 1998, these efforts recovered more than $480 million. Some funds recovered are used for the program, but 92% of the funds are returned to Medicare (DHHS & OIG, 1999).

All of these efforts at reducing costs have affected the health care system in areas other than cost containment. They have affected decision-making processes, power structures, the kinds of care provided, and the ways that individual health care providers practice. It is important to recognize the full impact that cost containment has had.

Critical Thinking Activity

What cost-control measures have you seen in places where you have had clinical practice? Analyze the effects of these cost-control measures on client care.

ACCESS TO HEALTH CARE

Access to health care refers to the individual's ability to obtain and use needed services. Access can be an economic, geographic, or sociocultural issue (Fig. 2-3).

Economic Access

Creating access for those who are economically disadvantaged requires that providers consider many factors. In addition to providing a family with a prescription, for instance, a provider must make sure there is a way to fill that prescription. It is not enough to prescribe a special diet without ensuring that the individual has the necessary knowledge and resources to follow that diet.

FIGURE 2–3 Despite the many different sources of health care financing, a family may face obstacles to obtaining effective health care.

Coverage by third-party payers also affects economic access. As more small businesses find their health care benefit costs escalating, they may eliminate these benefits. Individuals and families whose incomes are marginal may be unable to purchase insurance because of the high cost of individual policies. Although giving people an incentive to use services wisely is the stated goal of raising deductibles and copayments, the result for some families may be the delay or avoidance of timely care.

Some individuals are unable to obtain health insurance because of preexisting illnesses. These are often the people who are most in need of health care services. Another group concerned about being denied insurance coverage are those with the potential for serious health problems. As genetic testing for potential health problems has become more widespread and the information gleaned from it more exact, insurance companies have used the results of these tests as a basis for denying coverage to healthy individuals. As more tests become available, this issue is cause for growing concern, especially as it relates to access to health care (see Chapter 10 on bioethical issues).

Geographic Access

Geographic access to health care is a special concern for those in rural areas. As changes have occurred in the health care system, small rural hospitals have found themselves unable to compete or to manage financially. This has led to the closure of some small rural hospitals. When a rural hospital closes, residents lose emergency room care, hospital access, and diagnostic services. Travel for health care especially affects the elderly and poor (Reif, DesHarnais, & Bernard, 1999).

Communities without hospitals find it more difficult to recruit physicians and other primary care providers. Historically, most health care providers have preferred not to work in areas without hospitals available to provide diagnostic and treatment services; consequently, rural communities found it difficult to recruit health care providers. Many medical schools, with the support of both federal and state funds, developed programs to encourage medical students and residents to consider family practice as a specialty and practice in a rural location. Although successful in increasing the number of physicians entering rural practice, in some states they were unable to keep up with the number leaving rural practice. However, in 1998 the University of Iowa Medical School announced that for the first time, the number of physicians entering rural practice in Iowa was greater than those leaving.

Geographic access may be a concern for those in urban areas as well. Economically depressed areas of large cities have fewer health care providers, thus forcing the residents of those areas to travel long distances, often using inconvenient public transportation, in order to receive health care. The Healthy People 2000 Report (DHHS, 1992) recommended that health care services be made available in locations such as work sites and schools to improve access.

Access to health care also is affected by whether all services are available in one location. It is common for individuals to be required to visit several geographically separate locations to receive all needed health care. Some organizations now offer a single *point-of-service*, meaning one geographic location where providers can take care of all needs. A single point-of-service makes it unnecessary for an individual to go to one location to see a primary provider, to another to see a specialist, to still another for diagnostic tests, and to yet another location for procedures. The single point-of-service makes efficient use of the client's time, lessens the likelihood that the client will fail to follow through with recommended procedures, and simplifies communication between providers.

Sociocultural Access

Sociocultural differences also affect access. When individuals feel uncomfortable in a setting because of their socioeconomic status or because their cultural background and beliefs are not respected, they are reluctant to use the services provided. Making care culturally accessible may mean having translation services, materials in multiple languages, and care providers who understand and are sensitive to cultural differences.

Access to health care is discussed in more detail later in this chapter, in association with key indicators of system effectiveness (Fig. 2-4).

FIGURE 2–4   The pressure for change in health care delivery continues to grow.

MAINTAINING QUALITY IN THE HEALTH CARE SYSTEM

A wide variety of mechanisms are used to maintain quality in the health care system. Two of the most important are accreditation standards and evaluation processes.

Accreditation of Health Care Institutions and Agencies

Health care institutions may be approved by both governmental and nongovernmental agencies. Approval by a specific agency may be required for an agency to receive some types of third party payment. Therefore, accreditation is important for the agencies involved.

GOVERNMENTAL APPROVAL

Institutions and agencies providing health care usually must be approved by the governmental agency, often a department of health, in the state where they are located.

Approval may take the form of state licensing, which usually focuses on maintaining minimum standards to safeguard public health. For some agencies, this meets their needs.

Those agencies that seek Medicare or Medicaid funding must meet specific federal standards and be Medicare certified in addition to meeting the basic state standards. The Medicare standards relate to many aspects of care. By designating those to whom payment will be given, Medicare effectively exerts control. Because the costs of private care are so high, most people choose to receive care where it can be reimbursed. When care is not reimbursable, individuals may make other choices.

MEDICARE/MEDICAID CERTIFICATION

Health care institutions and agencies also may seek accreditation from nongovernmental bodies that set standards for high quality and provide guidelines to assist in developing policies and procedures. Medicare and Medicaid have granted several of these nongovernmental agencies what is called *deemed status*. This means that the standards of the agency are "deemed" to equal or exceed the Medicare standard. Therefore, a health care agency that has been accredited by the voluntary process described below is "deemed" to meet the standards set by Medicare and Medicaid, and is not required to pursue an additional accreditation process.

JOINT COMMISSION ON ACCREDITATION OF HEALTHCARE ORGANIZATIONS

Hospitals, nursing homes, and related organizations may seek accreditation from the Joint Commission on Accreditation of Healthcare Organizations (JCAHO). This nonprofit, voluntary organization originally was established by the American College of Surgeons and the American Society of Internal Medicine to set standards for hospital care. Today's organization has a board of directors with members from many health care and public occupations. The standards of the organization are comprehensive and involve evaluating the structural aspects of institutions, policies and procedures, and the outcomes of care provided. JCAHO has deemed status for federal programs. Historically, assisted-living settings have not had a standard accreditation, and in many states little regulation. In 1999 JCAHO announced that it will develop an accreditation process for assisted-living settings, with standards completed by 2000 and the first accreditations to be available in 2001 (Vickery, 1999).

COMMUNITY HEALTH ACCREDITATION PROGRAM

The Community Health Accreditation Program (CHAP) is a separate arm of the National League for Nursing that was established to provide a voluntary accreditation system for community health and home health agencies. This is a peer-reviewed process governed entirely by community health agencies with public representation. CHAP has deemed status for Medicare and Medicaid certification.

NATIONAL COMMITTEE FOR QUALITY ASSURANCE

The National Committee for Quality Assurance (NCQA) reviews and evaluates health maintenance organizations. It is a relatively new, independent nonprofit organization developed by the HMO industry. NCQA has established a set of statistical measures called Health Plan Employer Data and Information Set (HEDIS). This information is available from their Web site at www.ncqa.org. These data provide a standard set of information that both employers and consumers can use to compare and evaluate HMOs. Included in the HEDIS data set are nine indicators of quality, seven of which are related to processes and two of which are related to outcomes. Most of these data relate to prevention and not to the effective diagnosis and treatment of illness. The organization's plan is to expand this data set to include more clinical data. Because the data have been collected only for a short time and because all HMOs are not using the same methods for collecting data, the HEDIS statistics have limited value for comparison even though they do provide some important information (Brooks, McGlynn, & Cleary, 1996).

Evaluation of Health Care

A variety of evaluation mechanisms are used within the health care system. Some involve evaluating agencies providing care and others involve evaluating client outcomes.

PEER REVIEW AND QUALITY ASSURANCE

The first systematic evaluation of health care services was established through the Professional Standards Review Organization set up by Medicare and Medicaid. As part of the 1982 revisions of Medicare, the evaluation process was altered to require that hospitals contract with an external medical review organization, called a Utilization and Quality Control Peer Review Organization (abbreviated PRO). These organizations were established through contracts awarded by the Secretary of Health and Human Services through competitive bidding. Most of the PROs are statewide in scope and are required to have a substantial number of physicians represented in the organization to set standards and review care effectively.

Evaluation may include preadmission, preprocedure, concurrent, or retrospective reviews. The purpose of the reviews is to determine whether care given was necessary and whether it was given in the appropriate manner. For example, the reviews have resulted in an increase in the number of outpatient surgeries (day procedures) performed, and a subsequent decrease in the number of inpatient surgeries. These changes have resulted in significant economic savings. The PRO also is required to evaluate outcomes of care to ensure that the changes made do not jeopardize clients.

OUTCOME MEASUREMENTS

Outcome measures refer to actual health results in the clients and communities served. Outcomes now are measured in relationship to hospitals, long-term care facilities, and the population as a whole. Some outcomes have been designated *key indicators*, which are specific, measurable aspects of health care that show the effectiveness of the system and indicate whether access to services is available. These are a major factor in changes health care institutions are undertaking.

Hospital Health Care Outcomes. The federal government compiles statistics related to hospital health care outcomes. These include infection rates and morbidity and mortality rates associated with specific hospitals and procedures. In 1995 the federal government began releasing these figures to the public. These government statistics may be helpful in evaluating some aspects of care. One result of outcome studies has been the recommendation that only hospitals that perform a specified number of highly technical surgeries (for example, cardiac surgeries) each year should offer those procedures. Hospitals that perform fewer procedures per year have higher complication and mortality rates.

The Agency for Health Care Policy and Research created the Healthcare Cost and Utilization Project (HCUP) to identify a set of items that could be used as indicators of inpatient quality of care and community access to care. They identified three groups of quality indicators. The first group includes potentially avoidable adverse hospital outcomes (such as mortality rates for common surgeries, wound infection rates, and incidence of pulmonary complications). The second group includes potentially inappropriate use of hospital procedures (such as inappropriate use of cesarean section and hysterectomy). The third group includes potentially avoidable hospital admissions (such as pediatric asthma and immunization-preventable influenza in the elderly). The data for these items, collectively referred to as HCUP QIs (Healthcare Cost and Utilization Project Quality Indicators), are collected routinely by hospitals and states, then compared to targets such as Healthy People 2000, hospital peer groups, or the agency itself over time. The purpose is to identify areas in which there is potential for improvement and develop plans for that improvement (Quality Indicators, 1998).

Individual Institutional Outcomes Measurement. Individual institutions also are establishing ways to measure the outcomes of the care they provide. "Outcomes" here refers to data such as the number of clients admitted with a fractured hip who had uncomplicated recoveries leading to effective rehabilitation and the number of clients who had complications or did not recover. Knowledge of outcomes is essential for planning and, increasingly, for effective marketing. Often data have been collected but are scattered among many different records and are difficult to retrieve. Because data only become valuable for planning when they are organized in a useful framework for analysis, health care agencies have moved rapidly to the computerization of data and the implementation of standardized protocols for data collection.

One of the standardized tools hospitals use to monitor outcomes is called the *clinical pathway.* This is also referred to as a critical path, a care map, or an anticipated recovery path. The clinical pathway describes the optimum progression through the system of the individual with a particular health problem. By establishing the desired outcome for day 2 of the postoperative client with a fractured hip, it is possible to determine when an individual client is not meeting the desired outcome. The advantage for the individual is that care can be modified immediately to address the problem. The advantage for the system is the ability to aggregate data across all clients and examine what it is working well and what needs to be changed.

Long-Term Care Quality Indicators. Quality indicators also are used in long-term care as part of the regulatory process. HCFA has identified 11 areas of care in which they specified 24 quality indicators. HCFA states that these 24 indicators represent common conditions and items that are important to residents. These quality indicators serve as the focus for the state surveyors. Long-term care facilities are being encouraged to track these indicators themselves and use them as a focus of improvement (Gold, 1999).

National Health Indicators. In 1992 the Department of Health and Human Services and the Public Health Service published Healthy People 2000, National Health Promotion and Disease Prevention Objectives. The purpose of this document was to establish national goals to serve as a focus for health promotion and disease prevention activities by individuals, organizations, and the federal government. Achievement of these benchmarks could indicate the overall health status of the population being served. Unfortunately, achievement of these benchmarks has been a far more difficult task than originally envisioned.

In an effort to continue moving forward, the Healthy People 2010 project was developed. Five sets of indicators of the overall health of the population of the United States have been developed. These include health and disease outcomes (such as the incidence of specific preventable diseases), preventive health behaviors (such as the percentage of individuals who smoke), mental health indicators (such as psychological status), health system access (such as physical accessibility of health resources), and ecological indicators (such as firearms injuries and deaths). The specific indicators and measurable criteria for tracking the nation's progress are being refined through consultation with many interested groups (Display 2-4).

POWER IN THE HEALTH CARE SYSTEM

Part of trying to understand any system involves examining some of the unique sources of power and authority within it. If we define power as the capability of doing or accomplishing something, then understanding how power is distributed and used in the health care system can help us to function more effectively. Smith (1994) stated that as health services and educational preparation for health professions undergo systemic changes, we must give attention to the allocation of power in these services and education systems. Sources of power unique to the health care system are the authority to decide who may enter and leave the system, who may practice in it, and how funding is controlled.

Regulatory Power

The primary regulatory agencies in health care are governmental bodies. These agencies administer licensing laws that govern who is allowed to practice. Other agencies approve or accredit institutions that educate personnel for health care and licensing, or

Display 2–4

OUTCOMES FROM *HEALTHY PEOPLE 2010*

A. Health and Disease Outcomes
  1. General physical well-being
  2. Infant mortality
  3. Death rates from preventable causes
  4. Disability-free survivorship
  5. Self-reported health status
  6. Sexually transmitted diseases
  7. HIV
  8. Cancer
  9. Low birth weight
  10. Cardiovascular disease (CVD)
  11. Asthma or chronic obstructive pulmonary disease (COPD)
  12. Hip fractures or osteoporosis
  13. Injury
  14. Diabetes
  15. Disability days
B. Preventive Health Behaviors
  1. Unintended pregnancies
  2. Immunizations
  3. Tobacco use
  4. Physical activity
  5. Alcohol use
  6. Substance abuse
  7. Appropriate body weight
  8. Nutrition
C. Mental Health
  1. Psychological status
D. Health System Access
  1. Physical accessibility
  2. Poverty
  3. Health literacy
  4. Education levels
E. Ecologic
  1. Air quality
  2. Iatrogenesis
  3. Firearm death and injury rates
  4. Violence
  5. Homelessness
  6. Motor vehicle accident death and injury rates

approve those that provide services. Through regulation these agencies have a profound effect on how institutions operate.

The accrediting bodies (such as JCAHO, CHAP, and NCQA, as discussed earlier in this chapter) all have power to stimulate change in the system. If you have the opportunity to be in an institution when accreditation visitors are present, you will note that every aspect of the physical plant, the policies and procedures, and the competence of staff are examined. Preparing for an accreditation visit stimulates the agency to self-evaluate and correct any deficiencies.

Financial Power

Because they represent the financial interests of large groups of people and control payments for services, third-party payers have the power to demand changes in the health care system. When they were first established, these agencies did not see their role in health care as anything beyond a financial relationship. As health care costs rose, these agencies began looking for ways of controlling costs to maintain their competitive place in the insurance market. They have set increasingly rigid criteria for payment for services. The standard rates set for payment for procedures have tended to place some restraints on charges (although actual fees often are slightly ahead of payment schedules).

By determining whom they will pay for services, insurance companies reduce the choices available to those who carry insurance—and subscribers usually must select from the choices available if they wish to be reimbursed. Third-party payers therefore exert a more powerful influence over institutions and care providers than do individual subscribers.

Physician Power

Physicians historically had almost unlimited power within the health care system. They determined who entered the system and when. They decided if and when other services and personnel would be used, and they determined when clients would leave the system. As other agencies and professionals in the health care system have obtained some power and independence, the overall power of the physician has diminished. Payers are reviewing medical plans for care and refusing reimbursement when care does not follow their established guidelines. Many hospitals routinely review costs associated with care ordered by physicians, and sometimes restrict the physician's ability to order certain high-cost drugs and procedures. Prior approval of costly care may be required. Care pathways may demand that physicians provide standardized care that leads to quick discharge.

As a group, physicians have opposed changes that would disperse power in the system, arguing that they are the most educated and knowledgeable of all health care providers and that their professional judgment should be accepted. Those favoring increased distribution of power have argued that more competition, more choice for consumers, and input from a greater variety of health care providers and from consumers will make the system more balanced and more responsive. Despite changes, physicians are still powerful in the health care system.

Consumer Power

The sources of power previously discussed present problems for the client because the client is excluded from them. Clearly the client is involved in only the most basic aspect of entry into the system: determining that he or she needs care. The client cannot enter any institution without the express approval of a physician. The client has no control over who becomes a primary care provider, and, with the advent of HMOs and PPOs, may have limited choice in selecting providers. Funding usually is controlled by third-party payers, and the client is often powerless to determine who will be paid, how much will be paid, and when payments will be made.

Consumers do have rights in the health care system. These are stated in different ways by different institutions and groups, but all revolve around the recognition of the health care consumer as an adult with the ability and right to be self-determining. As a general rule, consumers are not aware of their rights, and even when they are aware, they may be reluctant to take advantage of them. Consumers are in a particularly vulnerable position in the health care system. Because they depend on those in the system for life itself, they are often reluctant to complain or request changes for fear of offending those on whom they depend. When consumers try to exert power in the system, they may meet with resistance. Consumers are most often effective in exerting power in the system by working in groups and through established committees and agencies.

A health care consumer bill of rights has been proposed as federal legislation. Although it did not pass in 1999, new bills are being proposed by each political party. Most of the areas of conflict involve rights related to financial aspects of care and whether consumers should have the right to sue a health plan for adverse consequences of denial of care.

Nurse Power

Nurses historically have had limited power in the health care system, a situation that has its roots in many of the traditional aspects of nursing. These are discussed in Chapter 4. Change may not occur as rapidly as desired, and nurses often are frustrated because of their inability to influence the system. Many new graduates are especially distressed to learn that, as individuals, they cannot affect the system. Somehow they expect that if they speak with a voice of reason and act in the best interest of their clients, others will respond positively. Nevertheless, things are changing in nursing. We discuss these issues throughout this text. Nursing organizations are working to provide nurses with a voice at higher decision-making levels in health care. By understanding the political realities and the ways in which decisions are made, and by working together to speak with a united voice, nurses can increase their power in the system (see Chapter 3). Nursing education programs increasingly try to educate nurses to act as client advocates and agents of change (see Chapter 6). Collective bargaining and shared governance have provided nurses with mechanisms for demanding recognition of the importance of their role and for being participants in decision-making processes (see Chapter 12) (Fig. 2-5).

FIGURE 2–5   Nurses working together have power to change the health care system.

Critical Thinking Activity

Nurses are actively seeking power in the health care system. How might nurses in the settings with which you are familiar increase their power?

CONTINUING CONCERNS IN THE HEALTH CARE SYSTEM

There are ongoing concerns in the health care system relating to the actual use of health care services by the public, and to the structure of the system itself.

The impetus for change continues to grow. Several states already have instituted efforts to create a more coordinated health care system for their citizens. In recent years, several bills for health care reform were considered by the United States Congress, but none passed. No one can predict the details of the future system with certainty, but we have tried to point out the major changes now occurring and the directions in which the new health care system is moving.

Nurses have continuing interest and concern in the direction in which health care moves. Nurses are most concerned about client well-being in the midst of a powerful system. As pressures to change increase, nurses continue to speak out for consumers. Who will help consumers cope with their health problems and those of their families? Who will assist them in negotiating the various parts of the health care system? Will the individual identities and unique needs of consumers be addressed, or will each person be treated as the mythical "standard client"?

Another important concern of nurses is whether that aspect of health care that we call "nursing," with its focus on the individual, will be maintained. Will the pressures for demonstrating cost-effectiveness result in a loss of caring because it is not always quantifiable? Will the system recognize the critical thinking skills and abilities of nurses as well as their technical skills? Will many educated and skilled nurses be replaced by unlicensed assistive personnel? The future poses many as yet unanswerable questions!

Critical Thinking Activity

Identify clients you have encountered from a variety of social, cultural, and economic backgrounds. Given these clients' needs and backgrounds, what type of practitioner would best meet their needs for primary care? What barriers might they meet in trying to gain access to primary care? What might you do to assist these individuals?

KEY CONCEPTS

- The financing of health care is complex and involves personal payment, insurance companies, health maintenance organizations, preferred providers, and governmental systems, each of which operates differently.

- Through control of financing, third party payers exert control over all aspects of health care.
- Cost increases have created stress in the health care system. Understanding the basis of these increases is essential to planning to contain costs.
- Mechanisms for controlling costs and improving patterns of care have been instituted. These have included changing methods of payment, controlling health care providers, and managing care. The federal government has played a major role in the development and implementation of these mechanisms.
- Access to health care must be considered in terms of economic, geographic, and sociocultural access. A major concern in the system is those who do not have access.
- Quality of care is maintained by a wide variety of mechanisms. Institutions and agencies providing care receive oversight in the form of governmental approval and accreditation by certifying organizations.
- Quality is evaluated through peer review and the use of outcome measures including key indicators and individual patient outcome standards.
- Power is exerted in the health care system by those who control finances, those who control access, and those with special knowledge. Historically, nurses and consumers have enjoyed little power in the system. Both are working to gain recognition and to affect more significantly the way the system functions.
- There are continuing concerns in health care regarding the effective use of health care resources and changing the health care system.

REFERENCES

American Medical Association, again on the offensive. Am J Nurs 95(8):64–67, 1995

Biordi DL. Accounting for nursing costs by DRG. J Nurs Admin 25(1):6–8, 1995

Brooks RH, McGlynn EA, Cleary PD. Quality of health care: Part 2: Measuring quality of care. N Engl J Med 335(13):966–970, 1996

Case Management Society of America. Standards of Practice for Case Management. Little Rock, AR: Author, 1995

Center for Health Economics Research. Access to Health Care: Key Indicators for Policy. Princeton, NJ: The Robert Wood Johnson Foundation, 1993

DRGs reflect nursing resources. Hospitals 59(19):56, 1985

Eroding care, cuts in RN staff anger AJN readers. Am J Nurs 96(7):69–73, 1996

Gold MF. Rewriting the book on quality (special section). Provider 25(7):2–4, 1999

Halloran E, Halloran DC. Exploring the DRG equation. Am J Nurs 85(10):1093–1095, 1985

Department of Health and Human Services (DHHS). Healthy People 2000: National Health Promotion and Disease Prevention Objectives, (DHHS Publication No. PHS 91-50212). Washington, DC: U.S. Government Printing Office, 1990

Department of Health and Human Services (DHHS) & Office of Inspector General (OIG). Health Care Fraud and Abuse Control Program 18 Month Outcomes, August 1999. Available at: www.dhhs.gov/progorg/oei. Accessed June 24, 2000.

How Good Is Your Health Plan? Consumer Reports 61(8)28–42, Aug 1996

McKibbon RC, Bimmer PF, Galliher JM, Hartley SS. Nursing Costs and DRG payments. Am J Nurs 85(12):1353–1355, 1985

Moccia P. Curriculum revolution: Agenda for change (p. 63). New York: National League for Nursing, 1988

Owens C. Managed care organizations. New York: McGraw-Hill, 1995

Quality Indicators from the Healthcare Cost and Utilization Project (HCUP QIs). Fact Sheet. Rockville, MD: Agency for Health Care Policy and Research, 1998. Available at: *http://www.ahcpr.gov/data/qifact.htm.* Accessed September 12, 1999.

Reif SS, DesHarnais S, Bernard S. Community perceptions of the effects of rural hospital closure on access to care. J Rural Health Spring;15(2):202–209, 1999

Smith GR. Power and health care reform. J Nurs Educ 33(5):194–197, 1994

Yasko JM, Fleck A. Healthcare reform and cost containment in oncology care: Prospective payment (DRGs). Oncol Nurs Forum Apr. 22(3):491–502, 1995

Vickery, K. JCAHO issues assisted living accreditation principles. Provider 25(6):16, 1999

FURTHER READING

Angell M, Kassierer JP. Quality and the medical marketplace: Following the elephant. N Engl J Med 335(12):883–885, 1996

Blumenthal D. Quality of health care: Part 1: Quality of care—what is it? N Engl J Med 335(12):891–894, 1996

Buxton FL Jr. Health care reform hits the laboratory. What (almost) happened in California. Laboratory Medicine 26(2):113–117, 1995

Drayton-Hargrove S, Woods JH. Ethical analysis of health care reform: Implications for diverse communities. Assoc. Black Nrsg Fac Jrnl 6(4):99–103, 1995

Infante MC. Legally speaking: The legal risks of managed care. RN 59(3):57–59, 1996

Keepnews D, Stanley S. Managed care and nursing's principles. Am Nurs 28(7):5, 1996

Porter-O'Grady T, Wilson CK. The leadership revolution in health care. Gaithersburg, MD: Aspen, 1995

Stahl, DA. Subacute care: Creating alternatives, maximizing reimbursement for subacute care (RUGS III). Nursing Management 26(4):16–17, 1995

Relevant web sites

Joint Commission on Accreditation of Healthcare Organizations (JCAHO) *www.jcaho.org*

National Committee for Quality Assurance (NCQA) *www.ncqa.org*

Health Care Financing Administration (HCFA) *www.hcfa.gov*

Foundation for Accountability (FACCT) *www.facct.org*

3

The Political Process and the Nursing Profession

The struggle for power is a pervading feature of politics; thus, politics in general as well as the politics of nursing requires the learning of power.

(Kalisch & Kalisch, 1982)

OBJECTIVES

After completing this chapter, you should be able to:

1. Explain the relevance of the political process to nursing.

2. Discuss seven ways you might influence the political process.

3. Outline the current U.S. federal governmental role in health care.

4. Discuss common state legislative concerns.

5. Discuss common local political concerns.

6. Explain the reasons for the existence of the large numbers of nursing organizations.

7. Identify the major purpose of each specialized organization presented in the chapter.

8. Analyze the ways that nursing organizations seek to affect the health care delivery system and the political processes that control it.

9. Explain how politics is relevant to your participation in organizations.

KEY TERMS

Allocation of resources

Americans With Disabilities Act (ADA)

Authorization Act

Conditions of participation

Department of Health and Human Services

Fiscal intermediary

Hatch Act

Lobbying

Minimum data set (MDS)

Nurse Practice Act

Occupational Safety and Health Act (OSHA)

Omnibus Budget Reconcilia-	Political action committees	Resident assessment
tion Act (OBRA)	(PACs)	protocols (RAPs)
Ontario Plan		Whistleblower

*P*olitics is the way in which people in any society try to influence decision making and the allocation of resources. Because resources (money, time, and personnel) are limited, it is necessary to make choices regarding their use. There is no perfect process for making optimum choices, because whenever one valuable option is chosen, some other option must be left out. Politics is a part of every organization and a part of government at every level. In a democratic society, all individuals can choose to be involved at some level in this decision-making process. This chapter presents the political process, discusses some of the current issues in regard to political decisions, and describes how you can play a role in the political arena and in nursing organizations.

RELEVANCE OF THE POLITICAL PROCESS FOR NURSES

Nurses always have been involved in politics. Florence Nightingale used her contacts with powerful men in government to obtain supplies and the personnel she needed to care for wounded soldiers in the Crimea (Woodham-Smith, 1983). Hannah Ropes was able to fight incompetence and obtain decent care for wounded Civil War soldiers because she understood who the influential people in Washington were and who would be receptive to her efforts on the soldiers' behalf.

Modern times are no different. With many voices competing to be heard in the decision-making circles of any nation, the person who understands power and politics is the one most likely to obtain the resources needed to accomplish desired ends.

Health care is costly, and public dollars can be and are spent in many ways to provide health care. What part of the federal budget should be allocated to health care? What part of the state budget? The local governmental budget? Of the money allocated, what part should be used for preventive health programs? What part for research? What part for care and treatment? What part for education? What diseases or conditions should be targeted for investigation? Who should receive those dollars? These questions are answered by legislation and administrative decisions of governmental agencies.

Decisions also must be made in health care agencies. What positions will be funded? What equipment purchased? What programs should be adopted and which of the current programs should be dropped? These questions are answered by committees, managers, and governing boards.

Nursing organizations are confronted with similar questions. What is the role of the organization? Should resources be spent on benefits for members? On activities relevant to the nursing profession as a whole? On activities related to general health care? In the political arena? How can nurses affect decision making? What is the individual's role as a nurse in the organization? These questions may be answered by representative assemblies, committees and commissions, and elected officers.

Knowing where the decision making occurs, who makes the decision, and being familiar with how you can influence that process is critical. Each governmental entity, agency, and organization has its own mechanism for operating. However, they have many similarities that can help you plan your activities.

Your practice as a nurse is controlled by a wide variety of governmental decisions. One of the most basic is the Nurse Practice Act of your state. In that document, nursing is defined legally, and the scope of nursing practice is outlined. This document affects what you do each day that you practice. All of the philosophic discussions about the role of the nurse must return to the reality of the nurse's role as legally defined in the state's practice act. Do you care what that role is now or what changes are made in it? Does it make any difference to you what education is required by that law, or if that law requires continuing education? Answering "yes" to any of these questions underlines the relevance of the political process for you.

Many decisions are made in the various nurses' organizations. These organizations speak for nurses in many settings. Are you happy with the way they are spending funds paid in dues? Do you agree with all of the public statements they make? Do you support their mechanisms for decision making? Are you happy with the image of nurses and nursing the public receives from these organizations? Do you care what these organizations do with their resources? The political process is an important part of their functioning, too.

 ## Critical Thinking Activity

Identify a current health care issue in your state or province. Investigate that issue and form a position that you can support with data. Examine your position for personal biases.

INFLUENCING THE POLITICAL PROCESS

You can have an effect on such things as what health care legislation is submitted, the content of the legislation, and what legislation is passed. However, this does not happen without effort and action. Historically, women have been less active in politics than men. This has been the result of a variety of societal factors. Gradually women are assuming a more active role in politics: more are running for and being elected to office, more work with policy-making bodies, and more vote. Because the majority of nurses are women, this changing social climate is important to nursing. Nurses, in particular, have demonstrated increasing political awareness.

Each person must determine his or her own level of personal involvement, but there is, in the broad realm of the political process, a way for everyone to find a suitable role. Some of these ways are outlined here and in Display 3-1.

Display 3–1
INFLUENCING THE POLITICAL PROCESS

- Become informed through a variety of sources.
- Vote for candidates or ballot issues that reflect your concerns.
- Vote for officers within professional or political organizations.
- Express your opinions through letters or in public forums.
- Communicate directly with legislators and public officials.
- Work for or contribute to nonlobbying nursing organizations or political action committees.
- Work for or contribute to candidates who represent your views.
- Testify before decision-making bodies.

Becoming Informed

To become informed about legislation and health care, you need to learn about the sources of information available. Each source of information is valuable to you, but should be weighed based on its known biases. Even the most objective-sounding report can be biased, not only in what is reported, but also in what is not reported. Identifying the groups that support and the groups that oppose a particular viewpoint might help you to recognize bias. Determine whether a group and its members would tend to gain or lose personally by the passage of proposed legislation. Are special interest groups voicing an opinion? When biases are evident, it is advisable to obtain information from groups with divergent viewpoints. Decisions must be based on firm factual data.

Once you are informed about the current issues in legislation or in an organization, you are better prepared to form personal opinions about them and to try to influence the outcome of the political process.

NEWSPAPERS

Your daily newspaper can be an excellent source of information about significant legislation being proposed, when an issue is controversial or of widespread interest. When you rely on the newspaper for information, however, you sometimes learn of legislation only after it has already been passed.

TELEVISION AND RADIO

Television and radio news reports are usually quite brief and give only an overview of a particular piece of legislation being introduced. This overview may be helpful in alerting you to something that you will want to study more intensively. Some television programs, such as those on public television, do discuss issues in depth. In an attempt to meet the Federal Communications Commission (FCC) rules regarding equal time, these programs usually make an attempt to present both sides of any issue.

PROFESSIONAL JOURNALS AND NEWSLETTERS

Professional journals usually devote some space to current legislative issues. This is done routinely in the American Journal of Nursing and in the American Nurse. When major issues are being debated, other nursing periodicals often contain articles of interest. The journals of other health care professions also may carry information regarding current issues. Newsletters and journals of organizations that have a political focus provide information on what they see as current issues. These organizations include consumer groups such as Common Cause, political groups such as Young Democrats and Young Republicans, and nonpartisan groups such as the League of Women Voters.

ORGANIZATIONAL MEETINGS

Nursing organizations and other health-related organizations sometimes hold open meetings to present and discuss legislative issues. Often knowledgeable speakers can help you to understand what is being proposed and the potential effects of a proposal. These organizations also may sponsor e-mail networks to get out information on important pending legislation. Nursing organizations can be excellent sources of information because they often are in touch with legislators and legislative staff.

GOVERNMENTAL PUBLICATIONS

Copies of legislation are usually available through your congressional representatives (for federal matters) and your state representatives (for state matters). Along with copies of the legislation, a legislator may send other informational material. Government agencies affected by proposed legislation also may provide information about its potential effects, although they are not allowed to try to influence legislation.

INTERNET WEB SITES

Internet Web sites are an increasingly useful source of information. In most states, the text of bills being introduced is available on a governmental Web site, where you can read the bill on the computer or print the document to read. Either of these can be done while online or the materials can be downloaded for later use. Nursing and health care organizations that maintain Web sites often have a site devoted to political issues affecting members of the organization or relevant issues that affect health care. Many news organizations (television stations, newspapers, and magazines) maintain Web sites with information on current issues. Any of these sites may provide links to still more sites that provide useful information.

Voting

Your individual vote on a ballot issue is significant, although it is a common practice to belittle the importance of the individual vote in any election. Recent major elections in this country, however, have demonstrated how important every vote can be. One of the unfortunate statistics in the United States is that only a very small percentage of eligible people in the United States are registered voters. Nurses, as a group, represent a high percentage of all people who vote. When legislators hear statistics such as "1 in 17 women voters is a nurse," or "1 in every 44 voters is a nurse," they pay attention to the opinions of nurses. Although you cannot vote directly on legislative issues, you can vote for candidates whose positions you support and who share your values. Absentee ballots are always available for those who cannot be present at their polling place on the day of an election. These ballots must be requested well in advance of the election, however (Fig. 3-1).

Voting for officers in organizations may be ignored by a large majority of members. They look at the ballot, cannot identify those running for office, and therefore do not vote. Most organizations do make an attempt to introduce members to the various candidates. If you do not know the candidates, you can seek information about them: read their prepared statements of position, and learn about their previous activities. Those elected to office usually determine the direction and priorities of an organization. If you are contributing your dues dollars, you want to have a voice in choosing those who are entrusted with making the decisions.

Shaping Public Opinion

Public opinion does influence the actions of legislators and regulatory bodies. As a registered nurse, you can help to shape public opinion; your judgment about matters that

FIGURE 3–1   Sharing your opinions is one avenue of political involvement.

affect health care can help others make their own decisions. Share the knowledge you have gained through your personal experience and research. Do not be afraid to state your own position, although you must be prepared to support your position with evidence if you want to be considered a thoughtful health care professional. Certainly, you will not want to make every social occasion an opportunity to share political positions, but you should take advantage of opportunities that arise to present your concerns to others.

Another means of shaping public opinion is writing a letter to the editor of a newspaper or news magazine. These letters are read by many people. The following suggestions will maximize your chances of appearing in print:

- Carefully follow the instructions provided by the publication for letters to the editor. These usually will refer to length, signature, address, and telephone number.
- Clearly present your opinion with well-reasoned arguments.
- Including personal experiences that illustrate health care concerns can be useful; however, you must be careful that health care examples do not violate the confidentiality of clients or divulge confidential information regarding your employer.

Additional information about writing effective letters is provided in Figure 3-2.

Within an organization, you may also influence opinion and action by clearly presenting reasoned arguments. You can discuss issues with other members, attend meetings, and voice your opinion. Remember that a viewpoint supported by strong, reasoned judgment and rationale will be better received than a simple statement of opinion.

Communicating With Legislators and Officials

Legislators are affected by the views of their constituents. The legislator's staff reviews letters sent to a legislator; views are tabulated, and letters with significant opinions or information are directed to the legislator for individual consideration. Although some groups encourage members to sign form letters or postcards, personal letters always have the greater impact.

Concern regarding the rules and regulations of a specific department of government can be addressed to the officials of that department. It is possible for officials to become insulated from the effects of their decision making. Communication from concerned citizens can be as important to them as it is to legislators. Letters to officials should reflect the same care and professional viewpoint as letters to legislators in order to be most effective.

A carefully written personal letter reflecting thoughtful and informed opinions on an issue that a person is competent to evaluate will receive the most attention from any governmental person or department. As a registered nurse, you have expertise in an area of health care and can provide a valuable viewpoint. Identify yourself as a registered nurse in your letter and outline why you are concerned about the issue in question. Legislators often appreciate personal anecdotes from your practice (with identities concealed, of course) that underscore your point. (See Figure 3-2 for information

HOW TO WRITE YOUR CONGRESSMAN

How to learn their names . . .
Call your public library, local newspaper, or chapter of the League of Women Voters to learn the names and addresses of your U.S. senators, your representative to congress, your state senator(s), and your state representative(s), (called assemblyman in California, New Jersey, New York, and Wisconsin; delegate in Virginia and West Virginia).

How to obtain a copy of a bill
For a Senate bill, write or visit (no telephone requests filled) the Senate Documents Office, Washington, DC 20510; for a House bill, write or visit the Doorkeeper of the House, U.S. Capitol, Washington, DC 20515.

Ask for the bill by number and enclose a self-addressed and gummed label for fastest service. There is no charge.

Requests are normally filled the day received, unless the bill is out of print, and sent via first class mail. There is a limit of six items per day per person, and of three copies of one bill per person (or of one copy per bill if the bill is 60 pages or longer).

Request a copy of a state bill from the appropriate state legislator.

Copies of a hearing record can be requested from the committee conducting the hearing although they usually are not ready for distribution until several weeks after the hearing.

An alternate to the above procedures, for federal bills and hearing records, is to request a copy from your appropriate senator or representative.

Fundamentals:
1. Address your letter properly: "Hon. _____, House Office Building, Washington, DC, 20515" or "Senator _____, Senate Office Building, Washington, DC 20510".
2. Identify the bill or issue. Try to give the bill number or describe it by popular title.
3. Watch your timing. Inform your congressman while there is still time to take effective action.

(Reprinted by permission of the N.A.A.C.O.G.)

Write to the right persons:
Concentrate on your own delegation. The representative of your district and the senators of your state cast your votes in the Congress and want to know your views.

Be brief:
Be reasonably brief. Your views and arguments stand a better chance of being read if they are stated as concisely as the subject matter will permit. It is not necessary that letters be typed—only that they be legible—and the form, phraseology, and grammar are not important.

Do:
1. Write your own views—not someone else's. A personal letter is far better than a form letter or signature on a petition. Form letters often receive form replies.
2. Give your reasons for taking a stand. The effects of a bill on a certain constituency will be far more helpful.
3. Be constructive. If a bill deals with a problem, but you believe the bill is the wrong approach, outline the correct approach. If you have expert knowledge, share it with your congressman.
4. Say 'well done' when it is deserved. Congressmen appreciate this from people who believe they have done the right thing.

Do not:
1. Don't make threats or promises.
2. Don't berate your congressman. If you disagree with him, give reasons for your disagreement.
3. Don't become a 'pen pal'. Quality is more important than quantity.
4. Don't demand a commitment before the facts are in. A bill rarely becomes law in the same form as introduced, it is possible for a writer to change his or her position once a bill reaches a floor.

The above material, excerpted from *Congressional Record, Nov. 2, 1977,* by Morris K. Udall, was prepared by the Washington office of The American College of Obstetricians and Gynecologists.

FIGURE 3–2   How to write your congressional representative.

on writing to members of Congress.) The names and addresses of your congressional representatives and of your individual state representatives are available online from the American Nurses Association. Go to www.nursingworld.org and link to "Capitol-Wiz." This page connects you to a list of members of Congress, their names, and addresses.

Many governmental agencies, both legislative and regulatory, have e-mail addresses that allow you to send messages electronically. As the "information highway" becomes more widely accessible, using this form of communication has become easier. E-mail has the advantage of being extremely timely. Although you may have e-mail access at your place of work, your employer may not allow you to use it for political activity. If you are employed by a government entity, such as a public health department, the law prohibits you from using governmental resources such as e-mail for political activity. Members of the U.S. Congress may be e-mailed by linking through the www.nursingworld.org Web site identified above. That Web site also gives you information about the legislative process and some tips for writing your message. An e-mail message should be composed as carefully as a letter, using the guidelines in Figure 3-2. One important point is to include your full name and home address in your e-mail. Staff members review the address, forward only those messages that are personally identifiable, and especially note those from a congressperson's own district. Do remember that e-mail is public. You should not say things on e-mail that you would be uncomfortable with presenting in public.

Telephone calls can be made to the legislator's office. Staff members keep a record of all calls, and the positions of callers are noted. To call a member of Congress, contact the U.S. Capitol Switchboard at (202) 224-3121, and ask for the individual's office. In some states a toll-free number is maintained for calls to state legislators during the legislative session. You will be asked to leave a message. Be sure to identify yourself fully, including both name and address. State the bill or issue about which you are calling and clearly state your position.

Telegrams are delivered by telephone within 5 hours of being sent. A mailgram is a less expensive type of telegram that is delivered in the regular mail on the next business day after it is sent. These are especially useful ways of communicating to legislators right before an important vote or committee deliberation.

Visiting congressional or state representatives also is an effective means of expressing your concerns. One of the best ways to arrange to speak with congressional representatives and senators is to contact their local offices. Through these offices you may receive assistance in arranging your visit. They may also help you to arrange other interesting and valuable activities such as attending committee hearings, taking tours, and visiting Congress in session. Appointments should be made well in advance, as representatives and senators often have busy schedules. If your time is limited, you may have to modify your expectations and meet with a staff member who will relay your concerns. Plan carefully for your visit. It is helpful to write out concerns and questions. Be sure to leave time for answers to the questions that you pose. Even when you disagree with the position taken by your legislator, be polite and present your concerns calmly. Rudeness will result in the legislator's unwillingness to listen to what you have to say.

These same activities may be useful in working within an organization. Those elected to office do not know the views of members unless communication occurs. For communication to be effective, you must know when and where boards meet, how to get information to board members, and the names of those responsible for specific aspects of the organization's operations.

Critical Thinking Activity

Identify a political issue about which you feel strongly. Write a letter to a governmental official that provides a sound rationale in support of your position.

Group Action

The political process in the nursing profession takes many forms. Nurses can be involved as individuals, but they are far more effective when they work in groups. Because nursing is the largest single health care occupation, nurses have many votes. For this reason, legislators pay attention to positions held by groups of nurses.

NONLOBBYING NURSING ORGANIZATIONAL EFFORT

Most traditional nursing organizations are nonprofit groups and therefore are limited in their political activity. The major role of nonprofit groups in politics involves testifying to facts, organizational positions, and concerns in the health care arena. The American Nurses Association (ANA) has an office in Washington, DC, and tries to keep the nursing profession informed about legislative matters of importance in health care. The ANA also provides experts in the nursing profession who testify before congressional and regulatory groups about proposed legislation.

The Tricouncil for Nursing is a collaborative effort of the ANA, the National League for Nursing (NLN), the American Organization of Nurse Executives, and the American Association of Colleges of Nursing. It represents the interests of nursing practice, research, and education. By working collaboratively, these organizations have strengthened the voice of nursing and its visibility in Washington, DC. This coalition has become the trusted spokesperson for nursing. Legislators rely on the information it provides and recognize it as a united voice for the nursing profession.

The ANA organized the Nurses Strategic Action Team (N-STAT) to provide nurses with a means to mobilize quickly to influence legislative policy. This organization promotes grassroots involvement in legislative issues, meets with members of Congress, and organizes letter writing and telephone campaigns. It involves thousands of nurses. You can imagine that receiving thousands of letters about a single topic might get the attention of a legislator.

Another effort by the ANA to inform nurses about legislative issues is the regular publication of *Capitol Update: The Legislative Newsletter for Nurses*. An individual can subscribe to this publication or read it online from the ANA Web site. This publication brings the latest in legislative concerns to your attention 20 times a year.

The Nurses' Coalition for Legislative Action is a group of 28 nursing specialty organizations that works to support the positions of its member organizations at the federal level. Specialty nursing organizations have joined this coalition to bring a larger voice to the support of issues that affect nursing specialty practice. Like the Tricouncil, the focus is on information gathering for member organizations and on testifying regarding education, research, and practice issues in nursing.

Most state and district nurses' associations have legislative committees that monitor legislative and regulatory actions in their areas. They may provide educational events for nurses in regard to current issues, and testify at hearings regarding health-related issues. They also may seek to mobilize letter writing or telephone campaigns.

POLITICAL ACTION COMMITTEES

To take a more active role in seeking the passage of desired legislation, the defeat of undesired measures, and the election of particular candidates, groups form organizations called political action committees (often referred to as PACs). These organizations are registered as political action groups and are free to try to affect the political process. They are not considered nonprofit organizations because their funds are used for political purposes; therefore, donations to them are not tax deductible (Fig. 3-3).

FIGURE 3–3 Nurses may lobby to get desired legislation passed by visiting legislators, by presenting information and arguments about the bill, and by writing letters.

The ANA political action organization is titled the ANA-Political Action Committee (ANA-PAC). ANA-PAC actually lobbies for the passage or defeat of bills and supports candidates for public office. Since the 1976 federal elections, ANA-PAC has raised funds to support candidates for the Senate and the House of Representatives based on their expressed and demonstrated stands on key health issues such as health care reform proposals, funding for nursing and biomedical research, extension and funding of nursing education, and third-party reimbursement for nurses. Not all candidates endorsed by ANA-PAC were supported financially because of the limited funds available. Candidates' successes are attributable to many factors, but the effect of nursing support has been demonstrated. Many state nursing associations also have political action organizations. These groups serve the same function on the state level as ANA-PAC does on the national level. Many candidates actively seek the endorsement of nursing organizations that are perceived as influential with voters.

Although these nursing political action groups have not grown rapidly in size, their growth has been steady. In addition, nurses are gaining more sophistication in their approach to the political process. Although nurses do not have high incomes, their combined financial contributions can significantly help a candidate or issue. All of these factors have resulted in nurses gaining increased power in the political sphere. There is still a long way to go before nurses have the same kind of power that is wielded by those in labor, education, and medicine, but change is occurring.

Critical Thinking Activity

Contact your state nurses' association and find out if your state has a political action organization. If it does, contact that organization and ask what the current issues are in the state. Investigate those issues.

OTHER POLITICALLY IMPORTANT GROUPS

Many organizations in addition to those specifically related to nursing are concerned about health and social issues. Some are official lobbying groups; others provide information resources. Groups such as Common Cause (a consumer lobbying group), AARP (formerly the American Association of Retired Persons), the League of Women Voters, and even church organizations often act to affect the political process. You may support these groups simply by donating money for their needs or by being actively involved in their work.

Testifying for Decision-Making Bodies

Many decisions affecting nursing and health care are made by committees and commissions at various levels of government. These decision-making bodies often hold hearings to gather information before decisions are made. As a nurse, your testimony may have particular value when certain areas of health care are considered. A nurse may testify as either an official representative of an organization or as an independent individual.

You may learn of opportunities to testify through announcements in the newspaper and through professional publications. In general, you must register in advance to testify. In some instances, there is registration at the door before a meeting begins, but for more formal situations, you will have to notify the committee in advance that you wish to testify.

If you have an opportunity to testify, be sure to make your position clear so that the decision makers know whether you speak for yourself or for a larger group. Prepare your testimony ahead of time, but try to avoid simply reading a statement. A less formal presentation is usually more interesting for the listener. Be prepared with sources for any facts or figures you present, and explain any technical terms you use. Find out whether there is a time limit for each testimony. If you are given a time limit, make sure that you present your most important arguments and facts first. Most committees will accept written testimony if you cannot be there in person, but the personal presentation is usually more effective.

Individual Support for Legislation and Candidates

You may choose to personally support a specific piece of legislation by contributing money for publicity and campaigning, or by working on a committee that is striving for the passage of a proposal. Funds are needed for printing and distributing literature, newspaper ads, and television and radio announcements. Workers may be needed for secretarial tasks, to contact people in a door-to-door campaign, and to speak on behalf of the issue.

Supporting a candidate for public office is accomplished in the same way. In our political system the reality is that those who have actively supported a candidate during an election campaign are listened to more closely when decisions are being made. Working for a candidate is one way to make your view known. It is also an excellent way to gain firsthand knowledge of the political process (Fig. 3-4).

Working in Policy-Making Agencies

Nurses have been appointed to major administrative positions in state and federal health agencies and to the staffs of several senators and representatives. The Robert Wood Johnson Foundation has provided one-year fellowships for nurses to study policy in Washington, DC. Nurses who complete these fellowships have the skills and abilities to be effective in influencing health care policy. Nurses have a promising future in the health policy arena.

Seeking Election to an Office

Those elected or appointed to an office, whether in a local nursing organization or the U.S. Congress, have considerable power to affect outcomes. Leaders in nursing organizations help to shape the direction and efforts of those organizations. Legislators have power to affect significant regulations and spending plans. Nurses in several states

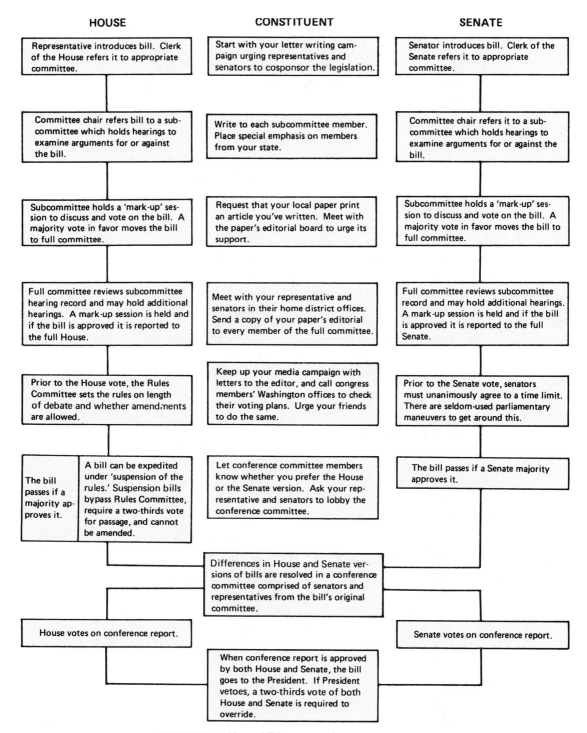

FIGURE 3–4 How a bill becomes a law.

have been effective in shaping health policy by seeking and being elected to office as members of their state legislatures. Eddie Bernice Johnson, elected as a Congresswoman from Texas in 1994, was the first nurse to hold an elective federal office. In the 1996 elections, four nurses were candidates for congressional seats, and of these, three were elected to office. As women in general have become more politically visible, nurses are a part of this growing political trend.

Limitations on Your Political Activity

If you are an employee of any governmental agency, such as a public health department or the Veterans Administration, your political activity is subject to restrictions that do not apply to the general public. Restrictions applying to federal government employees are defined in the Hatch Act. Prohibited activities are mainly those that have to do with supporting a particular political party by being an officer or party spokesperson. The Hatch Act also prohibits any political activity on the part of a government employee, on behalf of a party or in support of legislation that could be construed as representing his or her government agency.

The Hatch Act does not interfere with a private citizen's right to support parties and candidates financially, to join political parties, to work for or against measures that will appear on a ballot, or to participate in nonpartisan (ie, not connected with a political party) elections as a candidate. Each state has its own version of the Hatch Act. If you are employed by a governmental agency of any kind, you should investigate the limitations that your employment may place on your political activity.

THE FEDERAL GOVERNMENT'S ROLE IN HEALTH CARE

Federal legislation has affected nursing and health care in important ways. If you understand key concepts of the federal government's involvement in health care and how federal legislation has affected health care delivery, you will be more effective in the political arena.

Federal Agencies Related to Health Care

The federal government operates in the health care field in complex ways. Literally dozens of federal agencies are involved with health care in some way. The Department of Health and Human Services (DHHS) is a cabinet-level administrative unit of the federal government with four major service divisions (Display 3-2).

The Public Health Service, which includes the Centers for Disease Control and Prevention (CDC) is one agency with which you should already be familiar. The National Institutes of Health (NIH), the Food and Drug Administration (FDA), the Health Resources Administration (HRA), and the Health Care Financing Administration (HCFA) are all part of the DHHS. This agency has tremendous impact through its rules and regulations and the projects it funds.

Display 3–2
MAJOR SERVICE DIVISIONS OF THE DEPARTMENT OF HEALTH AND HUMAN SERVICES

Office of Human Development Services
Administration on Aging
Administration for Child, Youth, and
   Families
Administration for Native Americans
Administration for Public Service

Public Health Service
Centers for Disease Control and
   Prevention
Food and Drug Administration
Health Resources Administration
Health Services Administration
National Institutes of Health
Alcohol, Drug Abuse, and Mental Health
   Administration

Social Security Administration
Systems
Governmental Affairs
Family Assistance
Hearings and Appeals
Operational Policy and Procedure
   Assessment

Health Care Financing Administration
Health Standards and Quality Bureau
Bureau of Quality Control
Bureau of Program Operations
Bureau of Program Policy
Bureau of Support Services
Office of Child Support Enforcement

The Federal Budget Process

Because funding is a driving force in all decision making, you will find it useful to understand something of the federal budget process. The availability of government funding for each federal program depends on two separate legislative actions. The first action is the authorization act. This is a bill, passed by both the House of Representatives (where any revenue bill must originate) and the Senate, that describes a program and outlines the rules under which funds for the program can be expended. It also sets a ceiling on the amount of money that can be provided. It is under these authorization acts (often referred to by the "title" of the section of the authorizing act) that funds are dispensed for all the health-related activities described in this chapter.

The second necessary legislative action is the appropriations act. The appropriations process establishes the federal budget and the specific amounts of money appropriated for actual spending for each previously authorized program. Both the House and the Senate pass a budget appropriations act. Then a joint House and Senate committee meets to achieve a compromise that both will accept. The final result is called the "Omnibus Budget Reconciliation Act" (OBRA), which includes the compromises the budget committee has worked out between the House and Senate versions of the budget. Each budget act—for example, OBRA 1997—is identified by the year in the title. The amount appropriated for any program cannot exceed the amount originally authorized, but it can be, and often is, less. This is sometimes confusing because two monetary amounts, the authorized amount and the budgeted (or appropriated) amount, may be reported in connection with the same act.

The budget act also may place restrictions on the people and organizations receiving federal funds. It is under this authority that the federal government sets standards for nursing homes that receive reimbursement through Medicaid and Medicare. The rules and regulations for nursing homes, called the "conditions of participation," included in OBRA 1987 (the budget reconciliation act for 1987) were extensive. These rules and regulations did not take effect until October 1, 1990. This allowed the affected organizations to begin the process of change to meet the new requirements.

Historically, a third factor has affected the amount of money available for a specific federal program: the participation of the executive branch of government in decisions regarding how and when available funds will be spent. If money that has been authorized and appropriated has not been spent by the end of a budget period, it is lost. This money then must be reauthorized and reappropriated. The executive branch has used this mechanism to withdraw support for programs it opposes.

Funding for Nursing Education

Beginning in 1964, the federal government provided funding to support nursing education through what was first titled the Nurse Training Act and later called the Nurse Education Act. Initially the funding was generous and included money for buildings, classroom renovation, equipment, faculty development, and student scholarships and traineeships. As the shortage of nurses abated and priorities changed in Washington, DC, the amount of funding gradually declined.

Every two years, when the biennial budget is passed, nurses try to rally congressional support for additional funding for nursing education. Funds currently appropriated through the Nurse Education Act are limited and primarily used to support education for advanced nursing practice and graduate degrees. In fiscal year (FY) 1998 the Funding for Nurse Education Act was $65.38 million, and in FY 1999 the appropriation was raised to $67.85 million.

Nursing Research Support

A major advance for nursing research in the 1980s was the addition of a National Institute for Nursing Research (NINR) to the other major divisions of the National Institutes of Health. Nurses and nursing organizations lobbied long and hard for legislative authorization for this institute. It is now a major financial source of nursing research dollars. Funding for nursing research is increasing: in FY 1998 the appropriation was $63.597 million and in FY 1999 it increased to $69.834 million (Capitol Update, 1999, p 1).

Occupational Safety and Health

The Occupational Safety and Health Act (OSHA) mandates actions and prescribes safety equipment to improve the health and safety of the working environment. Many people think that the rules and regulations created by OSHA are too cumbersome. Nevertheless, concern for the safety of the working person is of considerable importance to nurses. Occupational injuries create major health problems for the adult population. They are costly not only in terms of health and personal loss but also in terms of lost productivity. Nurses also are affected by the provisions of OSHA in their own work environments. They, too, are subject to injury and accident on the job. The safety concerns of nurses in the workplace are discussed in Chapter 11.

Nurses in occupational health nursing also are involved in OSHA through educating workers about job safety. In some situations, safety precautions are time consuming and uncomfortable, and workers may be tempted to ignore them. Nurses may be able to help workers understand the importance of following health and safety regulations. Occupational health nurses also assist management in planning to make the environment safe and in establishing appropriate procedures for treating injuries.

OSHA regulations have required health care employers to provide the equipment, supplies, immunizations, and education to enable the implementation of CDC recommendations for "universal" precautions. The antiregulatory stance of Congress since 1994 has been reflected in the failure of OSHA to upgrade infection control requirements to the CDC recommendation for Standard Precautions.

More recently, OSHA has been investigating the effects of repetitive strain injuries, among which are back injuries in health care workers. Funds for National Academy of Sciences research related to the link between repetitive motions and workplace injuries were included in the 1999 fiscal year appropriation. The expectation is that the results of this research will guide OSHA regulations about workplace standards for lifting.

Another occupational concern to nurses is needle-stick injuries. OSHA has mandated that all health care agencies have in place a blood-borne pathogens prevention program. This includes both training for behaviors of staff and what are termed "engineering" controls. Engineering controls are the use of safe equipment that does not rely solely on the action of the individual to maintain protection. The FY 1999 appropriations bill included a requirement that employers record all injuries from potentially contaminated needles and other sharp instruments. The CDC, in November 1999, changed its recommendation to include the use of safe needles (NIOSH, 1999, www.cdc.gov/niosh). OSHA has not required safe devices; therefore, the efforts of health care workers have been aimed at legislation that would require OSHA to enact regulations regarding safe devices. A "Health Care Worker Protection Act" has been introduced in the past and will be reintroduced in 2000 in the 106th Congress. This Act would mandate safer needles and funding for training of health care workers. Many states have initiated legislation to deal with this concern.

A current safety concern of health care workers is violence in the workplace. Nurses in psychiatric settings have long recognized the hazards they face in working with aggressive, violent, and sometimes out-of-control clients. Emergency rooms are sites where the violence of society spills over into the health care setting. Even obstetric units may encounter violence by family members. Nurses are asking that OSHA mandate health care workplaces to provide safety from violence. (See Chapter 11 for a further discussion of violence in the workplace.)

Nursing Home Regulations

OBRA 1987, the federal budget bill passed for 1987, contained regulations that for the first time mandated a national standard for quality of care in long-term care facilities receiving federal money through Medicare or Medicaid. Although the provisions of this act were set to take effect in October 1990, there were delays because of legal challenges to the requirements and because of the extra time that was needed to establish monitoring mechanisms. This is not unusual when legislation requires difficult and costly implementation. Therefore, some of the provisions of OBRA 1987 took effect as late as 1994. Despite earlier concerns, it is now clear that these regulations have positively affected the care environment in nursing homes. The use of restraints has decreased, resident rights are more effectively supported, and basic care needs are being identified and met.

More recently, the budget bill for 1999 established a prospective payment system for skilled nursing facilities that resulted in decreased payments from Medicare and Medicaid. Because of widespread concern over the effects of this action, many groups lobbied Congress for change. Late in 1999, Congress amended the funding formula to restore some of the funds that had been cut. How this will affect care remains to be seen.

Future Federal Legislation

Many issues will come before Congress in the next two years. The ANA is preparing to support some strongly and to monitor the progress of others. Community Nursing Organizations (CNO) were authorized as a demonstration project in 1997. These organizations provide nurse-directed care in four states (Arizona, Illinois, Minnesota, and New York). ANA is developing a specific strategy to support the continued support for the development of this unique approach to care (Capitol Update, 1999, p. 2).

Pending Regulatory Changes

HCFA has proposed new regulations regarding conditions of participation of acute care hospitals in Medicare and Medicaid. These new regulations have been opened for comment. The ANA has expressed concern over the impact of some of these regulations. The final rules are expected to be completed in 2000.

STATE-LEVEL LEGISLATIVE CONCERNS

Many issues that vitally affect the health care arena are decided at the state level. Because the health care issues in each state are different, only some general areas of concern are outlined here.

State Agencies and Health Care

State institutions range from those that care for the mentally retarded and the mentally ill to penal systems and institutions of higher education. Health care is a consideration in all of these settings. When budgets are planned, topics as diverse as immunization and contraception may be part of the debate. Nurses often can advocate for those who are unable to speak for themselves about their own health care needs. Sometimes nurses who work in these settings are unable to deliver quality care because of severe budgetary deficiencies. All nurses can support efforts to provide quality health care in such settings.

Nurse Practice Acts

Nurse practice acts are being discussed and revised in many states. This process is long and difficult, and requires intense political effort by nurses to avoid creating problems for the profession. One current concern related to placing the act before a state legislature for action is the pressure to lessen the standards or allow unlicensed assistive personnel to perform more nursing tasks. Another concern is the implementation of multistate licensure. (See Chapter 6 for further discussion of licensure laws.)

State Legislative Concerns

Some of the major workplace concerns of nurses are emerging as topics of state legislation. Concerns about the nurse's vulnerability when unsafe care is part of an institution's practice have led to efforts toward achieving whistleblower protection. A *whistleblower* is a person who reports to authorities the wrongdoing of individuals in their own work setting or the organizations in which they are employed. The state of New Jersey was the first to pass legislation that protects from retaliation health care employees who refuse to participate in or who report unsafe practice (Whistleblower, 1997). The federal government encourages whistleblowing to reveal fraud in the Medicare and Medicaid programs (Polston, 1999).

As discussed above, the use of safe needles or protected devices for blood drawing and parenteral medication administration is being lobbied for in state legislative and regulatory arenas. These devices are being manufactured and do dramatically decrease the incidence of needlestick injury; however, they cost a great deal more than the needles they replace. For example, in one setting a needle that cost 34 cents was replaced with a needleless connector that cost $1.74. When computed system-wide that is a tremendous increase in costs. However, nurses are pointing out that the cost of surveillance and care of those who sustain needlestick injuries also must be added to the cost of using needles. What is the cost of a case of hepatitis C? Of hepatitis A? Of HIV?

Still another issue has been that of latex sensitivity in health care workers and in clients. As the use of protective barriers has dramatically increased over the years, exposure to latex has skyrocketed. This exposure involves skin contact and inhalation of latex proteins that are dispersed on glove powder. Developing mechanisms to decrease exposure has involved using nonpowdered gloves, nonlatex products in some situations, and latex-free environments for the seriously affected. Again, these products are more costly. As more and more care is financed by flat fees regardless of costs, institutions find it increasingly difficult to increase costs and remain competitive. Legislation requiring all institutions to have specific programs to decrease latex exposure would level the cost basis and make it more likely that reimbursement would be adjusted to meet this demand.

LOCAL POLITICAL CONCERNS

The budgetary process always seems to be at the root of most political and legislative concerns. Because only a limited amount of money is available, budgets always are developed through a series of compromises. To gain one objective, it is sometimes necessary to recognize that funds will not be available for achieving another. In most communities, budgets for public health departments, school nurses, and so forth are developed over a period of several months. Hearings are often held, at which members of the public may ask questions and address issues. Nurses often have found that involvement at this planning stage is most rewarding. Determining priorities for health care is essential, and nurses can speak with authority on these matters. Nurses actually employed in a public department undergoing review may be limited in making their views known because of regulations governing their action in the political sphere. For this reason, it is significant that nurses outside of government institutions recognize the importance of community health. It is not only the practice of the public health nurse that is affected by the priorities of the agency. For example, a nurse who is employed in a hospital may wish to refer a discharged patient to a public health nurse for follow-up, only to find that, owing to changes in the ordering of priorities, home visits for the identified purpose are no longer being made.

In many communities, decisions about the allocation of federal money are made at the local level. The most recent Congress had a goal of creating large block grants where priorities would be decided locally. Support for alternative health care centers, blood pressure screening, and senior citizen centers may depend on whether those who are knowledgeable about the benefits of these services are willing to voice their advocacy in local decision-making bodies.

HEALTH CARE REFORM

The United States is the only major industrialized country (other than South Africa) that does not provide some type of government-sponsored health care for all citizens. Through Medicare and Medicaid, and the widespread effects of the military, public health, and Native American health systems, the federal government already is deeply involved in the provision of health care. President Clinton's proposal for a national system of managed competition was defeated, pushing most of the impetus for reform to the states.

As each state debates this issues, common questions recur.

- Do people have a right to health care?
- If there is such a right, what level of health care can people expect to receive? Routine preventive services? Surgery and hospitalization for all conditions? Or treatment only for serious life-threatening conditions?
- Should catastrophic illnesses, transplantation, and experimental treatments be included?
- What about fertility-enhancing services? Should abortion services be included?

- How can health care be transformed into an effective, coordinated system?
- How will changes in the health care system be financed?

These are difficult philosophical and ethical questions, and there are no simple answers.

Nursing's Agenda for Health Care Reform

The ANA, the NLN, and almost 60 other nursing organizations cooperated in presenting Nursing's Agenda for Health Care Reform (American Nurses Association, 1991) to legislators, health care agencies, and the public. Nursing's agenda was based on the belief that any health care system must (1) provide quality health care, (2) allow access for all citizens, and (3) be cost effective. One aspect of the agenda was a federally defined standard package of essential health care benefits. The goal was to provide primary care and prevention financed by a combination of public and private sources. Nursing suggested improving access to health care, which is often affected by geographical, economic, and cultural factors, by delivering it in schools, workplaces, and the home. Nursing also suggested controlling costs through managed care, and implementing the plan in steps. When health care reform failed in 1992, many thought that nursing's agenda was also lost.

One key concern of nurses has been direct reimbursement of nursing care. This has been of special concern to primary health care nurses. The availability of funding for nursing care will, to a great extent, determine whether the public is able to use such services. Physicians (through the American Medical Association) have consistently supported provisions for direct payment only to physicians or for care ordered by physicians. Other organizations of direct care providers (social workers, nurses, psychologists, and so forth) are seeking greater breadth in reimbursement. If third-party payment is closed to nurses and other direct care providers, then their ability to provide services is severely curtailed. Physicians believe that controlling access to third-party payment will control health care costs. Limiting access also would preserve the physician's unique position of power in the health care setting.

Although planning for health care reform at the federal level was dropped as a result of political opposition, many of the issues that nursing supported are still being discussed, and proposals contained in nursing's agenda are being adopted at state and local levels. Nurses continue to support plans that allow comprehensive access to health care and provide mechanisms for nurses to work to the full extent of their abilities.

Many states are moving ahead toward health care reform at the state level. States instituting health care reform have asked for waivers from the federal rules governing Medicaid to incorporate all Medicaid funds into their planning. Nurses have been active in many states as the various issues are debated and priorities set.

Most of the health reform plans address concerns regarding malpractice suits and the cost to the system of litigation. Most include a dispute resolution mechanism as an alternative to court proceedings. Plans vary with respect to the presence of caps on awards, limits on attorney's fees, the approach to punitive damages, and the statute of limitations. The use of mid-level providers (advanced practice nurses and physician's assistants) to increase access and hold down costs has been an ingredient of health reform proposals in most states. The issues surrounding universal access to health care continue to be problematic.

Critical Thinking Activity

Identify an aspect of health care reform that concerns you. Analyze the various proposals currently before Congress or your state legislature in regard to that specific concern. Rank the proposals in order of your preference, providing rationale for your decision making. In a small group, hold a discussion in which you share your analysis of the various proposals.

NURSING ORGANIZATIONS

A student once said that it seems that every time nurses identify a problem, their first action is to form a new organization. Although this may be something of an exaggeration, it contains a bit of truth. When you first learn about the great number of nursing and nursing-related organizations, it all seems confusing and their purposes and functions may seem duplicative (Fig. 3-5).

FIGURE 3–5 The large number of nursing organizations may seem overwhelming.

The existence of a large number of diverse organizations for nurses is, in many ways, a reflection of nursing itself. The profession offers a wide variety of employment opportunities to its members, with distinct and varied contributions and interests in health care. When nurses become committed to a particular specialty group, they have a tendency to want to advance the purposes and interests of the people working in that area. For example, operating room nurses have more in common with other operating room nurses, in terms of interests and concerns, than they have with nurses working in hospice care. Likewise, nurses involved in hospice care would probably prefer to share concerns with one another than to discuss them with critical care nurses. With more than 2.2 million nurses in the United States, it is understandable that there are many different areas of nursing interest, and therefore many different nursing organizations.

The formation of a large number of nursing organizations has resulted in concern regarding the overlapping of function and interrelationships among some of the organizations. Unfortunately, there has often been a spirit of competition rather than cooperation among these groups in the past. Because nurses traditionally have not had high incomes, joining more than one organization has not been a desirable option for economic as well as philosophic reasons.

Nursing organizations recently have made a concerted effort to promote cooperation. Nurses are better informed about the various organizations and receive better salaries than in the past. However, these facts have not resulted in significantly greater participation by professional nurses in their organizations. Some people specifically do not join because of philosophical differences, but many nurses seem to be apathetic and do not recognize the importance of nurses acting together. Some, because they are combining a job with family and home responsibilities, feel they do not have the time or energy to become involved. Nurses need to recognize the potential for power that they possess as a group. As the nation moves toward health care reform, this has never been a more critical issue. (Appendix B is an overview of the many nursing and nursing-related organizations.)

 ## Critical Thinking Activity

> Do you believe that there are too many nursing organizations? Give the rationale for your answer. If you could develop a method for reducing the number of nursing organizations, what criteria would you suggest be used to support the continuation of existing groups? Provide the rationale for each criterion you suggest.

American Nurses Association

The ANA, the professional association for registered nurses, had its origins in a meeting of nursing leaders at the World's Fair in Chicago in 1890. Through their suggestions and efforts, the alumnae organizations of ten schools of nursing sent delegates in 1896 to form a committee to organize a professional association. The resulting organization was called the National Associated Alumnae of the United States and Canada. The name was changed in 1899 to the Nurses' Associated Alumnae of the United States and Canada. In 1901, Canada was dropped from the title because the state laws of New York (where the organization was incorporated) did not allow for representatives from more than one country. The name "American Nurses Association" was adopted in the United States in 1911; Canadian nurses formed their own organization.

The ANA has been identified as the organization for registered nurses. As such, it has always had as its primary interest the concerns of the nurses it represents. Throughout history, the organization has been active in issues relating to licensure (see Chapter 7), collective bargaining (see Chapter 12), nursing education (see Chapter 6), and a host of other concerns facing nurses and nursing.

MEMBERSHIP

The ANA membership comprises the 50 state nurses' associations and the 3 territorial constituent units. State nurses' associations (SNAs) comprise the district nurses' associations (DNAs). The individual nurse belongs to the ANA through the SNA. Prior to 1982, when the federation model was adopted, individual nurses were members of the ANA. The change to membership through the SNAs was made because it was thought that SNAs would be able to recruit more members and have greater control. However, there has not been an increase in membership. Each state is free to establish its own membership plans; however, membership is limited to registered nurses. The only exception to this rule is the admission to membership of some new graduates who have not yet passed the licensing examination.

It is regrettable that fewer than half of the registered nurses in the United States participate in the ANA. Those who do participate are often the leaders in the nursing profession. One reason for the low level of membership is the high cost of membership. Annual dues to the national association and the state and district associations are paid together, and in most parts of the country they are more than $300 combined. Another reason nurses have for not joining is a lack of time to participate in activities. Many nurses have the dual responsibilities of job and home and feel that they have no time left for involvement in a professional organization. Other nurses do not see how the benefits available through membership in the association are personally valuable. Some explain that they are just not interested in the issues and concerns of the organization. Finally, some nurses do not join because they do not agree with the position of the ANA on major issues; this has been especially true with regard to the role of the SNAs in collective bargaining and with regard to some of the ANA's positions on nursing education.

Those who are active in the ANA believe that its work is severely hampered by the low level of membership. The number of members limits the funds of the organization. Because some specific programs, such as the collective bargaining programs, are costly to the state association, there has been a strong move to require nurses to belong to the association if it serves as a bargaining agent. In some states, the state association has set a specific percentage of an agency's staff that must be members before they will become the bargaining agent for the nurses in that agency.

A current controversy involves differing views regarding the purpose of the professional organization. Many nurses believe that the organization primarily should be concerned with what it can do for the individual nurse. Others believe that a truly professional approach focuses on what the individual nurse can contribute to the profession through the organization. Some think that the organization should be an advocate in the realm of economic security. Another point of controversy is the organization's stand on political issues.

In 1995, the California Nurses Association experienced a great deal of internal turmoil because of a perceived lack of support from the ANA regarding the massive changes being created by health care reform (Costello, 1995). As a result the CNA delegate assembly voted to withdraw from the American Nurses Association and to establish itself as an independent "international" organization. This enabled the CNA to keep all of the dues in the state for its own purposes, but it also deprived CNA members of a voice and opportunities at the national level. Some nurses who did not support the separation of the CNA from the ANA joined ANA affiliate organizations in bordering states during the dispute. The ANA tried to resolve the problems, but was unsuccessful; instead, it subsequently established another organization called ANA-California. ANA is encouraging nurses in California who are interested in being part of the national organization and its efforts to join this new organization.

ACTIVITIES AND SERVICES

The ANA has been referred to many times throughout this book. As a professional association, it has been involved in all the issues that nursing has confronted. There has not been universal support in the nursing community for all of the activities that the ANA has championed or for the stands that it has taken. In any group as large as nursing, it is perhaps inevitable to have a wide range of viewpoints.

Advancement of the Profession. The ANA supports work on such policies as the ANA Social Policy Statement (American Nurses Association, 1980). These activities are ongoing efforts to support the advancement of nursing as a profession. The ANA also supports research on topics related to the profession itself, such as historical patterns of licensure (Snyder & LaBar, 1984).

One of the most significant services the ANA offers to members is certification through the American Nurses Credentialing Center. Recognition for expertise in a particular area usually is granted based on demonstration of knowledge through testing and clinical practice, although the criteria for certification vary among specialties.

Legislative Activity. The ANA is extensively involved in legislative activity. The organization often represents the profession in testimony before Congress on numerous issues affecting nursing. The need to be geographically closer to legislators in order to have greater participation in legislative efforts was the major reason for the relocation of the ANA offices to Washington, DC, in 1992. The organization provides testimony for or against legislation that will affect the profession, either directly or indirectly: legislative topics include funds for nursing education, collective bargaining issues, concerns for higher education, and human rights issues. It also testifies on health-related issues affecting the general public, such as the quality of care in nursing homes and health care reform. A newsletter, *Capitol Update*, is published monthly and provides information to the reader about issues currently being addressed in the Capitol. *Capitol Wiz* is available on the ANA Web site: www.nursingworld.org.

Collective Bargaining. An activity that has a major impact on the economic welfare of nurses is the organization's support of collective bargaining. This is also one of the most controversial services of the ANA. The SNAs are the official bargaining representatives in most instances (see Chapter 12). In 1999, the ANA restructured to create an arm titled United American Nurses that will represent nurses in workplace issues and provide a forum for the collective bargaining sections of the state associations.

Other Resources and Services. In addition to its activities, the ANA provides direct services to members. These include access to a group professional liability insurance plan and group insurance for health, disability, and accident coverage. From time to time the ANA also provides access to group travel arrangements and purchasing discounts.

Through its educational services, the ANA produces and distributes a wide variety of nursing educational materials, such as films, as well as a biennial report entitled "Facts About Nursing." This report provides basic statistical information that is used by many organizations and individuals. Reports of committees and commissions and special studies supported by the ANA also are published.

The *American Nurse* is the official publication of the ANA; official announcements of ANA business are published in this paper. The paper also contains current news relevant to nursing and health care, editorials, letters, and classified advertisements. The *American Journal of Nursing* is the official journal of the organization. It is published monthly and contains some current news, but its major focus is professional articles. It is published by Lippincott Williams & Wilkins, but retains autonomy over its own content.

The ANA also publishes many pamphlets and informational resources of value to nurses. A complete list of publications is available from the organization.

Organizations Related to the ANA

Because it is an official professional association, the ANA is related to other organizations in unique ways. These organizations operate autonomously, but are closely tied to the ANA.

INTERNATIONAL COUNCIL OF NURSES

The International Council of Nurses (ICN) is the international organization for professional nursing, with membership consisting of national nursing organizations. The ANA, as a constituent member of the ICN, sends delegates to its convention and participates in its activities. The ICN is interested in health care in general and nursing care in particular throughout the world. It works with the United Nations when appropriate, and with other international health-related groups, such as the International Red Cross.

The ICN concerns itself with such issues as the social and economic welfare of nurses, the role of the nurse in health care, and the roles of national nursing organizations throughout the world, and their relationships to their governing bodies. The primary governing body of the organization is the Council of National Representatives, which meets biennially.

The ICN has representatives from 104 national nurses' organizations. The Council of National Representatives governs the organization, which consists of all the presidents of the member organizations. Activities of the organization are carried out by its Board of Directors, the officers, volunteer nurse members of constituent organizations, and employed staff, including an executive director. The ICN maintains headquarters in Geneva, Switzerland.

Every 4 years a quadrennial congress is held. This meeting is open to all nurses and to delegates from the national organizations. Concerns addressed at recent congresses focused on such issues as career ladders, educational standards, research, human rights, and nursing's role in the planning of a national health policy.

AMERICAN NURSES FOUNDATION

In 1955, the ANA established the American Nurses Foundation (ANF) as a tax-exempt, nonprofit corporation for the purpose of supporting research related to nursing. It is independently financed and self-governing. The Board of Trustees is composed of members of the Board of Directors of the ANA, other nurse members, and non-nurse members from other health-related fields and from the public. To accomplish its varied objectives, the ANF solicits gifts and contributions from individuals and organizations. These gifts are tax deductible.

The ANF maintains a three-pronged approach to supporting research. The first objective is to conduct policy analyses to provide nursing leaders and public policy makers with the information they need for decision making. The second objective is related to developing "nurse scholars" who engage in study of such areas as journalism and public policy. Support is directed toward independent study, research, and doctoral and postdoctoral work for these nurse scholars. The third objective is to facilitate the research and educational activities of ANA. This includes providing consultation and funding for groups in the ANA that wish to initiate projects.

AMERICAN ACADEMY OF NURSING

The ANA established the American Academy of Nursing (AAN) in 1973 as an honorary association in the ANA. The Board of Directors of the ANA chose the original members. The AAN is now an independent organization, and new members are selected by those currently in the AAN. Those elected to the AAN are called fellows and may use the title "Fellow of the American Academy of Nursing" (FAAN). The purpose of this organization is to recognize nurses who have made significant contributions to the profession of nursing.

National Student Nurses' Association

The National Student Nurses' Association (NSNA) is a professional organization for students in schools of nursing and was started in 1952. Although it works with the ANA, it is a fully independent organization, run and financed by nursing students. It sponsors its own annual convention.

Although the NSNA is an autonomous organization, it has close ties with the ANA. Members of the NSNA serve on selected committees in the ANA, speak to the House of Delegates at the ANA convention to provide a student viewpoint, and work together with the ANA in regard to current issues.

Each state has a state nursing student association that operates in the same relationship to the state professional organization as the NSNA does to the national organization. State conventions and workshops are held in many states. State issues are addressed by the state association in the same way that national issues are addressed by the NSNA. Local nursing student organizations may or may not exist in individual schools of nursing. These local organizations may be closely tied to the state and national groups, or they may be independent. It is possible for an individual student to join the state and national student nurses' organizations even if no local counterpart exists.

A major project of the NSNA is "Breakthrough into Nursing," which is designed to recruit and maintain the enrollment of minorities in schools of nursing. The project has enlisted nursing students to speak to minority teenagers to interest them in nursing early in their scholastic careers, and to act as preceptors and tutors to increase the retention of minority students when they enroll in schools of nursing.

The NSNA often is asked to testify before congressional committees when issues relevant to nursing education are being considered. In this role, the organization becomes the public voice for all nursing students.

In 1975, the NSNA developed a Student Bill of Rights which was updated in 1991. This document carefully balances the rights of students with the responsibilities of students. It supports the view of students as competent adults who are engaged in an educational program. The rights that are outlined relate to educational programs, to the rules and policies of an institution, and to freedom in personal life and decision making (Fig. 3-6).

In the past it was common for schools of nursing to require membership in the student nurse organization at local, state, and national levels. With increasing emphasis on student rights and freedom of choice, this practice is no longer followed and has led to recruitment problems for many nursing student organizations. Students are busy, with full lives and limited funds. Some do not understand that the efforts of the organization benefit them in ways not immediately apparent. The activities of the student organization cannot occur without a wide membership base for funding and for credibility. Certainly, the profession of nursing and the situation of the individual nursing student would be adversely affected if the NSNA did not remain a viable and active force.

Bill of Rights and Responsibilities for Students of Nursing

An NSNA Student Bill of Rights and Responsibilities was initially adopted in 1975. The following updated version was adopted by the NSNA House of Delegates in San Antonio, Texas (1991).

Students should be encouraged to develop the capacity for critical judgment and engage in a sustained and independent search for truth.

The freedom to teach and the freedom to learn are inseparable facets of academic freedom: students should exercise their freedom in a responsible manner.

Each institution has a duty to develop policies and procedures which provide and safeguard the students' freedom to learn.

Under no circumstances should a student be barred from admission to a particular institution on the basis of race, creed, sex, color, national origin, handicap, or marital status.

Students should be free to take reasoned exception to the data or views offered in any course of study and to reserve judgment about matters of opinion, but they are responsible for learning the content of any course of study for which they are enrolled.

Students should have protection through orderly procedures against prejudiced or capricious academic evaluation, but they are responsible for maintaining standards of academic performance established for each course in which they are enrolled.

Information about student views, beliefs, political ideation, or sexual orientation which instructors acquire in the course of their work or otherwise, should be considered confidential and not released without the knowledge or consent of the student, and should not be used as a basis of evaluation.

The student should have the right to have a responsible voice in the determination of his/her curriculum.

Institutions should have a carefully considered policy as to the information which should be a part of a student's permanent educational record and as to the conditions of this disclosure.

Students and student organizations should be free to examine and discuss all questions of interest to them, and to express opinions publicly and privately.

Students should be allowed to invite and to hear any person of their own choosing within the Institution's acceptable realm, thereby taking the responsibility of furthering their education.

The student body should have clearly defined means to participate in the formulation and application of institutional policy affecting academic and student affairs, e.g., through a faculty-student council, student membership or representation.

The institution has an obligation to clarify those standards of behavior which it considers essential to its educational mission, its community life, or its objectives and philosophy.

Disciplinary proceedings should be instituted only for violations of standards of conduct formulated with significant student participation and published in advance through such means as a student handbook or a generally available set of institutional regulations. It is the responsibility of the student to know these regulations. Grievance procedures should be available for every student.

As citizens and members of an academic community, students are subject to the obligations which accrue to them by virtue of this membership and should enjoy the same freedoms of citizenship.

Students have the right to belong or refuse to belong to any organization of their choice.

Students have the right to personal privacy in their living space to the extent that the welfare and property of others are respected.

Adequate safety precautions should be provided by nursing programs, for example, adequate street lighting, locks, and other safety measures deemed necessary by the environment.

Dress code, if present in school, should be established with student input in conjunction with the school director and faculty, so the highest professional standards are maintained, but also taking into consideration points of comfort and practicality for the student.

Grading systems should be carefully reviewed periodically with students and faculty for clarification and better student faculty understanding.

Students should have a clear mechanism for input into the evaluation of nursing faculty.

National Student Nurses' Association, 1991. Available at http://www.nsna.org/pubs/billofrights/ Accessed November 15, 1999.

FIGURE 3–6   The NSNA Student Bill of Rights (Reprinted by permission of the National Student Nurses' Association).

National League for Nursing

Another major nursing organization is the National League for Nursing (NLN), which was established in 1952 and is often referred to as "The League." Its history and background are discussed in Chapter 4. The NLN achieves its missions through "collaborating, connecting, creating, serving, and learning" (NLN, 1995).

MEMBERSHIP

The NLN offers membership to individuals and agencies. It is unique among nursing organizations in offering membership and participation to consumers, to non-nursing members of health care teams, and to institutions concerned with nursing service and nursing education, as well as to registered nurses.

ACTIVITIES AND SERVICES

The NLN works in a complementary, rather than competitive, manner with the ANA. Whereas the ANA speaks as the official voice of nurses, the NLN seeks to unite the interests of nursing with those of the community, with special emphasis on nursing education.

Testing Services. Until 1982 the NLN produced the licensing examination for the state boards of nursing. Although it no longer has this responsibility, it does have a large testing service that produces standardized tests to be used in the nursing program admission process, achievement tests for various levels in a program, the NLN mobility examinations (which are used to provide advanced placement credit), and diagnostic examinations for those preparing for the NCLEX examinations.

Accreditation Services. Most students are aware of accreditation services, especially if they are attending a NLNAC-accredited school. Accreditation, which is voluntary, is one of the longest-standing services that the NLN provided. Initially accreditation was performed by the National Nursing Accrediting Service, which merged with other groups to form the NLN. Beginning in 1997, a separate but related organization, the National League for Nursing Accrediting Commission (NLNAC), has been charged with accrediting responsibilities. This change was necessary to meet the requirements of the Department of Education for a structure that clearly separated the accreditation process from any potential for conflict of interest in the organization. There were many changes in the accreditation process, when the National Advisory Committee on Institutional Quality and Integrity (NACIQI), which acts in an advisory capacity to the Secretary of Education, established a new framework for voluntary accreditation with many additional regulatory features (Tanner, 1996). Some changes continue today. The American Association of Colleges of Nursing has recently established another accrediting body for baccalaureate and higher degree programs, which will be discussed later in the chapter.

The goals of accreditation include providing the public with well-prepared nurses, guiding students in the selection of a program, ensuring the public of the quality of a school and its faculty, and stimulating the continued improvement in schools (Fig. 3-7).

FIGURE 3–7   Accreditation is designed to help ensure that the desired outcomes of education are achieved.

Recently there has been a significant push toward evaluating the "outcomes" of various educational programs rather than focusing more heavily on the process of education and its structure.

Program and Professional Development.   The NLN also offers consultation to schools that are seeking to improve their programs or that are initiating new programs, and to health agencies that are seeking to improve services. This consultation usually takes the form of personal visits to the school by paid staff and appointed members, but consultations at NLN headquarters or by telephone also are offered.

The NLN sponsors continuing education workshops and conferences throughout the country, often repeating a workshop in different locations to spare nurses and others the expense of travel. Subjects are determined in consultation with the councils and are geared to current needs and interests. Curriculum, research, accreditation, testing and evaluation, student recruitment and retention, political awareness and health care legislation, and a nurse executive series are regular subjects for continuing education. The NLN has developed and conducted workshops designed to assist the new graduate with the state licensing examination. The constituent leagues, which are grouped by regional assemblies, also offer workshops designed to meet the interests of particular areas of the country.

Like ANA, NLN also makes available such services and products as malpractice insurance and life insurance.

Division of Research.   When any group needs figures on nursing education, it cites data gathered by NLN's Division of Research. The division is a primary provider of statistics on nursing education, and each year surveys all schools of registered and practical nursing for enrollments, admissions, and graduations. It also conducts a yearly survey of newly registered nurses regarding the characteristics of their employment. Every 2 years, the nurse-faculty census is taken; every 3 years, data are gathered on men and minorities in schools of nursing.

Career Information and Publications. The career information service answers thousands of inquiries about nursing education that arrive each year by mail and by telephone. The NLN web site contains information for individuals interested in exploring nursing careers.

The NLN publishes annual lists of accredited schools of associate degree, baccalaureate, master's, diploma, and practical nursing programs, plus a list of doctoral programs and information on scholarships and loans. The data obtained through the research surveys are published in the annual *Nursing Data Book* and *State-Approved Schools of Nursing*. (Each of these booklets carries a nominal price.)

Through its journal, *Nursing & Health Care Perspectives*, and a newsletter, *NLN Update* (also available on the Web), members are kept informed about current issues. Sometimes NLN spokespersons offer testimony on legislation or rulings significant to the organization. The NLN publishes many texts and references about curriculum, ethics, public policy, nursing administration, long-term care, and other topics of interest to nursing. It also produces educational videos.

National Council of State Boards of Nursing

Although it is not a nursing organization like those previously discussed, our discussion would not be complete without mention of the National Council of State Boards of Nursing, Inc. (NCSBN). This organization was formed in 1978 to replace the Council of State Boards that had been part of the ANA. The purpose of this organization is to provide a forum for the legal regulatory bodies (whatever their particular state titles might be) of all states to act together in the developmentment of the licensing examinations, and in other matters of common concern. There is one delegate to this council from each state agency. The actions of this council are particularly important because its membership represents the legal authority for the control of nursing education and nursing practice.

Although each state agency must operate within its own laws, it does have authority to establish many specific rules and regulations. Working together, the state boards hope to promote uniform standards for the nursing profession. One of the agenda items they have addressed is the development of a Model Nurse Practice Act. Much energy has gone into the development, validation, and establishment of computerized testing for the licensing examination for both registered and practical nursing. Currently the organization is studying the methods used to approve and license advanced practice nurses and the concerns associated with multistate practice.

Organizations Representing Licensed Practical Nurses

Two nursing organizations are concerned primarily with advancing the interests of practical (vocational) nurses. These two organizations are the National Federation of

Licensed Practical Nurses (NFLPN) and the National Association for Practical Nurse Education and Service (NAPNES).

The National Federation of Licensed Practical Nurses (NFLPN) is one of the professional organizations for practical nurses. Founded in 1949, its membership is limited to licensed practical and vocational nurses. The NFLPN has assisted the ANA in some activities, and actively supports the need for the practical nurse in health care. State and local groups of the NFLPN are active in educational issues affecting the licensed practical nurse, and have supported the associate degree as the appropriate educational preparation for the responsibilities of the licensed practical nurse in the current health care system.

The National Association for Practical Nurse Education and Service was organized as the Association of Practical Nurse Schools in 1941. Its purpose was to address the needs of practical nursing education. The name was changed in 1942 to the National Association for Practical Nurse Education; in 1959, it added "and Service" to that title. The official publication of the organization is *The Journal of Practical Nursing*, which has been published since 1951. It also publishes a newsletter, *NAPNES Forum*, that keeps members alert to activities of the organization. Membership is open to licensed practical/vocational nurses, practical/vocational nursing students, faculty, directors, and others interested in promoting the purposes of the organization. It was the first organization to provide accreditation for practical nursing programs, although that role now rests with the NLN affiliate.

North American Nursing Diagnosis Association

The North American Nursing Diagnosis Association (NANDA) is open to individuals as well as group members. The purpose of this group is to work toward uniform terminology and definitions to be used in nursing diagnosis, and to share ideas and information regarding this topic. Members identify and research problems nurses manage, prepare documentation, and submit these to NANDA to be included in the consideration process. Committees then review the problems. Those that meet the basic criteria for nursing diagnoses are submitted to the membership. Defining characteristics are identified, and conditions that form the etiology or are related to the development of the diagnosis are identified. A national convention held every 2 years is the final forum for the debate and discussion of proposed new nursing diagnoses. The general outline of the taxonomy (classification system) was established by a group of nursing theorists and then accepted by the organization.

American Organization of Nurse Executives

According to their Web site, the American Organization of Nurse Executives (AONE) is the "national professional organization for nurses who design, facilitate, and manage care" (available at www.aha.org/resources/AboutAone.html). This organization provides the forum for nurses with managerial and executive responsibility to work collaboratively both with other nurses in similar roles and through the organization with other organizations. AONE is one of the members of the Tricouncil for Nursing, which serves as an information resource for legislative and governmental personnel.

Clinically Related Organizations

Some of the earliest specialty organizations were related to specific clinical practice areas of nursing. A major focus of these organizations now is continuing education related to a particular nursing specialty. Most groups also have some mechanisms, such as certification, for recognizing achievement in the field. One of the earliest specialty organizations, founded in 1941, was the American Association of Nurse Anesthetists, a group of approximately 24,000 members, of whom 40% are men.

Specialty organizations also include groups that began as auxiliaries to specialty physicians' organizations such as the AWHONN: The Association of Women's Health, Obstetric and Neonatal Nurses. This organization was started for nurses affiliated with physicians who were "fellows" of the American College of Obstetricians and Gynecologists. As more members joined and nurses became more active, groups such as this one became autonomous. (See Appendix B for a listing of the major specialty groups.)

The overlapping purpose and actions of the Councils on Practice of the ANA and the corresponding specialty organizations have caused some concern. One attempt to promote a more cooperative effort was the creation of the Nursing Organization Liaison Forum (NOLF), which operates as a forum in the ANA.

One of the newest nursing organizations is the National Alliance of Nurse Practitioners (NANP), organized in 1986. Its purpose is to promote the health care of the nation by promoting the visibility, viability, and unity of nurse practitioners. Its activities focus on advancing the role of the nurse practitioner in the health care delivery system. Issues related to the reimbursement of nurse practitioners are of major concern to this organization.

Groups Related to Ethnic Origin

As the movement for self-determination and preservation of identity arose within ethnic groups in the United States, nurses within various ethnic groups began to unite to achieve a greater voice in health care. Some ethnic groups are nationally organized; others are organized on a more local level. As these groups have become stronger and more organized, their interests have included the recruitment and support of nursing students from the particular ethnic groups they represent. These ethnic groups also encourage their members to become more politically involved in nursing and nursing leadership.

Honorary Organizations

Sigma Theta Tau is an international organization established in collegiate schools of nursing to recognize those with superior ability and leadership potential, and those who have made important contributions to nursing. Candidates may be asked to join during the senior year of a baccalaureate program, or any time thereafter. Sigma Theta Tau has established a nursing library at its headquarters in Indianapolis that has reference abilities to support advanced scholarship; the organization also provides the first online nursing journal that can be accessed by computer. Local chapters may maintain funds to support individual research projects, hold research conferences, and recognize those who have made significant contributions to nursing.

Alpha Tau Delta is a professional nursing fraternity. Students who are enrolled in baccalaureate nursing programs and demonstrate scholarship and personality characteristics in line with the organization's professional goals are eligible for membership.

Religiously Oriented Organizations

The National Council of Catholic Nurses and the Nurses' Christian Fellowship (primarily a nondenominational Protestant group) were organized to assist nurses in sharing concerns and integrating their work and their religious beliefs. These two organizations place special emphasis on meeting a patient's spiritual needs and on dealing with ethical issues.

Educationally Oriented Organizations

Since the 1960s, there has been a great deal of change and development in nursing education as it has moved from the hospital into the educational setting. During this time, there has been an increased emphasis on educational methods, curriculum development, and research

In several major geographical regions of the United States, educational organizations extending membership to schools of nursing, members of the state boards of nursing, and other interested individuals were developed to promote interstate and interinstitutional cooperation in seeking pathways to improved nursing education and scholarship. These organizations are the Western Institute of Nursing (WIN), the Council on Collegiate Education for Nursing of the Southern Regional Education Board (CCEN/SREB), the New England Organization for Nursing (NEON), the Midwest Alliance in Nursing (MAIN), and the Mid-Atlantic Regional Nursing Association (MARNA).

The National Organization for the Advancement of Associate Degree Nursing (NOAADN) has four purposes: to speak for associate degree nursing education and practice; to reinforce the value of associate degree nursing education and practice; to maintain endorsement of registered nurse licensure from state to state for the associate degree nurse; and to retain the registered nurse licensure examination for graduates of associate degree nursing programs. Membership is open to individuals, states, agencies, and organizations.

The American Association of Colleges of Nursing (AACN) was formed to assist collegiate schools of nursing in working cooperatively to improve higher education for professional nursing. Membership is limited to deans and directors of programs that offer a baccalaureate degree in nursing, with an upper-division nursing major, and that are part of a regionally accredited college or university. In 1996, this organization instituted planning to become an accrediting organization for baccalaureate and higher degree programs in nursing. A related organization, the Commission on Collegiate Nursing Education (CCNE), was formed to provide accreditation. This organization began accrediting activities in 1999 and applied to the National Advisory Committee on Institutional Quality and Integrity (NACIQI) of the Department of Education for approval as an accrediting organization. That approval process has began. Thus, there are now two separate specialized accreditation organizations for baccalaureate and higher degree nursing programs. The development of two organizations for accreditation of these programs has created concerns in some areas of nursing that it may create competition rather than foster cooperative efforts for excellence in nursing education.

Miscellaneous Organizations

The American Assembly for Men in Nursing was formed by those who believed that, as a minority in the profession, men needed to speak about issues with a united voice. The membership has expanded to include women who are concerned about gender issues in nursing. The organization has addressed the issue of discrimination toward men in nursing and seeks to present nursing as a profession in which both men and women can contribute and excel.

Nurses House, Inc. provides assistance for nurses in need. It originated from a bequest in 1922 from Emily Bourne, who donated $300,000 to establish a country home where nurses might find needed rest. As the need for this residence decreased, supporters of this endeavor sold the estate and invested the proceeds. Income from the investment and funds donated by nurses (and friends of nurses) are used to provide guidance and counseling for nurses with emotional and chemical dependency problems, encouragement to homebound nurses, and temporary financial assistance to nurses who are ill, convalescing, or unemployed. Nurses House seeks members and donations to assist in continuing these activities.

The Gay Nurses' Alliance was an outgrowth of the movement of homosexual individuals to be accepted without having to disguise their sexual orientation. This group primarily has focused on the issue of gay rights. They also provide a forum for gay individuals to address the difficulties they may face in the nursing profession.

Critical Thinking Activity

As a new graduate, assume you have $400 per year to spend on membership in a nursing organization. In trying to decide which organization to join, how would you go about learning the focus of several groups that have attracted your interest? What process could you use to ensure that you are joining the group that best serves your needs? Which organization would you join? Provide a clear rationale based on both economic and professional reasons for your choice.

KEY CONCEPTS

• Because scarce resources are allocated through the political process, nurses will find that understanding this process is essential to influencing the health care system.
• Every individual nurse has many opportunities to affect the political process. This can be done simply by keeping informed, by voting, or by trying to shape public opinion.

Communicating with legislators and officials can be done as an individual or as part of a group. Testifying presents issues of importance, and individual support can be given to those running for office. You may even decide to run for a public office.

- The federal government is active in health care through many existing agencies in the Department of Health and Human Services and in other branches of government. The federal budget process affects the health care services available through the many legislative acts affecting health care.

- Many factors are coming together in support of health care reform. Nursing organizations support efforts to reform health care access, quality, and cost control. The major reform proposals take different approaches to funding, managing reimbursement, malpractice reform, the role of the states, determining who should be covered, and determining what benefits should be included in new health care plans.

- A political process is part of any large organization, and nursing organizations are no exception. Understanding the political process can help you participate more effectively in a large organization.

- The variety of organizations in nursing is often confusing to the new nursing graduate and to the public. These organizations represent nurses and special interest groups in nursing.

- A major nursing organization is the American Nurses Association, whose membership is open to registered nurses only. It is recognized as the voice of professional nursing. It is also active in issues related to the economic welfare of nurses.

- The National Student Nurses Association addresses the interests and needs of nursing students. It is a fully autonomous organization open to nursing students only.

- Another major nursing organization is the National League for Nursing which, historically, has championed better nursing education. Membership is open to individuals and agencies interested in nursing. The NLN is responsible for the accreditation of all types of nursing programs throughout the United States.

- Two nursing organizations exist expressly to serve the needs of licensed practical (vocational) nurses. These groups are the National Federation of Licensed Practical Nurses and the National Association for Practical Nurse Education and Service.

- Organizations also exist that represent specialty groups in nursing. Members usually are drawn together by their common interests and concerns. The organizations provide continuing education and, in some instances, certification.

- Some organizations, such as Sigma Theta Tau, are honorary in their focus. These groups strive to bring recognition to nurses and nursing.

- A wide variety of other organizations meet the special needs of their membership. This may relate to social interests, ethnic background, or other common denominators.

REFERENCES

American Nurses Association. Nursing's Agenda for Health Care Reform. Washington, DC: American Nurses Publishing Co., 1991

American Nurses Association. Nursing: A Social Policy Statement. Kansas City, MO: American Nurses Association, 1980

ANA lobbying team named in top 100. Washington Watch. Am J Nurs 98(2):16, 1998

Bowles C. The NLN makes a new road: An interview with NLN CEO Patricia Moccia. NHC Perspectives on Community 17(2):82–87, 1996

Capitol Update. Appropriations (Health). 16(20):1, 1999

Costello K. ANA weak on protecting nursing practice. Calif Nurse 91(8):4, 16, 1995

Lasswell H. Politics: Who gets what, when, how. New York: Meridian Books, 1986, p. 3

NIOSH Alert: Preventing needlestick injuries in health care settings. DHHS (NIOSH) Pub # 2000–108. November 1999. Available at www.cdc.gov/niosh. Accessed June 24, 2000.

Polston MD. Whistleblowing. Am J Nurs 99(1):26, 1999

Tanner CA. Accreditation under siege. J Nurs Educ 35(6):243–244, 1996

Whistleblower law goes on the books in N.J. RN 60(8):12, 1997

Woodham-Smith C. Florence Nightingale. New York: Atheneum, 1983 (reprint of 1951 edition)

FURTHER READING

Cella KJ. Legislation: NAFTA, NIOSH & OSHA. Imprint 43(2):31–32, 1996

Chaffee M. Insider's viewpoint: The nurse in Washington internship (NIWI). Nurs Policy Forum 2(1):12–15, 18–19, 1996

Hall-Long BA. Nursing's past, present, and future political experiences. NHC Perspectives on Community 16(1): 24–28, 1995

Helms LB, Anderson MA, Hanson K. "Doin' politics": Linking policy and politics in nursing. Nurs Admin Quart 20(3):32–41, 1996

Huston CJ. Nursing and political action in the 20th century: From separation to fusion. Revolution 5(3):50–53, 1995

Keepnews D. Issues: ANA challenges Pew Health Profession's findings. Imprint 43(3):24–25, 1996

Keepnews D, Marullo G. Policy imperatives for nursing in an era of health care reform. Nurs Admin Quart 20(3):19–31, 1996

Rodwell CM. An analysis of the concept of empowerment. J Adv Nurs 23(2):305–313, 1996

Sharp N. Legislative effects: It's politics, not policy. Nurs Management 26(12):18–19, 1995

See the following regular publications

American Journal of Nursing, Washington Watch (a monthly column)
Legislative Newsletter
The American Nurse. Kansas City, MO: American Nurses Association, monthly newspaper
Capitol Update. A monthly publication published by the ANA
Capitol Wiz (available online at *www.nursingworld.org*)
See also the official publication of your state nurses' association.

Relevant web sites

American Nurses Association *www.nursingworld.org*
American Nurses Association/American Journal of Nursing/Lippincott Publishing *www.nursingcenter.com*
Centers for Disease Control and Prevention *www.cdc.gov*
National Student Nurses' Association *www.nsna.org*
National League for Nursing *www.nln.org*
Library of Congress: Access to current legislation in the "Spirit of Thomas Jefferson" *thomas.loc.gov/*
U.S. Congress Handbook (address and links) *www.congress-handbook.com*

UNIT II

Appreciating the Development of Nursing as a Profession

The purpose of Unit II is to provide an understanding of the events that brought nursing to where it is today. Having information about the history and development of the nursing profession helps the individual who is just starting a caring career to better appreciate and interpret the things that are presently occurring, and thus move into the new role more comfortably. Learning about the history and development of the profession can help you appreciate the heritage of the discipline and the events that resulted in nursing offering the opportunities and challenges that nursing provides today. This unit begins with a history of nursing that describes its growth from early times, to an era where preparation for nursing existed as apprentice-type training, to a profession that now encompasses doctoral and post-doctoral scholarship.

Many believe that nursing is a young profession. Others question whether it actually should be considered a profession. These debates are considered in this unit. Some of the studies that were conducted about nursing are described and their impact on the development of the profession is explored.

The educational processes by which we prepare nurses continue to experience change, modification, and refinement in response to changes that are occurring in the health care delivery system. The various routes to educational preparation for a nursing career are discussed, including a history of the various approaches. You will learn about some of the individuals who made significant contributions to the profession. The unit concludes with a discussion of the future of nursing education.

4

Exploring Nursing's Origins

History can open the door to storehouses of information that can be used to assist with the development of reasoned conclusions about specific phenomena. Critical thinking cannot help but be fostered and strengthened by the study of history.

(Donahue, 1993)

OBJECTIVES

After completing this chapter, you should be able to:

1. Summarize the health care practices and developments of early civilizations.

2. Analyze how the development of nursing as a profession has been influenced by each of the three historical images of the nurse.

3. Examine the implications of the "Dark Ages of Nursing" on the development of the nursing profession.

4. Discuss the contribution of Florence Nightingale to nursing and its development.

5. Explain the impact of wars on the development of nursing education.

6. Describe the early development of nursing schools in the United States.

7. Delineate the characteristics of early nursing programs.

8. Identify the first organizations created by and for nurses and discuss the purpose of each.

9. Discuss the history of hospitals and long-term care facilities in the United States.

10. Identify the factors that influenced the development of health care facilities and explain why each was important.

Almshouse	Folk image of nursing	Pesthouse
Ancient cultures	Hospitals	Religious image of nursing
"Dark Ages of Nursing"	Long-term care facilities	Servant image of nursing
Ebers papyrus	Materia medica	Training schools
Florence Nightingale	Nursing organizations	"Uncommon women"

There is no particular date or time period at which nursing came into being. Nursing, as we know it today, may go back less than 150 years. The early origins of nursing, however, are intertwined with the ancient civilizations and cultures of the world. The same is true of medicine. Our best speculations regarding their origins necessarily must be tied to our knowledge of cultures that existed in the past, and to the contributions these cultures left for future generations. As you might anticipate, these cultures were many and varied. They reflected the events and developments (or lack of the same) that characterized each period in history. In this chapter, we will review some of the various cultures and historical events that have contributed to nursing's history and to nursing's development as a profession.

HEALTH CARE IN ANCIENT CULTURES

The life of primitive societies was necessarily a nomadic one. Well-defined groups, built around the nucleus of family relationships, wandered in search of food, warmth, and an environment that supported life. Solidarity among these scattered groups, organized for the convenient management of human affairs, existed for purposes of mutual protection. Anthropologists believe that primitive groups originated in Africa and migrated across the world. Ice ages in the northern latitudes drove these groups back to the warmer climates found around the Mediterranean Sea, in India, and in China, where civilizations developed. Historians suggest that the movement of early tribes radiated from the interior of Europe and Asia toward the warm shores of the Mediterranean Sea, India, and China (Jamieson & Sewell, 1944).

The regions around the Mediterranean Sea were thought to occupy the center of the earth with all areas to the east known as "eastern" and all those to the west known as "western" (Donahue, 1996, p. 28). The sophistication of health care practices varied considerably from one culture to another, and were based largely on the ingenuity of the group. Consistent among most of them were strong beliefs in the power of gods, with sickness and suffering attributed to the presence of evil spirits. These evil spirits were dealt with in many ways, including noisy incantations and dances, making offerings and sacrifices, and working with medicine men who worked their "magic" to drive away the demons (Kalisch & Kalisch, 1995). The health care practices of some of the early cultures are highlighted in Table 4-1.

TABLE 4–1. **Highlights of Health Care Practices of Selected Early Civilizations**

Society	Contributions
Egypt	Provided the earliest medical records; included over 700 classified drugs
	Developed system of community planning that helped avoid public health problems
	Established strict rules regarding cleanliness, food, drink, exercise, and sexual relations
Palestine	Developed Mosaic Code, which included an organized method of disease prevention
	Isolated people with communicable diseases, differentiated clean from unclean
	Established rules that forbade eating meat past the third day after slaughter
Babylonia	Skilled mathematicians and astrologers; beliefs based on numbers and movement of the stars
	Believed illness a punishment for sin and used incantations and herbs for purification with surgery more advanced than internal medicine
	Developed Code of Hammurabi, which perhaps represents the first sliding scale for payment based on class
Assyria	A warlike group whose laws were severe and who made frequent use of death penalty
	Believed in good and evil spirits and in many gods. Ill health was a punishment for sin
Persia	Followed the preaching of Zoroaster, who introduced the concept of two creators: one good, one evil
	Established early schools for priest-physicians, from which evolved three types of physicians: those who healed by the knife, those who healed with herbs, and those who healed through exorcism
Greece	Society heavily steeped in mythology, animal sacrifice, and faith in the power of gods
	Placed much emphasis on healthy bodies; founded the Olympic games
	Built beautiful temples where learning and healing occurred
	Built institutions to care for sick and injured called *xendochium; iatrion* were built to offer ambulatory care
	The home of Hippocrates, born about 400 B.C., who became known as the Father of Modern Medicine
Rome	Borrowed medical practices from the countries they conquered; physicians were often slaves
	Clung to gods, superstition, and herbs when faced with illness
	Practiced fairly advanced hygiene and sanitation with emphasis on bathing
	Women enjoyed more independence that in other comparable societies
India	Civilizations highly developed, with systems of sanitation, bathrooms, public baths, and other amenities
	Vedic age (1500 B.C.) characterized by worship to Brahma, which resulted in segregation of society into castes
	Emphasized hygiene and prevention of sickness and described major and minor surgery, children's diseases, and diseases of the nervous and urinary system. Advanced surgery and materia medica.
	Buddhism emerged about 500 B.C. with an advanced understanding of disease prevention, hygiene and sanitation, medicine and surgery. Prenatal care emphasized for mothers and public hospitals constructed staffed with nurses (mostly men).
China	Followed the teachings of Confucius; patriarchal rule dominated with emphasis on whole family; women considered vastly inferior to men
	Developed concept of yin and yang and had elaborate materia medica using many drugs still used today
	Developed acupuncture skills still in practice today, studied circulation, and developed approach to examination: look, listen, ask, feel
	Baths used for reduction of fever, bloodletting to release evil spirits from the body

(continues)

Society	Contributions
TABLE 4–1.	**Highlights of Health Care Practices of Selected Early Civilizations** (*Continued*)
The Americas	Sun god of particular significance; health viewed as a balance between man, nature, and the supernatural
	Rites, ceremonies, herbal treatments, charms, and perhaps human sacrifice contributed to healing practices
	Medicine men (first known as shamans and later as priests) were responsible for curing ills of body and mind
Arabia	Populated by nomadic people who lived a difficult life in the hot, dry desert. Muhammad, born about 570 A.D., developed the religion of Islam that worshipped the god Allah. His teachings established strict rules of living, dictating habits of cleanliness, eating, and human interaction. Elevated the position of women

Egypt

The ancient Egyptians settled in the long, narrow valley that lay along the banks of the Nile River while other cultures were settling along the Indus, Euphrates, and Tigris rivers. The Egyptian community was considered to be much more advanced than others of the region. By the year 5000 B.C., stone implements had been developed to facilitate work, followed by the wheel and cart, and animals were domesticated to help with heavy burdens. A system of irrigation increased the productivity of the fertile soil.

In Egyptian culture, treating disease was considered the responsibility of priests. The Egyptians, like the people of all early cultures, looked on natural phenomena as the work of the gods. Health and security meant keeping the gods happy and sickness reflected the presence of some evil spirit in possession of the sufferer (Kalisch & Kalisch, 1995).

The oldest medical records so far discovered and deciphered are those from Egypt, dating back as far as 3000 B.C. Early records, sometimes in the form of hieroglyphics, were carved in stone or written on papyrus. The Egyptians developed an elaborate pharmacopoeia that classified more than 700 drugs, and a system of community planning was developed that helped to avoid public health problems, especially those related to disease transmitted through water sources. Egypt is credited with being one of the healthiest of the ancient countries, perhaps because of the progress it made in the fields of hygiene and sanitation. The Egyptians developed strict rules around such things as cleanliness, food, drink, exercise, and sexual relations. They also established a "house of death," which was located at a site away from civilization. Mummies that have survived to the present day clearly show that the Egyptians were skilled in wrapping and embalming their dead. It is also believed that they were accomplished in dentistry, often filling teeth with gold. The oldest medical books on record come from Egypt. These books outline surgical techniques and methods of birth control, describe disease processes, and suggest remedies. One of the books was purchased by Dr. Ebers of Germany in 1874. It became known as the "Ebers papyrus" and is considered to be the best of the Egyptian medical books (Jamieson & Sewell, 1944). Out of this culture came the first physician known to history, Imhotep (2900–2800 B.C.). He was recognized as a surgeon, an architect, a temple priest, a scribe, and a magician.

Although women in ancient Egypt received more respect than women in other Eastern countries, it is not clear whether nurses existed as such. Women most likely worked in the temples, along with priest-physicians, holding the rank of priestess or serving as midwives or "wet nurses."

Cultures of the Fertile Crescent

Several cultures made their homes in a crescent-shaped strip of land that extended from the Persian Gulf on the east to the Mediterranean Sea on the west. This area, known as the Fertile Crescent, enjoyed a warm, hospitable climate and rich soil, and benefited from the water provided by three great rivers: the Tigris, the Euphrates, and the Jordan. The Fertile Crescent often is referred to as the "cradle of civilization." Because the cultures that settled there were often warlike and took possession of land by conquering the empire in power, the boundaries of these early societies sometimes overlapped.

PALESTINE

The Hebrews made their home in the area called Palestine, at the western end of the Fertile Crescent and adjacent to Egypt. This region included what is now Israel, as well as some of the surrounding area. The land was mountainous, with narrow, gorge-like valleys that lacked the richness of minerals found in other areas and had inadequate rainfall. The society of the Hebrews was primarily an agricultural one as the people learned to cultivate the olive and the grape.

The Hebrews are credited with more democratic sharing of knowledge than any of the other ancient civilizations. Possibly, much of the knowledge of the Hebrews was learned from the Egyptians, who held them captive for many years. Under the leadership of Moses, the adopted son of the Egyptian Pharaoh's daughter, the Hebrews developed the Mosaic Code, which included an organized method of disease prevention. The code emphasized the isolation of people with communicable diseases, differentiated clean from unclean, and covered every detail of personal, family, and public hygiene. Thus, religion, law, and medicine combined to control the public health with the responsibility for enforcement given to the priest-physician, although kings ruled the country.

Bible scriptures, such as Leviticus 7:16–19 and 19:5–8, which forbade the eating of meat past the third day after an animal was slaughtered, were no doubt written because of the effects of the warm climate and lack of refrigeration. Similarly, Mosaic and Talmudic regulations regarding the slaughtering of animals, which included requirements for examination and inspection to check for diseases of the internal organs, were in keeping with the advanced sanitary ordinances of Hebrew society.

With regard to the treatment of women in Hebrew society, Nutting and Dock (1935) write:

All the stern and ungraciously sounding texts relating to the 'uncleanliness' of women, which when considered only in the abstract seem so needlessly humiliating, are in reality witnesses of the extreme care and solicitude of the Jews for the health of their women, and of the sanctity and beauty of their family life. These regulations secured to women the personal isolation and privacy, quiet, and consideration necessary on hygienic grounds, and especially made the time of childbirth a period of isolation and quiet, of cleanliness of body and clothing, and of rest for mind and body (pp. 62–63).

Hebrew culture recognized one god who had power over life and death. From this belief evolved the role of the priest as supervisor of medical practices related to cleansing and purification. Priest-physicians took on the function of health inspectors. The writings of the early Jewish rabbis taught that visiting the sick was a duty, even if the sick were not Jews.

BABYLONIA

The lifestyle of the Babylonians was entirely different from that of the Egyptians or the Hebrews. Babylonia was located in the southern part of present-day Iraq, although its borders differed from those of the modern country. At one time, it was known as Mesopotamia. Each city was an autonomous community governed by a divine ruler and a priest-king. Women never enjoyed much esteem in Babylonian society, with their role being primarily domestic, not unlike other cultures of the time.

The Babylonians are credited with being skilled mathematicians and astrologers. Many of the beliefs of the Babylonians were based on their study of nature, their belief in the potency of numbers, and their observations of the movement of stars and planets. The division of the year into months, weeks, days, hours, and minutes is said to have originated with the Babylonians (Donahue, 1996).

The Babylonians believed illness to be the punishment for sin and for displeasing the gods. Purifying the body brought about a cure, usually by incantations and the use of herbs. Temples, in which the purification occurred, became centers of medical care (Fig. 4-1). Preventive medicine consisted of doing what it was believed the gods desired. Babylonia is the source of the second oldest surviving medical records (Nutting & Dock, 1935). In Babylonian culture, surgery was more advanced than internal medicine, which concerned itself primarily with banishing demons and avoiding evil spirits.

In 1900 B.C., Hammurabi, King of Babylonia, developed the famous Code of Hammurabi. The principal source of our knowledge of this code is a stone monument found in 1901 and preserved today in the Louvre in Paris. This code, which may represent the first sliding scale for fee payment, divided the public into three classes. Those classified as "gentlemen" were expected to pay their surgeons in silver coins rather than in goods or services. A surgeon who bungled an operation on a "gentleman" risked paying a heavy price; the surgeon might have his hands cut off if the surgery was not successful. This puts the malpractice rates absorbed by physicians today in a different light.

ASSYRIA

The history of the Assyrians began around 2300 B.C. (Jamieson & Sewell, 1944). This nation was centered in the northern part of present-day Iraq, and extended into what is now Syria and southern Iraq as it conquered other nations. After ceaseless warfare, the Assyrians took possession of the land of Babylonia. The Assyrians are character-

FIGURE 4–1 In many early societies the practice of medicine involved the use of magical formulas that drove away demons that possessed the body.

ized as a hardened, warlike group whose one supreme god was a "god of battles." Their instruments of war were said to be stronger than those of other cultures. The Assyrians were the first to use weapons made of bronze. Their laws were severe, with mutilation and death inflicted on those who failed to follow the heavy mandates. Early Assyrians believed in good and evil spirits, in magic and superstition, and in many gods. Like many other early cultures, they also believed that ill health was a punishment for sin and that evil spirits could occupy a person's body. The practice of medicine developed around these religious beliefs as the Assyrians practiced only magic and empirical medicine consistent with their superstitions (Donahue, 1996).

Persia

Persia, one of the most extensive empires of the Near East, was located in what is now modern-day Iran and, at one time, extended throughout the Fertile Crescent. The Persians' quest for territory and power resulted in their conquest of much of that area. They believed in Zoroaster, a prophet who lived about 600 B.C. and wrote the sacred books of Persia. His writings introduced the world to the concept of two creators—one good, and one evil—and to the sacred elements of fire, earth, and water. The writings of Zoroaster also introduced the concept of immortality as a mental state. The

Persians adopted the cultural practices of the lands they conquered, including many of the medical and surgical practices of Egypt. They established early schools to prepare priest-physicians, from which evolved three types of physicians: those who healed by the knife, those who healed with herbs, and those who healed through exorcism.

Greece

Greek civilization developed on a peninsula that extended into the Mediterranean Sea from the southeastern part of Europe. The ancient Greeks are remembered in part for their worship of gods and goddesses and for their emphasis on healthy bodies, which led them to found the Olympic games. In Greek mythology, Asklepios (sometimes spelled Aesculapius or Asclepius), son of Apollo, was taught the healing arts by Cheiron, a wise centaur. Asklepios usually is represented as carrying a staff, to show that he traveled from place to place, around which is entwined a serpent, representing wisdom and immortality. Some people believe that when the army medical services fashioned the caduceus, the symbol of the medical profession, the staff and serpent that were incorporated into the symbol came from this legend.

Exquisite temples, located on beautiful sites, were built as shrines to Asklepios; these temples became social and intellectual centers as well as places to obtain cures. The curative process usually began with animal sacrifice and continued through various purifying rituals. In addition to these shrines, two other institutions, the xenodochium and the iatrion, offered care to the sick in ancient Greece. The xenodochium first offered care to travelers and later to people who were sick and injured. This may have been the forerunner of the city or county hospital as we know it today. The iatrion was a facility offering ambulatory care and would correspond to our outpatient clinics.

It is rather surprising that from this society, so heavily steeped in mythology, animal sacrifice, and faith in the power of the gods, came the Father of Modern Medicine. Hippocrates was born about 400 B.C. on the island of Cos. He stressed natural causes for disease, treated the whole patient with a patient-centered approach to care, and introduced the scientific method of solving patient problems. His teaching emphasized the necessity of accurate observations and careful record keeping. Rather than attribute ill health to an infliction by the gods, Hippocrates believed that health depended on equilibrium existing among the mind, the body, and the environment. From his philosophy evolved the humoral theory of disease, which has lasted for centuries.

Many other early physicians came from Greece, although some eventually practiced their skills in Rome after the Roman Empire conquered Greece. Some physicians, such as Aristotle (who distinguished arteries from veins), Galen (a physician to the gladiators and renowned medical writer who is credited with demonstrating that arteries when opened always gush blood), Asclepiades (who helped establish medicine in Rome and proposed an atomistic approach to disease), and Pedanim Dioscorides (whose *De Materia Medica* contained descriptions of over 600 herbal preparations) made such significant contributions to medicine that their names are remembered today (Kalisch and Kalisch, 1995).

Rome

At one time the Roman Empire was quite extensive, stretching across the entire northern border of Africa and Egypt. The medical advances of the ancient Romans fell short of those of the Greeks. Medical practices often were borrowed from the countries the Romans conquered, and the physicians from those countries were made slaves who provided medical services to the Romans. Although the Romans clung to gods, superstition, and herbs when faced with disease, their hygiene and sanitation were fairly well advanced. Their genius found its best expression in the area of public hygiene rather than in medicine per se. Many homes were equipped with baths, and cleanliness was valued. The Romans also constructed public baths.

Roman society was divided into two classes: the patricians, an affluent and privileged group; and the plebeians, who represented the poor or lower class and were denied citizenship. Patrician women in Roman society had more privileges than women of similar economic status in other ancient cultures. Women were quite independent and were allowed to own property, appear in public, and campaign publicly for causes they believed should be advanced. They could even entertain guests and sit with them at the table.

India

Located in the southern part of the Far East, India was essentially isolated by mountains from other parts of the ancient world. People who migrated from central Asia in ancient times traveled through the mountain passes. Excavations indicate that the first civilizations in India (3000–1500 B.C.) were highly developed, with systems of sanitation, bathrooms and public baths, and other amenities. The Vedic age began in 1500 B.C. and was characterized by worship of the eternal spirit Brahma. Brahmanism (also known as Hinduism) was to become a major religion in India, out of which developed the stratification of Indian society into four different castes and the concept of sacrifice to satisfy gods. Sources of information about health practices come from the Vedas, a sacred book of Brahmanism dating back to 1600 B.C. and considered by some to be the oldest known written material. Medicine, as described in the books of *Ayur Veda* (or the Veda of Longevity), emphasized hygiene and prevention of sickness and included discussions of major and minor surgery, children's diseases (including inoculation against smallpox), materia medica (the drugs and other remedial substances used in medicine), and diseases of the nervous and urinary systems (Nutting & Dock, 1935; Jamieson & Sewall, 1944). Their practice of surgery may have been the most highly developed of any ancient culture.

Siddhartha Gautama, who lived about 500 B.C., was a Hindu ascetic who, at age 29, left his wife and child to find salvation and to develop a more intimate relationship with the spiritual. He attained a state called "enlightenment," declaring himself Buddha and offering a new religious philosophy known as Buddhism. Buddhism emerged as the major religion of early India, although some would consider it more a moral discipline than a religion. Buddha aspired to bring peace and contentment (Nirvana) to all, which he believed could be achieved by freeing the self of all desires and worldly things. During the Buddhist period, under the rule of King Asoka, India developed an advanced understanding of hygiene and sanitation, disease prevention, medicine, and surgery. The importance of prenatal care to both mother and infant seemed well understood and practiced. Buddhism disregarded the caste system of the earlier religion, and made education and the right to peace possible for everyone. Public hospitals were constructed during this time, and some vital statistics were collected. These hospitals were staffed with nurses whose qualifications were similar to those expected of today's practical nurses. The main difference was that, in almost all cases, Indian nurses were men. In rare instances, old women were permitted to assume this role. Donahue (1996, p 48) states that three main qualities of character were required of these attendants: high standards, skill, and trustworthiness.

China

Ancient China was located far to the northeast of India, across the range of the Himalaya Mountains and, like India, was cut off from the Mediterranean world. The Chinese are thought to have come from central Asia around 3000 B.C. (Jamieson & Sewall, 1944). Chinese civilization developed along the banks of the Yellow River. The ancient Chinese followed the teachings of Confucius, who sought to relieve the country's oppression by reviving ancient customs as a basis for a government ideal. Patriarchal rule dominated, and emphasis was placed on the value of the family as a unit. Women were considered vastly inferior to men; the number of sons she could produce determined a woman's value. A daughter was always severed from connection with her family of origin when she married; her obligations and loyalties were automatically transferred to the family of her husband. Although young married women were treated almost as slaves, old women were received with love and given a position of high esteem in families. Ancestor worship attained great importance.

Great emphasis was placed on the value of knowledge in solving life's problems, and rules of etiquette were important. The early Chinese established the philosophy of the yang and the yin. The yang represented the active, positive, masculine force of the universe, and the yin represented the passive, negative, feminine force. The Chinese believed that these two forces operated in contrasting and complementary ways. Health practices based on this philosophy focused on prevention and good health was believed to result from a balance between the yang and the yin.

China's medical knowledge extends far back in history. Dissection was performed in China before 2000 B.C. The development of elaborate materia medica was of major significance; many of the drugs used by the Chinese in ancient times, such as ephedrine, are used in modern medicine. The Chinese developed acupuncture skills that continue to be practiced today. They also studied the circulation and emphasized the behavior of the pulse. Principles of examination were based on the following guideposts: "look, listen, ask, feel." Baths were used for the reduction of fever and bloodletting was used as a method of helping an evil spirit escape from the body.

The Americas

Early civilization in the Americas may have begun 10,000 or even 20,000 years ago (Donahue, 1996, p 64). It is thought that early inhabitants probably came from Central Asia, gaining access across a land bridge over the Bering Strait into Alaska. Like other early tribes, they were nomadic, wandering in search of food and shelter. Several groups, including the Mayas, Incas, Aztecs, and Toltecs, developed a high degree of civilization.

The sun god was particularly important to these cultures. Rites, ceremonies, herbal treatments, charms, and, in some instances, human sacrifice, contributed to healing practices. Health was a balance among man, nature, and the supernatural. Medicine, pharmacy, nursing, religion, and magic often were not viewed as separate entities. Medicine men (known first as shamans and later as priests) were responsible for curing ills of both the body and the mind, and disease was believed to result from displeasing the gods.

Little is known about the role of the nurse in these early civilizations, although the status enjoyed by Indian women was good and American Indians made significant contributions to modern-day medicine and medical practice. The Aztecs in particular had hospices for the care of the ill, used minerals as drugs, soporifics to decrease pain, and assisted women with childbirth (Donahue, 1996).

Critical Thinking Activity

> Given the lack of organized nursing, how do you believe the people of the early cultures received care? Who do you think provided that care? How did they know what to do?

HISTORICAL PERSPECTIVES OF NURSING

Writings about early health care make little or no mention of nursing or nurses. One might assume that a family member, particularly the wife or mother, provided needed care. Health practices varied depending on the level of development of a society. Ritualistic ceremonies and worship of gods were common and various individuals in the culture assumed the role of healer. Each primitive society had its own curative agents, taboos, and practices; some were more advanced than others. A sound theory of disease was absent from most early cultures.

Although ancient cultures developed medicine as a science and a profession, they showed little evidence of establishing a foundation for nursing, with the possible exception of the male attendants in early Buddhist hospitals in India, and of midwives, who had an established role in several cultures. It was not until the early Christian period that nursing as we think of it began to develop.

Muriel Uprichard identifies three heritages from the past that impeded the development of nursing as a profession. They are "the folk image of the nurse brought forward from primitive times, the religious image of the nurse inherited from the medieval period, and the servant image of the nurse created by the Protestant-capitalist ethic of the 16th to 19th century" (Uprichard, 1973, p 24). Whether or not they hampered progress, these concepts of the nurse have certainly had an impact.

The Folk Image of the Nurse

Since the time of the first mother, women have carried the major responsibility for nourishing and nurturing children, and caring for elderly and aging members of the family. It is difficult to pinpoint a particular time or place for the beginning of nursing, as we know it. It is reasonable to assume those early tribes and civilizations required health care. It is also reasonable to assume that in those tribes and civilizations were people who demonstrated adeptness and a special interest in meeting the needs of those who were sick, injured, or bearing children. These "nurses" received their education largely through trial and error, by advancing those methods that appeared to be successful and by sharing information. Superstition and magic played a significant role in treatment; folklore abounded, and a close relationship existed between religion and the healing arts.

Nursing skills primarily evolved from intuition. For example, while planning a diet for the family, an astute woman would have noticed that eating certain foods resulted in episodes of diarrhea and vomiting, whereas eating other herbs, roots, and leaves had a soothing effect on the body. Families developed recipes that were handed down from generation to generation; effective treatments and cures were recorded and shared.

The Religious Image of the Nurse

The first continuity in the history of nursing began with Christianity. Christ's teachings admonished people to love and care for their neighbors. With the establishment of churches in the Christian era, groups were organized as orders whose primary concern was to care for the sick, the poor, orphans, widows, the aged, slaves, and prisoners, all in the name of charity and Christian love. Christ's precepts placed women and men on parity, and the early church made both men and women deacons, with equal rank. Unmarried women had unprecedented opportunities for service. Although these opportunities represented positive changes, they also fostered certain limitations. Because nursing developed an image closely tied to religion and religious orders, strict discipline was expected. Absolute attendance to the orders of persons of higher rank (eg, priests or physicians) was demanded. This type of thinking for many years characterized nursing.

THE DEACONESSES

One group of particular significance to the history of nursing was the deaconesses of the Eastern Christian Church. These women, who were required to be unmarried or widowed, were often the widows or daughters of Roman officials, and thus had breeding, culture, wealth, and social position. Like the deacon, these individuals were ordained; and, as a church official, worked on an equal basis with the deacon. These dedicated young women practiced "works of mercy" that included feeding the hungry, clothing the naked, visiting the imprisoned, sheltering the homeless, caring for the sick, and burying the dead. The deaconesses were the earliest counterparts to the community health nurses of today. When they entered homes to distribute food and medicine, they carried a basket. It has been suggested that this was the forerunner of the contemporary visiting nurse's bag. No discussion of nursing history would be complete without mentioning Phoebe, who is often referred to as the first deaconess and the first visiting nurse. She carried Paul's letters and cared for him and many others. In the Epistle to the Romans, dated about A.D. 58, reference is made to Phoebe and to her work.

THE WIDOWS AND THE VIRGINS

Two other groups—the Order of Widows and the Order of Virgins—shared many common characteristics with the deaconesses and carried out similar responsibilities. Members of the Order of Widows may never have been married. It seems that the title of widow was used to designate respect for age. Those who were married, however, took vows never to remarry if widowed. The Order of Virgins emphasized virginity as essential to purity of life, and virgins were ranked as equals to the clergy. Because these women often visited the sick in their homes, they are sometimes recognized as the earliest organized group of public health nurses. The movement peaked in Constantinople in about A.D. 400, when a staff of 40 deaconesses lived and worked under the direction of Olympia, a powerful and deeply religious deaconess. The influence of the deaconess order diminished in the fifth and sixth centuries, when church decrees removed clerical duties and rank from the deaconess.

Although the position of deaconess originated in the Eastern Christian Church, it spread west to Gaul and Ireland. In Rome, women who served in comparable positions were known as matrons. Active during the fourth and fifth centuries, these Roman matrons held independent positions and had great wealth, which they contributed to charity and to nursing. Among these Christian converts were three women who contributed significantly to nursing. Their stories are told in Display 4-1.

THE ROLE OF THE MONASTIC ORDERS

The monastic orders also developed during this period, including the order of Benedictines, which still exists. The monasteries played a large role in the preservation of culture and learning as well as in offering refuge to the persecuted, care to the sick, and education to the uneducated. By joining a monastic order, young men and women were able to follow the career of their choice while living a Christian life. The learning of the classical period would have been lost when the Roman Empire fell were it not for the monks and monasteries.

One of the earliest organizations for men in nursing, the Parabolani brotherhood, was established at this time. Responding to needs created by the Black Plague, this group reportedly organized a hospital and traveled throughout Rome caring for the sick. At the same time, monastic nurses such as the famous St. Brigid, St. Scholastica (a twin sister of St. Benedict), and St. Hilda, founded schools, tended to the sick, and gave to the poor.

During this period (approximately A.D. 50 to 800), the first hospitals were established, usually as a part of a nearby monastery that included, in addition to the church, grain fields, gardens, orchards, farm buildings, and eventually, schools. Many of these hospitals are still standing. There were more than 700 hospitals in England by the middle of the 16th century. The Hotel Dieu in Lyons was established in 542 and the Hotel

Display 4–1
ROMAN MATRONS

FABIOLA

Fabiola, a charming and beautiful young woman, was born into an influential and wealthy Roman family. Growing up in a lavish home, she enjoyed a happy social life. However, her marriage to a worthless gentleman resulted in divorce. She married a second time, and was no happier in her second marriage. Under the influence of Marcella, she converted to Christianity and, after the death of her second husband, began her career of charity. Fabiola's new beliefs made marriage after divorce a sin. She publicly acknowledged this, committed her life to charitable work, and in 390 A.D. built the first public hospital in Rome described as a *nosocomium*. Here she cared for the sick and poor whom she gathered from the streets and highways, personally washing and treating wounds and sores that repulsed others. Later in her life she is said to have built a hospice for strangers at Ostia, a seaport of Rome. St. Jerome tells of some of her work and her attributes in his writings. She died about 399, and scores of Romans are said to have attended her funeral to show their respect for her.

MARCELLA

A Roman woman of means, Marcella made her luxurious home into a monastery for women. Here other matrons such as Fabiola and Paula became involved in Christian study. Much inspiration came to them through a great friend and teacher, St. Jerome. Marcella devoted her life to instruction, charitable work, and prayer and became recognized as an authority on interpretation of biblical passages. She assisted St. Jerome in his translation of the Hebrew prophets. During the sack of Rome, her home was invaded by warriors who expected to find valuables stored there. When they found little more than a bare building, they whipped Marcella, hoping she would reveal the hiding places of riches. After the assault she is said to have fled to St. Paul's church, which was nearby. There she died as a result of her injuries.

ST. PAULA

Learned, wealthy, and broken-hearted by the death of her husband, Saint Paula was also a scholar of Marcella. She is said to have assisted St. Jerome (whose lifetime exceeded that of all the women with whom he associated) in the translation of the writings of the prophets. St. Paula traveled to Palestine and devoted a fortune to the establishment of hospitals and inns for pilgrims traveling to Jerusalem. In Bethlehem she organized a monastery, built hospitals for the sick, and developed hospices for pilgrims, where tired travelers and the ill received care. Some credit her with being the first to teach nursing as an art rather than a service. She had a daughter, Eustochium, who joined her mother in the adoption of Christianity, and with her expressed its ideals through charitable work.

Dieu in Paris around 650. The Hotel Dieu in Paris was staffed by the first order specifically devoted to nursing, the Augustinian Sisters. The Santo Spirito Hospital in Rome, the largest medieval hospital, was established by papal order in 717.

The Crusades, which swept northern Europe, lasted for almost 200 years (1096–1291). The deaconess movement, suppressed by the Western Church, became all but extinct. Military nursing orders evolved as a result of the Crusades. The Knights Hospitallers of St. John was one such order. It was organized to staff two hospitals located in Jerusalem and had as its grand master a monk named Gerard. He drew up codes and introduced the black robe with a white Maltese cross that became the uniform for the brethren (Kalisch & Kalisch, 1995). The same cross was later used on a badge designed for the Nightingale School; this badge was the forerunner of the nursing pin as we know it today. (The symbolism of the pin is discussed later in this chapter.) The Knights, organized as a nursing order, soon became famous for their hospitality and care and their numbers, possessions, and wealth increased. At times they were required to defend the hospital and its patients. In Germany, a women's order called "consorores" was founded specifically to perform hospital work. Although they took vows, the women were not granted the same status as the Knights, and they lived outside the monastic precincts.

Two other monastic orders were founded during this period: the Knights Templars in 1118 and the Knights of the Teutonic Order in 1190. The Hospitallers and the Templars played significant roles during the Crusades. Secular orders of nurses also came into existence at this time. Operating much like the monastic orders, members of these groups could terminate their vocations at any time and were not bound to the vows of monastic life. Examples of the secular orders include the Order of Antonines (1095); the Beguines of Flanders, Belgium (1184); the Misericordia (1244); and the Alexian Brothers, founded during the bubonic plague epidemic of 1348. The only nursing education offered to these dedicated people was in the form of an apprenticeship; a newcomer to the organization would be assigned to a more experienced person for instruction.

The inquiring student is encouraged to seek greater depth of knowledge about the nursing orders, their purposes and goals, and the lives of those who devoted their energies to the care of the sick and the poor by consulting the nursing references given at the end of this chapter.

MUSLIM CULTURE

Miles from the western centers of civilizations, thousands of nomadic people living in tribes struggled for existence on the arid desert of Arabia. Subsistence was difficult, and occupation of an oasis often became the frequent basis for battle. They made pilgrimages for worship to the city of Mecca where a shrine in the form of a sacred, black stone was found. In this city, about 570 A.D., a child who was to be named Muhammad was born. At about age 40, he began to preach a religion that would later be identified by the name "Islam." Not well received by the people of Mecca, the ideas appealed to a nomadic tribe known as Bedouins. As the religion grew, mosques were built for worshipers. Civil and religious life both were given direction through the writings of Muhammad. Thirty years after his death these writings were incorporated into a book known as the *Koran*. Muhammad formulated rules for good living that excluded gambling, lying, wine drinking, uncleanness, and eating unclean food. He advocated kindliness, honesty, hospitality, forgiveness, almsgiving, cleanliness, and eating only prescribed foods. People prayed to the god Allah. Women in the society held little position, they were denied education, and their husbands were chosen for them. Their role was to bear children; if infertile, they could be beaten. Husbands could have as many as four wives at one time; however, women could have but one husband at a time. Although husbands were allowed to divorce their wives, the reverse was not true. In some respects Muhammad improved woman's position. Infanticide was forbidden and parents were required to include daughters in inheritances. A few women were even allowed to learn to read (Sewell & Jamieson, 1944).

As the Islamic culture grew, the writings of Hippocrates and Galen were translated into Arabic. Although Muslim beliefs regarding uncleanness forbade dissection, an extensive materia medica developed. Hospitals were built.

Little has been written in nursing history books about the role of nursing in early Muslim cultures. Recently, attention has been drawn to an 11th century Muslim "Nightingale" named Rufaida Al-Asalmiya, who was a nurse during the time of the Prophet Muhammad. Rufaido Al-Asalmiya lived in Al-Media (Yethreb), a region of what is now Saudi Arabia, where her father was a healer. While assisting her father, Rufaido developed many nursing skills. With the permission of the Prophet Muhammad, she began to train women and young girls in the art of nursing. She is said to have developed the first code of nursing conduct and ethics, long before it was introduced in the western world. When the holy war began, she is reported to have provided care to the Muslim army in battle, enjoining her Muslim nurses to assist her. She continued this care after the battle ended, setting up tents near the mosque of Nabvi where she provided care and health education. A building at the Aga Khan University School of Nursing has been named in her honor (Jan, 1996).

The Servant Image of the Nurse

The Renaissance and the Reformation (occurring from the 14th through the 16th centuries) followed the Middle Ages. During the Renaissance, also known as the Age of Discovery, a new impetus was given to education, and, to some extent, to medical education. For example, Ambroise Pare (1510–1590), a French surgeon, revived the method of tying blood vessels to stop hemorrhaging, believing that procedures based on acute observation were better than those based on ancient doctrines. Andreas Vesalium (1514–1564) published a treatise of surgery and anatomy that refuted the teachings of Galen, who up to that point had been the undisputed authority on medicine. Nursing education, however, was all but nonexistent during this period.

The Reformation, a religious movement inspired by the work of Martin Luther, began in Germany in 1517. It resulted in a revolt against the supremacy of the pope and the formation of Protestant churches across Europe. Monasteries were closed, religious orders were dissolved, and the work of women in these orders became almost extinct.

The Reformation brought about a change in the role of women. The Protestant Church, which stood for freedom of religion and thought, did not grant much freedom to women. During the Reformation, women were no longer revered by their churches and encouraged toward charitable activities, but were deemed subordinate to men. Their role was defined within the confines of the home; their duties were those of bearing children and caring for the home. Work in hospitals no longer appealed to women of high birth. Hospital care was relegated to "uncommon" women, a group comprising prisoners, prostitutes, and drunks (Fig. 4-2).

FIGURE 4-2 From the Middle Ages to the 19th century, nursing was often left to "uncommon women."

Women faced with earning their own living were forced to work as domestic servants, and although nursing was considered a domestic service, it was not a desirable one. The nurse was regarded as the most menial of servants. Pay was poor, the hours were long, and the work was strenuous. Nursing care was not subject to inspection and was not governed by standards. The same bed linen might be used for several patients, even though suppurating wounds were common. Thus began what may be called the "Dark Ages" of nursing.

Charles Dickens (1936) described the image of nurses and nursing during this time through the characters of Sairey Gamp and Betsy Prig in his book *Martin Chuzzlewit*, which was written in 1843:

She was a fat old woman, this Mrs. Gamp, with a husky voice and a moist eye, which she had a remarkable power of turning up, and only showing the white of it. Having very little neck, it cost her some trouble to look over herself, if one may say so, at those to whom she talked. She wore a very rusty black gown, rather the worse for snuff, and a shawl and bonnet to correspond. . . . The face of Mrs. Gamp—the nose in particular—was somewhat red and swollen, and it was difficult to enjoy her society without becoming conscious of a smell of spirits. Like most persons who have attained to great eminence in their profession, she took to hers very kindly; insomuch, that setting aside her natural predilections as a woman, she went to a lying-in or a lying-out with equal zest and relish (p. 318).

Mrs. Prig was of the Gamp build, but not so fat; and her voice was deeper and more like a man's. She had also a beard (p. 417).

The 16th and 17th centuries found Europe devastated by famine, plague, filth, and horror. In England, for example, King Henry VIII effectively had eliminated organized monastic relief provided to orphans and other displaced persons. Throughout Europe vagrancy and begging abounded, and those caught begging were often severely punished by being branded, beaten, or chained in galleys where they served as oarsmen. Knowledge of hygiene was insufficient; the poor suffered the most. Social reform was inevitable. Several nursing groups were organized. These groups gave money, time, and service to the sick and the poor, visiting them in their homes and ministering to their needs. Such groups included the Order of the Visitation of Mary, St. Vincent de Paul, and in 1633, the Sisters of Charity. The last group became an outstanding secular nursing order. They developed an educational program for the intelligent young women they recruited that included experience in a hospital as well as visiting in the home. Receiving help, counsel, and encouragement from St. Vincent de Paul, the Sisters of Charity expanded their services to include caring for abandoned children. In 1640, St. Vincent established the Hospital for Foundlings in Paris. Later, in 1809, the Sisters of Charity established a nursing order in the United States, under the direction of Elizabeth Bayley Seton. Other branches of this order were to follow, variously called the "Gray Sisters," the "Daughters of Charity," or the "Sisters of St. Vincent de Paul."

The Beginning of Change

Those countries in Europe that remained Roman Catholic escaped some of the disorganization caused by the Reformation. During the 1500s the Spanish and the Portuguese began traveling to the Americas. In 1521, Cortes conquered the capital of the Aztec civilization in Mexico and renamed it Mexico City. Early colonists to the area included members of Catholic religious orders, who became the doctors, nurses, and teachers of the new land. In 1524, the first hospital on the American continent, the Hospital of Immaculate Conception (Hospital de Nuestra Senora O Limpia Concepcion), was built in Mexico City. Mission colleges were founded. The first medical school in America was founded in 1578 at the University of Mexico, the second at the University of Lima before 1600.

Farther north, Jacques Cartier sailed up the St. Lawrence River in 1535 and established French settlements in Nova Scotia. Franciscan Friars, Jesuits, Dominicans, and other settlers and explorers followed. In 1639, three Augustinian nuns arrived in Quebec to staff the Hotel Dieu of Montreal, a hospital that opened that year. The Ursuline Sisters, an order of teaching nuns who accompanied the Augustinians from France, are credited with attempting to organize the first training for nurses on this continent. They taught the Indian women of the area to care for their sick during a smallpox epidemic. Jeanne Mance, who had been educated at an Ursuline convent, came to Montreal from France in 1642. She is considered to be the founder of the Hotel Dieu of Montreal as well as the co-founder of Montreal itself. She returned to France in 1657 to recruit financial support and staff, and returned with three French hospital nuns from the Society of St. Joseph de la Fleche to staff the Hotel Dieu (Donahue, 1996).

In Europe, outstanding men of medicine made vital and valuable contributions to medical knowledge. Among lay persons influencing social change during this time was a young minister in Kaiserwerth, Germany, Theodore Fliedner (1800–1864). With the assistance of his first wife, Friederike, Fliedner revived the deaconess movement by establishing a training institute for deaconesses at Kaiserwerth in 1836. During a fund-raising tour through Holland and England, Pastor Fliedner met Elizabeth Fry of England, who had brought about reform at Newgate Prison in London. Greatly impressed with Mrs. Fry's accomplishments, the Fliedners followed her example and first worked with women prisoners in Kaiserwerth. Later they opened a small hospital for the sick, and Gertrude Reichardt, the daughter of a physician, was recruited as their first deaconess. The endeavors at Kaiserwerth included care of the sick, visitations and parochial work, and teaching. A course in nursing was developed that included lectures by physicians.

Friederike, who played a large part in helping to bring Theodore's visionary plans to fruition, was herself deeply dedicated to the deaconess movement. While away from home promoting deaconess activities, she learned that one of her children had died. A second child died shortly after her return and she herself died in 1842 after the birth of a premature infant. His second wife, Caroline Bertheau, who had some nursing experience before her marriage, also assisted Pastor Fliedner in his work. In 1849 Pastor Fliedner traveled to the United States, where he helped to establish the first Motherhouse of Kaiserwerth Deaconesses in Pittsburgh, Pennsylvania. With the help of four deaconesses, the Motherhouse of Kaiserwerth Deaconesses assumed responsibility for the Pittsburgh Infirmary, which was the first Protestant hospital in the United States. The hospital is now called Passavant Hospital.

In England, at about the same time, Elizabeth Fry (1780–1845) organized the Institute of Nursing Sisters, a secular group often called the Fry Sisters. Two other groups followed shortly; the Sisters of Mercy, a Roman Catholic group formed by Catherine McAuley (1787–1841), and another Catholic group called the Irish Sisters of Charity, formed by Mary Aikenhead (1787–1858).

Critical Thinking Activity

Knowing what you do about the history of the image of nursing, how will you, as a nurse of the future, advance the image of nursing? What aspects of the role are most critical? Who are the people who most need to be influenced? What aspects of the profession should be changed?

THE NIGHTINGALE INFLUENCE

The three images of nursing discussed in the previous sections—the folk image, the servant image, and the religious image—all influenced the development of nursing. In the latter half of the 18th century, however, one woman dramatically changed the form and direction of nursing and succeeded in establishing it as a respected field of endeavor. This outstanding woman was Florence Nightingale.

Born on May 12, 1820, the second daughter of a wealthy family, she was named after the city in which she was born—Florence, Italy. Because of her family's high social and economic standing, she was cultured, well traveled, and educated. By the age of 17, she had mastered several languages and mathematics and was extremely well read. Through the influential people she met, she was expected to select a desirable mate, marry, and assume her place in society.

Florence Nightingale had other ideas, however. She wanted to become a nurse, but this aspiration was unthinkable to her family because of the hospital conditions of the day. She continued to travel with her family and their friends and, in the course of these travels, met Sidney Herbert and his wife, who were becoming interested in hospital reform. She began collecting information on public health and hospitals and soon became recognized as an important authority on the subject.

Through friends she learned about Pastor Fliedner's institute at Kaiserwerth. Because it was a religious institution under the auspices of the church, her parents would permit her to go there, although she could not go to English hospitals. In 1851 she spent 3 months studying at Kaiserwerth.

In 1853, she began working with a committee that supervised an "Establishment for Gentlewomen During Illness." She eventually was appointed superintendent of the establishment. As her knowledge of hospitals and nursing reform grew, she was consulted by reformers and by physicians who were beginning to see the need for "trained" nurses. Despite her growing reputation as a respected expert, her family continued to object to her activities.

When the Crimean War broke out later that same year, war correspondents wrote about the abominable manner in which the British Army cared for the sick and wounded soldiers. Florence Nightingale, by then a recognized authority on hospital care, wrote to her friend Sir Sidney Herbert, who was then Secretary of War, and offered to take a group of 38 nurses to the Crimea. (At the same time, he had written a letter requesting her assistance in resolving this national crisis. Their letters crossed in the mail.) Her achievements in the Crimea were so outstanding, despite the toll they took on her own health, that she was recognized in 1907 by the Queen of England, who awarded her the Order of Merit.

In 1856, Florence Nightingale returned to England, her health broken. Much has been written of her "illness," and many have suggested that it was, to a large degree, a neurosis. She retreated to her bedroom, and for the next 43 years conducted her business from her secluded apartment.

Throughout her lifetime, Florence Nightingale wrote extensively about hospitals, sanitation, health, and health statistics, and especially about nursing and nursing education. She crusaded for and brought about great reform in nursing education.

In 1860, she devoted her efforts to the creation of a school of nursing at St. Thomas' Hospital in London, financed by the Nightingale Fund. The basic principles on which Miss Nightingale established her school included the following:

- Nurses would be trained in teaching hospitals associated with medical schools and organized for that purpose.
- Nurses would be selected carefully and would reside in nurses' houses designed to encourage discipline and form character.

- The school matron would have final authority over the curriculum, living arrangements, and all other aspects of the school.
- The curriculum would include both theoretical material and practical experience.
- Teachers would be paid for their instruction.
- Records would be kept on the students, who would be required to attend lectures, take quizzes, write papers, and keep diaries.

In many other ways Florence Nightingale advanced nursing as a profession. She believed that nurses should spend their time caring for patients, not cleaning; that nurses must continue learning throughout their lifetime and not become "stagnant"; that nurses should be intelligent and should use that intelligence to improve conditions for the patient; and that nursing leaders should have social standing. She had a vision of what nursing could and should be.

Florence Nightingale died in her sleep at the age of 90. The week during which she was born is now honored as National Nurses Week. The enthusiastic student is encouraged to learn more about this fascinating woman in Cecil Woodham-Smith's book *Florence Nightingale*.

THE MILITARY INFLUENCE

Through her experience in the Crimean War, Florence Nightingale first brought attention to nursing as a career and profession and to needed changes in health care delivery. Similarly, other wars have brought advances in how care is provided; nursing has not always fared as well. In the following section we will highlight some of those areas; however, it is impossible, in the context of this book, to provide more than just an overview (Fig. 4-3).

The American Revolution

All of the English colonies scattered along the Atlantic Coast of the United States were involved in the American Revolution. The hastily organized army existed without the benefit of a medical corps or trained nurses. The nuns of the Catholic Church, who also cared for those who were ill with epidemic diseases such as scarlet fever, dysentery, and smallpox, nursed wounded soldiers. On the battlefield, women who had followed their husbands to the battlefield often nursed soldiers. Homes and barns near the battles were turned into hospitals. Other women contributed to the cause by making clothing and bandages or by helping to feed the soldiers from their own pantries.

When the war ended, the usual type of poverty existed, with invalids and cripples who needed care. However, the colonies were not sufficiently developed to have such services available. In response, a new type of institution evolved, which is perhaps the forerunner of today's clinic or hospital outpatient department. In 1786 the Philadelphia Dispensary was established and volunteer physicians treated those needing care at no charge. These dispensaries later became a major site for controlling disease. Vaccination against smallpox was one of the earliest preventive treatments offered.

FIGURE 4–3   Nurses were widely recruited for service in the military.

The Influence of the Civil War

The Civil War broke out in the United States in 1861. Although social reform was on the rise, the nursing profession was still in an embryonic, unorganized stage. There was neither an army nurse corps, nor an organized medical corps. There were no ambulance services or MASH units. Responding to the nursing needs created by the war, in which it is estimated that 618,000 men died (Donahue, 1996, p. 247), many women volunteered to help. After a brief training course, they performed nursing duties. Many religious orders also volunteered and provided service. A steamer, captured from the Confederates, was converted into a floating hospital and anchored near Vicksburg. Considered the first Navy hospital ship, the *Red Rover* was staffed through the volunteer efforts of the Catholic Sisters of Mercy, who became the first "Navy" nurses. An account of some of the contributions of nurses during the Civil War and afterward is found in Table 4-2. The serious need for trained nurses, created by the Civil War, was undoubtedly a significant factor in the development of nursing in the United States.

The Spanish-American War and the Boer War

These two conflicts occurred at about the same time in history. The United States entered the Spanish-American War in 1898, and the British went to war against the

TABLE 4–2.   Nurses of the Civil War and Their Contributions*

Nurse	Contribution
Sojourner Truth (1797–1883)	Born into slavery and named Isabella, this African American was sold three times by the time she was 13, the last time for $300. She married an older slave and bore him 5 children, some of whom were also sold into slavery. In 1843 she changed her name to Sojourner Truth. She nursed Union soldiers, worked for improvement in sanitary facilities, and sought contributions of food and clothing for black volunteer regiments. She supported her travel from sales of her *Narrative of Sojourner Truth: A Northern Slave* (1850) dictated to Olive Gilbert because she was illiterate. She continued her work as a nurse/counselor for the Freedmen's Relief Association after the war (Whitman, 1985, p. 814–816).
Dorothea Lynde Dix (1802–1881)	A Boston school teacher already known for her humanitarian efforts on behalf of the mentally ill, she was commissioned as Superintendent of Women Nurses for All Military Hospitals during the Civil War when she was past 60 years of age. Her authority was often challenged by the physicians.
Mary Ann Ball Bickerdyke (1817–1901)	Called "Mother" Bickerdyke by the troops, this Illinois woman challenged the work of lazy, corrupt medical officers. She served under fire in 19 battles. Her efforts were recognized by the government in the launching of the hospital ship, the *SS Mary A. Bickerdyke* in 1943.
Walt Whitman (1819–1892)	A well-respected poet who worked as a volunteer in hospital wards after searching for a brother who had been wounded. Dressed wounds, wrote letters, read to soldiers, brought gifts and food. Later wrote about the war and suffering of soldiers
Harriet Ross Tubman (1820–1913)	An abolitionist sometimes called "Conductor of the Underground Railroad," this black nurse was commended for caring for the sick and wounded without regard for color.
Mary Livermore (1820–1905)	Another untrained nurse of the Civil War, she later became a suffragist and advocated education for all women. Addressing the sixth annual convention of the Nurses' Associated Alumnae, she described the activities of the Civil War nurses.
Clara Barton (1821–1912)	Served as a volunteer with the Sixth Massachusetts Regiment. Independently operated a large-scale relief operation. Was instrumental in founding the American Red Cross in 1882. Called "little lone lady in black silk" (Donahue 1996, p. 255)
Kate Cummings (1828–1909)	A volunteer in the southern army, her diaries chronicled the work of the "matrons" who served in the Confederate hospitals.
Louisa May Alcott (1832–1888)	Served as a volunteer nurse during the Civil War. From these experiences she wrote a small book entitled *Hospital Sketches,* which described the work of the volunteer nurses of the Civil War. The nurse character of the book was Miss Tribulation Periwinkle.
Jane Stuart Woolsey (1830–1891)	One of three sisters from a cultivated and elite northeastern family with colonial ancestry, Jane served the Union Army as supervisor of the nursing and cooking department. She provided much narrative to describe the conditions of the day, authoring a book entitled *Hospital Days.* Later she served as the directress of the Presbyterian Hospital in New York.

(continues)

TABLE 4–2. Nurses of the Civil War and Their Contributions* *(Continued)*	
Nurse	**Contribution**
Abby Howland Woolsey (1828–1893)	A sister of Jane, she too served as a volunteer nurse for the Union Army and fought diligently for the abolition of slavery. Helped found the Bellevue Hospital Training School for Nurses and wrote one of the first books on the organization of nursing schools—*A Century of Nursing with Hints Toward the Organization of a Training School (1876)* (Whitman, 1985, pp. 904–906).
Georgeanna Muirson Woolsey (1833–1906)	Another Woolsey sister involved in war efforts, she benefited from a month-long nursing training experience in New York when selected by the Woman's Central Association of Relief as one of a group of a hundred for leadership potential. She wrote of her war experiences in a book entitled *Three Weeks at Gettysburg*. She later helped found the Connecticut Training School for Nursing in New Haven, enjoying the support of her husband, Dr. Francis Bacon (Whitman, 1985, pp. 903–906).
Susie King Taylor (1848–1901)	Born into slavery, as a young girl she secretly learned to read and write. While serving as a volunteer nurse for the Union Army, she also worked as a teacher.

*Much of the information contained in this table was gathered from the work of Kalisch and Kalisch, 1995, except as otherwise noted.

Boers of South Africa in late 1899. By this time the Red Cross had organized and the United States, Canada, and Great Britain all had nursing schools to prepare young women for nursing roles.

In the early days of the Spanish-American War, little attention was given to the selection of nurses to care for the wounded. Volunteers included nurses with training, those partly trained, the untrained, and both men and women. The entire system lacked organization; needed supplies were lacking. These conditions attracted the attention of both the government and the people. Among groups addressing the concern was the Nurses' Associated Alumnae of the United States and Canada, who offered to develop a process through which better skilled nurses might be secured. When Mrs. Isabel Hampton Robb, the group's president, visited Washington for this purpose, she found the department of army nursing already under the direction of Dr. Anita Newcomb McGee, a physician, who was setting up standards for selection. The management of the chosen nurses was given over to the Red Cross, which retained this role throughout the war.

Camp nursing became the predominant approach to care. Anna C. Maxwell, on leave from the Presbyterian Hospital in New York, was Chief Nurse at one such camp. Among problems she encountered were inadequate water facilities, lack of laundry and laundry services, and lack of medical supplies. In addition, many of her nurses became ill with typhoid fever.

When the war ended, nurse leaders exerted pressure to secure legislation to ensure an efficient army nursing service. A bill establishing the Army Nurse Corps was passed in 1901, and in 1908 the Navy Nurse Corps was established. Jane A. Delano was appointed Superintendent of the Army Nurse Corps. At about this time, the Red Cross began a complete reorganization, and William Howard Taft served as its president for eight years. He also became president of the United States during this time.

In South Africa, the situation was much the same as in the United States—the need for more efficient and educationally prepared nurses was apparent. The British Army Nursing Service, organized in 1881 as a result of the Crimean experience, recruited Canadian volunteers who functioned under the direction of Georgina F. Pope. Canada was the first country to accord military rank to women. Britain soon learned that it needed a group of nurses who could be called upon in an emergency, and the Queen Alexandra's Imperial Military Nursing Service came into being.

History honors the contribution of a special nurse, Clara Maas, from the Spanish-American War; a commemorative stamp was issued in her honor. This 25-year-old nurse was so moved by the suffering of her patients with yellow fever that she volunteered to be bitten several times by the disease-carrying mosquito in an effort to determine how the disease was transmitted. Although she survived the first bite, she died of yellow fever from a subsequent exposure.

A memorial in Arlington National Cemetery honors the memory of the women who gave their lives as Army Nurses in the Spanish-American War. It was erected by the Society of Spanish-American War Nurses.

World War I

In 1914 Austria declared war on Serbia, Germany invaded Belgium and France, and England became involved in the conflict. The United States would join them on April 6, 1917. Through Queen Alexandra's Imperial Military Nursing Service, England was prepared to meet the emergency needs for care. Navy and air force branches were added to that of the army. As the need for more nurses became greater, the British Red Cross organized a Voluntary Aid Detachment composed of laypersons. These individuals were given short emergency courses to prepare them for service. When the United States joined the conflict, nurses from the Army and Navy Nurse Corps were ready to provide care to the wounded; other experienced nurses were recruited and enlisted. Despite continuous efforts to provide an adequate supply of nurses in both civilian and army hospitals, the lack of qualified nurses became more marked as time went on. The influenza epidemic of 1918 was of major proportions; pneumonia and typhus also claimed many lives, including doctors and nurses.

Recognizing the demand for a long-term supply of military nurses, the Army School of Nursing was organized in 1918. Annie W. Goodrich served as its dean.

The experiences of the war also pointed to the serious need for uniformity in methods of nursing education. In response, England founded the Royal College of Nursing in 1916. Inspection and accreditation of schools became one of this group's major concerns.

Although there were many who made supreme efforts during World War I, Edith Cavell has been memorialized. An English nurse, Miss Cavell had organized the first school for nurses in Brussels, Belgium. During the battles that occurred in Brussels, the school and hospital offered care to the soldiers of all armies. As a result, Miss Cavell was arrested by the German soldiers and charged with helping Allied Soldiers escape from occupied Belgium. She was sentenced to death and executed at dawn the next day, October 12, 1915.

In 1938, a statue sculpted by Francis Rich from Tennessee marble, titled "Spirit of Nursing," was erected at Arlington National Cemetery among the graves of nurses who had served their country. The only one of its kind to honor nurses in all the services, it was rededicated in 1971 (Klein, 1997).

World War II

In response to Germany's invasion of Austria and Poland, England declared war against Germany in September 1939. The United States entered the war after Japan attacked Pearl Harbor on December 7, 1941. Thus began a conflict that was to be known as a "total war" because it affected every nation in the world. In the United States, the National Nursing Council for War Service was organized in July 1940 to help meet the increasing need for individuals at all levels of preparation who could care for the sick and wounded. The United States Cadet Nurse Corps was established under the Bolton act, which was authorized in June 1943. It provided funds for tuition, a monthly allowance, uniforms, and other expenses for women who would enter nursing and, upon completion of their education, serve in the military service. Volunteer nurse aides were given short, intensive training so that they might assist nurses in hospitals.

In the Second World War, nurses were given commissions as officers and had military rank, something that had not been true previously. This gave them a level of status and authority that supported their work. Nurses who were assigned to war zones, as opposed to working in military hospitals, often found themselves facing a serious dilemma. The army had done nothing to prepare them for battlefield medicine or for life in the field. Wounded men were treated in field hospitals close to battle lines with supplies and equipment that might be inadequate while bombs dropped around them. Although they were in the army, the nurses considered themselves healers, not soldiers. Elizabeth Norman (1999) poignantly describes the situation in her book *We Band of Angels*:

Then the shooting started, and they found themselves confronting as much danger and deprivation as any dogface in the field. The men who worked with them—doctors, medics, orderlies and attendants—were no longer "colleagues" and "staff," they were comrades in arms now, and "the girls," as so many referred to them, were no longer anomalies in the ranks, they were a military unit in the middle of battle. They were women at war (p. 39).

During this time, flight nursing came into existence as nurses were trained to assist with the air evacuation of sick and wounded soldiers and at ground medical installations. Nurses in these roles worked under extremely dangerous circumstances because the planes used to transport patients also were used to transport cargo. Because of this dual activity, the planes were not marked with the Geneva Red Cross or other insignia, and they remained fair game for enemy fighters.

Stateside, the country was involved in an industrial boom as defense plants mushroomed in response to military needs. Public health nurses moved into industry to carry out preventive health education and programs. Industrial nursing evolved on a national scale, with nurses employed in all types of manufacturing plants.

All of these activities left the country desperate for nurses. Serious shortages were felt in civilian hospitals and in military situations. Kalisch and Kalisch (1995) report that by the winter of 1944–1945, 65,000 nurses were enrolled in the army and navy and approximately 13,800 were employed in industry (p. 344). Nursing students began to carry much of the workload in hospitals that had nursing education programs.

The Korean and Vietnam Conflicts

On June 25, 1950, the Korean War broke out. Once again nurses were called into military service. Learning from the experiences of World War II, treatment centers located close to the front lines were established—the Mobile Army Surgical Hospital (MASH). Triage care evolved, made more effective by advances in antibiotics and medical technology. Flight nursing saw a significant resurgence, as the need for air evacuation of the wounded reached new heights.

The American troop commitment to Vietnam began about the same time as the Korean conflict. By 1963, approximately 15,000 military advisers were in South Vietnam and the first 13 nurses were placed on the staff at the Eighth Field Hospital in Nha Trang in March 1962 (Kalisch and Kalisch, 1995). Recruitment of nurses was once again a major activity; extraordinary incentives were offered because of widespread lack of support for the Vietnam conflict. Owing to the guerrilla tactics of the Viet Cong, no military front existed. The country was partitioned into separate field zones and semipermanent, air-conditioned hospitals were constructed. Fixed installations were assigned to area-support missions with ground evacuation of wounded almost impossible. Terrain and climate were tremendous obstacles. Advances in medical technology, however, permitted far better care than during any other combat situation. The contribution of nurses during this conflict was recognized publicly in a sculpture, designed by Glenna Goodacre, of three nurses and a wounded soldier erected near the Vietnam Memorial in Washington, D.C., in 1993.

On October 18, 1997, the Women in Military Service for America Memorial was dedicated at the Arlington National Cemetery. This marble, stone, and glass memorial is located at the gateway to the cemetery. The dedication included a special nurses ceremony in which wreaths were placed at the "Spirit of Nursing" statue (Klein, 1997).

Critical Thinking Activity

Select a nursing leader of the past whom you would like to interview. Why did you choose that person? What would you like to ask that individual? How would you use the information that person shared with you?

EARLY SCHOOLS IN THE UNITED STATES

After the establishment of the Nightingale School in England, nursing programs flourished and the Nightingale system spread to other countries. In the United States, much of the push for nursing education occurred shortly after the Civil War, during which the lack of trained nurses presented a serious concern.

The Establishment of Early Schools

As with many other significant events that have evolved from a variety of influences, it is difficult to pinpoint the first nursing program in the United States. As early as 1798, a pioneer physician, Dr. Valentine Seaman, is said to have initiated the first system of instruction for nurses at New York Hospital (Donahue, 1996, p. 235). A society was formed in 1839 under Quaker influence, called the Nurse Society of Philadelphia, and a combined Home and School were opened. Historical records show that before 1850, some intermittent preparation was provided to individuals who cared for the sick. A plan of instruction also had been developed for women who would supply maternity service in the home under the guidance of Dr. Joseph Warrington, who was obstetric physician to the Philadelphia Dispensary for the Medical Relief of the Poor.

In 1850, a commission of the Massachusetts Legislature recommended that institutions be formed to educate nurses. A plan for educating nurses was included in the formation of the New England Female Medical College, and a few nurses were educated through this institution. Other hospitals operated training programs, although the course of studies lasted only 6 months. The Woman's Hospital of Philadelphia, which operated under the direction of two female physicians, opened a training school in 1861, but it made little progress until endowed in 1872. Despite these efforts, the nursing services provided by most hospitals during the 1860s were disorganized and inadequate. In many cases, nursing care was provided by women who had been arrested for drunkenness or disorderly conduct and who were serving out 10-day sentences. The better hospitals benefited from the work of Catholic sisters or Protestant deaconesses, although most of them also were untrained.

In 1869, responding to the impetus given nursing during the Civil War, the American Medical Association established a committee to study the issue of training for nurses. The committee, chaired by Dr. Samuel D. Gross (1805–1884), was charged with identifying the best possible method to organize and manage institutions for training nurses. Their report concluded that every large hospital should have a nursing school; emphasized that the union between religious exercises and nursing would be conducive to the welfare of the sick; and recommended that schools be placed under the guardianship of county medical societies (Donahue, 1996, p. 265).

The efforts of several influential and socially prominent women of the time were significant in establishing structured training for nurses. An editorial written by Sarah J. Hale, editor of *The Godey's Lady's Book and Magazine*, entitled "Lady Nurses," advocated the elevation of nursing to the level of a profession. Ms. Hale further recommended providing an education "especially adapted for ladies who desire to qualify themselves for the profession of nurse" (Hale, 1871, pp. 188–189).

The New England Hospital for Women and Children is often credited with being the first hospital to establish a formal 1-year program to train nurses in 1872. It operated under the guidance of a female physician, Susan Dimock, who had received her medical education in Europe and had some knowledge of the work of Florence Nightingale. Five probationers started the program on September 1. It was from this school that Melinda Ann (Linda) Richards graduated in 1873 to become America's first trained nurse. This school was the alma mater for the first black nurse graduate, Mary Eliza Mahoney, in 1879.

By 1873, three additional schools had opened: the Bellevue Training School in New York City, the Connecticut Training School, and the Boston Training School. Typically, these schools did not admit males. In 1888 the Mills School of Nursing at Bellevue Hospital opened to train male nurses for patient care. Separate schools to educate black nurses also opened; among them Spelman Seminary in Atlanta in 1886; Hampton Institute in Virginia and Providence Hospital in Chicago in 1891; and Tuskegee Institute in Alabama in 1892 (Kalisch & Kalisch, 1995). Table 4-3 identifies some of the early schools.

Similar movements to establish nursing schools were occurring in other countries. In 1868, a school was organized in Sydney Hospital, Australia. In Edinburgh, Scotland, a program was started at the Royal Infirmary. The Mack Training School in St. Catherines, Canada, was started in 1884.

Characteristics of the Early Schools

The life of the nursing student at the turn of the century was not an easy one. The strong militaristic and religious influences over nursing were embodied in the expectations held for nursing students. "Monastic and military traditions heavily influenced not only the actual workings of the schools of nursing but also the public's conception of them. The nurse in training was expected to yield to her superiors obedience characteristic of a good soldier and actions governed by the dedication to duty derived from religious devotion" (Kalisch & Kalisch, 1995, p. 111).

Typically, nursing students were about 21 years of age, single, and female. The first weeks or months of their education were spent as probationers, or "probies," and their duties helped with the operation of the hospital but did little to educate them as nurses. For example, they spent much of their time washing, scrubbing, polishing, folding, stacking, and the like. Rules of conduct were rigid and unforgiving and early superintendents saw it as their responsibility to "discipline" pupils, ensuring that they possessed good morals, and were honest, conscientious, obedient, respectful, loyal, passive, and devoted to duty. Nursing students were expected to be unselfish, thinking not of themselves but of the happiness and well-being of others (Fig. 4-4).

Initially, nursing education was largely an apprenticeship and resulted in students providing much of the workforce of hospitals. The workday was long and arduous, often starting at 5:30 in the morning and ending with nursing prayers very late at night, and consisted primarily of work on the hospital wards. The superintendent or her assistants provided instruction. There was no standardization of curriculum and no accreditation. The few lectures that were part of the program were usually given by physicians and scheduled at 8 or 9 PM after a long day of work. A 7-day workweek was the standard and the help needed on the hospital units took precedence over the education of the young women. Lectures would be canceled if their services were needed.

As schools developed, facilities to house nursing students became necessary. Although some of the early programs provided sleeping quarters in the hospital, nursing students usually were housed in a building next to the hospital, often referred to as the "nurses' dormitory." A "housemother" often controlled the nurses' residence. In religious affiliations, a Deaconess or Sister served the same purpose. Housemothers

TABLE 4–3.   Early North American Training Schools for Nurses*

Date	Name and Place	Comments
1798	New York Hospital—New York	Dr. Valentine Seaman initiated a system of instruction for nurses. His lectures covered the topics of anatomy, physiology, maternal nursing, and care of children.
1839	Philadelphia Dispensary—Philadelphia	Dr. Joseph Warrington provided obstetrical training to a group of women who would work with families who would otherwise not receive care. The Nurse Society of Philadelphia grew out of this training.
1861	Bellevue Hospital—New York	Dr. Elizabeth Blackwell converted Bellevue Hospital into a training center for nurses. About 100 women were trained to provide care during the Civil War in an intensive 4-week course.
1861–1862	Women's Hospital of Philadelphia—Philadelphia	Opened a training school, but it progressed slowly until 1872 when it became endowed—the first endowed school of nursing in America. Organized and conducted by two female physicians.
1862	New England Hospital for Women and Children—Boston	Dr. Marie Zakrzewska, a colleague of Dr. Blackwell's, offered a 6-month program to nurses.
1872	New England Training School—Boston	An expansion of the New England Hospital Program has been identified as the first formal school for nurses, under direction of Dr. Susan Dimock. The first graduate was Linda Ann Richards. Mary Mahoney, the first black nurse, also graduated here.
1873—May	Bellevue Training School—New York	First of a trio of schools modeled after the Nightingale model—Lavinia Dock was one of the early graduates.
1873—October	Connecticut Training School—New Haven	Second of the trio of schools started in 1873—introduced first textbook, *New Haven Manual of Nursing,* which was written by a committee of nurses and physicians.
1873—November	Boston Training School—Boston (attached to Massachusetts General)	Third of the trio—Linda Richards became superintendent of nurses in November 1894. Idea for school initiated by the Woman's Educational Association. Medical staff did not support initiation of the school.
1874	St. Catharine's General and Marine Hospital—Ontario, Canada—later called the Mack Training School	Patterned after the Nightingale schools, this program included instruction in the art of nursing, chemistry, sanitary science, physiology, and anatomy.
1877	Training School of the New York Hospital—New York	Offered an 18-month course to prepare graduates for nursing
1878	Boston City Hospital Training School—Boston	Required graduates to complete a 2-year program of study
1884	Toronto General Hospital—Toronto, Canada	Mary Agnes Snively became superintendent of this school, which had early beginnings in 1877.
1884–1885	Farrand Training School for Nurses—Harper Hospital, Detroit	Considered one of the better schools, students had two annual series of lectures, approximately 20 hours total.
1886	Spelman Seminary—Atlanta, GA	The first separate school to educate black nurses, who were often denied admission to other schools.

(continues)

	TABLE 4–3. Early North American Training Schools for Nurses* *(Continued)*

Date	Name and Place	Comments
1888	Mills School of Nursing at Bellevue Hospital— New York	First school established for male nurses. Prepared them to give general patient care.
1889	Johns Hopkins School of Nursing—Baltimore	Program opened under direction of Isabel Hampton Robb. Mary Adelaide Nutting graduated in 1891.
1890	Montreal General— Montreal, Canada	Although wanting a nursing program as early as 1835, hospital conditions would not allow. Nora Gertrude Livingstone established school in 1890.

*Information for this table was gathered primarily from Donahue, 1996 and Kalisch & Kalisch, 1995.

assured that codes of behavior were adhered to and that curfews were enforced. Violations usually resulted in expulsion from the program or the loss of a part of the uniform, such as the bib section of an apron. This signified to all that some infraction had occurred. Young women, who were attracted to nursing because of the imagined glamour of wearing a long crisp white apron and ministering to sick (though handsome) young men, often became discouraged with the severe duties and routine. The attrition rate was high in the early schools.

Although there were some changes in the curriculum—work hours were decreased, the length of study was increased, and the theory component was organized into specific areas of care such as medical, surgical, and obstetrical nursing—hospital-based programs remained largely unchanged through the 1940s and 1950s. The following is a quote from a special publication developed on the occasion of the closing of a diploma school:

FIGURE 4–4   The duties assigned to probationers may have helped operate the hospital but did little to educate the nurse.

In 1921, a nurse was discharged for "cigarette habit." Skirts of nurses' uniforms were getting shorter but there was periodic measurement to be sure some were not too short.

The year 1924 would see Deaconess' first student protest. Student nurses were required to wear their hair long in those days. A number of them though made arrangements with a barber in the Victoria Hotel to stay open late one evening and they all went down and had their hair bobbed in the latest style. They were deprived of their caps for several weeks and ordered to wear switches and what-nots, their punishment comparatively slight, since "banks and other business regularly dismissed employees for social offense" (Deaconess Hospital School of Nursing 1980, p. 10).

Students provided the majority of care given and were seen as such a valuable commodity to the hospital that even small hospitals established nursing programs. This proliferation of schools became a serious concern as early as 1905. Early pioneers and advocates for nursing championed programs that offered a sound educational foundation and reasonable working hours. During the time Isabel Hampton was "Principal" of the Johns Hopkins Training School (a position she accepted in 1889 and continued until her marriage to Dr. Robb in 1894), she arranged for a regular period of 2 hours of free time during a day that was limited to 12 hours. She would have liked to limit the workday to 8 hours, however. Time was allowed for recreation and for meals (Jamieson & Sewell, 1944, p. 432).

Early Textbooks and Journals

There were few textbooks prior to 1900, a factor that complicated the learning process. Many of the lectures presented by physicians were given from notes they had taken while medical students. The first nursing textbook was reportedly the *Handbook of Nursing for Family and General Use*, written by a committee composed of physicians and nurses associated with the Connecticut Training School at New Haven Hospital. Other books followed over the next 2 years. Table 4-4 describes some of the early textbooks.

Nursing journals also appeared toward the end of the 19th century. Five different journals for nurses were published before 1901. The first appeared in 1886 and was entitled *The Nightingale*. In 1889, under the direction of Mary E.P. Davis, a company was formed with 550 cash subscriptions, and a new journal called the *American Journal of Nursing* made its debut in October 1890 (Fig. 4-5). The journal continues to be published today (Kalisch & Kalisch, 1995, pp. 115–116).

 ### Critical Thinking Activity

Imagine that you are an instructor in an early nursing program. There are no textbooks. There are no nursing journals from which you can assign reading. How would you go about teaching the students for whom you are responsible? What would you see as the major concerns? How would the classes differ from those you are in today?

THE AMERICAN JOURNAL OF NURSING

VOL. I OCTOBER, 1900 NO. I

CONTENTS

PUBLISHED MONTHLY BY
J. B. LIPPINCOTT COMPANY
624 CHESTNUT STREET, PHILADELPHIA, PENNA.
FOR THE
ASSOCIATED ALUMNAE OF TRAINED NURSES OF THE UNITED STATES

SUBSCRIPTION PRICE, $2.00 A YEAR SINGLE COPY, 20 CENTS

FIGURE 4–5 Cover of the first issue of the American Journal of Nursing.

TABLE 4–4. Early Nursing Textbooks*		
Date	**Author**	**Title/Topic**
1878	A committee of physicians and nurses	*Hand-book for Family and General Use*
1885	Clara Weeks Shaw	*A Textbook of Nursing for the Use of Training Schools, Families and Private Students*
1890	Lavinia Dock	*The Textbook on Materia Medica for Nurses*
1893	Diana Kimber	The first anatomy book for nurses, *Anatomy and Physiology*
1889 (about)	Isabel Hampton	*Nursing: Its Principles and Practices for Hospital and Private Use*
1894 (about)	Isabel Hampton Robb	*Nursing Ethics*

*Information for the table was gathered primarily from Donahue, 1996 and Kalisch & Kalisch, 1995.

THE BEGINNING OF NURSING ORGANIZATIONS

By the end of the 19th century, conditions had reached a point at which changes were accomplished most effectively through organizations. Nursing pioneers saw this as an opportunity to bring about changes in nursing practice and nursing education.

Nursing Organizations in England

In England, the establishment of an organization for nursing was driven by the energies of Mrs. Bedford Fenwick (Ethel Gordon Manson), a prominent leader who, in 1887, campaigned for nurse registration. She believed that standards were necessary to improve nursing. Although her ideas for nurse registration were not well accepted, she founded the British Nurses' Association in 1888. It grew rapidly to 1000 members by the end of the first year. It later became the Royal British Nurses' Association.

The American Society of Superintendents of Training Schools for Nurses

In 1893, the World's Fair and Columbian Exposition was held in Chicago to celebrate the 400th anniversary of Columbus' arrival in the United States. The Fair provided the meeting place for many professions and artisans. The first nurses' meeting was held in the Hall of Columbus from June 15–17, 1893, as part of the International Congress of Charities, Corrections, and Philanthropy. The nursing meeting was chaired by Isabel Hampton and was attended by American and Canadian nurses. Attendees included such individuals as Lavinia Dock—suffragist, nurse activist, historian, and educator—who spoke on the relation of training schools to hospitals. An address sent by Florence Nightingale was presented to the group. The papers presented were later compiled in a publication, *Nursing the Sick, 1893*. The day after the meeting, Isabel Hampton arranged a meeting of a small group of leaders to discuss the possibility of starting a nursing organization. This meeting resulted in the formation in 1896 of the American Society of Superintendents of Training Schools for Nurses, so named because most of the attendees were directors of nursing schools and the membership was restricted to those nurses associated with nurse training. Concern for the standards of nursing education was primary, and a committee to study nursing education was quickly appointed. In 1907, the Canadian members formed their own organization, the Canadian Society of Superintendents of Training Schools. The American organization changed its name in 1912 to the National League for Nursing Education (Donahue, 1996, p. 326).

In 1952, the National League for Nursing Education became the National League for Nursing when six organizations merged into one. The organizations involved in the merger were the National Organization for Public Health Nursing (est. 1912), the Association of Collegiate Schools of Nursing (est. 1933), the Joint Committee on Practical Nurses and Auxiliary Workers in Nursing Services (est. 1945), the Joint Committee on Careers in Nursing (est. 1946), the National Committee for the Improvement of Nursing Services (est. 1949), and the National Nursing Accrediting Service (est. 1949).

Nurses' Associated Alumnae of the United States and Canada

As the number of nurses increased throughout the United States and as hospitals formed individual alumnae groups, the need arose for an organization of trained nurses. At the third meeting of the American Society of Superintendents of Training Schools in 1896, a committee prepared a constitution and bylaws for such an organization with the delegates representing the various alumnae associations. The constitution was accepted a year later, and the Nurses' Associated Alumnae of the United States and Canada was formed. The first president was Isabel Hampton Robb. The purposes of the group were:

1. To establish and maintain a code of ethics;
2. To elevate the standards of nursing education;
3. To promote the usefulness and honor, the financial and other interests of the nursing profession (American Nurses' Association, 1941, p. 2).

When it was discovered that New York law would not permit foreign membership in an incorporated association, the words "and Canada" were dropped from the title in 1901 and Canadian participation was prohibited. In 1911, the name of the organization in the United States became the American Nurses Association.

In 1908, the Provisional Organization of the Canadian National Association of Trained Nurses was formed, which was renamed the Canadian Nurses Association in 1924. This group also had as its primary concerns the education of nursing students, the improvement of nursing care, the amelioration of conditions for nurses, and state registration of nurses to protect the public.

The International Council of Nurses

The International Council of Nurses, the oldest of all international nursing organizations, was formed in 1899. Founded by Mrs. Bedford Fenwick, it held its first meeting in Buffalo, New York, at the World Exposition in 1901. Mrs. Fenwick was the first president of the organization. The membership originally was composed of self-governing national nurses' associations rather than individual members, although until 1904 individual members could belong because few countries had organized nursing associations. Its purpose was to encourage communication between nurses of all nations and to provide opportunities for nurses from all over the world to meet and discuss concerns about the profession and about patient care. At the present time, the International Council of Nurses meets once every 4 years.

An overview of the major organizations is found in Chapter 3. A quick review of Appendix B can give you insight into the tremendous number of specialty and special interest groups that now exist in nursing. The information provided in this Appendix can help you to research individual organizations that may be of interest to you. As you review Appendix B, you can understand why some critics suggest that nursing has too many organizations working in too many different directions.

Critical Thinking Activity

Research a particular nursing specialty organization. Why did you choose that organization? Compare and contrast the philosophy of that organization with your own.

THE DEVELOPMENT OF HOSPITALS IN THE UNITED STATES

The history of hospitals in the United States can be traced back to the mid-1700s when most cities built *almshouses*, also called poorhouses at the time. Almshouses provided food and shelter for the homeless poor, and served as homes for the aged, the disabled, the mentally ill, and the orphaned. *Pesthouses* also were built at this time to isolate people with contagious diseases, especially those diseases contracted aboard ship. These facilities housed people suffering from cholera, smallpox, typhus, and yellow fever, and the more common communicable diseases such as scarlet fever. Pesthouses would open and close as needed.

Neither almshouses nor pesthouses were institutions from which most individuals would want to seek or receive care. They were crowded and unsanitary, with insufficient heat and ventilation. Cross-infection was common and mortality was high. Those with the financial means were cared for in their homes.

The first hospital founded in what was to become the United States was started in Philadelphia in 1751, at the urging of Benjamin Franklin. Franklin believed that the public had a duty to provide care to the poor, friendless, sick, and insane. A bill, passed that year, authorized the establishment of the Pennsylvania Hospital (Kalisch & Kalisch, 1995). The New York Hospital in New York City was established in 1773, primarily to prevent the spread of infectious diseases brought by sailors and immigrants. Massachusetts General Hospital in Boston opened its doors in 1816, and New Haven Hospital in Connecticut in 1826.

The early hospitals cared for people with acute illnesses and injuries, but did not admit the mentally ill. Several separate hospitals were established for this purpose. The first such facility was established as a department of the Pennsylvania Hospital in 1752. The second was founded in Williamsburg, Virginia, in 1773; the third, known as Friends Hospital, was located in near Philadelphia in 1817. By 1840, eight hospitals to treat the mentally ill had been established (Kalisch & Kalisch, 1995). The cruel and inhumane treatment of patients in the early mental hospitals is legendary. Dorothea Dix, mentioned in Table 4-1, campaigned vigorously for and brought about much reform in the area of mental health treatment. Although never educated as a nurse (she was a schoolteacher), Dix volunteered as a nurse during the Civil War and is included in the Nursing Hall of Fame because of her significant contributions to the profession.

The earliest hospitals left much to be desired. Most were housed in large buildings that had been converted into temporary quarters. Often they were dirty, rank with infection, and poorly ventilated. Linen was used for several patients before it was laundered, even though draining, suppurating wounds were common. The stench was overwhelming, and it is said that nurses used snuff to make working conditions more tolerable (Kalisch & Kalisch, 1995). Hospitals constructed during the early 19th century often followed a block plan in their design, and the buildings resembled large barns. In the 1850s, Massachusetts General Hospital constructed a facility divided into wards or pavilions, each one a separate building with high ceilings and good ventilation. The buildings were built of wood because it was believed they would need to be replaced after 20 years because of contamination (Kalisch & Kalisch, 1995, p 22).

Factors Affecting the Development of Hospitals

Six developments can be cited as major forces that each played a unique role in the continued development of hospitals and patient care:

- Advances in medical science
- The development of medical technology
- Changes in medical education
- The growth of the health insurance industry
- Greater government involvement in health care delivery
- The emergence of professional nursing

ADVANCES IN MEDICAL SCIENCE

By the end of the colonial period, two medical schools had been established in the United States. Before that time, physicians learned their skills through an apprenticeship with a practicing physician. As medicine became more of a science, advances occurred. One of the most significant was the discovery of anesthesia and the rapid advances in surgery that followed. The germ theory also did much to advance the practice of medicine because it inspired the development of agents or techniques that would sterilize or serve as antiseptics. The growth of hospitals in the United States was a direct result of such advances, which made hospitals safer and more desirable. The discovery of sulfa in the mid-1930s and antibiotics in the mid-1940s heralded even greater changes.

THE DEVELOPMENT OF MEDICAL TECHNOLOGY

The development of specialized medical technology was a natural successor to the advances in medical science. The first hospital laboratory was opened in 1889, and x-rays were used in diagnosis in 1896. The electrocardiogram (ECG) was invented in 1903 and the electroencephalogram (EEG) in 1929 (Haglund & Dowling, 1993).

CHANGES IN MEDICAL EDUCATION

Advances in medical education also had a significant impact on the development of health care in the United States. The Flexner Report (see Chapter 5) was completed in 1910, and it led to changes in the structure and content of curricula in medical schools. It also expanded the role of hospitals to include education and research and resulted in internships and residencies for medical students.

GROWTH OF THE HEALTH INSURANCE INDUSTRY

The growth of the health insurance industry is another factor responsible for the development of hospitals. Although there were some antecedents, most sources indicate that the first hospital insurance plan was initiated at Baylor University Hospital in 1929 to serve the needs of schoolteachers in Dallas, Texas (Raffel & Raffel, 1989). The approach used there was to form the model for Blue Cross plans around the country.

Today, figures vary as to what percentage of the population is protected against the costs of medical care by some type of insurance. A report based on the findings from *The Commonwealth Fund 1999 National Survey of Workers' Health Insurance* found that lack of insurance is a significant and growing problem. The study found that nearly one of five (19%) working-age adults lacked health insurance, and that two of five (41%) with incomes less than $20,000 lacked insurance (Millions of Working, 1999). There is great concern for the millions of individuals who have no protection.

GREATER INVOLVEMENT OF THE GOVERNMENT

In early times the government was involved in health care delivery primarily at a local level, building almshouses and facilities for the insane. By 1935, the government was providing grants-in-aid to assist in the establishment of public health and other programs to furnish health assistance to citizens. The Hospital Survey and Construction Act of 1946 (also called the Hill-Burton Act) resulted in the construction of many hospitals and other health facilities. The initiation of Medicare and Medicaid in 1965 made another significant impact on the health care industry because the legislation encouraged capital construction and the development of hospitals through the manner in which the system of reimbursement was structured.

THE EMERGENCE OF PROFESSIONAL NURSING

Another force that significantly influenced the growth of hospitals was the development of professional nursing. Haglund and Dowling (1993, p. 139) cite two ways in which advances in nursing contributed to the growth of hospitals (Fig. 4-6). First, they "increased the efficiency of treatment, cleanliness, nutritious diets, and formal treatment routines" that resulted in patient recovery. Second, they resulted in considerate, skilled patient care that made hospitals acceptable to all people, not just the poor. The role of the nurse and nursing influences the health care delivery system more today than ever before.

HISTORY OF THE NURSING HOME

Like our acute care facilities, the nursing home had a rather harsh beginning. In the 19th century, the government constructed almshouses and poorhouses to shelter the destitute elderly. These facilities attracted a strange mixture of residents, including those who needed asylum and detention, as well as the poor, the chronically disabled, and the mentally ill. According to the moral perspective that prevailed at the time, poverty and disability were viewed as indications of an undisciplined, improvident, and even profligate life. A person who was housed in a "county poorhouse" often had no financial resources and no family to provide care and assistance, and

FIGURE 4–6 The growth of hospitals was significantly influenced by the emergence of modern nursing.

endured a certain social stigma. In time these almshouses became the community "dumping grounds" for all of society's cast-offs. The early facilities for the country's dependent elderly offered the same grim surroundings as the early hospitals. They were unsanitary, overcrowded, and poorly ventilated. Residents were expected to work to assist with their keep if they were able. Individuals who provided care sought employment there usually as a last resort. Appropriations to manage these facilities were meager because most citizens did not identify with the institutions that housed the poor and the transient, who probably had no history of contributing to the community.

As the United States grew as a society, various groups became concerned about the conditions that existed in the poorhouses. Eventually, patients were separated according to their condition and the mentally and chronically ill were reassigned to different hospitals. An increasing number of churches and fraternal organizations started homes to care for their elderly members. As a result of the Social Security Act of 1935, private (for-profit or proprietary) nursing homes emerged during that decade. Raffel and Raffel (1989, p. 205) state, "The original exclusion of benefits for patients in public institutions (since repealed) apparently stemmed from congressional concern about conditions in county poorhouses and a desire to get them closed."

In the postwar period, the Hill-Burton Act of 1946, which supported hospital construction, was expanded to include voluntary (nonprofit) nursing homes, and some states also developed grant programs. Since 1950, government funding for nursing home care has increased steadily, and culminated in the 1965 Medicaid program, which by 1991 covered 40% of all nursing home costs (Callopy et al., 1991). Governmental regulation of nursing homes has become increasingly involved and complex.

As changes in funding occurred and as short-term acute care hospitals became increasingly specialized, the role of the nursing home changed. In the 1950s and 1960s the deinstitutionalization movement, which saw large numbers of the elderly population discharged from mental hospitals, also affected nursing homes. Nursing homes began to assume the role of providing specialized care for the elderly. By the 1960s, this role was well established, but the nursing home industry was plagued by constant reports of substandard and negligent care and, in some instances, charges of absolute abuse of patients and misuse or embezzlement of their funds. This resulted in even greater scrutiny and regulation by the government.

Today, *nursing home* is a broad term that encompasses a wide spectrum of facilities ranging from special units in acute community hospitals to those that are a part of the campus of care retirement centers. Only about 6% have 200 beds or more. The facilities are licensed by the state in which they operate, and each state has its own definitions and requirements. Approximately 75% are certified by Medicare as "skilled nursing facilities," a necessary qualification if Medicare funds are to pay for the care. An even greater percentage are certified to care for Medicaid patients. All facilities receiving federal funds must meet federal as well as state standards. The major reason for admission to a nursing home is functional dependency rather than medical diagnosis. The use of nursing homes will continue to grow in the future as the population grows older, with an estimated national expenditure of $131 billion anticipated by the year 2000 (Williams & Torrens, 1993).

THE AMERICAN HOSPITAL ASSOCIATION

The American Hospital Association was founded in 1899 as the Association of Hospital Superintendents with a membership of nine. Its purpose was to establish and maintain high standards of hospital service, care of the sick, and control and prevention of disease. Nurses who held positions as hospital administrators were instrumental in the early development of this organization, although their roles might have been somewhat passive. It has been suggested that "this passivity cast a negative influence over nurse training standards" (Kalisch & Kalisch, 1995, p. 132). Today's American Hospital Association is an extensive organization with many activities. (See *http://www.aha.org/*)

Critical Thinking Activity

If you had the power to change one single event in the history of nursing, what would it be? Why would you make that change? How do you think it would have affected nursing today?

KEY CONCEPTS

• Nursing has its roots in all endeavors to care for the sick and injured; therefore, it is difficult to pinpoint a particular period in history when nursing first began.
• Nursing's history has influenced the way the profession is recognized by the public. There were three significant images of the nurse in the past: the folk image, the religious image, and the servant image.
• The "Dark Ages of Nursing" occurred during the Reformation, when only those individuals who could not find other employment cared for the ill.
• Florence Nightingale had a significant impact on the form and direction of nursing and established it as a respected field of endeavor. Many of her precepts are still a part of nursing.
• During times when the United States was at war, the serious need for trained nurses to care for the sick and wounded became a public concern.
• Early nursing schools were developed in the United States for the purpose of nursing service as much as for educating young women. The programs were rigorous; often a 7-day workweek consisted of 14-hour workdays.
• Nursing organizations, the forerunners of today's associations, began to emerge toward the end of the 19th century as the pioneers of early nursing saw the need for change in nursing education and nursing practice.
• Acute care hospitals have a history reaching back into the ancient past. Advances in medical science, the development of medical technology, changes in medical education, the growth of the health insurance industry, government involvement,

and the emergence of professional nursing all affected the development of modern hospitals.
- Long-term care facilities have histories similar to that of acute care hospitals; both often started as facilities to house the poor and indigent. Today's nursing homes provide specialized care to the elderly or disabled and rehabilitation services to others.

REFERENCES

Collopy B, Boyle P, Jennings B. New directions in nursing home ethics (A Hastings Center Report Special Supplement, March-April). Hastings Center Rep 21(2):1–16, 1991

Dickens C. Martin Chuzzlewit. *In* The Works of Charles Dickens, vol II. New York: Books Inc, 1936

Deaconess Hospital School of Nursing. Eighty-One Years of Nursing: 1989-1980. Spokane, WA: Deaconess Hospital, 1980

Donahue MP. Why nursing history. In MM Styles & P Moccia (Eds.): On Nursing: A Literary Celebration (p 147). New York, National League for Nursing, Pub. No. 14-2513, 1993

Donahue MP. Nursing: The Finest Art, 2nd ed. St Louis: CV Mosby, 1996

Jan R. Rufaida Al-Asalmiya, the first Muslim nurse. Image: Journal of Nursing Scholarship. 28(3):267–268, 1996

Haglund CL, Dowling WL. The hospital. *In* Williams SJ, Torrens PR: Introduction to Health Service, 4th ed. New York: Delmar Publishers, Inc., 1993:135–176

Hale S. Lady nurses. Godey's Lady's Book and Magazine 82:188, 1871

Jamieson EM, Sewall M. Trends in Nursing History, 2nd ed. Philadelphia: W.B. Saunders Co., 1944

Kalisch PA, Kalisch BJ. The Advance of American Nursing, 3rd ed. Philadelphia: J.B. Lippincott Co., 1995

Klein JA. Honoring female military nurses. BRAVO Veterans Outlook, August-September 1997. Available at: *http://www.nursingnetwork.com/veterans.htm*. Accessed January 14, 2000.

Millions of working Americans can't afford to get sick. The Commonwealth Fund Quarterly, Fall 1999. Available at: *http://www.cmwf.org/publist/quarterly/index.asp*. Accessed January 9, 2000.

Norman, EM. We Band of Angels. New York: Random House, 1999

Nutting MA, Dock LL. A History of Nursing. New York: GP Putnam's Sons, 1935

Raffel MW, Raffel NK. The U.S. Health System: Origins and Functions, 3rd ed. New York: John Wiley & Sons, 1989

Uprichard M. Ferment in nursing. In Auld E, Birum LH: The Challenge of Nursing. St Louis: CV Mosby, 1973:24–31

Whitman A. American Reformers. New York: H.W. Wilson Co., 1985

Williams SJ, Torrens PR. Introduction to Health Service, 4th ed. New York: Delmar Publishers, Inc., 1993

FURTHER READING

Aaronson LS. A challenge for nursing: Reviewing a historic competition. Nurs Outlook 37(6):274–279, 1989

Backer BA. Lillian Wald: Connecting caring with activism. Nurs & Health Care 14(3):122–129, 1993

Bunting S, Campbell JC. Feminism and nursing. Adv Nurs Sci 12(4):11–24, 1990

Calhoun J. The Nightingale Pledge: A commitment that survives the passage of time. Nurs & Health Care 14(3):130–136, 1993

Carnegie ME. The Path We Tread: Blacks in Nursing 1854–1990, 2nd ed. New York: National League for Nursing Press, 1991

Christy T. First fifty years. Am J Nurs 9(9):1778–1784, 1971

Dickson HP. The Badge of Britannia: The History and Reminiscences of the Queen Elizabeth's Overseas Nursing Service, 1886–1966. Edinburgh: Pentland Press, 1990

Dolan JA. Nursing in Society: A Historical Perspective, 14th ed. Philadelphia: WB Saunders, 1978

Griffin GJ, Griffin JK. Jensen's History and Trends of Professional Nursing, 7th ed. St Louis: CV Mosby, 1973

Kalisch BJ, Kalisch PA. Heroine out of focus: Media images of Florence Nightingale: I. Popular biographies and stage productions. Nurs Health Care 4(4):181–187, 1983

Kalisch BJ, Kalisch PA. The nurse-detective in American movies. Nurs Health Care 3(3):146–153, 1982

Kalisch BJ, Kalisch PA, Scobey M. Reflections on a television image. Nurs Health Care 5(5):248–255, 1981

Larisey MM. Attic treasures: A look at nursing history. Nurs Forum 25(1):20–24, 1990

Lewenson S. Taking Charge: Nursing Suffrage and Feminism in America, 1873–1920. New York: Garland, 1993

Mellish JM. A Basic History of Nursing. 2nd ed. Durban: Butterworths, 1990

Melosh B. Not merely a profession: Nurses and resistance to professionalization. Am Behav Scientist 32(6):668–679, 1989

Norman, EM. Women at War: The Story of Fifty Military Nurses Who Served in Vietnam. New York: Random House, 1999

Parsons M. The profession in a class by itself. Nurs Outlook 34(6):270–275, 1985

Pennock MR. Makers of Nursing History. Portraits and Pen Sketches of One-hundred and Nine Prominent Women. New York: Lakeside Publishing Co., 1941

Roberts MM. American Nursing: History and Interpretation. New York: Macmillan, 1954

Schorr TM, Kennedy MS. Celebrating a Century of Caring: 100 Years of American Nursing. Philadelphia: Lippincott, Williams & Wilkins, 1999

Sofer D. On the battleground. Am J Nurs 99(9):33–35

Woodham-Smith C. Florence Nightingale. New York: McGraw-Hill, 1951

Relevant web sites

American Association for the History of Nursing *www.aahn.org*
   (See especially the Internet Resources.)
American Association of Men in Nursing *AAMN.org*
American Hospital Association *www.aha.org*
Army Nurse Corps-History Web Page *www.army.mil/cmh-pg/anc/anchhome.html*
Center for Nursing Historical Inquiry *www.nursing.virginia.edu/center/history.html*
Center for the Study of the History of Nursing *www.nursing.upenn.edu/history*
Florence Nightingale Museum Trust *www.florence-nightingale.co.uk*
History of Nursing Archives *www.bu.edu/speccol/nursing.html*
Margaret M. Allemang Center for the History of Nursing *www.allemang.on.ca*

5

The Development of Nursing as a Profession

Only when we grant love, passion, feeling, and imagination the same legitimacy that we grant reason, logic, and techniques; only when we restore our sense of community and reclaim our place as active participants in our world; only then will we be healthy as individuals, a profession, and a world community.

(Moccia, 1988)

OBJECTIVES

After completing this chapter, you should be able to:

1. Analyze the reasons the profession has had difficulty defining nursing.

2. Discuss the ways in which nursing differs from medicine.

3. Formulate a personal definition of nursing and identify a theorist who defines nursing similarly.

4. Identify the seven characteristics against which social scientists have evaluated professions and examine the ways they can be applied to nursing.

5. Compare and contrast the terms profession and professional.

6. Explain how the image others hold of nursing affects the profession and the role of nurses.

7. Analyze areas of nursing about which studies have been conducted and discuss why each is important.

8. Discuss the concept of a universal language for nursing and describe why nursing classifications are important.

9. Describe some of the traditions in nursing and provide the rationale for why they became traditions.

KEY TERMS

Body of specialized knowledge
Classification
Code of ethics

Formal characteristics
Image
Institutions of higher education

Lifetime commitment
Medicine
North American Nursing Diagnosis Association (NANDA)

Nursing Interventions Classification (NIC)	Profession	Service to the public
	Professional	Studies about nursing
Nursing Outcomes Classification (NOC)	Professional activity	Taxonomy
Occupation	Professional policy	Traditions

What is nursing? Is nursing an art or a science? If it is both, which category should receive the primary emphasis? How can "hunches," "gut feelings," and "intuition" be useful in a world of practicality surrounded by scientific rationale, steeped in protocol, and immersed in critical thinking and clinical pathways? Should nursing be considered a profession or an occupation? What factors are affecting the emergence of nursing as a profession? Does nursing possess a unique body of knowledge? Is the nurse a professional? If so, what educational background qualifies the nurse for professional standing? Should the educational preparation for nursing occur in a variety of settings that award different degrees? How will the skills of graduates from various programs be differentiated in practice? Do different levels of competence exist in the practice of clinical nursing? What is the position of the nurse in relation to other members of the health care team? What is the language of nursing? Is a single language adequate? What is the role of the nurse in preventive care? What is the exclusive role of the nurse? What forces have had a hand in the development of that role? What is the future of that role? What should we remember from our past that can assist in the development of nursing in the future?

These are but a few of the questions being asked by nurses today. Not all the questions have clear or obvious answers. Some of the answers result in debate and dialogue among nurses, health care providers, and health care consumers. As a novice joining the ranks of those who have preceded you, you will want a grasp of the issues that have challenged, and in some instances plagued, nurses over the years. Most novice nurses develop an appreciation of nursing's heritage by gaining an understanding of the nurses who helped to shape the profession. As a nurse in the 21st century, you may have many opportunities to directly influence the answers to these questions.

NURSING DEFINED

When you entered the nursing program in which you are now enrolled, what was your perception of nursing as a profession? Has that perception of nursing been changed by the experiences you have had as a nursing student? Some might ask, "So why spend so much time and effort trying to define nursing?" Chitty (1997, p. 143) helps answer that question. She states, "They [ie, definitions] are a good place to begin in attempting to understand any complex enterprise such as nursing." Defining nursing can be difficult. Nurses themselves cannot agree on a single definition, partly because of the history of nursing. Little is known about the work of the nurse in prehistory; however, Donahue (1996, p. 2) writes, "From the dawn of civilization, evidence prevails to support the premise that *nurturing* has been essential to the preservation of life. Survival of the human race, therefore, is inextricably intertwined with the development of nursing."

A major factor that has made it difficult to define nursing is that it is taught as encompassing both theoretical and practical aspects, but it is pursued (and continues to be defined) primarily through practice, a little studied area. Benner (1984) states, "Nurses have not been careful record keepers of their own clinical learning. . . . This failure to chart our practices and clinical observations has deprived nursing theory of the uniqueness and richness of the knowledge embedded in expert clinical practice." She further discusses the differences between "knowing that" and "knowing how." When attempting to define nursing we often stumble over these two concepts and how to combine the distinct and unique aspects of both.

Early Definitions of Nursing

A nurse is a person who nourishes, fosters, and protects; a person who is prepared to care for the sick, injured, and aged. In this sense "nurse" is used as a noun and is derived from the Latin *nutrix*, which means "nursing mother." The word "nurse" also has referred to a woman who suckled a child (usually not her own)—a wet nurse. Dictionary definitions of nurse include such descriptions as "suckles or nourishes," "to take care of a child or children," "to bring up; rear." In this way "nurse" is used as a verb, deriving from the Latin *nutrire*, which means "to suckle and nourish." With such an origin it is understandable that people generally have associated nursing with women.

References to "the nurse" can be found in the Talmud and in the Old Testament, although the role of the nurse in these references is not clearly defined. The nurse in these texts was probably more similar to the wet nurse than to someone who cared for the sick.

And Deborah, Rebekah's nurse died, and she was buried under an oak below Beth-el: so the name of it was called Allon-bacuth. (Gen. 35:6–8, Revised Standard Version of the Bible)

Over the centuries, the word "nurse" has evolved to refer to a person who tends to the needs of the sick. Florence Nightingale, in her *Notes on Nursing: What It Is and What It Is Not*, described the nurse's role as one that would "put the patient in the best condition for nature to act upon him" (Nightingale, 1860, p. 133), a definition that often is quoted today.

It is more than just a coincidence that the development of nursing as a profession has been inextricably tied to the role of women in society at various times in history, and to the forces that have had an impact on society. We need to remember that it was 1916 when Margaret Sanger opened the first birth control clinic in the United States. And in 1919, after 40 years of campaigning, women in the United States were granted the right to vote through the 19th Amendment to the Constitution. In the past, nurses undoubtedly were more concerned about carrying out their responsibilities than about defining the role of the nurse. Through the years, we have seen the concept of the nurse grow and evolve from the nurse as mother, nourishing and nurturing children, to the nurse, without specific reference to gender, with responsibilities encompassing ever-expanding and challenging services to people needing health care.

Distinguishing Nursing from Medicine

The formulation of clear and concise definitions of nursing also has been hampered by the lack of an obvious distinction between nursing and medicine. For example, it is not unusual to hear a prospective nursing student say, "I've always been interested in the medical field, so I decided to go into nursing." Something of an interdependence exists between medicine and nursing, and they have somewhat paralleled one another in historical development. However, anyone who has been involved in the profession of nursing for any period of time will be quick to assure you that distinct differences exist. The primary differences are the purpose and goal of each profession, and the education needed to fulfill each role. Also, we must acknowledge that historically medicine has been perceived as a profession for men, and nursing a profession for women. Though we can dismiss these stereotypes today, they had an influence on the development of both professions. Finally, the subservient role of the nurse in relationship to the physician in the past has been significant in shaping the definition of nursing.

In general, medicine is concerned with the diagnosis and treatment (and cure, when possible) of disease. Nursing is concerned with caring for the person in a variety of health-related situations. The caring aspects of nursing are well documented in nursing literature (Benner & Wrubel, 1989; Bevis & Watson, 1989; Carper, 1979; Watson, 1979). We think of medicine as being involved with the cure of a patient, and nursing with the care of that patient. The role of the nurse in patient care (today we often refer to this as client care) also involves teaching about health and the prevention of illness, and caring for the ill individual. Nursing takes place in the community and the home, in hospice centers, ambulatory care environments, schools and day care centers, and rehabilitation facilities; in all environments, nurses play a key role in promoting higher standards of health.

With advancing technology in the health care fields, the diverse areas of specialization, the different routes to educational preparation, and the distinct practice settings and roles occupied by the nurse, it is critical that nurses provide clear information for themselves and for the public. To state that you are a registered nurse says little about what you do. It conveys nothing about where you are employed or your educational background. For example, as a registered nurse, you might be employed in a community hospital or in a long-term care facility; you might have a significant role in a critical care unit; you might have earned additional credentials and be working in advanced practice; or you might be a nurse educator.

Thus, you can see that the words "nurse" and "nursing" have been applied to a wide variety of health care activities, in many different settings, performed by people with a variety of different educational backgrounds. The old adage "A nurse, is a nurse, is a nurse" is out of place in a highly technical health care delivery system that struggles to keep "high touch" and "high tech" compatible.

The Effect of Technology on the Definition of Nursing

Technological advances have significantly affected the definition of nursing and the role of the nurse. Also, the methods by which care is delivered have been reshaped significantly. The acute care hospital provides care to patients who are much more acutely ill and who are diagnosed with conditions they would not have survived 25 years ago. Today, recovery is anticipated after careful evaluation and treatment that can require diagnostic procedures (eg, angiography, sonography, or tomography), delicate medical procedures, and specialized critical care nursing that requires a host of variously prepared health care providers. Critical thinking skills are needed to perform the diverse tasks expected of a nurse. Nurses in many positions have been required to assume ever-greater levels of responsibility. Only recently have nurses been given the official authority, autonomy, and recognition that should accompany those responsibilities.

Definitions of Nursing Theorists

Many would stress that any definition of nursing must indicate that it is both an art and a science. It is an art in the sense that it is composed of skills that require expertness and proficiency for their execution. It is a science in the sense that it requires systematized knowledge derived from observation, study, and research. As nursing has grown into a profession, many nursing theorists developed definitions of nursing consistent with their conceptual frameworks. Table 5-1 presents the definitions of some of the theorists.

In 1958, Virginia Henderson, a nurse educator, author, and researcher, was asked by the nursing service committee of the International Council of Nurses to describe her concept of basic nursing. Hers is still one of the most widely accepted definitions of nursing:

The unique function of the nurse is to assist the individual, sick or well, in the performance of those activities contributing to health or its recovery (or to peaceful death) that he would perform unaided if he had the necessary strength, will or knowledge. And to do this in such a way as to help him gain independence as rapidly as possible (Henderson, 1966, p. 15).

TABLE 5–1.   Definitions of Nursing by Major Theorists

Theorist	Major Theme	Definition
Florence Nightingale (1859)	Environment/ Sanitation	The goal of nursing is to put the patient in the best condition for nature to act upon him, primarily by altering the environment.
Hildegard Peplau (1952)	Interpersonal Process	Nursing is viewed as an interpersonal process involving interaction between two or more individuals that has as its common goal assisting the individual who is sick or in need of health care.
Faye Abdellah (1960)	Nursing Problems	Nursing is a service to individuals, families, and society based on an art and science that molds the attitudes, intellectual competencies, and technical skills of the individual nurse into the desire and ability to help people cope with their health care needs, and is focused around twenty-one nursing problems.
Ernestine Wiedenbach (1964)	Nursing Problems Model	Nursing is a helping, nurturing, and caring service rendered with compassion, skill, and understanding, in which sensitivity is key to assisting the nurse in identifying problems.

(continues)

TABLE 5–1.   Definitions of Nursing by Major Theorists *(Continued)*

Theorist	Major Theme	Definition
Virginia Henderson (1966)	Development/Needs	Nursing's role is to assist the individual (sick or well) to carry out those activities . . . he would perform unaided if he had the necessary strength, will, or knowledge.
Myra Levine (1969)	Conservation and Adaptation	Nursing means the nurse interposes her skill and knowledge into the course of events that affect the patient. When influencing adaptation favorably, the nurse is acting in a therapeutic sense. When the nursing intervention cannot alter the course of adaptation, the nurse is acting in a supportive sense.
Ida Jean Orlando (1972)	Interpersonal Process	Nursing's unique and independent role concerns itself with an individual's need for help in an immediate situation for the purpose of avoiding, relieving, diminishing, or curing that individual's sense of helplessness.
Dorothea Orem (1980)	Self-Care	Nursing is concerned with the individual's need for self-care action, which is the practice of activities that individuals initiate and perform on their own behalf in maintaining life, health, and well-being.
Dorothy E. Johnson (1980)	Systems Approach	Nursing is an external regulatory force that acts to preserve the organization and integration of the patient's behavior at an optimal level under those conditions in which the behavior constitutes a threat to physical or social health, or in which illness is found.
Imogene M. King (1981)	Open Systems Approach	The focus of nursing is the care of human beings resulting in the health of individuals and health care for groups, who are viewed as open systems in constant interaction with their environment.
Betty Neuman (1982)	Systems Approach	Nursing responds to individuals, groups, and communities who are in constant interaction with environmental stressors that create disequilibrium. A critical element is the client's ability to react to stress and factors that assist with reconstitution or adaptation.
Sister Callista Roy (1984)	Adaptation	The goal of nursing is the promotion of adaptive responses (those things that positively influence health) that are affected by the person's ability to respond to stimuli. Nursing involves manipulating stimuli to promote adaptive responses.
Martha E. Rogers (1984)	Science of Unitary Man	Nursing is an art and science that is humanistic and humanitarian directed toward the unitary human, and concerned with the nature and direction of human development.

Nursing as Defined by Organizations

Both the American Nurses Association (ANA) and the National Council of State Boards of Nursing have made efforts to define nursing.

AMERICAN NURSES ASSOCIATION DEFINITIONS OF NURSING

In 1965, the American Nurses Association published the "First Paper on Education for Nursing" which identified significant aspects of nursing. It stated that "essential components of professional nursing practice include care, cure, and coordination" (American Nurses Association, 1965, p. 107).

In 1980, the ANA, through its Social Policy Statement, provided yet another definition of nursing: "Nursing is the diagnosis and treatment of human responses to actual or potential health problems" (American Nurses Association, 1980, p. 9). That definition had a widespread effect, and we see its application in the language used in nursing diagnoses today.

NURSING AS DEFINED BY THE NATIONAL COUNCIL OF STATE BOARDS OF NURSING

In 1994, the National Council of State Boards of Nursing (NCSBN) again revised the Model Nurse Practice Act that was first developed in 1982 and revised in 1988. The single most important part of any nurse practice act is the legal definition of nursing practice (see Chapter 7). This legal definition is critical because it provides the foundation and guidelines for education, licensure, scope of practice, and, when necessary, the basis for corrective actions against people who violate the practice act. Although early publications of the Model Nurse Practice Act reflected the difficulty the committee experienced in arriving at a precise and succinct definition, the 1994 revision was clear. It stated, "The 'Practice of Nursing' means assisting individuals or groups to maintain or attain optimal health, implementing a strategy of care to accomplish defined goals, and evaluating responses to care and treatment" (Model Practice Act, National Council of State Boards of Nursing, 1994).

Defining Nursing for the Future

As the profession grows and responsibilities change, undoubtedly we will continue to redefine and refine our definition of nursing. By being responsive to changes, nursing has become more closely aligned with professions such as law, theology, and education, in which changing practices have required greater precision and refinement of definitions of the profession. Recent challenges facing the Task Force on Workforce Regulation of the Pew Health Professions Commission regarding the scope of nursing practice as defined in state practice acts also will encourage examination and clarification of nursing's definition.

Critical Thinking Activity

Analyze the definitions of the major nursing theorists. Develop your own definition of nursing and compare it to those of the theorists and to those of your classmates.

CHARACTERISTICS OF A PROFESSION

The meaning of professionalism has been a subject of debate for many years. The *Flexner Report*, issued in 1910, was one of a series of papers issued by the Carnegie Foundation about professional schools. The Flexner Report, which focused on medicine, provided the incentive for many future efforts to define and discuss the characteristics of a profession (Table 5-2).

When nursing and nursing education were evolving in the United States, no one questioned whether nursing qualified as a profession or whether it was more occupational in nature. As a matter of fact, evidence suggests that from an early date the word "profession" was associated with nursing. Strauss (1966) gives as an example a magazine article entitled "A New Profession for Women" that appeared in 1882. The article described nursing reform, and carried with it a picture of Isabel Hampton. Strauss (1966) also refers to the writings of Lizabeth Price, published in 1892, in which nursing was discussed as a profession.

From approximately the 1950s through the 1970s or mid-1980s, nursing periodically was reviewed against the characteristics of a profession that had been established in the sociological literature. The activities for which nurses were responsible, the legal ramifications of practice, and particularly the education of future nurses were subjected to the scrutiny of sociologists and nursing leaders who found it challenging to examine nursing against established standards.

Some critics challenge that nursing falls short of meeting these criteria. Some of nursing's leaders also would claim that nursing falls short of fulfilling a professional role (Schlotfeldt, 1987; Newman, 1990). Amid these challenges, other nurses are working to advance the standing of nursing through the development of a code of ethics, standards of practice, and peer review. In light of the challenges, it might be helpful to explore how major criteria could be applied to nursing (Fig. 5-1).

A Body of Specialized Knowledge

A primary criticism leveled at nursing is that it has no "body of specialized knowledge" that belongs uniquely to nursing. Critics state that nursing borrows from biologic sciences, social sciences, and medical science, and then combines the various skills and concepts and calls it "nursing." Nursing leaders and theorists disagree whether nursing is a unique profession or one borrowed from other disciplines. In fact, this amalgamation and synthesis of some areas with application to another may be one of the unique qualities of nursing. Nursing researchers also are working to develop an organ-

TABLE 5–2. Criteria for a Profession

Flexner (1915)	Bixler & Bixler (1959)	Pavalko (1971)
• Activities must be intellectual (as opposed to physical) • Activities, because they are based on knowledge, can be learned • Activities must be practical rather than academic • Profession must have teachable techniques • Must have a strong internal organization of members • Practitioners must be motivated by altruism (a desire to help others)	• Utilizes a specialized body of knowledge • Enlarges the body of knowledge it uses and improves its techniques of education and service by the use of the scientific method • Entrusts the education of its practitioners to institutions of higher education • Applies its body of knowledge in practical services which are vital to human and social welfare • Functions autonomously in the formulation of professional policy and in the control of professional activity • Attracts individuals of intellectual and personal qualities who exalt service above personal gain and who recognize their chosen occupation as a lifework • Strives to compensate its practitioners by providing freedom of action, opportunity for continuous professional growth, and economic security	• Work is based on a systematic body of theory and abstract knowledge • Work has recognized social value • Requires a special amount of education to attain specialization • Provides service to the public • Group has freedom to regulate and control its own work behavior (autonomy) • Members are committed toward work as a lifetime or long-term pursuit rather than a stepping stone to another profession • Members share a common identity and possess a distinctive subculture • There exists a code of ethics

ized body of knowledge that is unique to nursing. Nursing theorists are challenging one another to identify and describe the general principles that govern nursing practice. (See Chapter 6 for more information on nursing theories.)

Similarly, nursing leaders are developing a language of nursing, which is discussed later in this chapter. As a result of these efforts, nursing is emerging as a profession with an established body of knowledge.

Use of the Scientific Method to Enlarge the Body of Knowledge

Critical to any profession is its ability to grow and change as the world changes. Equally important is the method by which those changes occur. Changes cannot take

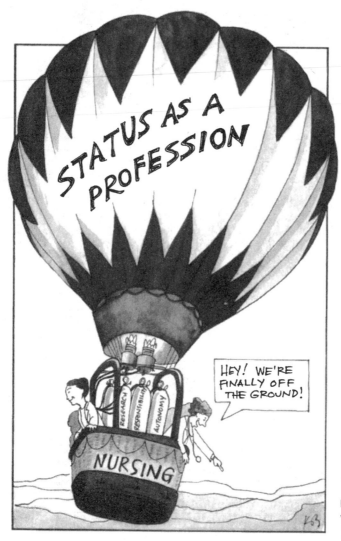

FIGURE 5–1 Some continue to question whether nursing truly can support the title of "profession."

place in a haphazard, random, or hit-or-miss fashion; they must be well thought out. Data must be systematically gathered and carefully analyzed, the problem(s) must be correctly identified, alternative solutions must be sought, the best approach selected and implemented, and the results thoroughly evaluated. As a student of nursing, you already recognize that this has been applied to nursing practice through the nursing process and through critical thinking. Tangible proof of this growth is the quick turnover in nursing textbooks. In a quality program, one seldom finds a clinical text in use that has not been published within the last 4 years. Accreditation criteria set down for nursing programs by the national accrediting agencies require that libraries be stocked with up-to-date references and periodicals. Nursing knowledge also increases because of nursing research and nursing practice. The number of nurses involved in nursing research is growing. Similarly, the number of nursing journals devoted to reporting nursing research results continues to grow. All of this reflects the continued growth of the body of knowledge in nursing through the use of the scientific method.

Education Within Institutions of Higher Education

Perhaps no issue in nursing has been more controversial than the education of its practitioners. Nursing's heritage, like that of medicine, was founded in apprenticeship. Students were assigned to experienced practitioners who taught the skills with which they were familiar. Once those skills were acquired, the student moved into the world of employment. Our earliest programs of education were located in hospitals rather than colleges or universities. (See Chapter 4 for more information on the history of nursing education.)

Over time, the settings in which nurses are educated have changed. Today, most nursing programs preparing registered nurses are located in collegiate settings (at either community colleges or senior colleges or universities). However, not all nurses today are educated in institutions of higher learning. Hospital-based programs still provide an avenue to nursing education. Controversy over the length of nursing education programs (2 versus 4 years) and the "technical" aspects of patient care continues.

Control of Professional Policy and Professional Activity

Most critics reviewing professions against professional standards emphasize the ability of any group to develop its own policy and to function autonomously. Some would suggest that this is an area in which nursing always has been weak, although current health care reform may assist the profession in achieving the full autonomy it has been seeking. Traditionally, the nurse worked under the direction of the patient's physician, often in a hospital setting. The physician wrote the orders for medical care to be implemented by the nurse, and the agency or hospital set the policies under which that care was delivered. Only in the last 50 years has nursing made significant inroads in defining the unique role of the nurse in "care" as opposed to "cure" of the patient. Today, nurses are responsible for planning and implementing the nursing care patients receive, and nurses are also accountable for the care provided. Nursing committees establish policies and protocols. Nursing diagnosis, once challenged as an inappropriate responsibility for nurses, has become a standard of good nursing care. In some practice settings, nurses are eligible for third-party payment; that is, insurance companies reimburse them for the care they have provided. One can anticipate that this situation will continue to improve with health care reform. Although nurses still carry out the medical regimen outlined by physicians, a more collaborative relationship is beginning to occur, and the contribution of the nurse is receiving more recognition. The practice acts of an increasing number of states provide prescriptive authority to nurses who have completed the necessary educational preparation. The number of nurses seeking preparation and working in advanced nursing practice roles is increasing.

All health care professions are changing in response to public demand. Consumers are represented on licensing and accreditation boards, protocols exist for managing conditions and situations, and fees may be established by outside groups. Society is no longer willing to give any profession total autonomy.

A Code of Ethics

The general standard for the professional behavior of nurses in the United States is the ANA Code for Nurses. This document was developed by the ANA and periodically is revised to address current issues in practice. The International Council of Nurses, housed in Geneva, Switzerland, also has developed a code for nurses that reiterates many of the behaviors outlined in the ANA code. The international code sets the standards for ethical practice by nurses throughout the world. Copies of both codes and more discussion regarding the ethical conduct of nurses are found in Chapter 9.

Nursing as a Lifetime Commitment

Bixler and Bixler (1945) emphasized in their list of criteria for professions that a profession should attract people of certain intellectual and personal qualities, who exalt service above personal gain and who consider their chosen occupation to be their life work. Pavalko (1971) also identified as a significant criterion the commitment members have toward work as a lifetime or at least a long-term pursuit rather than a stepping stone to another profession. Studies indicate that most people who prepare for a career in nursing remain in the profession. However, the "burnout" that occurs from stress (see Chapter 11) has become a concern. Most individuals who have been nurses continue to identify themselves as nurses long after they have retired. Today there is a greater likelihood that individuals who enter the profession of nursing at one educational level will continue to advance in practice and education by pursuing additional degrees (and experience). The concept of "articulation" between variously positioned degree-granting institutions is in the forefront of nursing today. More discussion of articulation in nursing education is found in Chapter 6.

Service to the Public

Many theorists list altruism, service to the public, and dedication among criteria for professions. Some suggest that altruism, or the desire to provide for the good of society, must be the worker's motivating force. Nurses have long struggled with the ambiguity that can result from this concept. Possessing a history with a strong religious heritage, the giving of oneself at all costs helped frame the image of nursing and nurses. As nursing has come of age as a profession, we have recognized that "giving away" one's services should not be considered professional. Because nurses expect appropriate remuneration for services rendered does not suggest that they are less than dedicated to the patients for whom they are caring. Providing service to the public should not mean sacrificing one's financial security. Medicine, law, dentistry, and engineering are some examples of professions in which practitioners are amply rewarded financially for the services they provide. Collective bargaining, once viewed as antithetical to professionalism, is becoming an acceptable method of negotiating work-related issues for many professions. Greater discussion of nurses and collective bargaining is included in Chapter 12.

Critical Thinking Activity

> Select one of the characteristics of a profession that you believe nursing does not completely meet. Describe the actions that you believe should occur in the profession that would result in the profession fully meeting that criterion.

DIFFERENTIATING BETWEEN THE TERMS "PROFESSION" AND "PROFESSIONAL"

Nursing involves activities that may be performed by many different caregivers. These people include nurse aides or assistants, practical nurses, and registered nurses prepared for entry into nursing through any of several educational avenues (see Chapter 6). Each of these caregivers contributes to nursing as a profession. To meet the nursing needs of the public, it is essential that caregivers function at various levels of practice. This has led to confusion about the use of the terms *profession* and *professional*. Is there a difference between looking at the practice of nursing in its totality and the "professional" practice of nursing?

A popular view of a professional involves the approach a person has to the role that is required. Most professionals approach their activities earnestly, strive for excellence in performance, and demonstrate a sense of ethics and responsibility in relationship to their careers. Such people consider their work a lifelong endeavor rather than a stepping stone to another field of employment. They place a positive value on being termed professional, and perceive being termed nonprofessional or technical as an adverse reflection on their status, position, and motivation.

Certain people suggest that professionalism has a great deal to do with attitude, dress, conduct, and deportment. The attributes that are considered professional vary according to the personal values and stereotypes of the person doing the evaluating. For example, an early concept of the "truly professional" nurse was that of a person dressed in a starched white uniform and cap, whose hair was off her collar, and whose shoes were freshly polished. Some individuals would continue to support this concept of the "professional nurse." Others might perceive the "professional nurse" as one who is open and kind in interpersonal relationships, who focuses on the needs of others, and who is tactful and skillful in interview techniques.

In at least one instance, federal legislation has helped to establish a list of the characteristics of a professional. Public Law 93-360 (Labor Management Relations Act, 1947 [amended, 1959, 1974]), which governs collective bargaining activities, defines the professional employee as follows:

(a) any employee engaged in work (i) predominantly intellectual and varied in character as opposed to routine mental, manual, mechanical, or physical work; (ii) involving the consistent exercise of discretion and judgment in its performance; (iii) of such a character that the output produced or the result accomplished cannot be standardized in relation to a given period of time; (iv) requiring knowledge of an advanced type in a field of science or learning customarily acquired by a prolonged course of specialized intellectual instruction and study in an institution of higher learning or a hospital, as distinguished from a general academic education or from an apprenticeship or from training in the performance of routine mental, manual, or physical processes; or

(b) any employee, who (i) has completed the courses of specialized intellectual instruction and study described in clause (iv) of paragraph (a), and (ii) is performing related work under the supervision of a professional person to qualify himself to become a professional employee as defined in paragraph (a).

The sociological and legal definitions are much more restrictive than the popular concept associated with the term professional. A communication block can result from people using the term in different ways. When one person is using a restrictive, sociological definition and the other person responds from a standpoint of personal belief and feeling, agreement is almost impossible. Styles offers a refreshing approach. She has used the word *professionhood* rather than professionalism and suggests that nurses would be better served by a set of internal beliefs about nursing (that force us to pay attention to our own image as the dominant figure) than by a set of external criteria about professions (Styles, 1982).

THE IMAGE OF NURSING TODAY

During the late 1970s and early 1980s, much time and energy were invested in studying the image of nursing. Much of this work was done by Beatrice and Philip Kalisch, who have written prolifically about the topic. Their writing focuses on segments of an overall study of the image of the nurse in various forms of mass media, including radio, movies, television, newspapers, magazines, and novels. They believe that popular attitudes and assumptions about nurses and what nurses contribute to a patient's welfare can greatly influence the future of nursing. It is their contention that since the 1970s, the popular image of the nurse not only has failed to reflect changing professional conditions, but has been based on derogatory stereotypes that have undermined public confidence in and respect for the professional nurse. Nurses should be concerned about negative or incorrect images because such images can influence the attitudes of patients, policy-makers, and politicians. Negative attitudes about nursing also may discourage many capable prospective nurses, who will choose another career that offers greater appeal in stature, status, and salary.

Television and Motion Pictures

An important source of information in this country is television and motion pictures. From studing nurses on television, Kalisch and Kalisch found that nurses often had no substantive role in the television stories they investigated, with nursing being a part of the hospital background in programs that focused on physician characters. The role of the physician was viewed as more important and physicians scored high on such attributes as ambition, intelligence, rationality, aggression, self-confidence, and altruism. When a nurse was the focus of a program, the story line involved the nurse's personal problems, rather than her role as a nurse. The nurse often was portrayed as the "handmaiden" to the physician, and scored high on such attributes as obedience, permissiveness, conformity, flexibility, and serenity. It is interesting to note that nurses ranked lower than physicians on such items as humanism, self-sacrifice, duty, and family concern, all of which are values traditionally ascribed to nurses (Kalisch & Kalisch, 1982a). This may be changing as the 1990s saw the debut of television shows such as "ER" and "Chicago Hope" that depict nurses as responsible decision-makers.

Kalisch and Kalisch found a rise and fall in the image of nurses in motion pictures, with the high point occurring during the war years of the 1940s and the low point occurring in the 1970s, when the nursing profession was denigrated and satirized in many films (Fig. 5-2). Because the largest proportions of moviegoers each year are adolescents, the image of nurses in movies will have an impact on the attitudes of students who are prospective nurses. The earlier, positive images of nurses usually came from films that were biographies of outstanding nurses such as Sister Kenny, who worked with polio patients, or Edith Cavell, a World War I heroine (who was discussed in Chapter 4). For a time the nurse-detective was a popular character in films; such nurses were portrayed as intelligent, perceptive, confident, sophisticated, composed, tough, and assertive. During the 1970s, however, nurses often were portrayed as malevolent and sadistic (eg, the roles of Nurse Ratched in *One Flew Over the Cuckoo's Nest* and Nurse Diesel in *High Anxiety*). This was the lowest point for the image of nurses in the history of film; nurses in film were lacking in such values as duty, self-sacrifice, achievement, integrity, virtue, intelligence, rationality, and kindness. Few films centered on the

FIGURE 5–2 Nurses should be concerned about negative or incorrect images because these are sure to influence the attitudes of patients, policymakers, and politicians.

individual achievement or personal autonomy of the nurse. When compared with the physician's role, the nurse's role was seen as less important (Kalisch & Kalisch, 1982b). There is hope that this trend is reversing, however. The film, "The English Patient," which received the Oscar as Best Picture of the Year in 1997, added credibility to the role of the nurse by portraying the nurse character as caring, thinking, and involved.

The Image of the Nurse in Print

To study the image of nursing in novels, Kalisch and Kalisch analyzed 207 books. As with film and television, they found that the nurse in the novel was almost always female, single, childless, white, and younger than the age of 35.

Because nurses almost always were depicted in novels as women, traditional female roles (ie, wife, mistress, mother) were emphasized. Three nurse stereotypes have resulted:

1. The nurse as man's companion
2. The nurse as man's destroyer
3. The nurse as man's mother or the mother of his children

The man in the novel is often a physician. Novelists of the 1970s and 1980s often maligned their nurse characters, ignoring the nurses' professional motivations and health care perspectives (Kalisch & Kalisch, 1982c).

Muff (1988) analyzed feminine myths and stereotypes and has elaborated on nursing stereotypes. After reading books about nurses written for school-aged children (eg, Cherry Ames, Sue Barton, Kathy Martin, and Penny Scott), she drew the following conclusions:

* Nursing is described as glamorous.
* Medicine and nursing are imbued with a sense of mystery and elitism.
* Nursing is simplistic.
* Nurses move from job to job.
* Nurses are subservient and deferential, following orders, running errands, and idolizing physicians for whom they work.

All of the nurses in these books were educated in hospital-based diploma programs, earning the "R.N." only after hours of hospital service, even though the Martin and Scott series were both written in the 1960s.

Muff (1988) also examined the role of the nurse as it is captured in the romance novel. In many instances appearances (eg, the color and condition of the nurse's hair) were most important, and the nurse was portrayed as a "pure" girl, dressed in white, whose main aim was to get a man, usually a doctor. Women who were not looking for husbands were in nursing for altruistic reasons, and duty and self-sacrifice were glamorized. Muff also found that the image of the nurse in the novel usually could be placed into one of the following categories: ministering angels, handmaidens, battle-axes, fools, and whores. She stated that the stereotypes of nursing presented in television and film also usually fit one of these categories. When reviewing the nurse image on get-well cards, she had to add a new category, that of "token torturer."

Only newspapers and newsmagazines tended toward realism rather than fantasy. News articles examined the shortage of nurses, discussing reasons for it (such as working conditions, salaries, benefits, and hardships). Special feature articles also provided information about new or unique nursing roles, such as those of nurses in Vietnam (Muff, 1982). With the outbreak of war in the Middle East in 1991, nurses received positive recognition by the media. Nurses serving in reserve status with branches of the military were among the first called up when the conflict began. As our society recognizes the need to honor women as well as men for their contributions, nurses are often singled out for special recognition—especially during wartime. (See Chapter 4 for discussion of recognition honoring nurses.)

As we moved into the 1990s, it was hoped that the image of nursing would improve; to some extent that has been true. Suzanne Gordon, a journalist who is not a nurse, became interested in the profession and has written about nurses and nursing. In *Life Support: Three Nurses on the Front Lines*, she realistically captures the challenges to the profession and addresses concerns about the undermining of nursing and of patients' healing through a health care system that is replacing caring with profit margins. However, the books have received more attention from nurses than from the people who most need to read them. In 1999, *Wit*, a play written by first-time playwright Margaret Edson after leaving a unit clerk job in a cancer research hospital, opened on Broadway. In this play, the nurse is the hero (Gordon, 1999).

In 1997, the University of Rochester conducted a study of nurses in the media, titled the *Woodhull Study on Nursing and the Media: Health Care's Invisible Partner.* It was named for Nancy Woodhull, the founding editor of *USA Today*, who became concerned about the lack of media coverage of nurses when she received care for lung cancer, which claimed her life in 1997. Commissioned by Sigma Theta Tau International, the study analyzed health care media coverage occurring in a single month. It examined over 20,000 articles for content, of which 2,500 health care-related articles were studied in depth. The study found that nurses are "virtually invisible in media coverage of health care." It further found that "The few references to nurses or nursing were mostly in passing, with no in-depth coverage" (Sieber et al., 1998).

Although some might argue that nurses have better things to do than to worry about how the nurse is portrayed in the media, a consistently misrepresented image can negatively affect how the public thinks about nurses. Therefore, nurses have responded to television advertisements or programs that portray nurses and nursing in a negative light with letters and telephone calls. Boycotts on the purchase of products that present nurses poorly in advertisements have proved to be an effective way to bring about change. They have resulted in the cancellation of a television show that cast nursing in an inaccurate and demeaning light. In addition, various nursing organizations have waged campaigns to enhance the image of nursing by emphasizing nursing as a prestigious, desirable, and respected career.

Following the Woodhull Study, the American Nurses Association (ANA) initiated a program titled "RN = Real News," which was a media outreach program to showcase nurses as experts in the area of health care. This initiative included a media speaker program and a media-training tool to help nurses gain the basic skills and confidence necessary for dealing effectively with the media (Stewart, 1999). More information about this program can be obtained by contacting ANA's Web site, *http://www.nursingworld.org* and clicking on "Nurses' Toolkit."

Critical Thinking Activity

Interview five of your friends who are not nurses. What is their image of nursing? What do they understand of the role of the nurse? Do they view nursing positively?

STUDIES FOR AND ABOUT NURSING

Early in the 20th century, the quality of many nursing schools and their graduates was poor, and many of Florence Nightingale's admonitions regarding nursing education were forgotten. Nurses, doctors, friends, and critics of nursing became concerned about the inadequate preparation being offered. Before the problem could be corrected, it was necessary to learn more about the programs and how nurses were being used in the employment market. To accomplish this, studies about nursing and nurses were initiated.

We recognize that many students in nursing are not excited by studies, especially not by those conducted years ago. However, they have affected the development of nursing as a profession, and it is important to discuss significant studies (Fig. 5-3). We think you will recognize some recurring themes that remain relevant today.

Although the first nursing studies were not begun until the early 1900s, the number of studies since the 1950s has been voluminous. It is impossible to look at any professional nursing publication and not find mention of some new study in progress. In an effort to classify and catalog references to these studies, Virginia Henderson prepared *A Nursing Studies Index*. In 1952, a group of nurses, under the sponsorship of the Association of Collegiate Schools of Nursing, launched a new journal called *Nursing Research*, which was designed to disseminate information about nursing research.

A single individual conducted many of the early studies with a particular purpose in mind. Over the years, studies often took the form of a "report" by a special group of individuals, often appointed by a governmental or professional agency. Although by no means inclusive of all studies and reports, Table 5-3 highlights some of the major significant studies of nursing that have provided benchmarks to the profession. Following is a discussion of some of the major studies and their impact on nursing.

Early Studies

One of the earliest nursing studies was carried out under the guidance of M. Adelaide Nutting in 1912. Published by the U.S. Bureau of Education, it was entitled "The Educational Status of Nursing." The study investigated what and how nursing students were taught, and under what conditions students lived. Although it did not receive the attention it probably deserved, it began to establish nursing as a profession, suggesting

FIGURE 5–3   The development of nursing as a profession has been affected by the many studies about nursing.

that schools of nursing be independent from hospitals and leading the way to more studies.

The Winslow-Goldmark Report, sometimes called the Goldmark Report, followed in 1923. It was also referred to as "The Study of Nursing and Nursing Education in the United States" (Winslow-Goldmark Report, 1923) and was the work of a committee composed of physicians, nurses, and lay people. The report focused on the preparation of public health nurses, teachers, administrators, the clinical learning experiences of students, and on the financing of schools. Subsequently, the Yale University School of Nursing and the Vanderbilt University School of Nursing were established, funded by an endowment from the Rockefeller Foundation.

A three-part study, sponsored by the Committee on the Grading of Nursing Schools (a 21-member group of representatives from many nursing and medical professional organizations), was conducted between 1928 and 1934. The first part, which was socioeconomic in nature, was entitled "Nurses, Patients, and Pocketbooks." It attempted to determine if there was a shortage of nurses in the United States. The second part, "An Activity Analysis of Nursing," examined those nursing activities that could be used as a basis for improving the curricula in nursing schools. Part three, "Nursing Schools Today and Tomorrow," described the schools of the period and made recommendations for professional schools.

TABLE 5–3.   Major Studies About Nursing

Date	Name of Study	Primary Investigator/Sponsor	Focus and Recommendation
1912	*The Educational Status of Nursing*	M. Adelaide Nutting/ U.S. Bureau of Education	What and how students were being taught and conditions under which they were living. Began to establish nursing as a profession
1923	*Winslow-Goldmark Report on Nursing and Nursing Education in the United States*	Josephine Goldmark/ Rockefeller Foundation	The educational preparation of students including public health nurses, teachers, and supervisors. It pointed out fundamental faults in hospital training schools and resulted in the establishment of the Yale University School of Nursing.
	Committee on the Grading of Nursing Schools—a three-part study	Francis Payne Bolton and contributions of thousands of nurses	
1928	*(1) Nurses, Patients, and Pocketbooks*	May Ayres Burgess/ statistician	An inquiry into the supply and demand for nurses. Demonstrated that there was an oversupply of nurses
1934	*(2) An Activity Analysis of Nursing*	Ethel Johns and Blance Pfefferkorn	Looked at the activities that constitute nursing as a basis for improving curricula
1934	*(3) Nursing Schools Today & Tomorrow*	Ethel Johns	Described the nursing schools of the period and made recommendations about professional schools
1937	*A Curriculum Guide for Schools of Nursing*—Not truly a study of nursing, but often referred to as one because of its far reaching effects	National League for Nursing Education	A revision of a 1917 publication, it outlined the curricula for a 3-year course, emphasizing sound educational teaching procedures. Followed by many schools of the time
1948	*Nursing for the Future*	Esther Lucille Brown/ Carnegie Foundation, the Russell Sage Foundation, and the National Nursing Council	Done to determine society's need for nursing. Described inadequacies in nursing schools. Resulted in recommendations that nursing education be placed in universities and colleges and encouraged recruitment of large numbers of men and members of minority groups into nursing schools
1948	*The Ginzberg Report or A Program for the Nursing Profession*—a report of the discussions of the Committee on the Functions of Nursing	Eli Ginzberg/Columbia University	Reviewed problems centering around the shortage of nurses. Recommended that nursing teams consisting of variously educated nurses be developed

(continues)

TABLE 5–3.   Major Studies About Nursing *(Continued)*

Date	Name of Study	Primary Investigator/Sponsor	Focus and Recommendation
1950	*Nursing Schools at the Mid-Century*	Margaret Bridgman/ National Committee for the Improvement of Nursing Services— Russell Sage Foundation	Studied the practices of over 1000 nursing schools (including organization, costs, curriculum, clinical resources, and student health) and stimulated improvement in baccalaureate schools
1955	*Patterns of Patient Care*	Francis George and Ruth Perkins Kuehn/ University of Pittsburgh	Assessed the amount of nursing service needed by a group of medical/surgical patients and determined how much of that care could be delegated to nursing aides and other nonprofessional people
1958	*Twenty Thousand Nurses Tell Their Story*	Everett C. Hughes/ANA and American Nurses Foundation	Looked at nurses, what they were doing, their attitudes toward their jobs, and job satisfaction. Formed basis for development of nursing functions, standards, and qualifications
1959	*Community College Education for Nursing*	Mildred Montag/Institute of Research and Service in Nursing Education— Teachers College, Columbia University	Reported the findings of a 5-year study of eight 2-year nursing programs. Led to the establishment of more Associate Degree programs
1963	*Toward Quality in Nursing: Needs and Goals*	W. Allen Wallis— Consultant Group on Nursing—a panel of nurses in the health field/ U.S. Public Health Service	A report requested by the U.S. Surgeon General to determine funding priorities. Advised on the need for nurses, recruitment concerns, need for nursing research, and improvement of nursing education
1970	*An Abstract for Action* (a report of the National Commission on Nursing and Nursing Education)	Jerome Lysaught/ANA, ANF, NLN, Mellon and Kellogg Foundations	Looked at current practices and patterns of nursing. Suggested joint practice committees, master planning for nursing education, funding for nursing education and research
1979	*The Study of Credentialing in Nursing*	Inez Hinsvark/ANA	A review of credentialing—especially of nursing. Resulted in the appointment of a Task Force. Supported a freestanding credentialing center for nursing
1983	*National Institute of Medicine Study*	Katherine Bauer/DHHS	Required by the Nursing Training Act of 1979, determined the need for continued outlay of federal money for nursing education. Resulted in 21 specific recommendations. Found that the shortage of nurses of the 1960s and 1970s no longer existed, that federal support of nursing education should focus on graduate study, and that the federal government should discontinue efforts to increase "generalist nurses"

(continues)

TABLE 5–3.   Major Studies About Nursing *(Continued)*

Date	Name of Study	Primary Investigator/Sponsor	Focus and Recommendation
1988	*Secretary's Commission on Nursing*	Lillian Gibbons/DHHS	Responded to serious nursing shortage. Validated the shortage. Recommended increased financial support of education and improved status and working conditions for nurses
1990	*Secretary's Commission on the National Nursing Shortage*	Caroline Burnett/DHHS	Appointed for 1 year to advise on implementation of 1988 report. Had three main foci: recruitment and retention, restructuring of nursing service, and use of nursing personnel and information systems
1991	*Report of the National Commission of Nursing Implementation Project (NCNIP)*	Vivian De Back/ANA, NLN, AACN, AONE, Kellogg Foundation	Looked at nursing education, practice, management and research and developed recommendations for the future of nursing
1993	*Health Professions Education for the Future*	E.H. O'Neill/Pew Health Professions Commission— Pew Charitable Trusts	Reinforced the belief that the education of health professions was not adequate to meet the health needs of America. Identified competencies for 2005 and emphasized the need for nurse-midwives, nurse practitioners, and the role of nurses in health promotion
1995	*Reforming Health Care Workforce Regulation*	Pew Health Professions Commission	Had as its mission assisting schools preparing health professionals to understand the changing nature of health care, the needs for the future, and how to design and implement the programs preparing these workers. Recommended reform of the licensing process, specifically elimination of exclusive scopes of practice

In 1932, the National League for Nursing Education (later to become the National League for Nursing) conducted its first study, a comparative study of the bedside activities of graduate and student nurses. The study indicated that nursing care should be given by graduate nurses rather than students, and provided information about the number of tasks assigned to nursing students that had nothing to do with acquiring a nursing education.

The last of the early nursing studies that we mention was not really a study, but often is referred to as one because of its far-reaching impact. *A Curriculum Guide for Schools of Nursing*, published in 1937, was a revised version of a document published in 1917. It outlined the curricula for a 3-year course, emphasizing sound educational teaching procedures. It was read and followed by many schools that were operating programs at that time.

Midcentury Studies

By the 1950s studies about nurses and nursing were numerous and dealt with many aspects of the profession. Only a few of those studies are mentioned here.

Of particular significance was a study published in 1948 entitled "Nursing for the Future." Conducted by Esther Lucille Brown, a social anthropologist, the study is also known as the Brown report. Funded by the Carnegie Foundation, the study was done to determine society's need for nursing and nurses, and recommended higher education for nurses. It prompted serious examination of professional education and pointed out weaknesses in the existing educational programs. The investigators recommended that basic schools of nursing be placed in universities and colleges, and encouraged the recruitment of large numbers of men and minorities into nursing schools. This report set the stage for studies of nursing education that followed in the 1950s and 1960s, and for recommendations that were to continue into the 1990s.

The Ginzberg report was published the same year. A report rather than a study, it reviewed problems centering on the current and prospective shortage of nurses. The conclusions and recommendations were published in the book entitled *A Program for the Nursing Profession*. The report recommended that nursing teams consisting of 4-year professional nurses, 2-year registered nurses, and 1-year practical nurses be developed. This would ease the nursing shortage by enabling each member of the team to function in the role for which he or she was educationally prepared. Today we continue to struggle with the utilization of graduates according to their educational preparation.

In 1958, a study entitled *Twenty Thousand Nurses Tell Their Story* was published. It was part of a 5-year research project that was conceived by the ANA and financially supported by nurses throughout the country. The study looked at nurses, what they were doing, their attitudes toward their jobs, and their job satisfaction. As a result, nurses learned a great deal about themselves.

Another significant study was initiated by Mildred Montag and was published in 1959. This study on "Community College Education for Nursing" resulted in the creation of associate degree nursing education (see Chapter 6).

Significant Studies of the 1960s and 1970s

In 1961, the Surgeon General of the U.S. Public Health Service appointed a 25-member panel called the Consultant Group of Nursing. This group was to advise him on nursing needs and identify the role of the federal government in assessing nursing services to the nation. In 1963, this group presented a report entitled *Toward Quality in Nursing*, which recommended a national investigation of nursing education that would place emphasis on the criteria for high-quality patient care.

After publication of *Toward Quality in Nursing*, the ANA and the NLN appropriated funds and established a joint committee to study ways to conduct and finance a national inquiry of nursing education. Later the study was expanded to reflect on probable requirements in professional nursing that would occur over several decades to come, and to examine changing practices and educational patterns of the present time. Financing was obtained from the American Nurses Foundation, the Kellogg

Foundation, the Avalon Foundation, and an anonymous benefactor. To conduct the study, the National Commission for the Study of Nursing and Nursing Education was set up as an independent agency and functioned as a self-directing group. The 12 commissioners were chosen for their broad knowledge of nursing, for their skills in related disciplines, or for their competencies in relevant fields, with no commissioner representing a particular interest group or position.

The study focused on the supply and demand for nurses, nursing roles and functions, nursing education, and nursing as a career. The commission found it necessary not only to examine these key concerns but also to relate these issues to the social system that provides care to the public.

The final report of the commission, *An Abstract for Action*, was published in 1970. It included 58 specific recommendations and concluded with four central recommendations. It also listed three basic priorities:

1. Increased research on both the practice and education of nurses
2. Enhanced educational systems and curricula based on research
3. Increased financial support for nurses and for nursing

In 1973, a progress report from the National Commission for the Study of Nursing and Nursing Education concerning the implementation of the recommendations of the original report was published under the title *From Abstract into Action*. The commission believed that it was imperative that nursing achieve the goals established in the recommendations so that nursing could emerge as a full profession and assist in providing optimal health care for this country.

Studies of the 1980s

One of the major studies of nursing conducted in the 1980s was that of the National Commission on Nursing. This group was composed of 30 commissioners from disciplines such as nursing, hospital management, business, government, education, and medicine—all of whom were concerned about the current nursing-related problems in the health care system, especially the apparent shortage of nurses. The American Hospital Association, Hospital Research and Educational Trust, and the American Hospital Supply Corporation sponsored the commission. The group began its work in September 1980 and focused on areas that dealt primarily with the environments in which nurses worked, the relationship between nursing education and nursing practice, nursing issues, and the status of nursing as a profession (National Commission on Nursing, 1981).

The commission began systematically to examine and evaluate data sources, including journal articles, state studies, and policy documents. A series of public hearings held in six major cities across the nation and two open forums provided the opportunity for input about nursing issues from each region of the country. The highlights of the findings, along with the commission's recommendations and future action plans, were published in the initial report of the group in September 1981. The final recommendations were published in 1983. Although the findings and recommendations are too lengthy to be included in this chapter in their entirety, it is important to mention the five major categories of issues identified by the study (National Commission on Nursing, 1981, p. 5):

1. The status and image of nursing, which includes changes in the nursing role
2. The interface of nursing education and practice, including models of education for preparing to practice
3. The effective management of the nursing resource, including such factors as job satisfaction, recruitment, and retention
4. The relationship among nursing, medical staff, and hospital administration, including nursing's participation in decision-making
5. The maturing of nursing as a self-determining profession, including defining and determining the nature and scope of practice, the role of nursing leadership, increasing decision making in nursing practice, and the need for unity in the nursing profession

Many of the commission's findings were not surprising to people who were involved with nursing. Included were findings indicating that physicians and health care administrators often did not understand the role of nurses in patient care, and that traditional and outdated images of nurses (including Victorian stereotypes and traditional male-female relationships) impeded acceptance of current roles. Some physicians and administrators thought that nurses were overeducated, and did not support an increase in the nurse's authority to make decisions concerning health care.

The findings that individuals and nursing groups are not unified in defining fundamental, professional goals for nursing, and that nursing, as a profession, lacks cohesiveness and a clear understanding of its role and direction, were not a revelation to many seasoned nurses. These same nurses also were not astonished to learn of the numerous and diverse associations that represent nursing but lack a way to determine common goals for nursing education, practice, and credentialing. The disagreement and confusion about educational preparation for nurses, and the controversy about entry into practice, were identified as further obstacles to the advancement of the profession. Clearly there is a need for a system of nursing education that promotes realistic expectations, provides appropriate support for practice and advancement, and includes educational mobility in nursing. As we begin the 21st century, nursing continues to grapple with many of these issues. A number of the issues are one with which nursing has struggled for years; most of them will not be completely resolved in the next decade. As a new graduate, you will have the opportunity to influence their outcome.

Following in the footsteps of the National Commission of Nursing was the National Commission on Nursing Implementation Project, which began in 1985. Funded by the W. K. Kellogg Foundation for 3 years, the project was cosponsored by the NLN, the ANA, the American Organization of Nurse Executives, and the American Association of Colleges of Nursing. Administered by the American Nurses' Foundation, its purpose was to provide leadership in seeking consensus about the appropriate education and credentialing for basic nursing practice, effective models for the delivery of nursing care, and the means for developing and testing nursing knowledge. The aim of this project was to lay the groundwork and take action wherever possible to support effective, high-quality nursing care delivery in the immediate and long-range future.

The results of another nursing study were released in January 1983. This 2-year study, mandated under the 1979 Nurse Training Amendments, was conducted by the Institute of Medicine Committee on Nursing and Nursing Education and was funded by the Department of Health and Human Services at a cost of $1.6 million. The objectives of the study were:

- To provide advice regarding federal support for nursing education
- To gain more information about nurses; to learn, for example, why they do not seek employment in medically underserved areas and why they leave the profession
- To make recommendations regarding measures to improve the supply and use of nursing resources.

The study made 21 specific recommendations to Congress. Because the study found that the shortage of nurses in the 1960s and 1970s had largely disappeared, it was recommended that the federal government discontinue efforts to increase the supply of "generalist nurses." (I.O.M. study, 1983).

The fallacies in these findings soon became apparent. Across the nation, nursing enrollments plummeted in the late 1980s. This drop in enrollment occurred at a time when nurses were assuming expanded roles and more nurses than ever were needed for the delivery of health care throughout the nation. The result was a serious national shortage of nurses, especially in certain settings and in specific areas of care, such as long-term care.

Studies of the 1990s

Responding to the need for more nurses, many studies of the early 1990s focused on the roles of nurses in the delivery of health care, on educational patterns that would encourage capable individuals to choose nursing as a career, and on programs that would facilitate educational mobility. Issues related to the nurse's image and the nursing shortage merged. A new Commission on the National Nursing Shortage replaced the Federal Commission on Nursing, and $275,000 was budgeted to assist in its function. This commission developed strategies to decrease the nursing shortage, which focused on recruitment, retention, restructuring of nursing services for the most effective use of nursing personnel, and gathering data about nursing and the information systems used in nursing.

Another group whose work has significantly affected nursing is that of the Pew Health Professions Commission (see Chapter 1). Although issued in the form of reports rather than a study, per se, the recommendations that have come from the Commission caused many nursing organizations to take a serious look at themselves and their activities. The reports of the Commission addressed issues related to nursing education, to credentialing, and to the supply of health care professionals. The recommendations in the first report regarding nursing education included the following:

- Recognizing the value of the multiple entry points of professional practice
- Consolidating professional nomenclature so that there is a single title for each level of nursing preparation and service

- Determining the practice responsibilities associated with different levels of nursing education
- Reducing the size and number of nursing education programs (with the suggestion that the reductions occur in associate degree and diploma programs)
- Expanding the number of masters level nurse practitioner programs.

The second report dealt with credentialing issues and recommended that scopes of practice be eliminated and that unlicensed personnel be employed in health care (see Chapter 7 for more detail). It also addressed the need to ensure competence among today's licensed health care practitioners.

 Critical Thinking Exercise

Identify at least three areas in nursing that you believe need further study, and describe how you would begin to conduct those studies. Whom would you involve?

DEFINING A LANGUAGE FOR NURSING

For many, the development of a special language for nursing is a fairly new development. It began as an effort to develop a language that would describe the clinical judgments made by nurses that are not in medical language systems. However, as early as 1909, nurses with a strong eye to the future and professionalism recognized that nursing would someday need a language of its own. Ninety years ago, Isabel Hampton Robb wrote the following after attending a meeting of the newly formed International Council of Nurses.

While attending a special meeting of the ICN in Paris, I was naturally at once struck by the fact that the methods and the ways of regarding nursing problems were . . . as foreign to the various delegations as were the actual languages, and the thought occurred to me that . . . sooner or later we must put ourselves upon a common basis and work out what may be termed a "nursing esperanto" which would in the course of time give us a universal nursing language (Hampton-Robb, 1909).

Defining a language for nursing primarily involves the development and refinement of *nursing nomenclatures* and *classification systems* that communicate information and guide data collection about nursing activities. The term "nursing nomenclature" refers to the words by which we name or describe phenomena in nursing. A "classification" is the systematic arrangement or a structural framework of these phenomena. As we move toward an international network of health care, the development of a language unique to nursing is viewed as critical to communication and decision making. Proponents of a specialized language for nursing emphasize the need for objective, science-based information to use in decision making. These data also provide the basis for accountability and the documentation supporting processes and outcomes of care. The data can be used further to answer research questions about nursing and nursing actions. In the age of information technology, uniform, accurate, and automated patient care data are required to conduct analyses that will result in improving the quality of care and costing out that care (Table 5-4). At present, the language of nursing primarily addresses nursing diagnoses, implementation activities, and nursing outcomes. Some would suggest that the existing systems are not adequate to reflect the entire scope of nursing practice and urge further development. We discuss the four currently most popular systems, and summarize others that have gained attention (Table 5-5).

North American Nursing Diagnosis Association

The first steps toward a common language for nursing started in 1973 when Kristine Gebbie and Mary Ann Lavin of St. Louis University called the First National Conference on Classification of Nursing Diagnosis. National Conferences have been held regularly since then. The National Group for the Classification of Nursing Diagnosis became a formal organization after the fifth conference and was renamed the North American Nursing Diagnosis Association (NANDA). The Association has two main purposes: to develop a diagnostic classification system (also known as a *taxonomy*) and to identify and approve nursing diagnoses. The list of nursing diagnoses (concepts that are given word labels) continues to grow as nurses encounter diagnoses in clinical practice that have not been included and submit these to NANDA for consideration. As a student, you have some familiarity with nursing diagnoses from the nursing care plans you develop for patient care and in the case studies you discuss in your classes.

McCormick and Jones (1998) point out that a taxonomy refers to a hierarchical system that includes vocabulary and terms. After the first meeting of the 100 participants, 29 conceptual areas were identified with approximately 100 terms. The current classification system contains 71 conceptual areas and 143 terms (Gordon, 1998).

The following is the definition of a nursing diagnosis accepted by the NANDA:

Nursing diagnosis is a clinical judgment about individual, family, or community response to actual or potential health problems/life processes. Nursing diagnoses provide the basis for selection of nursing interventions to achieve outcomes for which the nurse is accountable (North American Nursing Diagnosis Association, 1997).

TABLE 5-4.   Rationale for the Development of a Classification for Nursing

- Permits recognition and communication with others by giving a name to the things nurses do
- Provides a uniform legal record of care
- Supports clinical decision making
- Lays the groundwork for nursing research
- Captures the cost of nursing services for billing and accounting purposes
- Generates a structured retrieval data base for quality assurance

TABLE 5–5. Major Classifications for Nursing Care Recognized by the American Nurses Association		
Title	**What It Is**	**Characteristics**
North American Nursing Diagnosis Association (NANDA)	A clinical judgment about an individual, family, or community response to actual or potential health problems that provides a basis for selecting a nursing intervention	Currently contains 71 conceptual areas and 143 terms
Nursing Intervention Classification (NIC)	A comprehensive standardized language, describing treatments that nurses perform in all settings and in all specialties	Includes 433 interventions, each with a definition and a detailed set of activities, organized in 27 classes and 6 domains
Nursing Outcomes Classification (NOC)	A variable concept that represents a patient or family caregiver state, behavior, or perception that is measurable along a continuum and responsive to nursing interventions	Contains 218 outcomes, each of which has a list of indicators in the evaluation of patient status, a measurement scale, and a short list of references
Home Health Care Classification	Adapted, revised, and expanded NANDA to include additional home health care nursing diagnostic conditions	Consists of 145 home health care nursing diagnoses, 50 of which were major nursing diagnostic categories and 95 subcategories. Designed for use in the home health care setting
The Omaha System	A system of client problems, interventions, and client outcomes, referred to as the Problem Classification Scheme, the Intervention Scheme, and the Problem Rating Scale for Outcomes	Includes domains, problems, modifiers, and signs/symptoms; intervention categories, targets, and client-specific information; and outcome rating scales for knowledge, behavior, and status
Nursing Management Minimum Data Set	Establishes a standardized language to identify and collect those factors needed to manage nursing care across care settings	Defines 17 management variables that enable economic analyses and comparisons. Focuses on unit level data aggregation (Delaney & Huber, 1996)
Patient Care Data Set (PCDS)	Codifies patient problems and actions delivered by all caregivers during a hospital stay	Information gathered from hundreds of terms in patient records
Perioperative Nursing Data Set	Standardized language for documenting and evaluating perioperative nursing care	Designed for use in the perioperative nursing area
Systematized Nomenclature of Medicine (SNOMED)	Comprehensive system for indexing the entire medical record, including signs and symptoms, diagnoses and procedures	Allows full integration of all medical information in electronic medical record into a single data source

Nursing Interventions Classifications

In 1996, work done at the University of Iowa on the classification of nursing interventions received attention. The Nursing Interventions Classification (NIC) is a comprehensive, standardized language describing treatments that nurses perform in all settings and in all specialties, and includes both physiological and psychosocial interventions. The interventions are numbered to facilitate computerization. There are 433 interventions, each of which contains a definition and a set of detailed activities that describe what a nurse does. The interventions are organized into 27 classes and 6 domains. They have been linked with NANDA and are in the process of being linked with the Nursing Outcomes Classification (University of Iowa, 1999).

Nursing Outcomes Classification

Also developed at the University of Iowa, the Nursing Outcomes Classification (NOC) was published in 1997. Listed in alphabetical order, the classification includes 218 outcomes, 27 of which were developed after publication of the book. An outcome is defined as a variable concept representing a patient or family caregiver state, behavior, or perception that is measurable along a continuum and responsive to nursing interventions. Project developers believed that stating the outcomes as variable concepts rather than goals would allow the identification of positive or negative changes (or no changes at all) in the patient's status. Each outcome has a definition and a list of indicators that assist in evaluation of patient status. Outcomes thus far developed are at the individual patient or family caregiver level; outcomes for families and communities are beginning to be developed.

The outcomes are organized into 24 categories, called classes. Classes are grouped in six domains. The domains are Functional Health, Physiologic Health, Psychosocial Health, Health Knowledge and Behavior, Perceived Health, and Family. Because the work on outcomes is so new, you can anticipate that it will experience additions, refinements, and revisions (University of Iowa, 1999).

The Omaha System

The Omaha System, another example of early classification efforts, is based on federally funded research conducted by the Visiting Nurse Association of Omaha from 1975 to 1993 (Martin & Scheet, 1992). It was designed as a three-part, comprehensive yet brief approach to documentation and information management for multidisciplinary health care professionals who practice in community settings. It offers terms and codes to classify the client's health-related concerns or problems, the interventions that nurses and other health care professionals use, and the client's outcomes (Zielstorff, 1998). Client problems can be identified for individuals, families, and groups. The interventions describe both plans and interventions for specific client concerns. The outcome scales evaluate a client's health-related changes through the use of problem-specific knowledge, behavior, and status ratings. The Omaha System is recognized by the American Nurses Association and has been translated into numerous languages. Automation and technology advances and health care delivery changes have markedly expanded its use nationally and internationally (Martin, 1999).

Other Classification Systems

In 1988 a Nursing Minimum Data Set (NMDS) was developed by Werley and Lang. It identified the four nursing elements of nursing diagnosis, nursing interventions, nursing outcomes, and nursing intensity (Clark, 1998). These elements have set the stage for classification activities by many other groups.

The Patient Care Data Set was developed at the University of Virginia in 1994 in work done by Ozbolt, Fruchtnicht, and Hayden. They gathered hundreds of terms from patient's records, from which they developed the Patient Care Data Set. It codifies patient problems and the actions of all caregivers during a patient's hospital stay (Zielstorff, 1998).

The Home Health Care Classification (HHCC) of Nursing Diagnoses and Interventions evolved from the work of Virginia K. Saba and associates at Georgetown University School of Nursing. It was developed to provide a structure for coding and categorizing home health care nursing services. It identifies 20 Home Health Care Nursing Components to classify. Working with NANDA Nursing Diagnoses, a list of 104 diagnoses were adapted, revised, and expanded to include additional home health care nursing diagnostic conditions. In its final format, it includes 145 diagnoses—50 major nursing diagnostic categories and 95 subcategories. The diagnosis statements also collected the actual outcome for each nursing diagnosis, which were used to measure the outcome of home health care (Saba, 1996).

Another nursing classification recently developed is the Perioperative Nursing Data Set (PNDS). It was developed by the Association of Operating Room Nurses to provide perioperative nurses with standardized language they could use for documenting and evaluating the care they provide. It was their intent to develop a unified language that would allow nursing care to be systematically quantified, coded, and captured in a computerized format in the perioperative setting. It consists of nursing diagnoses, nursing interventions, and patient outcomes related to delivery of nursing care in the perioperative setting (AORN Online, 1999).

The Systematized Nomenclature of Medicine-Reference Terminology (SNOMED-RT) represents an additional classification of terms. Although SNOMED-RT was developed in 1998, its development started as early as 1965 with the development of a Systematized Nomenclature of Pathology (SNOP). In 1976, the Systematized Nomenclature of Medicine (SNOMED) listed 44,587 terms, and in 1993 SNOMED International expanded to 130,580 terms (SNOMED, 1999). Although focusing primarily on medicine, SNOMED-RT is recognized by the American Nurses Association.

The National Information and Data Set Evaluation Center

The National Information and Data Set Evaluation Center (NIDSEC) was established in 1995 by the American Nurses Association to review, evaluate against defined criteria, and recognize nursing information systems. Their mission is to "develop and disseminate standards pertaining to information systems that support the documentation of nursing practice, and evaluate voluntarily submitted information systems against these standards" (NIDSEC, 1999, p. 1). Within the framework of the NIDSEC, four dimensions of nursing data sets and systems are evaluated:

- Nomenclature (terms used)
- Clinical Content (the linkages among terms)
- Clinical Data Repository (how the data are stored and made accessible for retrieval)
- General System Characteristics (such as performance and attention to security and confidentiality)

Groups or vendors wishing to be recognized by ANA submit materials to a five-member review panel who, after examining the application, submit a recommendation to the NIDSEC Committee. If accepted by the Committee, the recognition extends for

3 years, after which a new application must be submitted. At this writing, nine groups are recognized by NIDSEC.

The International Classification for Nursing Practice Project

The International Classification for Nursing Practice Project (ICNPP) is an effort of the International Council of Nurses (ICN). The goal of the Project is to provide "a unifying framework for existing systems and a system which can be used in countries which have none" (Clark, 1998). Although the United States has been involved in the development of classification and information systems for some time, the need for a unified language is now recognized internationally. Because cultural and language differences exist, many of the classification systems currently employed in the United States are not useful in other countries. For example, the concept of self-care reflects the cultural values and norms of American society but may be perceived quite differently in other cultures. In 1989 the ICN was asked to encourage member National Nurses Associations (NNA) to become involved in developing information and classification systems and nursing data sets that could be used by nurses in all countries to identify and describe nursing. The project began a year later. In 1996, an alpha version of the Classification of Nursing Phenomenon and Nursing Interventions was field tested, and a beta version was launched June 1999 at ICN's Centennial Conference. Many challenges face the group working on this project.

Critical Thinking Exercise

> Analyze the history of the development of a classification and nomenclature specific to nursing. Describe possible future developments, and provide a rationale for your answer. What do you see as major impediments, and why? What do you believe will be the long-term benefits, and why?

TRADITIONS IN NURSING

Because of its history, nursing has developed many traditions. Some of them are being questioned or eliminated, primarily because they are not practical in today's workplace (eg, the wearing of a nursing cap). It is worthwhile, however, to reflect just a little on the development of these traditions and to discuss their relationship to nursing. Earle P. Scarlett (1991, p. 119), a Canadian physician, writer, and medical historian, would support such discussion. He wrote:

The truth of the matter is that any profession worthy of the name must forever be strengthening and re-creating its traditions. A profession is a sensitive organic growing thing, not a static order. And it is particularly important that we should remember this at the present time.

The Nursing Pin

The nursing pin may date back to the time of the Crusades, when Crusaders marched to Jerusalem to recover the Holy Land. Among the Crusaders were the Knights Hospitalers of St. John of Jerusalem. Their uniform, introduced by a man named Gerard, included a black robe with a white Maltese cross. The Maltese cross became a familiar sight on the battlefields of the Holy Land. Following the capture of Jerusalem in 1099, some of the Crusaders noted the excellent nursing care provided by the Hospital of St. John and decided to join the nursing group. The Maltese cross is an eight-pointed cross formed by four arrowheads joining at their points. The eight points of the cross signified the eight beatitudes that knights were expected to exemplify in their works of charity. When the Knights Templars and the Knights of the Teutonic Order were formed in 1118 and 1190, respectively, this symbol was carried forward. The Maltese cross later became a symbol of many groups who cared for the sick, including the United States Cadet Nurse Corps.

The actual symbolism of the pin relates to customs established in the 16th century, when the privilege of wearing a coat of arms was limited to noblemen who served their kings with distinction. As centuries passed, the privilege was extended to schools and to craft guilds, and the symbols of wisdom, strength, courage, and faith appeared on buttons, badges, and shields. It was probably this spirit that Florence Nightingale attempted to capture when she chose the Maltese cross as a symbol for the badge worn by the graduates of her first nursing school.

As nursing developed as a profession, each school chose a unique pin, awarded on completion of the program as a public symbol of work well done. Many of the early schools, particularly those associated with hospitals supported by religious groups, incorporated the cross into their pin. The first Nightingale School of Nursing in the United States was at Bellevue Hospital and is credited with developing the first school badge or pin, which was presented to the class of 1880 (Kalisch & Kalisch, p. 82). A crane in the center symbolized the nurse's vigilance, an inner circle of blue suggested constancy, and an outer circle of poppy capsules symbolized mercy and the relief of suffering.

The Nursing Cap

The history of the nursing cap is less certain. Several explanations of the origin of the cap have been suggested. It probably evolved during the period of time when nursing was greatly influenced by religion. It may have originated in the habit worn by the Sisters of Charity of St. Vincent de Paul, who established the first modern school of nursing in Paris in 1864. Another opinion suggests that the cap was influenced by the Institute of Protestant Deaconesses, founded by Pastor Theodore Fleidner at Kaiserwerth in Germany, and the institution where Florence Nightingale studied. The white cap of the deaconesses of the early Christian era and the nun's veil of the Middle Ages have been said to be the forerunners of the nursing cap as we know it today (Mangum, 1994). The veil was modified to become a cap and was associated with service to others. We need to remember, also, that in Florence Nightingale's day, every lady wore a cap indoors. If you look at pictures of Queen Victoria, you notice the cap of plain white stiffened muslin framing her face. It was considered proper for women to keep their heads covered; thus, the cap would be viewed as the proper dress for a young woman of the day. The cap worn by students at Kaiserwerth when Florence Nightingale was a student was hood shaped, had a ruffle around the face, and tied under the chin. A final conjecture is that the cap originally was designed to cover and help to control the long hair that was fashionable in the late 19th century, when short hair cuts were not acceptable for women.

As women's hair styles changed and hair was worn shorter, the head covering became smaller and lost its scarf or veil in the United States and Canada. (The hair-covering aspect remained a part of the cap in many areas of Europe.) As hospitals developed nursing education programs, they each created their own cap and nursing pin as a symbol of that particular hospital and nursing school. Some of these were rather "frilly" and were fashioned after the ether cone through which ether was dropped. As hair styles changed, the size of the cap also changed, until it became one of individual taste or preference. A "capping" ceremony was part of the ritual of the nursing student and is discussed later.

As the role of nurses changed and as high technology became a significant part of the hospital work environment, nurses found that caps were bothersome as they tried to carry out their duties. They were knocked askew by curtains, equipment, and tubing. By the 1980s, many hospitals no longer required the cap as a part of the uniform. Nursing programs responded by dropping the cap as a required article of dress. If students wished to have a cap, it was purchased from a local uniform store and had no particular identification with the program (Fig. 5-4).

The Nursing Uniform

Like the nursing cap, which is actually a part of the early nursing uniform, the requirement for special dress came from the religious and military history of nursing and has always been significant in nursing. This is due to the fact that dress provides a strong nonverbal message about one's image. The nurse attired in a white uniform, at least in the 1950s and 1960s, communicated an impression of confidence, competence, professionalism, authority, role identity, and accountability. As nurses have adopted more casual dress, some of this identity has been lost, and hospital committees, nursing programs, and nurses have spent considerable time discussing appropriate attire.

Early uniforms were long, usually stiffly starched, and had detachable collars and cuffs. A full uniform often included a long cape that would cover the uniform. Kalisch and Kalisch (1995, pp. 80–81) credit the New York Training School for Nurses at Bellevue Hospital with being the first school to adopt a standard uniform for student nurses in 1876. The uniform consisted of a gingham apron worn in the morning and a white apron worn in the afternoon over a dark woolen dress. A well-bred young woman, Euphemia Van Rensselaer, is credited with updating the basic uniform, which students were opposed to wearing. Given two days' leave of absence to have a uniform made for herself, she created a tailored uniform consisting of a long gray dress for winter and a calico version for summer, both worn with a white apron and cap. The attractiveness of her appearance resulted in other students accepting the uniform as standard

FIGURE 5–4 By the 1980s, many nurses were no longer wearing the cap as part of the nursing uniform.

dress. Later, a more easily laundered dress that could be worn throughout the year replaced the gray dress for winter.

A regulation uniform became a distinguishing mark of each nursing school by the end of the 19th century. Typically the uniform consisted of a bodice and skirt of white material, adjustable white cuffs, a stiff white collar, and a white cap. To maintain the feminine hourglass image popular at the time, a tightly laced corset was worn beneath the uniform and ankles were to be hidden from view. Some suggest that the adoption of a distinctive and attractive uniform played a significant role in developing a professional image for nursing, giving it status, respect, and authority.

By the 1900s, the uniform became more functional and the hemline was raised. By the mid-1960s, pantsuits became accepted and nurses in certain settings, particularly psychiatric and pediatric units, were challenging the appropriateness of uniforms, especially white uniforms. By 1970, significant changes were occurring in uniforms, with the acceptance of styles that were designed to "make the nurse more approachable." In psychiatric settings, "no uniform" became the standard of the day. Today, athletic shoes are acceptable in many institutions, and "scrubs" have become so accepted that they are featured in pamphlets advertising uniforms. In 1987, the Springhouse Corporation conducted a survey of nurses throughout the United States and found that most nurses prefer scrubs or lab coats worn over street clothes. The result of this change has been that nurses today are no longer identifiable by uniform. The stethoscope worn around the neck gives the consumer some clue to a person's position (ie, that the person is a health care worker rather than a maintenance person), and hospital identification badges provide further information, but sometimes do not include the person's full name.

Today there is still controversy over the appropriate attire for nurses. Mangum, Garrison, Lind, Thackeray and Wyatt (1991) recommend that nurses wear clothing that clearly distinguishes them as professional nurses. Although they do not suggest that nurses wear a cap, they have advocated the more traditional white dress or pantsuit. Others argue that what nurses wear matters less than what they know. Perhaps compromise is necessary.

Ceremonies Associated With Nursing Programs

Long-standing traditions embraced by nursing include the ceremonies that mark various points along the educational paths of nursing students. Primary among these are the "capping" and the "pinning" ceremonies.

Capping ceremonies are not as common today as pinnings, probably because most nurses and nursing students no longer wear caps. Historically, the cap was awarded to students after they completed a certain part of the program. In some schools it was awarded on completion of the probationary period, but more often it was given after the completion of the first year. Often held in a nearby church, a special ceremony was planned, to which students invited family and others who were interested in their progress. The director of the school, assisted by other school dignitaries and faculty, solemnly placed the cap on the head of each student. Students proudly wore the cap throughout the remainder of the program. Often a stripe was added to one corner of the cap to signify completion of the second year of study, and a black band was added at the time of graduation.

The second traditional ceremony in nursing, the pinning, was of even greater significance, and is continued by many schools today. The pinning heralded the completion of the program. Amid much pomp and circumstance, family and friends gathered to watch as the nursing director ceremoniously "pinned" each new graduate. Graduates often recited, in unison, the Nightingale Pledge (Display 5-1), written in 1893 by Lystra E. Gretter, superintendent of Harper Hospital School in Detroit (Calhoun, 1993). This tradition is often repeated in nursing schools today, although the original pledge in some cases is modified. Some schools include additional tradition through the "passing of the lamp." A representative of the graduating class hands a lamp (symbolizing the lamp carried by Florence Nightingale) to a representative of the next graduating class, thus reinforcing the concept of the continual caring represented in nursing.

As nursing education moved into institutions of higher education, some of the traditional ceremonies were discontinued. Some argue that the ceremony recognizing program completion in the collegiate environment is the college commencement, and that "special" celebrations for students of particular areas of study are not appropriate. However, in many large universities, the various disciplines now have separate ceremonies or an additional ceremony for their members. In other cases, the tradition is continued, although there is some tendency for graduates not to purchase a pin.

Display 5–1
THE NIGHTINGALE PLEDGE

I solemnly pledge myself before God and in the presence of this assembly:

   To pass my life in purity and to practice my profession faithfully;

   I will abstain from whatever is deleterious and mischievous and will not take or knowingly administer any harmful drug; I will do all in my power to maintain and elevate the standard of the profession, and will hold in confidence all personal matters committed to my keeping and all family affairs coming to my knowledge in the practice of my calling;

   With loyalty will I endeavor to aid the physician in his work, and devote myself to the welfare of those committed to my care.

Gretter, 1893

Critical Thinking Exercise

Review the traditions established in nursing. Which is the most meaningful to you, and why? Which is the least meaningful to you, and why? Do you believe traditions should be continued in nursing? Provide a rationale for your answer.

KEY CONCEPTS

- In its development as a profession, nursing has struggled with its definition, its image, and its role in the health care delivery system. The role of the nurse in the health care delivery system has probably never been more important than it is today.
- The position nursing occupies as a profession is often judged against sociologically developed characteristics of a profession. Not everyone agrees that nursing meets those standards.
- The standards of a profession typically include seven requirements: (1) possess a well-defined and well-organized body of knowledge; (2) enlarge a systematic body of knowledge and improve education; (3) educate its practitioners in institutions of higher learning; (4) function autonomously in the formulation of policy; (5) develop a code of ethics; (6) attract professionals who will be committed to the profession for a lifetime; and (7) compensate practitioners by providing autonomy, continuous professional development, and economic security.
- Nursing also has struggled with the terms "profession" and "professional." At times the characteristics of the "professional" become confused with the formal concept of a profession.
- Nursing has struggled with its image. Various groups have waged campaigns to improve the image of nursing and thus make it a more attractive profession. One

part of a recent campaign of the ANA is to help prepare nurses develop the basic skills and confidence to work with the media.

- Since the beginning of the 20th century, nursing has been a much-studied profession. Early studies dealt with nursing education; later studies dealt with the image of nursing, nurses themselves, and with nursing's role in health care delivery.
- As nursing has developed as a profession, more attention has been directed to establishing a unique classification and nomenclature for nursing. Efforts are being made to do this on an international basis.
- Nursing as a profession has many traditions, some of which are being challenged today. Among the traditions are the pin, the cap, the uniform, and nursing ceremonies.

REFERENCES

Abdellah FG. Patient-Centered Approaches to Nursing. New York: Macmillan, 1960

American Nurses Association. Nursing: A Social Policy Statement. Kansas City, MO: American Journal of Nursing Co, 1980

American Nurses Association. First Position on Education for Nursing. Am J Nurs 65(12):106–111, 1965

AORN Online Research. Perioperative Nursing Data Set. Available at: *http://aorn.org/research/pnds.htm*. Accessed November 1, 1999.

Benner P, Wrubel J. The Primacy of Caring. Menlo Park, CA: Addison-Wesley, 1989

Bevis EO, Watson J. Toward a Caring Curriculum; A New Pedagogy for Nursing. New York: National League for Nursing, 1989

Bixler GK, Bixler RW. The professional status of nursing. Am J Nurs 45(9):730, 1945

Calhoun J. The Nightingale Pledge: A commitment that survives the passage of time. Nurs Health Care 14(3):130–136, 1993

Carper BA. The Ethics of Caring. ANS 3:11–19, March, 1979

Clark J. The International Classification for Nursing Practice Project. 1998 Online Journal of Issues in Nursing. Available at: *http://www.nursingworld.org/ojin/tpc7tpc7_3.htm*. Accessed October 31, 1999.

Delaney C, Huber D. A Nursing Management Minimum Data Set (NMMDS): A report of an invitational conference. Chicago, IL: American Organization of Nurse Executives, 1996

Donahue MP. Nursing: The Finest Art, 2nd ed. St Louis: CV Mosby, 1996

Flexner A. *In* Bernard LA, Walsh M: Leadership: The Key to Professionalism of Nursing. NewYork: John Wiley & Sons, 1981

Gordon M. Nursing Nomenclature and Classification System Development. Online Journal of Issues in Nursing. Available at: *http://www.nursingworld.org/ojin/tpc7/tpc7_1.htm*. Accessed October 4, 1999.

Gordon S. Viewpoint: Nursing and Wit. Am J Nurs 99(5):9, 1999

Hampton-Robb I. Report of the third regular meeting of the International Council of Nurses. Geneva: ICN, 1909

Henderson V. The Nature of a Science of Nursing. New York: Macmillan, 1966

I.O.M. study sees need for funds in graduate, specialty areas. Am J Nurs 83(3):343, 344, 454, 1983

Johnson D. The behavioral system model for nursing. *In* Riehl JP, Roy C: Conceptual Models for Nursing Practice, 2nd ed. East Norwalk, CT: Appleton-Century-Crofts, 1980:207–216

Kalisch PA, Kalisch BJ. Nurses on prime-time television. Am J Nurs 82(2):264, 1982a

Kalisch PA, Kalisch BJ. The image of the nurse in motion pictures. Am J Nurs 82(4):605, 1982b

Kalisch PA, Kalisch BJ. The image of nurses in novels. Am J Nurs 82(8):1220, 1982c

King IM. A Theory for Nursing: Systems, Concepts, Process. New York: John Wiley & Sons, 1981

Labor Management Relations Act (1947) as amended by Public Laws 86-257 (1959) and 93-360 (1974), Section 2

Levine ME. Introduction to Clinical Nursing. Philadelphia: FA Davis, 1969

Mangum, S. Uniforms and caps: Do we need them? In Strickland OL, Fishman DJ: Nursing Issues in the 1990s. Albany, NY: Delmar Publishers, 1994:46–66

Mangum S, Garrison C, Lind C, Thackeray R, Wyatt M. Perception of nurses' uniforms. Image: The Journal of Nursing Scholarship 23:127–130, 1991

Martin KS. The Omaha System: Past, present and future. On-line Journal of Nursing Informatics, Volume 3(1), 1999. Available at: *http://cac.psu.edu/~dxm12/art1v3n1art.html*. Accessed November 22, 1999

Martin KS, Scheet NJ. The Omaha System: Application for Community Health Nursing. Philadelphia: Saunders, 1992

McCormick KA, Jones CB. Is one taxonomy needed for health care vocabularies and classifications? Online Journal of Issues in Nursing. Available at: *http://www.nursingworld.org/ojin/tpc7/tpc7_2.htm*. Accessed October 4, 1999

Moccia P. Curriculum Revolution: Agenda for Change. New York: National League for Nursing, Inc., 1988

Muff J. Handmaiden, battle ax, whore. *In* Muff J: Socialization, Sexism and Stereotyping. Prospect Heights, IL: Waveland Press, Inc. 1988:113–156

National Commission for the Study of Nursing and Nursing Education: Summary, Report and Recommendations. Am J Nurs 70(2):279, 1970

National Commission on Nursing. Initial Report and Preliminary Recommendations. Chicago: Hospital Research and Educational Trust, 1981

National Council of State Boards of Nursing, Inc. Model Practice Act. Chicago, Il: The Council, 1994

Neuman B. The Neuman System Model: Application to Nursing Education and Practice. East Norwalk, CT: Appleton-Century-Crofts, 1982

Newman MA. Professionalism: Myth or reality. *In* Chaska NL: The Nursing Profession: Turning Points. St Louis: CV Mosby, 1990:49–52

Nightingale F. Notes on Nursing: What It Is, and What It Is Not. (An unabridged republication of the first American edition, as published by D. Appleton and Company in 1860.) New York: Dover Publications, 1954

North American Nursing Diagnosis Association, 1997–1998. NANDA nursing diagnoses: Definitions and classification. Philadelphia: Author, 1997

Nursing World NIDSEC: home page. Available at *http://www.nursingworld.org/nidsec/index.htm*. Accessed November 1, 1999.

Orem D. Nursing: Concepts of Practice, 2nd ed. New York: McGraw-Hill, 1980

Orlando IJ. The Discipline and Teaching of Nursing Process. New York: GP Putnam's Sons, 1972

Pavalko RM. Sociology of Occupations and Professions. Itasca, IL: Peacock Publishers, 1971

Peplau HE. Interpersonal Relations in Nursing. New York: GP Putnam's Sons, 1952

Rogers ME. Science of Unitary Human Beings: A Paradigm for Nursing. Paper presented before the International Nurse Theorist Conference, Edmonton, Alberta, May 1984

Roy C. Introduction to Nursing: An Adaptation Model, 2nd ed. Englewood Cliffs, NJ: Prentice-Hall, 1984

Saba V. Home Health Care Classification (HHCC): Nursing Diagnoses and Nursing Interventions. Available at: *http://www.dml.georgetown,edu/research/hhcc*. Accessed October 31, 1999.

Schlotfeldt RM. Resolution of issues: An imperative for creating nursing's future. J Prof Nurs 3:136–142, 1987

Sieber JR, Powers CA, Baggs JR, Knapp JM, Sileo CM. Missing in Action: Nursing in the media. Am J Nurs 98(12):55–56, 1998

SNOMED. The History of SNOMED. Available at: *http://www.snomed.org/what/sld005.htm.* Accessed November 1, 1999.

Stewart, M. Issues update: ANA puts nursing in media spotlight. Am J Nurs 99(5):56–59, 1999

Strauss A. The structure and ideology of American nursing: An interpretation. *In* Davis J: The Nursing Profession. New York: John Wiley & Sons, 1966:60–108

Styles M. On Nursing: Toward a New Endowment. St. Louis: CV Mosby, 1982

University of Iowa. Nursing Interventions Classification (NIC): Overview. Available at: *http://www.nursing.uiowa.edu/nic/overview.htm.* Accessed October 21, 1999.

University of Iowa. Nursing Outcomes Classification (NOC): Overview. Available at: *http://www.nursing.uiowa.edu/noc/overview.htm.* Accessed October 21, 1999.

Watson J. Nursing the Philosophy and Science of Caring. Boston: Little, Brown, 1979

Wiedenbach E. Clinical Nursing, A Helping Art. New York: Springer Publishing Co., 1964

Winslow-Goldmark Report. The Study of Nursing and Nursing Education in the United States. New York: Macmillan, 1923

Zielstorff RD. Characteristics of a Good Nursing Nomenclature from an Informatics Perspective. 1998 Online Journal of Issues in Nursing. Available at: *http://www.nursingworld.org/ojin/tpc7/tpc7_4.htm.* Accessed October 4, 1999.

FURTHER READING

Aaronson LS. A challenge for nursing: Reviewing a historic competition. Nurs Outlook 37(6):274–279, 1989

Backer BA. Lillian Wald: Connecting caring with activism. Nurs Health Care 14(3):122–129, 1993

Bunting S, Campbell JC. Feminism and nursing. Adv Nurs Sci 12(4):11–24, 1990

Bullough VL, et al. The Emergence of Modern Nursing. New York: Macmillan, 1969

Delaney C, Huber D. Clinical testing of a national standardized minimum data set designed to capture the management context of health care delivery. In D Masys (Ed). Proceedings of the 1997 conference of the American Medical Informatics Association (CD-ROM), Philadelphia, PA: Hanley & Belfus, Inc., 1997

Dolan JA. Nursing in Society: A Historical Perspective, 14th ed. Philadelphia: WB Saunders, 1978

Gamer M. The ideology of professionalism. Nurs Outlook 27(2):108–111, 1979

Griffin GJ, Griffin JK. Jensen's History and Trends of Professional Nursing, 7th ed. St Louis: CV Mosby, 1973

Hanson KS. The emergence of liberal education in nursing education, 1893–1923. J Prof Nurs 5(2):83–91, 1989

Huber D, Delaney C. Nursing management data for nursing information systems. In Series on Nursing Administration (SONA), Information Systems Innovations: New Visions, New Ventures. Vol 10 (pp 15-29), 1998

Johnson M, Maas M. Nursing outcomes classification (NOC). St. Louis: Mosby, 1997

Kalisch PA, Kalisch BJ. The Advance of American Nursing, 3rd ed. Philadelphia: J.B. Lippincott Co., 1995

Kalisch BJ, Kalisch PA. Heroine out of focus: Media images of Florence Nightingale: I. Popular biographies and stage productions. Nurs Health Care 4(4):181–187, 1983

Kalisch BJ, Kalisch PA. The nurse-detective in American movies. Nurs Health Care 3(3):146–153, 1982

Kalisch BJ, Kalisch PA, Scobey M. Reflections on a television image. Nurs Health Care 5(5):248–255, 1981

Larisey MM. Attic treasures: A look at nursing history. Nurs Forum 25(1):20–24, 1990

McCloskey J, Bulecheck G. Nursing intervention classification (NIC), 2nd ed. St. Louis: Mosby, 1996

Melosh B. Not merely a profession: Nurses and resistance to professionalization. Am Behav Scientist 32(6):668–679, 1989

Parsons M. The profession in a class by itself. Nurs Outlook 34(6):270–275, 1985

Roberts MM. American Nursing: History and Interpretation. New York: Macmillan, 1954

Sleeper R, et al. Issues in Health Care: The Edna A. Fagan Health Care Lecture Series. Publication No. 14-1599. New York: National League for Nursing, 1976

Werley H, Lang N. Nursing minimum data set. New York: Springer, 1987

Woodham-Smith C. Florence Nightingale. New York: McGraw-Hill, 1951

Relevant Web Sites

Center for the Study of the History of Nursing *www.upenn.edu/nursing/facres_history.html*
ICNP® Beta version *icn.ch/icnpupdate.html*
National Council of State Boards of Nursing *www.ncsbn.org*
NursingNet *www.nursingnet.org*
Online Journal of Issues in Nursing *www.nursingworld.org/ojin*
University of Iowa College of Nursing *www.coninfo.nursing.uiowa.edu/index.htm*

6

Educational Preparation for Nursing

Strong educational preparation in the biological and psychosocial sciences, and in nursing arts and science, is the necessary base for advanced skill acquisition, because this knowledge provides the basis for safe care and gives the most advantageous position for gaining a sense of salience.

(Benner, 1984)

OBJECTIVES

After completing this chapter, you should be able to:

1. Compare the educational preparation of the nursing assistant, the licensed practical (vocational) nurse, the graduate of a hospital-based program, the associate degree graduate and the baccalaureate degree graduate.

2. Explain the purposes of other forms of nursing education including external degree programs, registered nurse baccalaureate programs, master's preparation, doctoral studies, nondegree programs, and articulated programs.

3. Identify factors that have prompted change in nursing education, including studies and sociopolitical events, and analyze the effect of each.

4. Analyze the effects the ANA Position Paper on Nursing Education would have on nursing licensure if adopted nationwide.

5. Discuss the concept of differentiated practice and provide a rationale for its development.

6. Discuss the impact of technology on nursing education.

7. Identify factors that have influenced changes in nursing education and analyze the effect of each.

8. Analyze the ways in which nursing theories serve to advance the profession.

9. Define the continuing education unit, critique the major points supporting both mandatory and voluntary continuing education, and the mechanisms for documenting and recording continuing education.

Accreditation	Diploma	Nursing assistant
Advanced placement	Doctorate	Position paper
Advanced practice	Educational mobility	Postsecondary education
Articulation	Entry into practice	Practical (vocational) nurse
Associate degree	External degree	
Baccalaureate degree	Grandfather clause	Registered nurse
Career ladder	Home health aide	Scope of practice
Community-based	Hospital-based program	Theorist/theory
Competencies	Internship	Titling
Continuing education unit (CEU)	Interstate endorsement	Virtual university
	Mandatory continuing education	Voluntary continuing education
Differentiated practice		

Most professions provide a single route of educational preparation. However, the development of nursing as a profession has resulted in three major educational routes that prepare graduates to write the National Council Licensure Examination (NCLEX) for registered nursing. These circumstances have resulted in alternatives and opportunities for prospective students. The benefits of these options for students and the public resulted in the Pew Commission identifying in their 1995 report (see Chapter 1) the multiple-entry points to professional nursing practice as a strength of nursing (Pew Commission, 1995).

Multiple-entry points have resulted in confusion for both consumers and employers. Health care consumers often find it difficult to understand the various nursing credentials—and probably have little interest in credentials as long as the care they receive is satisfactory. Employers have difficulty differentiating among the three major types of registered nurse graduates who, at least initially, enter the work environment performing similar behaviors. This confusion led to another recommendation from the Pew Commission: that nursing distinguish between the practice responsibilities of the graduates educated in each of the different educational environments. (Pew Commission, 1995).

An educator is charged with the responsibility of graduating a "safe" practitioner, but may not have a clear understanding of how the professional preparation provided by the various educational routes ought to differ in purpose, structure, and outcome. You will find that nursing leaders often vigorously debate aspects of nursing educational preparation, such as where it should take place, what content should be included in which programs and to what depth, which tests should measure the various competencies, and which credentials should be awarded.

The three educational avenues that prepare men and women for registered nursing are hospital-based diploma programs, 2-year associate degree programs (primarily found at junior and community colleges), and baccalaureate programs (offered at 4-year colleges and universities). It is also possible for students to begin their nursing education in programs that culminate in a master's degree, and several programs now exist in which a student can earn a doctorate before being eligible to write the state licensing examination for registered nursing. The following section discusses the various educational routes to nursing.

At least two other groups of caregivers are identified with nursing: the nursing assistant, who is certified, and the practical (vocational) nurse, who is licensed through a separate and different examination from that taken by the registered nurse. We briefly discuss the education of each group of caregivers.

THE NURSING ASSISTANT

For years, individuals called nursing aides or assistants have provided care to patients in hospitals and long-term care facilities. In the past, these caregivers were hired without formal preparation for their responsibilities and were provided "on-the-job training." The use of the nursing aide likely started during World War I, and certainly was reinforced during World War II when approximately 150,000 trained volunteer nursing aides served in wartime hospitals. Nursing aides or assistants have always provided the majority of care in nursing homes.

In 1987, Congress passed the Omnibus Budget Reconciliation Act (OBRA), which regulates agencies receiving federal funds, and includes regulating the education and certification of nursing assistants who work in nursing homes. This act stipulated that by October 1, 1990, all people working as nursing assistants in nursing homes (hospitals and assisted-living units were not included) would be required to complete satisfactorily an approved course of study and competency testing. Certification falls under state jurisdiction, but is guided by federal regulations. These regulations require that an individual complete a minimum of 75 hours of theory and practice, and pass both a theory and practice examination to be certified. In many states, the hours of preparation required exceed the 75 hours established by law. Following the federal legislation, the National Council of State Boards of Nursing Inc. developed the Nurse Aide Competency Evaluation Program (NACEP), which identifies the minimum skills a nursing assistant must attain and can be used to guide programs registering or certifying nursing assistants. The state agency responsible for certifying and maintaining the list of nursing assistants varies from state to state; most commonly it is the board of nursing or the state department of health services.

The certified nursing assistant (CNA) functions under the direction of the registered nurse or the licensed practical (vocational) nurse. Each state determines the skills that may be performed by the nursing assistant. Typically, these include basic nursing skills, such as changing bed linens; taking temperature, respiratory, and blood pressure readings for patients; bathing patients and helping with personal care; helping patients with eating, walking, and exercise programs; and supporting patients when they are allowed to get out of bed. The preparation of the certified nursing assistant emphasizes the importance of a safe environment and includes instruction in the use of side rails and restraints, and patients' rights. Some states also require a designated number of hours per year of continuing education. The training occurs in many settings, including high schools, long-term care facilities, hospitals, community colleges, regional occupational programs (ROPs), and privately operated programs. Some consider this preparation the first rung on the ladder of nursing education, and, in some states, the nursing assistant may be exempt from certain classes required in licensed practical (vocational) nursing programs.

The criteria for hospital accreditation established by the Joint Commission on Accreditation of Healthcare Organizations now requires that hospitals assure the competence of all employees, including nursing assistants. This led hospitals to the practice of hiring only those who were certified as nursing assistants in long-term care facilities and to the development of courses to prepare individuals as nursing assistants in acute care settings.

PRACTICAL NURSE EDUCATION

The practical nurse is no newcomer to the health care delivery system. In the past, the practical nurse was the family friend or community citizen who was called to the home in emergencies. This person, usually self-taught, learned by experience which procedures were effective and which were not. She would perform basic care procedures, such as bathing, and also would cook and perform light housekeeping duties for the family, much as the home health aide does today. Although controls on the licensing of practical nurses and the accreditation of their curricula were slower to evolve than those regulating professional nursing, states gradually enacted licensure laws governing practical nursing. By 1945, 19 states and one territory had licensure laws, but licensure of the practical nurse was mandatory in only one state (Kalisch & Kalisch, 1995). When more states began adopting mandatory licensure laws for practical nurses, many individuals who had been functioning in this capacity were granted a license by waiver, and were excused from any formal training (see Chapter 7 on credentialing). Most, if not all, of these people are now retired from nursing practice.

It is not clear when formal preparation for practical nursing began. Some suggest training programs were started in 1897 (Kalisch and Kalisch, 1995). A more popular belief is that the first programs were initiated through the YWCA in Brooklyn, New York, around 1892. The school established through the YWCA was known as the Ballard School, after Lucinda Ballard, who provided the funding to operate it. The course of study lasted approximately 3 months, and the students, called "attendants," were trained to care for invalids, the elderly, and children in a home setting.

A YWCA may seem to many of us to be a strange place for a practical nursing program. In fact, however, YWCAs were an important source of inexpensive housing for many young women who, in the late 1890s and early 1900s, traveled from their homes to large cities in search of new careers and better lives. Because most of these women were untrained and had no marketable skills, the YWCA was a natural site for a school.

The Thompson School, founded in Brattleboro, Vermont, in 1907; the American Red Cross, beginning in 1908; and the Household Nursing Association School of Attendant Nursing, begun in Boston in 1918, offered other early practical nursing programs.

Although only 11 schools were in existence by 1930, the number of programs expanded rapidly during the 1940s. During World War I, and especially during World War II, the need became crucial for people who had some basic nursing skills—and, more importantly, who could be prepared quickly. As the need intensified, the practical nurse, who until then had practiced primarily in the home, moved out into the world.

In 1941, the Association of Practical Nurse Schools was founded; in 1942, membership was opened to practical nurses and the name was changed to the National Association of Practical Nurse Education and Service (NAPNES). The first planned curriculum for practical nursing was developed in 1942, and in 1945, NAPNES established an accrediting service for schools of practical nursing. The National Federation of Licensed Practical Nurses (NFLPN) was organized in 1949. In 1957, the NFLPN, working with the American Nurses Association (ANA), attempted to clarify the role and function of the practical nurse, just as groups throughout the nation have worked at delineating the roles of other nursing program graduates. The National League for Nursing (NLN) established the Council on Practical Nursing in 1957, and in 1966, the Chicago Public School Program became the first practical nurse program to be accredited by this organization.

The general curriculum for practical nurses, which typically takes one year to complete, varies considerably from state to state and even from school to school. In many instances the education is measured in clock hours instead of credit hours, as in the professional registered nursing programs. Most of today's practical nursing educational programs stress clinical experience, primarily in structured care settings such as hospitals and nursing homes. Basic therapeutic knowledge and introductory content from biologic and behavioral sciences correlate with clinical practice; usually one third of the time is spent in the classroom and two thirds in clinical practice.

The educational preparation of the practical nurse takes place in a great variety of settings. High schools, trade or technical schools, hospitals, junior or community colleges, universities, or independent agencies may offer programs. If the rules and regulations of the state board(s) of nursing allow it, practical nursing and associate nursing degree programs could be incorporated in the community college, as part of a *career ladder* approach to nursing education. These programs sometimes are referred to as one-on-one programs; one year of preparation for practical nursing, followed by one more year qualifying the graduate to take the licensure examination for registered nursing. All nursing students in these colleges are grouped together for *core* courses during the first academic year. At the end of this time, a student has the option of stopping the educational program to seek licensure as a practical nurse, or continuing for an additional year to become a registered nurse. Many students opt to do both. Graduates of these core programs in practical nursing usually have a broader and more in-depth understanding of the biologic sciences, and sometimes the social sciences (often also a part of the core curriculum), especially if these are college-level courses that are transferable to a 4-year institution. Because issues related to *educational mobility* and *articulation* between programs have received much attention (discussed later in this chapter), these combined programs have become popular.

Graduates of practical nursing programs take the NCLEX-PN; if they pass the exam, they use the title "licensed practical nurse" (LPN) or, in California and Texas, the title "licensed vocational nurse" (LVN). Their scope of practice focuses on meeting the health care needs of clients in hospitals, long-term care facilities, clinics, and the home. Typically, LPNs or LVNs care for clients whose conditions are considered stable, giving direct patient care; observing, recording, and reporting; administering treatments and medications; and assisting in rehabilitation procedures. A registered nurse or a licensed physician directs their work.

As with the associate degree and hospital-based diploma programs for registered nurses, the educational preparation for practical nurses and the future of practical nursing have been topics of much discussion. Some advocate two levels of nurses: the practical nurse prepared with an associate degree and the registered nurse prepared with a baccalaureate degree. Others would eliminate practical nursing altogether. In 1987, North Dakota became the first state (and to date the only state) to require all candidates taking the licensure examination for practical nursing to have completed an associate degree in practical nursing (see discussion later in this chapter). With the "graying" of America, and the growing need for nurses in home health care and in long-term care facilities, practical nurses will continue to play a significant role in health care delivery.

DIPLOMA EDUCATION

The earliest type of nursing education in the United States took place in diploma programs administered by hospitals. The first hospital with a nurse training school was the New England Hospital for Women, which accepted five probationers on September 1, 1872 (Kalisch and Kalisch, 1995). The characteristics of these early schools were discussed in detail in Chapter 4.

By the late 1940s and early 1950s, many hospital-based nursing schools had affiliated with nearby colleges and universities; these schools adopted general education requirements such as anatomy, physiology, sociology, and psychology as part of the curriculum. During this time the National League of Nursing Education (later to become the NLN) assumed an active role in curriculum guidance and accreditation. Nursing programs gained a stronger educational foundation because they were required to align themselves more closely with other types of *postsecondary education,* that is, education occurring after the completion of high school.

Thus, diploma schools in operation today have sound educational programs that meet the criteria necessary for accreditation. They employ qualified faculty who have developed clinical learning experiences that meet the student's learning needs rather than the hospital's service needs (which often took priority in the past). These programs vary in length from 27 to 36 months. Many diploma schools are affiliated with a college or university so that postsecondary credit can be awarded formally. Graduates are provided with a foundation in the biologic and social sciences, and may have taken some courses in the humanities. There is a strong emphasis in diploma programs on client experiences. The course of study also includes experience in nursing management (for example, being in charge of a nursing unit). Graduates work in acute, long-term, and ambulatory health care facilities fulfilling the responsibilities established by the scope of practice for registered nurses as defined by the state in which they are licensed.

During the mid-1960s, there was a significant decline in enrollment in diploma schools. As more nursing education programs were moved to institutions of higher education, many hospital-based schools elected to discontinue their programs. Some merged with a local community college or university that assumed administrative responsibility for managing the nursing program, and awarded an associate or baccalaureate degree when graduation requirements were satisfied. The elimination of hospital-based programs has occurred most extensively in the western part of the United States.

Finances also played a role in this change. With increasing constraints on funding, many hospitals found that the costs associated with supporting a nursing program were too great. Many diploma programs existing today have strong endowments and private funding support.

ASSOCIATE DEGREE EDUCATION

Associate degree nursing programs prepare more graduates for licensure as registered nurses than do any of the other programs. The movement toward associate degree education began in 1952. Associate degree nursing (ADN) programs have the distinction of being the first (and, to date, the only) type of nursing education established on the basis of planned research and experimentation. Four events undoubtedly influenced their beginning. First, these programs followed in the wake of the organization and growth of 2-year community colleges in the United States. Community colleges were organized specifically to offer the first 2 years of a traditional 4-year college program and bring many vocational and adult education programs to the community. The goal of the community college was to make some form of college education available to everyone. Second, the cadet nurse program, which was created during World War II, demonstrated that qualified students could be educated adequately in less than the traditional 3 years. Third, the development of associate degree education was influenced by the studies conducted on nursing education in the United States, as discussed in Chapter 5. The final factor influencing the development of associate degree education was the critical national nursing shortage of the 1950s, which occurred because nurses employed during World War II returned home to raise families. It was anticipated that the 2-year program would produce nurses faster, thus helping reduce the shortage of nurses while, at the same time, helping to move nursing education into the overall system of higher education in America.

Associate degree programs have helped to solve the nursing shortage of the 1960s and the 1980s. These programs, which focused on preparing graduates skilled in bedside nursing, rapidly increased in number. Associate degree programs particularly appealed to men, minorities, and older students, who had not traditionally pursued educational preparation in nursing. Because most programs were located in community colleges, they tended to be more geographically accessible than the baccalaureate programs located in 4-year colleges and universities.

Characteristics of Associate Degree Education

Associate degree education began with the Cooperative Research Project in Junior and Community College Education for Nursing at Teachers College, Columbia University. The original 5-year research project, which was directed by Mildred Montag, included seven junior and community colleges and one hospital school, located in six regions of the United States. This type of nursing education has expanded from these original programs in 1952 to approximately 885 in 2000.

The four basic characteristics of associate degree education originally included (NLN, 1973):

1. Encompassing the nursing program as an integral part of the college that controls and finances the program
2. Ensuring the members of the nursing faculty the same privileges and responsibilities granted to other faculty
3. Organizing a curriculum with a clearly stated philosophy, rationale, and conceptual framework, designed to be completed in 2 years
4. Ensuring that nursing students are treated the same as other community college students with regard to admission, progression, and graduation requirements. The programs are designed to award an associate degree on completion, and graduates are eligible to write the state licensing examination for registered nursing.

In a typical program, approximately half of the credits needed for the associate degree must be fulfilled by general education courses such as English, anatomy, physiology, speech, psychology, and sociology; the other half must be fulfilled by nursing courses. Clinical learning experiences are carefully selected to correspond with the content delivered in classroom lectures; the pre- and post-conferences help to reinforce the relationship between the two. Some modifications in this structure are occurring as associate degree educators strive to meet the expectations of employers and the community while remaining true to the concept of associate degree education.

Competencies of the Associate Degree Graduate

In 1978, the Council of Associate Degree Programs (CADP) of the National League for Nursing (NLN) published a document entitled "Competencies of the Associate Degree Graduate" that was intended to describe the behaviors the associate degree graduates demonstrate on graduation. This document was revised and retitled as "Educational Outcomes of Associate Degree Nursing Programs: Roles and Competencies," in 1990. The revision condensed what were previously five roles into three. The roles identified in 1990 included: Role as Provider of Care, Role as Manager of Care, and Role as Member Within the Discipline of Nursing. It further expanded the competencies to reflect those that the graduate is expected to demonstrate 6 months following graduation. Many programs used these competencies as guidelines in the structure of the curriculum. Again, in 1999, a Task Force of CADP revisited the competency statements. The 1999 revisions reflected a much more comprehensive look at nursing and the role of the associate degree graduate and were less specific regarding particular skills. How these new statements might be used for curriculum development remains to be seen.

The advent of associate degree education in nursing has brought greater diversity in the students who enroll in nursing programs (Fig. 6-1). Nursing students were traditionally a homogeneous group—typically single white women, ranging in age from 18 to 35, who graduated in the upper third of their high school classes. Associate degree programs (although they sometimes impose selective admission policies on the "open door" philosophy of the community colleges) attract older people, married women, minorities, men, and students with a wider range of educational experiences and intellectual abilities. People who already possess baccalaureate or higher degrees in other fields sometimes seek admission to an associate degree program, often because it can be completed in a shorter period of time than would be needed to earn another baccalaureate degree.

Concerns Facing Associate Degree Education

Associate degree education, like other educational programs, has experienced change. With these changes have come some concerns.

PRESSURE TO INCREASE CREDITS

As programs have developed, there has been a growing tendency to place more emphasis and time on nursing courses than on general education courses. Faculty members, prepared with master's degrees in nursing, and nursing advisory committee members from service settings have difficulty defining *essential content*. Faculty members often try to comply with requests from advisory committees for graduates who will need

FIGURE 6–1 Associate degree programs attract older people, married women, minorities, men, and students with a wider range of educational experiences and intellectual capabilities.

shorter orientation programs, and who will possess greater knowledge in certain specialty areas (eg, coronary care). The 1990 changes in the role of the graduate as defined by the Council of Associate Degree Programs of the National League for Nursing established the need for courses in the curriculum to include management principles and skills. Changes that some colleges have made in the basic requirements for all associate degrees have increased the number of non-nursing credits nursing students must complete; the concept of "core courses" that are taken by all students who graduate from a college has become popular. More content and a greater number of credit hours, selective admission criteria (that give preference to students who have completed general education course work), long waiting lists for entry, and students who cannot attend school on a full-time basis are all factors that have contributed to programs that can take as many as 3 to 5 years to complete.

The recent shift to community-based practice also offers a challenge to associate degree educators. What part of the current curriculum should be cut to provide community experiences? How are community experiences to be supervised? What should be the balance between inpatient care and community experiences? Faculty members who have spent the greater part of their clinical nursing careers in acute care settings are sometimes reluctant to divert even an hour from the time students spent on acute care hospital units.

According to the interpretive guidelines for NLNAC accreditation, the maximum number of credits for an associate degree in nursing is 108 quarter hours or 72 semester hours (NLNAC, 1999). Many schools have struggled to meet this criterion.

THE SELECTIVE ADMISSION PROCESS

Another concern educators struggle with is the process used in selecting students for a nursing program. This challenge becomes more difficult to meet as the number of students seeking admission either increases dramatically or drops significantly, a phenomenon many programs have experienced over the last 15 to 20 years. As the demographics of students seeking admission become more diverse, the task of bringing to the program students who can realize success in their endeavors represents additional challenges to nursing faculty. In response to this problem, faculty members have developed selective admission processes. Some schools use a "waiting list," which honors the concept of "first come, first served." Other schools use systems similar to a lottery. Also popular are "factoring" or "point" systems that award numerical scores for courses completed, past work experience, cumulative grade point average, or a combination of all of these. These factoring systems often require that a student spend at least a year in college to secure a position in the beginning nursing class.

MISUNDERSTANDINGS ABOUT ASSOCIATE
DEGREE EDUCATION

For many years, associate degree education was poorly understood by employers, the public, and to some extent, nursing educators in baccalaureate and higher degree programs. Although this route to nursing education is now firmly established as credible preparation for a nursing career, it has continued to receive some opposition—with rumors surfacing periodically that the programs will be discontinued. The controversy regarding "entry into practice" and the preparation needed for "professional" nursing (which will be discussed later in this chapter) is renewed intermittently, although this issue has lost much of its original passion and dissension because of the nurse shortage of the late 1990s. Thus, advocates for associate degree education continue to find themselves clarifying facts and emphasizing the contributions made by graduates of the programs.

BACCALAUREATE EDUCATION

The first school of nursing to be established in a university setting was started at the University of Minnesota in 1909. The program existed as a quasi-autonomous branch of the university's school of medicine. The program was not very different from the 3-year hospital-based program; nothing was required in the way of higher general education, and graduates were prepared for the registered nurse certificate only. Education took place predominantly through apprenticeship, and students provided service to hospitals in exchange for education. However, nursing education did become a part of an academic organization, with 16 colleges and universities having developed programs by 1916.

Many of the early programs offering a baccalaureate degree in nursing extended over a 5-year period. This allowed for 3 years of nursing school curriculum similar to that of the hospital-based programs, and for an additional 2 years of liberal arts. In 1924, the Yale School of Nursing became the first to be established as a separate department within a university; Annie W. Goodrich was its dean. However, the proliferation of these schools was not rapid.

Although the development of baccalaureate education for nurses may not seem like a major step to young people today, you need to remember that it was not until 1920 that the 19th Amendment to the Constitution of the United States granted women the right to vote. Many people considered nursing to be a less than desirable occupation: vocational in its orientation; overshadowed by militaristic, religious, and technical characteristics; and confined to women. Liberal education, scholarship, and knowledge were thought to be incompatible with the female personality, and capable of interfering with marriage. The nursing curriculum, with its emphasis on the performance of skills rather than on the philosophical and theoretical approaches used in the humanities, was not well accepted by universities. Opposition to collegiate education for nurses also came from physicians, who argued that nurses would be "overtrained." Physicians were not certain that a sound knowledge base was as important as the technical skills and manual dexterity that could be acquired with brief training at the bedside. Physicians also argued that a baccalaureate education would make nursing services too expensive.

Many nursing leaders have advocated for baccalaureate education as the minimum educational preparation for supervisory and administrative nursing roles. Baccalaureate education also provides the background needed for public health positions, including school nursing, and the educational base for entry into graduate education in nursing. In 1965, the ANA recommended baccalaureate preparation in nursing as the minimum educational preparation for entry into professional nursing practice, an issue discussed later in this chapter. The American Nurses' Credentialing Center, which offers certification in 24 specialty areas, now requires a baccalaureate degree for initial basic certification in a nursing specialty, and requires a master's degree for initial certification as a clinical specialist or nurse practitioner. Those certified before these new requirements took effect are permitted to maintain their certification. Although some of the other nursing specialty organizations that provide certification do not require a baccalaureate degree for certification, that situation also is changing in favor of more education.

Characteristics of Baccalaureate Education

Baccalaureate nursing programs are located in 4-year colleges and universities. A university nursing program is termed a *basic* or *generic* baccalaureate program when the program of studies includes an upper division (junior and senior years) nursing major that is built onto 2 years of liberal arts and science courses taken during the freshman and sophomore years.

Applicants to such programs must meet the entrance and graduation requirements established by the university, and those of the nursing school. The admission requirements usually specify academic preparation at the high school (or preadmission) level, including courses in foreign language and higher-level mathematics and science, and a high cumulative grade point average. Relatively high scores on college admission tests also may be required.

During the freshman and sophomore years, students who pursue a nursing education take humanities, social, life, and physical science courses with college students who are preparing for other majors. In some schools, these courses may be completed on a part-time basis; however, this extends the overall course of study beyond 4 years. The number of required liberal arts and science courses may vary from program to program, but usually constitutes about one half the total number of credits specified for graduation—typically 120 semester credits or 180 quarter credits. Students usually begin their study of nursing content in their junior year, thus the term "upper-division major" in nursing. Nursing theory can be taught so that it builds on an understanding of the physical and biologic sciences and liberal arts studied the previous 2 years.

Until the 1980s most schools offering the baccalaureate degree in nursing required sophomore level nursing courses. Curriculum restructuring and economic pressures gradually led many baccalaureate programs to eliminate sophomore level courses with all nursing being taught in the last two years. More recently, some schools offering a baccalaureate degree in nursing have resumed introducing nursing content in the sophomore year of study. Nursing courses offered at this point often include an overview of the nursing profession and some of the fundamental nursing skills.

Students in baccalaureate nursing programs learn basic nursing skills. They also learn concepts of health maintenance and promotion, and disease prevention; supervisory and leadership techniques and practices also are taught, along with an introduction to research. Clinical course work includes experience in public health nursing, community health settings, and leadership responsibility within the acute care hospital. Emphasis is placed on developing skills in critical decision-making, on exercising independent nursing judgments that call for broad background knowledge, and on working in complex nursing situations in which the outcomes are often not predictable. Acting as a client advocate, the graduate with a baccalaureate degree in nursing collaborates with other members of the health care team in structured and unstructured settings, and supervises those with lesser preparation. Baccalaureate graduates often work with groups as well as with individuals. Baccalaureate programs face some of the same pressures faced by associate degree programs with a demand for additional content to be added to an already full curriculum.

Changes in Baccalaureate Education

In recent years, the nature of baccalaureate education has changed. Some schools, seeking to add an advanced component, have included courses that permit a degree of specialization at the baccalaureate level (eg, supplemental courses in coronary or critical care nursing). Other schools are providing more grounding in research, either as preparation for graduate school or for a more varied role in nursing. There is another interesting variation in baccalaureate education in California. In that state, the rules and regulations for schools of nursing stipulate that all courses required by the Board of Nursing for licensure as a registered nurse be offered within the first 36 months of full-time training, the first six academic semesters, or the first nine academic quarters, whichever is shortest (California Board of Registered Nursing, 1994). This means that all educational preparation required for application for licensure in California must be completed by the end of the junior year. The senior year is then open for specialty experience, preceptorships, or whatever a school might deem appropriate education. This variation in the licensure law has caused problems. Some students complete their junior year and successfully pass the licensing examination; these students may elect to drop out of school and work as registered nurses. Although they are licensed in the state of California in the category of "nongraduate" allowed by that state, these students have no educational credentials. This creates problems if they seek licensure in another state, because all other states (at the present time) require a degree or diploma for licensure. Table 6-1 provides a comparison of the major avenues to registered nurse licensure.

MASTER'S AND DOCTORAL PROGRAMS THAT PREPARE FOR LICENSURE

Our discussion of the various educational programs for registered nursing would be incomplete without mention of the generic master's program. The concept of the master's degree in nursing developed at Yale and several other schools of nursing, where students admitted with a baccalaureate degree in another area were granted a master's degree in nursing after completing an established 2-year program of study that prepared them for registered nurse licensure. Case Western Reserve University initiated the first program in which the student earns a doctorate in nursing (ND) before being eligible to write the licensing examination. Most of the graduates of these programs are engaged in teaching and research.

TABLE 6–1.   Educational Opportunities for Registered Nursing: A Comparison

	Diploma	Associate Degree	Baccalaureate
Location	Is usually conducted by and based in a hospital	Most often conducted in junior or community colleges, occasionally in senior colleges and universities	Located in senior colleges and universities
Length of Study	Requires generally 24–30 months but may require 3 academic years	Requires usually 2 academic or sometimes 2 calendar years	Requires 4 academic years
Requirements for Admission	Requires graduation from high school or its equivalent, satisfactory general academic achievement, and successful completion of certain prerequisite courses	Requires that applicants meet entrance requirements of college as well as of program	Requires that applicants meet entrance requirements of the college or university as well as those of program
Program of Learning	Includes courses in theory and practice of nursing and in biologic, physical, and behavioral sciences. May require that certain courses in the physical and social sciences be taken at a local college or university	Combines a balance of nursing courses and college courses in the basic natural and social sciences with courses in general education and the humanities	Frequently concentrates on courses in the theory and practice of nursing in the junior and senior years. Provides education in the theory and practice of nursing and courses in the liberal arts as well as the behavioral and physical sciences
Clinical Component	Provides early and substantial clinical learning experiences in the hospital and a variety of community agencies; these focus on an understanding of the hospital environment and the interrelationship of other health disciplines	Requires as a significant part of the program supervised clinical instruction in hospitals and other community health agencies	Provides clinical laboratory courses in a variety of settings where health and nursing care are given
Opportunity for Educational Advancement	Little or no transferability of courses unless affiliated with a community college or university	Is structured so that some credits may be applied to baccalaureate degree	Provides the basic academic preparation for advancement to higher positions in nursing and to master's degree

(continues)

These programs reflect the thinking of some nursing leaders that the minimum preparation for professional nursing should be the master's degree. These programs also provide a higher degree to those people who possess basic baccalaureate preparation in another area of study and are making a career change. With increasing emphasis on the need for a baccalaureate degree for professional practice, this type of program provides a credible opportunity to those with baccalaureate degrees in another

		TABLE 6–1. Educational Opportunities for Registered Nursing: A Comparison *(Continued)*		
	Diploma	**Associate Degree**	**Baccalaureate**
Competency on Graduation	Graduate is prepared to plan for the care of patients with other members of the health care team, to develop and carry out plans for the care of individuals or groups of patients, and to direct selected members of the nursing team. Has an understanding of the hospital climate and the community health resources necessary for the extended care of patients	Graduate is prepared to plan and give direct patient care in hospitals, nursing homes, or similar health care agencies and to participate with other members of the health care team, such as licensed practical nurses, nurses aides, physicians, and other registered nurses, in rendering care to patients.	Graduate is prepared to plan and give direct care to individuals and families, whether sick or well, to assume responsibility for directing other members of the health care team, and to take on beginning leadership positions. Practices in a variety of settings and emphasizes comprehensive health care, including preventive and rehabilitative services, health counseling and education, and care in acute and long-term illnesses. Has necessary education for graduate study toward a master's degree and may move rapidly to specialized leadership positions in nursing as teacher, administrator, clinical specialist, nurse practitioner, and nurse researcher
Licensure	Must successfully complete state licensing examination	Must successfully complete state licensing examination	Must successfully complete state licensing examination

area of study. When programs of this type are not available, many students with degrees in other disciplines choose to pursue a 2-year associate degree in nursing. Even when other options are available, some people with degrees in other disciplines opt for the 2-year degree because it requires less time and expense.

A generic master's degree program or generic doctoral program is not without its problems for the graduate. Although the newly licensed individual is truly a novice in the field, the expectation of most employers is that the graduate degree represents an expert level of practice. Thus, the graduate must carefully discuss expectations with any employer and clarify his or her own preparation for the role.

SIMILARITIES AMONG ENTRY-LEVEL PROGRAMS

Currently there are as many similarities in the various avenues to nursing education as there are differences. These similarities may be grouped into several broad classifications, including academic standards, administrative concerns, and areas relating to students.

Academic Similarities

In the academic realm, several similarities stand out:

1. All graduates write the NCLEX for registered nursing in their state. All writers must meet the same minimum cutoff score to pass the test and become licensed.
2. All schools preparing graduates for RN licensure must meet the criteria established for state board approval.
3. Most schools preparing for RN licensure (both associate degree and baccalaureate degree) have a similar number of credits of basic nursing education. Baccalaureate degree programs add credits for research, community health nursing, and leadership components.
4. All faculty are pushed to develop curricula responsive to the needs of today's health care delivery system, which demands greater efficiency, an ability to work in a highly technical environment, knowledge of new protocols, community experiences, and greater responsibility and accountability. A knowledge explosion and the emphasis on evidence-based practice challenges nurse educators to remain current of the newest developments and flexible when it comes to change.
5. All programs are placing a greater emphasis on critical thinking skills especially as related to decision making in the clinical area. Much energy is invested in finding the best method(s) to measure such thinking as an outcome of undergraduate education. These activities have been brought to the fore by changing standards for accreditation developed by the National League for Nursing Accreditation Commission in the 1990s.
6. The recruitment of faculty possessing master's and doctoral degrees is ongoing. Salaries in education have lagged behind those in practice. The graduate with a master's degree can find interesting and challenging positions in hospitals, clinics, and even in private practice that offer salaries far better than those offered in colleges and universities.
7. Members of the faculty are pushed to meet the increasing demands of education, clinical excellence, tenure, and possibly vocational certification or research. The workload and the time invested in performance of professional responsibilities often are greater than for instructors in other disciplines, even though they are considered colleagues in the educational setting.

Administrative Similarities

From an administrative perspective, three similarities are noted among entry-level programs:

1. Adequate financial support is a major concern. All nursing programs are relatively expensive to operate in comparison with other forms of education provided in colleges and universities. Federal and state agencies, as well as colleges and universities, are limiting funding and demanding greater accountability. In tough economic times, the nursing program—like the one at the University of

California, Los Angeles (UCLA)—may be the one chosen to be phased out. Less financial assistance is available to students in the form of scholarships and loans than in the past. Tuition costs are rising. Lindeman (The Future of, p. 5) summarizes the situation ". . . nurse educators will work in a market driven, highly competitive, system of higher education preparing the next generations of nurses to work in a market driven, highly competitive, health care system."

2. Finding appropriate learning experiences is a challenge. Most programs find themselves competing with other schools for learning experiences in clinical agencies. To some extent, this competition is caused by changes in societal values and in the health care delivery system. Families are electing to have fewer children and, more recently in some areas, to deliver these children at home. The result has been fewer clients in the obstetric units of hospitals. Pediatric clients are managed on an outpatient basis as much as possible, and hospitalization, when required, is kept to a minimum. The management of the client with psychiatric disturbances is moving from institutions to community mental health centers whenever feasible. The increase in the number and size of schools in urban areas creates a high demand for clinical facilities. Finally, there have been changes in the attitudes of the consumer and the agency toward having students provide care. The concept of the "teaching" hospital is not as viable as it once was. Consumers paying for the high cost of care want that care provided by qualified nurses rather than by students who are still learning.

3. Decisions regarding national accreditation. Many schools wrestle with the decision of whether to seek recognition of their program through national accreditation. Historically that recognition was granted through the National League for Nursing. When, in the mid-1990s, NLN experienced challenges to their accreditation procedures and policies, the American Association of Colleges of Nursing (AACN) developed a process by which 4-year programs could be recognized through AACN. In 1996 it established the Commission on Collegiate Nursing Education (CCNE) as an autonomous arm of the AACN and officially began its accreditation review activities in 1998. At the present time, the work of this organization is devoted exclusively to the evaluation of baccalaureate and graduate programs in nursing education. Today, programs located in 4-year colleges and universities must choose from which of these two organizations they wish to seek recognition. At all levels, programs wrestle with the cost and additional work such recognition involves.

Similarities Relating to Students

Three similarities relating to students are noted:

1. Recruitment and selection of students is a major task. All schools must develop sound educational programs while balancing student enrollments against recruitment and retention factors. In some years, the number of applications significantly exceeds the positions available in beginning classes; at other times, the number of applicants is lower than is desirable. At the same time, schools must be responsive to an increasingly diverse population that at times is not

prepared for college-level studies. This has resulted in the development of selective admission policies that must be scrutinized carefully by school officials, and in some areas reviewed by the school's attorney for correct legal form and legal ramifications, before being accepted by the school's policy-making group.

2. Legal concerns are demanding more time and attention. Programs are caught up in more legal concerns than in the past, because applicants and students are seeking their "rights as individuals" and challenging admission and dismissal policies. The National Student Nursing Association Student Bill of Rights and Responsibilities is widely accepted by schools of nursing in the United States. It sets forth the students' basic rights and establishes grievance procedures if a student believes that these rights have been violated (see Chapter 3, Fig. 3-6). Another legal concern relates to malpractice coverage for students. Some collegiate programs, now removed from the umbrella coverage of the hospital, ask that students purchase malpractice insurance as protection against any lawsuits that might arise as the result of errors committed in the learning process.

3. There is greater diversity in the student body. All programs are finding more diversity in the characteristics of applicants seeking admission. Programs are receiving more applications from men, minorities, older adults, and persons who possess degrees in other fields of study. Students with English as a second language present new challenges to nursing faculty in all types of programs. One usually finds nursing educators united in their efforts to create quality programs that will graduate students who can function satisfactorily in a changing and challenging health care delivery system (see Table 6-1).

Critical Thinking Activity

Imagine that you could restructure nursing education for an ideal world. Where would you begin? How many levels of nursing education would you incorporate in your model? Would each level be terminal or articulated with others? Where would general education fit into your model? How would you see the graduate of each program functioning on the health care team? How would you see each level reimbursed for services?

OTHER FORMS OF NURSING EDUCATION

The expansion of higher educational offerings in nursing results partly from the changing role of the nurse in health care delivery, and thus the need for more adequate education to meet the requirements of that role. Another contributing factor is the continuing push to make nursing truly professional. To increase nursing's professional component, there is a need for nurses who are interested and competent in research techniques and skills. A third significant reason for advancing nursing education relates to the need for leadership in nursing administration and education. Nurse educators, joining the ranks of other professionals in the academic environment, are required to possess equivalent educational backgrounds. Nurses who assume roles in nursing administration have found the need for a solid understanding of management and finance. Thus registered nurses seek baccalaureate, master's, and doctoral degrees to support the complex roles into which they move.

Registered Nurse Baccalaureate Programs

Recently there has been an increase in the number of registered nurse baccalaureate (RNB) programs. These programs are designed for the registered nurse, with either a diploma or an associate degree, who wishes to return to school to complete a baccalaureate degree in nursing. There are also master's degree programs that admit registered nurses with associate degrees who will graduate in 3 years with a master's degree in nursing, receiving a baccalaureate degree partway through the program. Still other master's degree programs in nursing admit registered nurses with associate degrees in nursing and a baccalaureate degree in another field (see discussion below). Some schools also have added programs designed to admit the licensed practical (vocational) nurse, who will emerge with a baccalaureate degree in nursing. These programs carry different names in different parts of the country, including baccalaureate registered nurse (BRN) programs, two-on-two programs, and, in the Midwest, capstone programs.

There are many reasons for the increase in this form of nursing education, several of which were discussed above. In addition, many highly qualified young men and women enter associate degree programs because of cost and time factors and plan for more education several years after completing the original program. The nursing profession is aiming to increase the number of nurses prepared with baccalaureate and higher degrees.

The RNB programs vary greatly throughout the United States. In some instances they exist in universities that already offer the generic baccalaureate program. The students may be completely integrated with generic baccalaureate students, partially separated from them, or in a totally separate program. Another form of RNB preparation is the two-on-two approach, in which registered nurse students transfer into the college or university with junior standing and complete an additional 2 years of upper-division nursing classes. In some instances, this is the only nursing program offered by a college or university; that is, the college may not offer a basic program that prepares a graduate for licensure. Some schools offer nurse practitioner preparation in conjunction with the baccalaureate degree, although the current trend is to place this at the master's level.

Another general trend is to allow the transfer of credits in the natural and biologic sciences, and in basic courses such as psychology and sociology earned at junior and community colleges. Often some transfer of credit is allowed for nursing courses (eg, 45 quarter credits or 30 semester credits), but the courses may be challenged by examination. Distribution requirements of the particular college or university must be satisfied, and upper-division nursing courses must be completed in such areas as physiologic nursing, community health, understanding nursing research, and supervision. A minimum of 2 years usually is required for completion of the program, although the time may be shorter or longer, depending on the number of requirements satisfied at the time of entry.

Some nurse educators criticized programs offering baccalaureate education to registered nurses when they were first launched; the ladder concept in nursing education was slow to develop. The criticism seemed to have three central themes. First, many nurse educators perceived associate degree education as terminal (ending at the associate degree level), and did not accept it as a stepping stone to baccalaureate education.

The second concern related to the problems associated with evaluating and granting credit for previous education. How should nursing process taught at the freshman level in a community college be compared with nursing process taught at the junior level in a 4-year college or university?

A third problem was determining whether additional courses designed specifically for the registered nurse should be offered. Educators seriously questioned whether the standards, program objectives, and educational structures that had been developed for the generic student were appropriate for the registered nurse. What learning experiences could be included that would help to "socialize" the student for the role of a baccalaureate graduate? What additional nursing courses were needed to form the upper-division major in nursing that would provide a foundation for graduate education? How was this student the same and how was this student different than the generic student?

Because the skills of the various graduates were not clearly delineated, it was difficult to develop a curriculum that would enable the RNB graduate to demonstrate specific outcome behaviors. When attempts were made to develop such programs, baccalaureate educators were confronted with another concern: they were working with adult students. This required them to rethink teaching and learning principles to provide effective education. Students were seeking a learning program that allowed for part-time study, provided more evening and weekend classes, and permitted part- or full-time employment—in other words, a program tailored to their life circumstances.

Recently, RNB education and two-on-two educational programs have gained greater acceptance. Schools operating both basic and RNB programs may report graduating more RNB students than basic graduates. At least four factors are responsible for the change in attitude toward RNB education. First, the ANA Commission on Nursing Education has provided a push to increase the availability of baccalaureate programs for registered nurses. Nursing educators are challenged to create and accept more innovative educational strategies.

The second factor comes from pressure within each state itself. Several states have enacted legislation, sometimes in response to the nursing shortage, that requires the development of a statewide plan for articulation between various types of nursing education programs. In most instances the legislation establishes a date by which the plan will be implemented.

The third factor influencing the development of RNB programs has been a call for increased educational mobility from organizations in the health care arena. The American Medical Association (AMA) House of Delegates has suggested career mobility as one way to alleviate the nurse shortage. The Pew Commission recommended strengthening existing career ladder programs to make movement through these levels of nursing as easy as possible (de Tornyay, 1996). Some of the RNB programs currently in operation provide for part-time study or for studies completed through evening courses. The desirability of such an approach for nurses who must work to support their education is obvious. Other innovative RNB programs provide baccalaureate education to people living in areas geographically remote from colleges or universities. These programs use new technologies for distance learning, including the electronic transmission of information.

A final factor influencing the development of RNB programs relates to the allocation of federal dollars to assist students who are seeking to advance their preparation in nursing. Many of the scholarships and traineeships, once available to all students, have been directed largely to students who wish to continue their education in the area of advanced practice in nursing.

The External Degree

The concept of an external degree is not new. Universities in Australia, the Soviet Union, and England have long recognized independent study validated by examination. The University of London has awarded college degrees earned in this fashion since 1836. The major difference between the external degree and the traditional educational experience is that students awarded an external degree are not required to attend classes or follow any prescribed methods of learning (however, they may choose to take some classes). Learning is assessed through highly standardized and validated examinations. This approach to education was not developed in the United States until about the mid-1950s, and then only in selected areas. New York's Empire State College and the University Without Walls consortium were the first schools in the United States to recognize the value of self-directed learning.

The New York Regents External Degree (REX) Program of the University of the State of New York has become part of this movement. The New York Board of Regents established the College Proficiency Examination Program in 1961. Similar to the College-Level Examination Program tests developed by the Educational Testing Service, the examinations allow students to gain credit and meet the regents' external degree requirements without attending classes.

In 1971, the New York Board of Regents authorized an external associate degree program in nursing; the external baccalaureate degree in nursing was to follow in April 1976, with the first baccalaureate degrees awarded in 1979. The W. K. Kellogg Foundation provided funds to support the initiation of the program. The programs have grown in popularity.

The nursing program, like other external degree programs in arts, science, and business, uses an assessment approach and is primarily—although not exclusively—designed for those with some experience in nursing. It is philosophically based on principles of adult learning, which advocate flexible and learner-oriented education. Specifically, the responsibility for demonstrating that learning has occurred is placed on the student, and the responsibility for identifying the content to be learned and objectively assessing that this has occurred rests with the faculty. The nursing major is divided into cognitive and performance components. Cognitive learning is documented through nationally standardized and psychometrically valid written examinations. Clinical skills are evaluated through four criteria-referenced performance examinations at regional performance assessment centers throughout the country.

Despite objections, alternative and nontraditional avenues to nursing education appeal to the learner, and these programs continue to evolve. Nursing education, like nursing care, should be tailored to fit the consumer's needs. There are some limitations on the use of external degree programs. Some states do not accept New York Regents degrees for initial licensure because their laws mandate that the educational process include supervised clinical practice. Some states will admit to the licensure examination for registered nurses only those external associate degree graduates who were licensed practical nurses and therefore have had supervised clinical practice in addition to clinical examinations.

NURSING EDUCATION AT THE GRADUATE LEVEL

The critical need for nurses with additional preparation to work in educational settings, in supervisory roles, as clinical specialists, and to fulfill the expanded role of the nurse has resulted in more programs at the graduate level.

Master's Preparation

There are a variety of models of master's preparation in nursing. Some less traditional approaches include outreach programs; summers-only programs; RN-to-MSN tracks (that provide a direct route to the master's degree for registered nurses who have graduated from diploma or associate degree programs); programs for students with special needs (such as registered nurses with non-nursing baccalaureate degrees, or those seeking preparation as technical nurse educators); and programs that admit non-nurses and foreign graduates. Some schools offer off-campus classes, at times rotating sites, and some deliver core content by way of television or through other distance learning technology. In at least one school, all classes are on Fridays. Several unique programs (eg, those at Yale University, Pace University, and the University of Tennessee at Knoxville) offer a master's degree in nursing after completion of a baccalaureate degree in another field. Such programs, called generic master's degree programs, were discussed earlier in the chapter.

Most programs require at least a full year for completion; many have been expanded to 2 years. Master's programs in nursing typically are found in senior colleges and universities that have baccalaureate programs in nursing. They have the option of seeking voluntary accreditation from the NLN.

Doctoral Studies

The number of requests for admission to doctoral study in nursing has increased greatly since the early 1980s. The impetus for this movement stems from the need for advanced study for academic advancement or tenure in the educational setting, and reflects the need in nursing research for the advancement of the profession as a whole.

Before doctorates in nursing were offered, doctoral study in other fields allowed nurses to benefit from post-master's preparation. A doctorate outside the area of nursing was often the only doctorate available to the person seeking further education; doctorates in nursing are relatively new to the educational milieu, as opposed to such degrees in psychology, sociology, anthropology, or physiology. Certainly nursing can and has benefited from other disciplines.

Doctoral programs in nursing offer various degrees such as the doctor of nursing science (DNSc), the doctor of science in nursing (DSN), the doctor of nursing education (DNEd), and the doctor of philosophy (PhD) in nursing. Other types of doctorates are available to nurses, such as the doctor of education (EdD) and the doctor of public health (DPH).

The difference in the preparation and function of graduates possessing the various degrees is confusing; typically, the nurse with a doctorate assumes a leadership role in education, often serving as a faculty member or the dean or director of a nursing program. These nurses also may choose to be involved in the research and development of a body of nursing knowledge.

An "Annual Guide to Graduate Nursing Education," which provides a listing of Post-Master's Certificate Programs, RN to Master's Programs, Nurse Practitioner Programs, and Doctoral Programs, is published each year by Jones and Bartlett, who do much of the publishing for the National League for Nursing.

Critical Thinking Activity

If nurse practitioners are to work in a collaborative way with physicians, and as primary care providers, what type and level of education do you believe they should complete? How would you ensure that this would occur? What standards regarding continuing education should be mandated for those involved in advance practice? Should it be more stringent than that required at the registered nurse level? Defend your position.

ARTICULATED PROGRAMS

Today, as increasing numbers of graduates seek additional education beyond the associate degree or diploma, the "ladder" concept in nursing education is growing in popularity. This has resulted in more registered nurse baccalaureate and "two-on-two" programs. Programs have been developed that provide direct articulation between lower-level and higher-level programs. In some states legislation has been passed strongly encouraging, and in some instances mandating, articulation plans.

The purpose of an articulated program is to facilitate opportunities for students to start nursing education, stop when some goal is achieved, or keep moving up the educational ladder. Several states (California, Colorado, Florida, Maryland, Minnesota, Missouri, New Mexico, North Dakota, Texas, Utah, and others) have established statewide articulation plans that provide the opportunity for registered nurses from associate degree programs to transfer to RNB programs. Many allow most of the work completed at the lower level to meet the requirements of the baccalaureate degree. The University of Washington, and some other schools, have formalized R.N. to master's pathways.

Similar plans exist for articulation between practical (vocational) nurse programs and associate degree programs. Again, the articulated program allows students to move up the career ladder from practical nurse to associate degree nurse, to the nurse with a baccalaureate degree. Students in an articulated licensed practical nurse/ associate degree program spend a year preparing to be an LP(V)N, and another year completing the associate degree. If they want to continue after this 2-year period, they can earn a baccalaureate degree at another institution after 2 more years of study. From that point, a student may continue to work toward a master's degree (Fig. 6-2).

Such programs usually involve planning between two or more institutions, but, depending on start and stop points, they may exist within a single institution. Of concern to nurse educators today is whether nursing assistants should be included in this ladder approach and, if so, how they can be accommodated. Some state boards of nursing already have stipulated that a mechanism be established to recognize the previous knowledge acquired by the nursing assistant.

The multiple-entry, multiple-exit programs are not without problems. Initially they are difficult to develop because of the tremendous amount of joint planning they require. Leveling of content in both nursing and in the supporting areas of the natural and behavioral sciences is critical. Understanding what has been taught and determining how to evaluate current knowledge is also important. This is particularly relevant to articulation between practical nurse programs and registered nurse programs, where

FIGURE 6–2 Among innovations occurring in nursing education over the past decade are programs that provide direct articulation between lower-level and higher-level programs.

graduates of the practical program may know how to perform many of the nursing skills but may lack the theory base of registered nurses. Educators need to speak the same language and develop mutual respect.

NONDEGREE PROGRAMS

Specialized programs have been developed to help individuals to prepare for roles of increased breadth and scope. Some programs are incorporated into the preparation leading to a particular degree; others exist as part of a school's continuing education program.

The registered nurse anesthesia and midwifery programs both award a certificate after completion of a standardized and rigorous course of study lasting from 18 months to 2 years. At one time, admission requirements stipulated licensure only; however, the trend is toward making a baccalaureate degree in nursing an admission requirement, and toward awarding a master's degree on completion of the program. Some states require a master's degree for the nurse anesthetist or nurse midwife.

More recent programs offer nurse practitioner and nursing specialist preparation in areas of nursing practice such as pediatrics, gerontology, family health, genetics, and women's health care. Recent health care reform has resulted in an increased emphasis on the role of advanced nursing practice in health care delivery, and more demand for educational programs to prepare these practitioners. The Pew Commission has encouraged the growing number of master's level nurse practitioner training programs (de Tornyay, 1996). Lipman and Deatrick (1994) stipulate that advanced skills in clinical decision making, and coordinating care from the hospital to the community and home, are essential parts of this preparation. Programs that prepare nurse practitioners concentrate study in specific areas over a period lasting from several months to a year or more. Requirements for admission vary tremendously. Most require licensure and a baccalaureate degree, and still others require that the education occur at the post-master's degree level. The American Nurses' Credentialing Center requires the master's degree for all those seeking initial nurse practitioner certification, and some states now require the master's degree for those seeking initial licensure as a nurse practitioner.

The proliferation of such programs has been so great that a complete listing is impossible. A student interested in pursuing such preparation is encouraged to write to the college or university of choice for information about available programs.

RESIDENCIES AND STRUCTURED ORIENTATION FOR THE NEW GRADUATE

When nursing education moved from hospital-based diploma programs into higher education, a new problem was created. Employers of the new graduates, who expected these graduates to function as experienced and qualified professionals on the day after graduation, complained that the graduates were not prepared to assume staff nurse positions within their institutions.

As nursing education moved into institutions of higher education, all clinical time was recognized in credit hours. If students worked on hospital units on weekends, they did so as hospital employees, not as a requirement of their education. As a result, students spent less time in the clinical area. Many graduates of diploma schools in the 1950s would have had as much as 4000 clock hours of clinical experience, albeit more as apprenticeship and service to the hospital than as a learning experience. Graduates of associate and baccalaureate degree programs, with integrated curricula and objective-based learning experiences, joined the work world with clinical learning time of 800 or fewer clock hours. Hospital-based programs also decreased their clinical hours as curricula were reorganized.

Those employed in nursing service, who were accustomed to a graduate who had spent the last three months of education running a unit, were critical of this new type of graduate who could think, analyze, and synthesize, but who was inexperienced in "doing." Individuals graduating today need orientation to the work facility and to their new role, and time to become efficient in using their newly learned skills. Although few would question the need for internships and residencies for new physicians, the need for similar experiences for new nursing graduates has been disputed. The new graduates, unable to live up to expectations placed on them, often became frustrated and discouraged; some opted for less stressful situations, sometimes even outside nursing. Nursing educators, in defending the education provided, cited other professions, such as law and engineering, in which graduates needed time to adapt to the world of work.

As a result of efforts to address this concern, orientation programs, internships, and residencies for new graduates were instituted by hospitals. The programs were intended to ease the transition from the role of student to that of staff by providing the opportunity to increase clinical skills and knowledge, as well as self-confidence. These programs can last from several weeks to a year, and are designed for graduates of all nursing programs—associate degree, diploma, and baccalaureate. They often include rotations to various units in the hospital, including specialty areas, and they accommodate different shifts. Usually some formal class work is associated with the experience, but the majority of the time is spent in direct patient care, often under the supervision of a preceptor.

Institutions receive some direct benefits from such programs in addition to securing a better prepared employee who remains in employment. Inadequacies in policy and procedure books have been uncovered and, as a result, these books have been rewritten. Performance evaluation tools that are more objective in format have emerged. Nursing practice throughout some agencies has become more standardized. Job satisfaction has increased. It is no longer unusual for hospitals to advertise planned orientation and internships as benefits offered to the new graduate seeking employment.

The major disadvantage voiced by hospitals is the cost of operating such programs. When cost containment is crucial, hospitals are not anxious to deal with the additional costs of such programs. Another problem is that some employees who benefit from such programs may resign from their positions soon after completing an internship. This has resulted in hospitals stipulating a period of required employment following the orientation or internship.

FACTORS INFLUENCING NURSING EDUCATION

During the 20th century, society experienced tremendous change. Nursing, as a part of that society, has also experienced enormous change. A number of factors influenced nursing education.

The Brown Report

In 1948, Esther Lucille Brown, who was not a nurse (see Chapter 5), conducted one of the important early studies of nursing. She was concerned that young women were not choosing nursing as a profession, and believed, as a result of her study, that the majority of nursing schools failed to provide a professional education. In "Nursing for the Future," Brown (1948) recommended that nursing education move away from the system of apprenticeship that predominated at the time (see earlier discussion of hospital-based programs in Chapter 4), and move toward a planned program of education similar to that offered by other professions. She recommended that the schools be operated by universities or colleges, hospitals affiliated with institutions of higher learning, medical colleges, or independently. She also recommended that programs periodically be examined or reviewed, and that a list of accredited schools be published and distributed.

The Brown report attracted the attention of many nursing leaders who shared her concerns about recruiting qualified women into nursing. The study took place shortly after World War II, and nurses who had been involved in the military had a new sense of autonomy and independence that they were not willing to leave behind. Committees were formed to respond to the suggestions put forth in the Brown study, particularly those related to the accreditation of programs. At the same time, the National League for Nursing Education (NLNE), later to become the National League for Nursing (NLN), recommended that hospital schools of nursing consider transferring control and administration of their programs to educational institutions. The NLNE also urged that federal grants be provided to nursing schools to allow for their improvement.

Development of the State Board Test Pool Examination

Along with the push for the improvement of nursing education, licensing authorities were pressured to establish a uniform licensing examination. The development and adoption of uniform testing throughout the United States is discussed in Chapter 7. The development of the State Board Test Pool Examination helped all schools to focus on common goals, and laid the foundation for interstate endorsement of licenses.

National Accreditation of Nursing Programs

By 1952, the NLN had a temporary accreditation program in place, and was helping schools to find ways to improve their programs of instruction. The accreditation of programs had a noticeable effect on standards of nursing education. As a result of accreditation activities, schools were forced to look at the educational preparation of faculty, the workload of faculty and students, the structure of clinical teaching, withdrawal rates, and the state board examination scores. This system of program assessment enhanced the quality of education, and graduation from a nationally accredited school meant added opportunities for advanced education or certain types of employment.

Changes in Nursing Service

While changes were occurring in the education of nurses, nurses in the workplace also experienced significant changes. With the advent of antibiotics and other major advances in medical protocols and medical technology during the mid century, the public was receiving care in hospitals rather than treatment in the home. Infants previously born at home were now being born in hospitals. Federal funds were allocated for the construction of hospitals. Increased hospitalization drove the need for qualified nurses to a new high. Hospitals were desperate to find nurses to fill needed positions, and nurses represented half of all hospital personnel.

The role of the nurse changed in response to changes in the workplace. Nursing staff began assuming responsibilities formerly associated with physicians. Unfortunately, they were also assuming responsibilities that could have been assumed by housekeeping, dietary, laboratory, and pharmacy departments. Nurses began spending more time managing personnel, delegating responsibilities, and carrying out other administrative duties. Nurses at higher levels in the organization needed higher levels of education (ie, baccalaureate and master's degrees).

The Report of the Surgeon General's Consultant Group

In 1961, the Surgeon General of the United States Public Health Service appointed a group to advise him of the federal government's role in providing adequate nursing services to the country. This group was known as the Surgeon General's Consultant Group on Nursing, and they published their report in 1963.

The report emphasized the need for more nurses, and identified the lack of adequate financial resources for nursing education as a major problem. Several other major concerns also were reported. Of critical importance were the reports that too few schools were providing adequate nursing education, that too few college-bound young people were being recruited into the profession, and that more nursing schools were needed in colleges and universities. Educational preparation at the baccalaureate degree level was recommended as the minimum preparation for nurses assuming leadership roles (U.S. Public Health Service, 1963).

The Surgeon General's Consultant Group on Nursing also recommended that federally funded low-cost loans and scholarships be made available to students in both professional and practical nursing programs. It advocated the use of federal funds to construct additional nursing school facilities and to expand educational programs. The Nurse Training Act of 1964 was an outgrowth of these recommendations.

The American Nurses Association Position Paper

In the early 1960s, the educational preparation of nurses became a major concern of the American Nurses Association (ANA). The ANA believed that the improvement of nursing practice depended on the advancement of nursing education. In 1962, a committee was appointed to study the issue. In 1965, this activity culminated in the development and publication of "A Position Paper on Educational Preparation for Nurse Practitioners and Assistants to Nurses."

The paper took four major positions:

1. The education of all those who are licensed to practice nursing should take place in institutions of higher education.
2. Minimum preparation for beginning professional nursing practice at the present time should be baccalaureate degree education in nursing.
3. Minimum preparation for beginning technical nursing practice at the present time should be associate degree education in nursing.
4. Education for assistants in the health service occupations should be short, intensive pre-service programs in vocational education institutions, rather than on-the-job training programs (American Nurses Association, 1965, p 107).

RESPONSES TO THE ANA POSITION PAPER

No other single action or position affected nursing as much as the ANA position paper. For almost 40 years, the profession has been divided over the issues it brought forth. A basic concern related to the fact that the roles, functions, and responsibilities (competencies) were not clearly differentiated for graduates of programs offering three different routes to preparation for registered nursing. All graduates took the same examination and performed similar activities when hired as new graduates in acute care facilities. That situation has not changed since the publication of the position paper.

Associate degree nursing programs in community colleges and hospital-based diploma programs took serious exception to the paper. Both groups saw their graduates as "professionals" and were unwilling to compromise title or licensure. As a result, many individuals associated with these two groups dropped their membership in ANA because they could not support this position.

Because of the dissension the position paper created among nursing groups, little immediate action followed. In 1974, New York became the first state association to support the ANA position; however, attempts to change the licensure law were unsuccessful. By 1986, 48 state nurses' associations had taken positions supporting the change. In January 1986, the North Dakota Board of Nursing published and put into effect administrative rules that required nursing programs to develop specific curricula leading to the associate degree for practical nurse programs and to the baccalaureate degree for registered nurse programs. The requirement became effective January 1, 1987. Thus North Dakota became the first, and to date the only, state to require graduates from colleges within the state to have a baccalaureate degree to take the licensure examination for registered nurse licensure and an associate degree for the licensure examination for practical nurse licensure (North Dakota Rule, 1986). Graduates from other states seeking licensure in North Dakota are given a specified period of time in which to meet this educational requirement.

Other nursing organizations also reviewed the tenets of the position paper and endorsed it. The first was the National Student Nurses' Association, which voted in favor of the paper at its 1976 convention. Soon other groups took positions supporting a baccalaureate degree as the minimum educational level for future entry into professional practice. In 1979, the following organizations endorsed this position: the Association of Operating Room Nurses, the Emergency Department Nurses' Association, The Association of Rehabilitation Nurses, the American Association of Occupational Health Nurses, and the Executive Board of the Nurses' Association of the American College of Obstetricians and Gynecologists (now called the Association of Women's Health, Obstetric, and Neonatal Nursing).

Several other groups have had more difficulty establishing a position regarding this issue. Because members of the NLN include educational councils representing practical, diploma, associate degree, baccalaureate, and higher degree programs, the organization has voiced support for all types of programs. At the 1987 biennial convention, the membership "postponed indefinitely" resolutions addressing this issue, and in 1989 instructed the NLN to put its energies into activities that would promote upward mobility in nursing.

The National Council of State Boards of Nursing and the National Federation of Licensed Practical Nurses (NFLPN) also made decisions about the education required for entry into practice. At an August 1986 meeting, representatives of the state boards voted without debate or opposition to take a "formal position of neutrality on changes in nursing education requirement for entry" (Hartung, 1986, p 124). In August 1984, the membership of the NFLPN voted to support increasing the period of study in the practical nurse program to 18 months, and to support awarding an associate degree at the completion of the program of study. To date only North Dakota has begun to implement these NFLPN recommendations.

Problems Associated with Changing Educational Requirements for Licensure

Several problems are associated with making any changes in educational requirements for licensure. Four major problems are related to titling, scope of practice, grandfathering, and interstate endorsement.

TITLING

One of the most controversial problems associated with changing requirements for licensure involves the use of *titles*. The RN title has a long history and is clearly recognizable to the public and to the health care community. Some states advocated using "RN" for the baccalaureate graduate and "LPN" for the 2-year associate degree graduate. Needless to say, this is unacceptable to associate degree graduates and students, who currently use the RN title if successful on state licensing examinations. It is also upsetting to graduates of current diploma schools, from which no degree is granted. They feel their contribution is being ignored. Others have suggested that the graduates of 2-year programs be titled "associate nurse" or "registered associate nurse." When a tertiary care hospital in South Dakota implemented differentiated nursing practice, the terms "associate nurse" for the associate degree graduate and "primary nurse" for the baccalaureate graduate were used. This approach again overlooks the diploma graduate. It is not likely that this issue can be resolved easily even as we make strong efforts to move toward differentiated practice (discussed later in this chapter).

SCOPE OF PRACTICE

Of equal concern is the description and delineation of the *scope of practice* for the two levels of caregivers. The scope of practice (discussed in Chapter 7) is that section of the Nurse Practice Act that outlines the activities a person with a particular license may legally perform. This would mean the separate testing of each level as currently exists between the registered nurse and the practical nurse licensure examination. This problem might be of less concern if the nursing profession could agree on an approach to differentiated practice. As some states have moved toward plans for two levels of practice, the process of making nursing diagnoses and developing nursing care plans sometimes has been included in the scope of practice of the baccalaureate-prepared nurse only, a position totally unacceptable to associate degree advocates. Again, the diploma graduate is left out of the discussion.

THE GRANDFATHER CLAUSE

The application of the *grandfather clause* presents another challenge to nurses. Historically, when a state licensure law is enacted, or if a current law is repealed and a new law enacted, the grandfather clause has been a standard feature that allows persons to continue to practice their profession or occupation after new qualifications have been enacted into law. The legal basis for the process is found in the 14th Amendment to the U.S. Constitution, which says that no state may deprive any person of life, liberty, or property without due process of law. The Supreme Court has ruled that the license to practice is a property right. The grandfather clause has been used in nursing at various times in the past. For example, when psychiatric nursing became a requirement of all programs, nurses who graduated and were licensed without psychiatric nursing experiences were "grandfathered" into the new role. In other words, they continued to practice as registered nurses without taking a formal course in psychiatric nursing, and without being required to write a psychiatric examination to maintain their licenses. If nursing began to require a baccalaureate degree for individuals using the registered nurse title, under the provisions of the grandfather clause, all associate graduates licensed prior to the implementation date for the change would continue to use the title "registered nurse." Those licensed after the change would use whatever new title was established. Although this serves to "protect" the title of currently licensed nurses, it does not prevent employers from writing job descriptions stipulating a baccalaureate degree as the minimum educational preparation acceptable for a particular position.

Complicating this matter is the fact that some nurses believe the grandfather clause should be conditional. If it were conditional, nurses licensed before the changes in the licensure law would continue to use their current title for a stipulated period of time—

for example, 10 years. At the end of that period, if they had not completed the education mandated in the changes (or any other conditions that might have been added), they would have to use the title stipulated in the new law for nurses with their educational preparation. Because of the complexity and the difficulties associated with implementation, it is unlikely that conditional "grandfathering" will ever become a reality.

INTERSTATE ENDORSEMENT

A fourth concern is that of *interstate endorsement*. Nursing is one of the few professions to have developed a process whereby national examinations with standardized scores are administered in each state or jurisdiction. This allows a nurse who has passed the licensing examination in one state to move to another state and seek licensure, without the need to retake and pass another examination. Because nurses have been highly mobile, this has been a great advantage. Changes in one state without similar changes in other states affect nursing mobility. For example, if a graduate of an associate degree program in New Jersey, who has passed the National Council Licensing Examination for registered nursing (NCLEX-RN), seeks licensure in North Dakota, additional education is required. North Dakota would issue the graduate a temporary permit to work as a registered nurse in North Dakota under the condition that the graduate enrolls in a baccalaureate program. The temporary permit is renewable as long as progress is made toward the degree. A permanent license is issued only when the baccalaureate degree is awarded. However, if this same New Jersey nurse moved to any other state, licensure as a registered nurse would be granted immediately without the need to meet the requirement of attaining an additional degree.

As the profession examines multistate licensure (see Chapter 7) this issue takes on new dimensions.

Critical Thinking Activity

> Take a stand on the ANA Position on Nursing Education. Provide a rationale for the position you have taken. What do you see as the outcome of the position paper? How would your position be implemented in the future? What implications might it have for nursing practice? Do you believe the salaries of nurses educated at different levels and practicing at differentiated levels should differ? Why or why not? If so, how?

DIFFERENTIATED PRACTICE

In the beginning of the 1990s, some nursing leaders began to reassess the entry-into-practice issue. Although the nursing shortage of the late 1980s and the push toward cost cutting in the 1990s may have encouraged its reevaluation, the review also may reflect a new thinking regarding the role of nurses and nursing and the role of all education in the United States. Many nursing leaders encouraged recognition of the need for different types of practitioners prepared with different types of education, or differentiated practice. *Differentiated nursing practice* can be defined as "the practice of structuring nursing roles on the basis of education, experience, and competence" (Boston, 1990, p. 2). It also has been defined as "practice expectations that are consistent with expected competencies of graduates from different kinds of education programs" (Harkness, Miller and Hill, 1992, p. 26). Today many groups support the concept of differentiated practice. The report of the Pew Commission (1995) advised that nursing distinguish between the different levels of nursing. The Commission recommended associate degree preparation for the entry level hospital setting and nursing home practice, baccalaureate degree preparation for hospital-based care management and community-based practice, and master's degree preparation for specialty practice in the hospital and independent practice as a primary provider. The National Commission Nursing Implementation Project (NCNIP) also strongly supported differentiated practice.

The American Association of Colleges of Nursing and the American Organization of Nurse Executives established a Task Force on Differentiated Competencies for Nursing Practice funded by the Robert Wood Johnson Foundation. This group was later expanded to include representatives from The National Organization for Associate Degree Nursing. Their goals focused on instituting five to ten differentiated education-practice demonstration projects across the country, developing a core of leaders for the projects, developing a value-neutral language to describe differentiated nursing practice and education, and disseminating the work completed in the project (American Association of Colleges of Nursing, 1995). That work continues today.

Competency Expectations and Differentiated Practice

The task of describing and differentiating the competencies and the scope of practice of nurses graduating from various types of programs is one of the major challenges facing nursing today. As stated earlier, graduates of baccalaureate nursing programs, associate degree programs, and hospital-based programs all write the same licensing examination, designed to assure minimum safe practice. This approach fails to recognize the broad range of functions in nursing, and the potential for improving the quality of care given, if different roles and responsibilities were identified. In the work environment of acute and long-term care facilities, little differentiation exists in beginning staff nurse positions.

Realistic statements about competencies of each level or category of nursing education are necessary so that each category of graduate can be used effectively and efficiently within the health care delivery system. Validated competencies also will provide a basis for the development of curriculum patterns to ensure adequate preparation of each category of caregiver, without running the risk of overeducating or undereducating at any one level. The competencies also can serve as a foundation for educational mobility patterns in the profession, job descriptions in the health care system, and responsive reimbursement packages.

The Work of Organizations in Defining Competencies

Some work has been done toward describing the competencies of graduates of different programs in nursing. Recently the Council of Associate Degree Programs has been revising a 1990 publication of the NLN titled "Educational Outcomes of Associate Degree Nursing Programs: Roles and Competencies," which was a revision of a 1978 statement. The "Characteristics of Baccalaureate Education in Nursing," revised by the Council of Baccalaureate and Higher Degrees of NLN in 1994, accomplishes a similar purpose for baccalaureate education. Similarly, the Council of Diploma Programs and the Council of Practical Programs of NLN have developed competencies for graduates.

Since 1986, the National Council of State Boards of Nursing has conducted several studies aimed at role delineation and job analysis of entry-level registered nurses, the most recent for registered nurses being done in 1996 and for practical nurses in 1997. The purpose of these studies was to validate the NCLEX-RN. During 1997, the National Council developed a protocol for conducting a study to identify similarities and differences in the practice of all levels of licensed nurses within and across employment settings; they conducted the study in 1998 (National Council, 1998). In 1999 they published the *Role Delineation Study*, which describes the similarities and differences in the roles of nurse aides, licensed practical/vocational nurses, registered nurses, and advanced practice nurses.

Some of the most recent work related to defining competencies has come from the Pew Health Professions Commission's Final Report. The fourth report, which continued the theme of reforming health professions, addressed skills needed to function in health care in the 21st century. Twenty-one competencies were identified as critical to practice (Display 6-1) (Bellack & O'Neil, 2000).

Special Projects to Differentiate Practice

Several projects have been conducted throughout the United States in an effort to achieve a regional consensus among nursing service persons and educators on differentiated statements of scope of practice for each level of graduate.

THE MIDWEST ALLIANCE IN NURSING PROJECTS

Two projects sponsored by the Midwest Alliance in Nursing (MAIN) have focused on defining competencies. The W.K. Kellogg Foundation funded one, entitled "Defining and Differentiating ADN and BSN Competencies and Facilitating ADN Competency Development." The second, entitled "Continuing Education for Consensus on Entry Skills," was funded by a grant from the Division of Nursing of the Department of Health and Human Services. These studies resulted in the development of general statements on roles and the delineation of specific competencies in the area of direct care, communication, and management (Primm, 1987).

THE HEALING WEB PROJECT

Following in the steps of the MAIN work on competencies, the Healing Web Group was composed of representatives of nursing education and practice from six midwestern and western states. These individuals had as their goal the design, implementation, and evaluation of a variety of educational and practice differentiation activities. The projects were to serve as models for differentiation in both practice and education, and

Display 6–1

TWENTY-ONE COMPETENCIES DEFINED BY THE PEW HEALTH PROFESSIONS COMMISSION

1. Embrace a personal ethic of social responsibility and service.
2. Exhibit ethical behavior in all professional activities.
3. Provide evidence-based clinically competent care.
4. Incorporate the multiple determinants of health in clinical care.
5. Apply knowledge of the new sciences.
6. Demonstrate critical thinking, reflection, and problem-solving skills.
7. Understand the role of primary care.
8. Rigorously practice preventive health care.
9. Integrate population-based care and services into practice.
10. Improve access to health care for those with unmet health needs.
11. Contribute to continuous improvement of the health care system.
12. Advocate for public policy that promotes and protects the health of the public.
13. Continue to learn and help others learn.
14. Practice relationship-centered care with individuals and families.
15. Provide culturally sensitive care to a diverse society.
16. Partner with communities in health care decisions.
17. Use communication and information technology effectively and appropriately.
18. Work in interdisciplinary teams.
19. Ensure care that balances individual, professional, system, and societal needs.
20. Practice leadership.
21. Take responsibility for quality of care and health outcomes at all levels.

to provide the model for collaboration between nursing education and practice. One project site has been in operation for over 9 years.

THE SIOUX FALLS EXPERIENCE

One of the sites for the Healing Web Group was Sioux Falls, South Dakota. Here a detailed project was implemented to differentiate educational design. For one year, nursing students in associate and baccalaureate degree programs are provided nursing education simultaneously in concurrent clinical laboratory experiences in which they work as a team with differentiated roles. A differentiated curriculum provides learning experiences specifically targeted to the competencies of the two levels of students. Team learning is directed at establishing the unique goals for the differentiated roles. This is reinforced in joint seminars involving hospital staff, faculty and students. The success of this project is supported by the small number of nursing programs in South Dakota and the fact that the ADN program is located at the University of South Dakota.

Sioux Valley Hospital has reported a significant cost savings with this differentiated practice model, including decreased length of stay, decreased intensive care days, and decreased number of readmissions. The hospital was identified by *Modern*

Hospital as among the "100 Top U.S. Hospitals—Benchmarks for Success" (Modern Hospitals, 1994).

THE COLORADO EXPERIMENT

In 1988, the State of Colorado developed two sets of recommendations. First, they asked for a statewide plan to facilitate articulation of nursing education programs, to allow nurses to move from one educational credential to another without unnecessary replication of learning or curricular experience. The second recommendation called for a differentiated model for nursing practice that would facilitate appropriate use of nurses with varying educational credentials and degrees of experience. This would be accompanied by a differentiated pay scale to allow appropriate compensation of nursing personnel as career advancement or growth occurred. Movement from one role to another required completion of the appropriate additional degrees, although growth within each role was possible without acquiring formal education.

A complex and detailed set of competency statements, job descriptions, and evaluative tools was developed as a part of this project. The project also facilitated movement from one role to another. Wide-scale implementation of this model has not yet occurred.

Critical Thinking Activity

> Given the situation we have today, with three routes to preparation for registered nursing, how would you differentiate the skills of the graduate of each program? How should that influence nursing practice? How would you implement differentiated practice on the unit on which you currently are working? Do you believe there should be a difference in salary? What is the rationale for your answer?

FORCES FOR CHANGE IN NURSING EDUCATION

As the nursing profession advances, and as education remains responsive to the changes that occur, it is imperative that nursing education undergo modifications. A discussion of some of the most significant challenges follows.

Incorporating Computer Technology in Nursing Education

It is safe to say that in the last 10 years, nursing education has experienced no transformation more dramatic than the incorporation of computer technology into all aspects of teaching, learning, and health care. These changes encompass activities covering everything from entire degrees that can be earned in on-line courses, to separate courses that are taught on-line, to the incorporation of computer technology in the classroom and learning laboratory. In the health care setting, computers are used for patient records, business functions, and increasingly as a support to effective decision making.

COMPUTER TECHNOLOGY IN THE CLASSROOM

The computer plays a major role in nursing education. It is as essential to the operation of colleges and universities as it is to the operation of hospitals. Additionally, it is an important instructional tool. The computer offers a variety of approaches to instruction that are appealing and helpful to a diverse student population. Classroom lectures and presentations are augmented by computer-assisted instruction (CAI) in the form of interactive and linear video programs, patient simulations, drill and practice routines, problem-solving programs, and tutorials, to name a few examples. Faculty use computers for word processing, literature review, and the development and scoring of tests. Some faculty use computers in the classroom to augment their lectures and discussions through Power Point presentations and other computer technology. E-mail and the Internet are also a part of most teaching environments. Some instructional programs are delivered to sites far from the main campus through distance learning modalities using computer technology. At the end of their program of study, all students demonstrate their ability to practice safely on computerized licensing examinations in the form of computerized adaptive testing (CAT).

Computer literacy among students and faculty is no longer an issue—it is the current state of the art. Nursing educators express concern about the initial cost of the equipment and programs needed for this instruction, as well as the increasing cost of keeping both equipment and programs current. At a time when the budgets of educational institutions are experiencing severe cuts, people responsible for purchasing supplies and equipment increasingly must find creative ways to acquire needed items. Another challenge to faculty is finding time to evaluate the existing software and integrate it into the approved curriculum.

COMPUTERS IN THE HOSPITAL ENVIRONMENT

Today's health care settings could not operate without computers and computerized equipment. Computers are used for business operations, medical records, and collection of clinical data such as vital signs and hemodynamic values. Computers may be voice activated for charting at the bedside, used for nursing care plans, for communication from the physicians' office to nursing stations, to regulate the administration of medications, and for many other facets of operation and patient care. Most of the equipment used in today's modern hospital is computerized. New graduates move into a highly technical world when they seek their first nursing positions (Fig. 6-3). The education they receive to prepare them for these positions also must include the skills necessary to work in this highly computerized environment.

DISTANCE LEARNING OPTIONS

Many students, who are geographically bound and unable to relocate to a community offering baccalaureate or master's education in nursing, have found *distance learning*

FIGURE 6–3 CAI can include interactive and linear programs, patient simulations, drill and practice routines, problem solving programs, and tutorials.

to offer convenience and flexibility. It also appeals to the nurse who cannot quit work to attend school. Essentially, distance learning refers to a teaching/learning situation in which the student and the teacher are not present in the classroom. Distance education may be accomplished through on-line courses, through courses broadcast to distant sites, and through courses taught in areas distant from the campus. Formats include on-line courses, videos, learning situations augmented by e-mail, television broadcasts, or interactive telecommunication that can be sent to a single site or to several sites at the same time.

For on-line courses, sometimes referred to as a *virtual university*, students register for a class and are given passwords and access to the system. They work with an instructor and other class members, discussing issues, sharing ideas, and testing theories without the need to commute to another area. These on-line programs use the power of the Internet to deliver learning that is independent of time and location. Often individuals in the group share a mailbox, which serves as an "electronic classroom" facilitating a group forum among students. Research material is available through an electronic library. Students usually concentrate on one subject at a time, with courses being sequenced but offered outside the constraints of established times. Students may sign on at any hour, day or night. The instructor may have posted a short lecture and provided discussion questions. Students complete reading and written assignments as in traditional learning situations, except the written assignments are sent to the instructor, graded, and returned on-line. Computer conferencing allows the student to participate in class discussion, ask questions, and receive feedback. After completing one course, the students move to the next until degree requirements are met.

Although these programs offer much flexibility to students, they also demand a great deal of discipline on the part of the student. A single course may require as much as 15 to 20 hours of study time per week. A student attempting such a program needs to be an independent learner. Sufficient faculty time also must be provided for students to receive effective feedback regarding their efforts. Library resources are always a concern for distant learners, and colleges need to provide access to appropriate learning resources for distance learners. Mechanisms for evaluating the learning must be developed thoughtfully to ensure the integrity of resulting credentials.

Establishing Programs That Provide for Educational Mobility

One of the challenges to nursing educators has been the growing emphasis on educational mobility in nursing. Students begin their education at one level and wish to continue into a program that prepares them for a higher level of client care and responsibility. They want to advance from one level to another with minimal repetition of course work. Educational mobility has received impetus in some states from legislative mandates that stipulate that plans for articulation from one type of nursing program to another must be developed and implemented within a given period of time. More recently, one of the recommendations of the Pew Commission (1995) included strengthening the existing career ladder programs to make movement through these levels of nursing as easy as possible. Thus we see associate degree programs articulated with practical (vocational) nursing programs, increased efforts to facilitate transfer of associate degree graduates into baccalaureate programs, and the emergence of LPN to BSN and ADN to Master's pathways.

Increasing Community-Based Practice Experiences

Another significant change in nursing practice is the trend toward community-based practice. Most nursing programs, especially hospital-based and associate degree programs, have a history of being strongly oriented toward the hospital as the primary clinical teaching environment. "Community," as it was used in nursing education, was associated with public health nursing and was to be found in baccalaureate education only.

Earlier hospital discharge to the home and an increasing emphasis on prevention has created new demands on nursing. Nurses are expected to provide care in clients' homes, the workplace, schools, nursing homes, community health agencies, clinics, shelters, and community gathering places. As the arena in which nursing is practiced begins to shift, nursing educators are challenged to define what part of the nursing curriculum should be taught in a community setting. Often this requires different clinical teaching strategies and approaches. Faculty, who received most if not all of their education in acute care hospitals, believe that students do not spend enough time on hospital clinical units and are therefore unwilling to further shorten the amount of time. Many are uncertain how a community experience should be provided and evaluated. Others worry about the legal ramifications associated with having students in many different environments and in less controlled situations. Tremendous strides have been taken in developing innovative approaches to community-based nursing; more will follow.

Increasing Emphasis on Nursing Theories and Research

As the nursing profession continues to grow, one of the areas receiving more emphasis is nursing theory and research. This emphasis will undoubtedly continue. As nursing education keeps pace with the advancement of nursing knowledge, there is a push to develop curricular patterns that respond to the work of nursing theorists. Most approval bodies, state and national, now stipulate that a nursing program must have a coherent organizing or conceptual framework around which the program of learning is developed. Some programs have chosen to select the approach of a particular nursing theorist, and structure the program of learning around that theorist's work. The program in which you are enrolled may reflect this trend. Perhaps one of the hospitals to which you are assigned for clinical experience also uses the principles of a nursing theory to structure the delivery of care, although this is less common than using a theory in curriculum development.

A theory is a "scientifically acceptable general principle which governs practice or is proposed to explain observed facts" (Riehl and Roy, 1974, p 3). Because nursing as a developing profession is seriously involved in research, to build a sound body of nursing knowledge, theories are valuable to us. They provide the bases for hypotheses about nursing practice. They make it possible for us to derive a sound rationale for the actions we take. If the theories are testable, they then allow us to build our knowledge base and to guide and improve nursing practice (Fig. 6-4).

Today, there are many published nursing theories. In an attempt to structure and organize those theories, various authors have categorized or classified them. Not all are classified similarly. Included are general classifications such as the art and science of humanistic nursing, interpersonal relationships, systems, and energy fields. Other categories include growth and development theories, systems theories, stress adaptation theories, and rhythm theories.

Examples of growth and development theories with which you are probably familiar are those of Maslow, Erikson, Kohlberg, Piaget, and Freud. Most basic nursing texts incorporate a discussion of the concepts developed by these theorists. The theories are so named because they focus on the developing person. They have the common characteristic of arranging this development in stages through which a person must pass to reach a particular level of development. They allow nurses to monitor progress through the stages and evaluate the appropriateness of that progress. You will recognize Maslow for his approach to self-actualization, Erikson for his psychosocial development, Kohlberg for his theories of moral reasoning, Piaget for his approach to cognitive development, and Freud for psychosexual theories on which medicine later based the school of psychoanalysis. These theories are not truly theories of nursing, however, because they were not developed for the purpose of explaining, testing, and changing the practice of nursing. They represent some of the "borrowed" knowledge around which we build our profession.

FIGURE 6–4   Nursing is in the process of building a body of scientific knowledge.

Most nursing theories are developed around a combination of concepts. Among these concepts, four approaches usually are included:

1. An approach to the human person
2. An approach to health and illness
3. An approach to the environment (or society)
4. An approach to nursing

Nursing theories usually are classified according to the structure or approach around which they are developed. Theories that speak to the art and science of humanistic nursing were among the earliest pure nursing theories developed. Some authors have looked back at the contributions of Florence Nightingale and have included her work in that grouping. Among others are Virginia Henderson and her *Definition of Nursing*; Faye Abdellah and the *Twenty-one Nursing Problems* (which is often cited as one of the early attempts at classification of nursing behaviors); Lydia Hall and her *Core, Care, and Cure* model; and Madeleine Leininger's *Transcultural Care Theory*.

Interpersonal process theories deal with interactions between and among people. Many of these theories were developed during the 1960s. Included in this grouping could be Hildegard Peplau's *Psychodynamic Nursing*, Joyce Travelbee's *Human to Human Relationship*, Ernestine Wiedenbach's *The Helping Art of Clinical Nursing*, and Imogene King's *Dynamic Interacting Systems* model, although the last also could be classified as a systems theory.

Systems theories are so named because they are concerned with the interactions between and among all the factors in a situation. A system usually is viewed as complex and in a state of constant change. It is defined as a whole with interrelated parts and may be a subsystem of a larger system as well as a suprasystem. For example, a person may be viewed as a system composed of cells, tissue, and organs. The person is a subsystem of a family, which in turn is a subsystem of a community. In a systems approach, the person usually is considered as a "total" being, or from a "whole" being viewpoint. Systems theories also provide for "input" into the system and "feedback" within the system. The systems approach became popular during the 1970s. Included in this group of theorists are Dorothy Johnson, Sister Calista Roy, and Betty Neuman.

Stress adaptation models are based on concepts that view the person as adjusting or changing (adapting) to avoid situations (stressors) that would result in the disturbance of balance or equilibrium. The adaptation theory helps to explain how balance is maintained and therefore directs nursing actions. Included in this group one often finds Sister Calista Roy's adaptation model and Betty Neuman's work, but both also may be considered systems models, as mentioned above.

One of the most recent classifications of theories is by energy fields. These theories, although developed earlier, received growing recognition during the 1980s. Included in this group are the works of Myra Levine, Joyce Fitzpatrick, Margaret Newman, and Martha Rogers.

It is not our purpose to discuss and critique the many approaches to nursing theory. The student who wants to pursue nursing theorists further is encouraged to consult the section on further reading at the end of the chapter. Table 6-2 outlines the approaches of several recognized nursing theorists.

 Critical Thinking Activity

> Select one nursing theorist. Describe what you find interesting and attractive about her nursing theory. Give a rationale for your decision, and describe how using her theory might affect your practice of nursing.

CONTINUING EDUCATION

Continuing education in nursing is defined as "planned learning experiences beyond a basic nursing educational program. The learning experiences are designed to promote the development of knowledge, skills, and attitudes for the enhancement of nursing practice, thus improving health care to the public" (American Nurses Association, 1974). Continuing education programs are widely publicized in today's nursing literature. They often are presented just before and during major nursing conventions. Some professional meetings carry continuing education credit. Other continuing education programs exist as extensions of nursing programs at colleges and universities.

TABLE 6-2. Nursing Theories and Theorists	
Theorist	**Theory or Model**
Lydia Hall	Viewed illness and rehabilitation as learning experiences in which the nurse's role was to guide and teach the patient through personal caregiving. Role involves therapeutic use of self (core), the treatment regimen of the health care team (cure), and nurturing and intimate bodily care (care)
Dorothy Johnson	A behavioral systems approach that focuses on health viewed as a state of equilibrium that the nurse assists in maintaining or balancing
Imogene King	A model in which three open systems interact with the environment: personal, individual, and social. Nurse's role is to assist individual to perform daily activities and includes health promotion and maintenance. Involves goal attainment
Madeleine Leininger	Focused on a caring model that must be practiced interpersonally. Emphasized a transcultural approach
Myra Levine	Developed around the four concepts of conservation of energy, structural integrity, personal integrity, and social integrity. Supports a holistic approach to nursing based on recognition of the total response of the person to the interaction between the internal and external environment
Betty Neuman	A systems model influenced by Gestalt theory, stress, and level of prevention. Employs lines of resistance and lines of defense in creating a healthy being. Nurses are to identify the stressors and assist the individual to respond. Involves primary, secondary and tertiary prevention
Dorothea Orem	Recognized as a self-care theory of nursing, supports the concept that each person has a need for the provision and management of self-care actions to achieve "constancy." When the individual is unable to provide these, a self-care deficit exists. The role of the nursing system is to help eliminate the self-care deficit through wholly compensatory, partially compensatory, or supportive-educative actions
Martha Rogers	Includes complicated approaches to health that involve helicy, resonancy, and complementarity. The holistic individual moves through time and space as part of an expanding universe with potential states of maximum well-being. Nurses act to promote symphonic interaction between man and environment by repatterning the human and environmental fields
Sister Calista Roy	Identified as an adaptation model that conceives of the individual as being in constant interaction with a changing environment, thus requiring adaptation. Four adaptive modes, or ways in which a person adapts, are identified through: (1) physiological needs; (2) self-concept, (3) role function, and (4) interdependence relations. The nurse's role is to assess a patient's adaptive behaviors and the stimuli that may be affecting the person to manipulate the stimuli in such a way as to allow the patient to cope or adapt

Like so many other areas of nursing, continuing education is not new. In an article entitled "Nursing the Sick," written around 1882, Florence Nightingale wrote:

Nursing is, above all, a progressive calling. Year by year nurses have to learn new and improved methods, as medicine and surgery and hygiene improve. Year by year nurses are called upon to do more and better than they have done. It is felt to be impossible to have a public register of nurses that is not a delusion (Nightingale, as cited in Seymer, 1954, p 349).

The first continuing education courses for nurses probably would be considered postgraduate instruction today. In 1899, Teachers College at Columbia University instituted a course for qualified graduate nurses in hospital economics. Nursing institutes and conferences were first offered to nurses in the 1920s; often these were given to make up for deficiencies in basic nursing curricula. Hospital in-service or staff development programs also were beginning to be discussed in nursing literature around this time. Today most hospitals employ someone who is responsible for the staff education program. By 1959, federal funds became available for short-term courses, giving much thrust to continuing education. In 1967, the ANA published "Avenues for Continued Learning," its first definitive statement on continuing education; and in 1973, the ANA Council on Continuing Education was established. The Council, which is responsible to the ANA Commission on Education, is concerned about standards of continuing education, accreditation of the programs, transferability of credit from state to state, and development of guidelines for recognition systems within states. In 1974, "Standards for Continuing Education in Nursing" was published by the ANA, and the federal government altered the Nurse Traineeship Act of 1972 to include an option that would provide continuing education as an alternative to placing more students into programs receiving federal capitation dollars.

By the 1970s, most nursing publications had something to say about continuing education for nurses. Practically all states were organizing or planning to organize some method by which the nurse could receive recognition for continued education. These systems were called continuing education approval and recognition programs, or continuing education recognition programs, and most state systems followed the guidelines and criteria prepared by the ANA.

The continuing education unit (CEU) became a rather uniform system of measuring, recording, reporting, accumulating, transferring, and recognizing participation in nonacademic credit offerings. The National Task Force on the Continuing Education Unit, which represented 34 educational groups, developed the definition of a CEU. Although nursing was not one of the groups, the profession has accepted the definition. Ten hours of participation in an organized continuing education experience under responsible sponsorship, with capable direction and qualified instruction, is equal to one CEU. Many states and organizations, however, simply report clock hours of instruction (Fig. 6-5).

A system for accreditation and approval of continuing education in nursing was developed and implemented by the ANA in 1975. Accreditation was awarded for a period of 4 years and assured the public that the continuing education offerings provided consistent quality. A new system, put into operation August 1, 1987, allowed organizations that offer continuing education to seek accreditation as either a provider or an approver. A provider is any organization responsible for the development, implementation, and evaluation of courses. An approver can be the state nurses' association, a specialty organization, or a federal nursing service designated to approve the continuing education process. Organizations can be both approvers and providers. This program made the system more accessible to groups seeking approval of courses or classes by bringing the process closer to the membership and to those offering the programs.

FIGURE 6–5 Today, colleges, universities, hospitals, voluntary agencies, and private proprietary groups are all offering continuing education courses to registered nurses.

Today colleges, universities, hospitals, voluntary agencies, and private proprietary groups all offer continuing education courses to registered nurses. The cost of this education varies tremendously. Nurses can earn continuing education credits for merely attending meetings and conferences. Little attempt is made to assess whether learning has occurred. Professional journals include sections of programmed instruction that can be completed in the comfort of one's living room. These have an evaluation mechanism. Telecourses are offered by television. Workshops, institutes, conferences, short courses, and evening courses abound. Courses are available on the Internet. Yet some nurses do not feel the need to keep up with these current offerings.

An issue today is whether continuing education should be mandatory or voluntary. Mandatory continuing education affects licensure; that means that any nurse renewing a license in a state requiring (mandating) continuing education will have to satisfy that requirement. Voluntary continuing education is not related to relicensure. Government agencies and state legislatures are exerting pressure on nurses, as they have on physicians, attorneys, dietitians, dentists, pharmacists, and other professionals, to provide evidence of updated knowledge before license renewal.

A position supporting mandatory continuing education raises some questions. How should the learning be measured? Who should accredit the programs? How can quality be ensured? By whom and where should records be retained? Who should bear the cost? What should be the time frame for continuing education? How many hours, courses, and credits should be required?

You can write directly to a state board of nursing for information on specific requirements for that state (see Appendix A for addresses).

Critical Thinking Activity

> Do you believe continuing education should be a mandatory requirement for the renewal of one's license? Why or why not? If your answer is no, how would you ensure competence? If you believe it should be mandatory, what kind of record-keeping would you require? Who do you believe should keep the records?

KEY CONCEPTS

- Three major avenues to preparation for licensure as a registered nurse exist in the United States: the hospital-based diploma, the university-based baccalaureate degree, and the associate degree (usually offered in community colleges). Many similarities exist among these programs. In addition, various nontraditional approaches to nursing education have evolved.
- Educational programs prepare nursing assistants and licensed practical (vocational) nurses for roles in the health care delivery system. As these programs have grown, greater oversight of the programs by approval bodies has occurred.
- The nursing shortage of the 1990s has resulted in decreased dissension regarding educational preparation for nursing and greater creativity and collaboration in educational approaches.
- Master's and doctoral programs that prepare nurses for leadership positions in the profession continue to grow, with more emphasis on the master's degree for advanced practice. The actual degree awarded at the end of doctoral studies varies.
- One of the most rapidly growing areas is that of advanced practice; this growth was accelerated by health care reform. Recommendations from major commissions have urged continued expansion of advanced practice programs.
- Many changes are occurring in nursing education. These include more emphasis on articulation and career ladder programs and a shift in educational settings from acute care facilities to community-based experiences.
- No change has affected nursing education as greatly as has the computer age. Entire programs can be completed on-line. Computer technology has changed the structure of the typical nursing classroom, and instructors prepare graduates who will be able to function in a health care environment that makes heavy use of computerized services.
- Nursing theories continue to influence nursing and nursing education. Nursing theories assist us in building a body of nursing knowledge and describing and defining nursing practice.

- Nursing education has been influenced by the ANA Position on Nursing Education that advocated the baccalaureate degree as the minimum educational preparation for professional practice. Many nursing educators, particularly those in diploma and associate degree programs, disagreed with this position.
- Models for differentiated practice are being encouraged; these models recognize and use graduates according to the competencies inherent in the program from which they graduated.
- Continuing education, whether further education that results in a higher degree, or whether in the form of classes, seminars, or workshops that update and increase expertise, is being encouraged by more and more organizations. Staying current in practice is critical to safe client care.

REFERENCES

American Nurses Association's first position on nursing education. Am J Nurs 65(12):106–111, 1965

American Nurses Association. Standards for Continuing Education for Nursing. Kansas City, MO: American Nurses Association, 1974

Bellack JP, O'Neil EH. Recreating nursing practice for a new century. Nursing and Health Care Perspectives 21(1):14–21, 2000

Benner P. From Novice to Expert. Menlo Park, CA: Addison-Wesley Publishing Co., 1984

Boston C. Differentiated practice: An introduction. *In* Boston C: Current issues and perspectives on differentiated practice (pp 1–3). Chicago, IL: American Organization of Nurse Executives, 1990

Broad-based research agenda addresses regulatory issues faced by member boards. Issues 17(1):1, 4–6, 1996

Brown EL. Nursing for the Future. New York: Russell Sage Foundation, 1948

California Board of Registered Nursing. Laws Relating to Nursing Education Licensure: Practice with Rules and Regulations. Sacramento: California Board of Registered Nursing, 1994

de Tornyay R. Critical challenges for nurse educators. J Nurs Ed 35(4):146–147, 1996

Hartung D. Organizational positions on titling and entry into practice: A chronology. *In*: Looking Beyond the Entry Issue: Implications for Education and Service, NLN Publication No. 41-2173. New York: National League for Nursing, 1986

Kalisch PA, Kalisch BJ. The Advance of American Nursing, 3rd ed. Philadelphia: JB Lippincott, 1995

Lindeman CA. The future of nursing education. J Nurs Educ 39(1):5–12, 2000

Lipman TH, Deatrick JA. Enhancing specialist preparation for the next century. J Nurs Educ 33(2):53–58, 1994

National Council of State Boards of Nursing. National Council Update. Issues 19(4):10–11, Chicago: Author, 1998

National League for Nursing Accreditation Commission. Interpretive Guidelines for Standards and Criteria 1999: Associate Degree Programs in Nursing. New York: Author, 1999

National League for Nursing. Educational Outcomes of Associate Degree Nursing Programs: Roles and Competencies. Publication No. 23-2348, Council of Associate Degree Programs. New York: National League for Nursing, 1990

National League for Nursing. Characteristics of Associate Degree Education in Nursing. Publication No. 23-1500, Council of Associate Degree Programs. New York: National League for Nursing, 1973

Nightingale F. Nursing the sick. *In* Seymer LR: Selected Writings of Florence Nightingale. New York: Macmillan, 1954

Pew Health Professions Commission. Critical challenges: Revitalizing the health professions for the twenty-first century. San Francisco, CA: UCSF Center for the Health Professions, 1995

Primm PL. Differentiated practice for ADN- and BSN-prepared nurses. J Prof Nurs 3(4):218–225, 1987

Riehl JP, Roy SC. Conceptual Models for Nursing Practice. New York: Appleton-Century-Crofts, 1974

100 Top U.S. hospitals—benchmarks for success. Mod Hosp 24(3):8, 14, 1994

U.S. Public Health Service. Toward quality in nursing: Needs and goals. Report of the Surgeon Generals Consultant Group on Nursing. Washington, D.C.: U.S. Government Printing Office, 1963

Valuing difference—Creating community: A model for differentiated nursing practice. American Association of Colleges of Nursing: Washington, D.C., 1995

FURTHER READING

A call for reform of our nursing education system. The AONE update. Nurs Management 24(1):33, 1993

American Nurses Association. A Case for Baccalaureate Preparation in Nursing, ANA publication No. NE-6 15M. Kansas City, MO: American Nurses Association, 1979

Bersky AK, Yocum CJ. Computerized clinical simulation testing: Its use for competence assessment in nursing. Nurs & Health Care 15(3):120–127, 1994

Bramble K. Nurse practitioner education: Enhancing performance through the use of the objective structured clinical assessment. J Nurs Educ 33(2):59–65, 1994

Brubaker BH. A faculty learns to make self-pacing work. Nurs Health Care 11(2):74–77, 1990

Cross utilization of nursing staff. The AONE update. Nurs Management 24(7):38–39, 1993

Davids SL, Laeger E. Developing a BSN program across two institutions: Arizona State University West Campus/Glendale Community College—the adjuvant model. Nurs Health Care 11(2):84–87, 1990

Fishman DJ. Nursing informatics: The electronic information revolution in education and practice. *In* Strickland OL, Fishman DJ: Nursing Issues in the 1990s. Albany, NY: Delmar Publishers, 1994:471–488

Frik SM, Pollack SE. Preparation for advanced nursing practice. Nurs Health Care 14(4):190–195, 1993

Heller BR, Oros MT, Curney-Crowley J. The future of nursing education: 10 trends to watch. Nursing and Health Care Perspectives 21(1):9–13, 2000

Koerner J. Differentiated practice: The evolution of professional nursing. J Nurs Ed 8:335–341, 1992

Koerner J, Karpiuk K. Implementing Differentiated Nursing Practice: Transformation by Design. Gaithersburg, MD: Aspen, 1994

Kurzen CR. Contemporary Practical/Vocational Nursing, 3rd ed. Philadelphia: JB Lippincott, 1997

Lambert C, Lambert VA. Relationships among faculty practice involvement, perception of role stress, and psychological hardiness of nurse educators. J Nurs Educ 33(4):171–179, 1993

Montag ML. Community College Education for Nursing. New York: McGraw-Hill, 1959

Pruitt RH, Campbell BF. Educating for health care reform and the community. Nurs Health Care 15(6):308–311, 1994

Seymer LR. The Nightingale training school: One hundred years ago. Am J Nurs 60(5):658–661, 1960

Sharp N. Second license for the advanced practice nurse? Nurs Management 23(9):28–29, 1992

Simpson RL. The new careers in nursing informatics. Nurs Management 23(10):26–27, 1992

Tanner CA, Hartshorn J, Rosenfeld P. Critical care nursing in baccalaureate programs. Nurs Health Care 10(9):482–488, 1989

Town J. Changing to computerized documentation—plus! Nurs Management 24(7):44–48, 1993

Trofino J. Voice-activated nursing documentation: On the cutting edge. Nurs Management 24(7):40–42, 1993

Yoder ME. Preferred learning style and educational technology: Linear vs. interactive video. Nurs Health Care 15(3):128–132, 1994

Relevant web sites

American Association of Colleges of Nursing *www.aacn.nche.edu*
Commission on Collegiate Nursing Education *www.aacn.nche.edu/Accreditation*
National League for Nursing *www.nln.org*
National League for Nursing Accreditation Commission *www.nlnac.org*

Legal and Ethical Responsibility and Accountability for Practice

I t is critical that newcomers to a profession have a well-grounded understanding to the legal and ethical dimensions of practice. This is especially true in nursing. This unit begins by exploring the issue of credentials for health care providers. It discusses the basic concerns related to credentialing, provides a rationale for credentials, and emphasizes the responsibility of health care providers (especially nurses) to the public.

The unit continues with a discussion of the legal ramifications of practice. Case examples are used to emphasize an understanding of the rights and responsibilities of consumers and health care providers. The role of the nurse as a witness concludes this chapter.

Ethical and bioethical issues associated with health care constantly challenge us as professionals and as members of society. Each new technological advance brings additional questions and concerns to our attention. The unit concludes with a discussion of these major questions and provides an understanding of the basis of ethical decision making and the factors that significantly affect it. Some of the specific problems are explored in the hope that considering them before you become directly involved will help you to address the issues more comfortably as you move into a professional role.

7

Credentials for Health Care Providers

We must be willing to identify the unnecessary, ineffective, and burdensome parts of our (licensing) system and strive to correct the problems.

(Schowalter, 1995)

OBJECTIVES

After completing this chapter, you should be able to:

1. Define and discuss the concept of credentialing in the health professions.

2. Differentiate between a diploma, certification, accreditation, and licensure as credentials.

3. Identify and analyze the major concerns addressed by nursing practice acts.

4. Outline the role of the State Board of Nursing or other state regulatory authority.

5. Differentiate between licensure by examination and licensure by endorsement.

6. Discuss the disciplinary process in regard to a nursing license.

7. Discuss issues in licensure including assuring continued competence, multistate licensure, and licensure for graduates of foreign nursing schools.

8. Explain the various uses of certification in nursing.

9. Discuss current trends in credentialing within the health care workforce.

KEY TERMS

Accreditation
Advanced practice
Certificate
Certification
Computerized adaptive testing (CAT)
Computerized simulation testing (CST)
Credentialing
Criticality
Degree
Diploma
Disciplinary action

254

Enacted (statutory) law	Multistate licensure	Remote state
Grandfathering	NCLEX-PN	Revocation
Home state	NCLEX-RN	Rules and regulations
License	Nurse practice act	State Board of Nursing
Licensure by endorsement	Party state	Sunset laws
Mandatory licensure	Permissive licensure	Telenursing

The public needs and wants an effective mechanism for verifying the abilities of health professionals. Health professionals want a mechanism that identifies their abilities and demonstrates their credibility to the public. The various health care credentials meet those expectations. Credentials are written documents that communicate to others the nature of one's competence and provide evidence of one's preparation to perform in a specific occupation. The basic rationale for legal credentials in health care occupations is that providing a standard mechanism for judging competence protects the safety of the public. Further, those who are engaged in careers in health occupations want to be assured that the standards of practice in their discipline remain high. They do not want to be replaced by people with less educational preparation who are willing to work for lower wages (Fig. 7-1). Credentials also are used by organizations or institutions to demonstrate their competence or quality to the public.

TYPES OF CREDENTIALS IN HEALTH CARE

There are many types of health care credentials; examples include diplomas, certificates, degrees, accreditation, and licenses. Each of these serves a different purpose. Not all are available for each different health occupation.

Diplomas, Degrees, and Certificates of Completion

A school or business offering instruction awards a *diploma* or *certificate* to those who complete a designated program of study. An example is the diploma awarded on graduation from high school or college. A business that provides instruction in using computer programs might present certificates to those who complete the course. When only a diploma or educational certificate is available, it is necessary to know about the educational institution and the specific educational program to evaluate the person's abilities. In nursing, diplomas have always been offered by nursing education programs. Licensed practical nursing programs offer a certificate of completion. Hospital-based programs preparing registered nurses offer only the diploma. College-based nursing programs offer academic *degrees* such as the associate, baccalaureate, or higher degree that require the fulfillment of certain general education courses and course work that prepares you for a particular career, such as nursing.

FIGURE 7–1 Various forms of credentialing ensure the public of qualified caregivers.

Accreditation

Accreditation is a process whereby educational institutions or programs are surveyed and evaluated. Some accreditation recognizes the entire educational institution, such as the accreditation offered by regional bodies for colleges and universities. If an institution's programs meet published standards, it is awarded accreditation. An associate, baccalaureate, or master's degree awarded by this institution then would reflect a standard of postsecondary education approved by the accrediting organization. Although a non-accredited institution might award a degree, there is no guarantee that the degree meets educational standards; therefore, the degree might not be accepted as adequate evidence of qualifications. Many educational credentials are acknowledged only if offered by an accredited educational institution. You may have experienced the need for this type of accreditation if you transferred academic credits from one college to another. A regionally accredited college or university usually limits direct transfer of coursework to that which was completed at an accredited institution.

Some academic accreditation is "specialized," meaning that it applies only to a particular special program in an institution, or to a particular type of technical-professional education. This accreditation requires that the specific program meet professional standards for excellence. An educational institution might have general accreditation for its degrees, but still not have specialized accreditation. Sometimes this is because of the cost of the accreditation process, or because of a philosophical stance that additional accreditation is not needed if the institution has general accreditation. Certain educational organizations are not degree-granting institutions, and therefore are not eligible for general accreditation, but they are still eligible for specialized accreditation. This is true of hospital-based diploma schools of nursing.

The national accreditation of nursing programs is a specialized accreditation. The National League for Nursing Accrediting Commission (NLNAC), a subsidiary organization related to the National League for Nursing, accredits nursing programs at all levels, practical nursing, hospital diploma nursing education, associate degree nursing education, and baccalaureate and higher degree educational programs. The Collegiate Commission on Nursing Education (CCNE), a subsidiary organization of the American Association of Colleges of Nursing, also began accrediting baccalaureate and higher degree nursing programs in 1999. Advanced practice nursing organizations such as the American Association of Nurse Anesthetists provide specialized accreditation for institutions offering advanced practice/nurse practitioner programs.

Licensure

A *license* is a legal credential conferred by an individual state. A wide variety of health professionals are licensed in different states. Most states require licensing only of those who have more direct contact with clients. Physicians, dentists, pharmacists, and nurses are licensed in all states. The licensing of other health care workers varies. An individual state or province determines eligibility for licensure and the type of testing required.

Mandatory licensure is a requirement that all individuals must obtain a license in a particular jurisdiction to practice. There is mandatory licensure for physicians and dentists in all states. Mandatory licensure is instituted when there is a compelling public interest in licensure to protect the public.

Permissive licensure is a system whereby an individual may choose to become licensed to provide evidence of competence, but a license is not required to practice. Permissive and mandatory licensure are discussed in greater detail later in this chapter.

Most licensing laws specify completion of a state-approved educational program, and require successful completion of a written examination prescribed by the state. Some professions, such as dentistry, require candidates to pass both a practical examination and a written examination. Nursing is unique in having a standard licensure process in every state and territory in the United States. This was developed through the cooperative action of the state boards of nursing. A national examination may exist for other professions, but its application may vary. For example, there is a national licensing examination for pharmacy, but California prepares and administers its own examination and does not use the national pharmacy examination. There are national medical board examinations, but some states administer independent medical examinations. Even when the same examination is used for licensure, as in pharmacy, some states require that a person new to the state retake the licensing examination when applying for a license in that state.

Some states require completion of continuing education to renew a health care license. Pharmacists were one of the first groups required to pursue continuing education to remain licensed. Continuing education is required for relicensure of nurses and physicians in many states. The cost of monitoring continuing education has been a barrier to its adoption in some states (see Chapter 6).

Licensure language and requirements for health professionals differ from state to state. In 1995 the Council on Licensure, Enforcement and Regulation (CLEAR) proposed a uniform language to be used in all state licensing regulations. Several national associations of professional regulatory boards also have suggested that greater uniformity of language and requirements would be a service to the public (Parkman, 1997).

Certification

For some groups a standard credential is available in the form of *certification* provided by a nongovernmental authority, usually a professional organization. Workers with this credential are referred to as "certified" or sometimes as "registered." This type of credential should not be confused with a legal license. Certification usually is granted on completion of an educational program and the passing of a standardized examination, both of which are prescribed by a professional organization.

Some organizations provide certification for several related occupational groups. One such organization is the National Accrediting Association for Clinical Laboratory Sciences (NAACLS). Members of the various professional groups involved in laboratory science cooperated in setting up this association. The organization is incorporated as a private, voluntary entity and is not a governmental institution or department. The purpose of this organization is to make the laboratory science credentialing system more independent and as objective as possible. This organization awards the title medical laboratory technician (MLT) or medical technologist (MT) to those who have met the educational standards and passed the certification examination. All groups in the field of laboratory science recognize these as professional credentials. Some states have made certification by this body the required criterion for practice in clinical laboratory sciences.

While some professional organizations conduct their own certification, in most instances they have established an independent national entity with the sole purpose of credentialing. There are several reasons for this. First, the public generally has not trusted the objectivity of professional groups that do not have consumer input; the creation of an independent credentialing body ensures that those currently practicing a profession are not the sole arbiters in determining who enters the field. Secondly, by setting up a separate organization, which must be self-supporting through fees for its services, professional groups are relieved of the financial burden that can result when an accrediting program grows rapidly and costs escalate. The third justification for creating an independent credentialing body is to provide a broader base of support from many related organizations for the credentialing process. A fourth reason relates to the complex federal laws governing nonprofit organizations and their tax-exempt status.

Critical Thinking Activity

> Choose an allied health occupation found in a health care facility in which
> you have clinical practice. Investigate the credentials needed for that
> occupation and how they would be obtained in your state. Analyze a way in
> which you could work collaboratively with an individual in this health
> occupation.

THE HISTORY OF CREDENTIALING IN NURSING

Nursing leaders historically have maintained an ethical position that accountability to the public for quality nursing care is essential. The public, however, often has no method for evaluating the competence of an individual nurse. Therefore, in the United States the nursing profession has tried to ensure that nurses have credentials that can be recognized by everyone.

Recognizable credentials were not always available for nurses. Before the Nightingale schools became prevalent in England, and nursing schools were established in the United States, little training was available to those who wanted to provide nursing care. Nurses with some training and those without any typically worked side by side. After schools of nursing became common, a rudimentary means of identifying the qualifications of a caregiver was the certificate of completion that was issued by the nursing school. This was the first true nursing credential.

However, because the quality of education offered in the nursing schools varied greatly—programs varied in length from 6 weeks to 3 years—it became apparent that a completion certificate was not an adequate guarantee of competence. Nursing leaders were concerned about this situation; they believed that clients had no way to judge a particular nurse's competence, or whether they might suffer from the care administered by a poorly prepared nurse.

In 1896, the Nurses' Associated Alumnae of the United States and Canada was created. This organization later evolved into the American Nurses Association (ANA). One of the major concerns of the association was the establishment of legal licensure for nurses. The route toward legal licensing for credentialing was long and difficult. Nurses, legislators, and the public had to be educated about the value of licensure for the profession and encouraged to support it. Display 7-1 presents a chronology of nursing licensure. An interesting historic note is that Florence Nightingale was opposed to nursing licensure. She believed that only continuing education and practice could assure competence and that a license approved at one time could not.

Permissive Licensure for Nursing

The ANA campaigned vigorously for the adoption of state licensing laws. These early laws provided for permissive licensure. The requirements for permissive licensure

Display 7–1
THE HISTORY OF NURSING LICENSURE

1867	Dr. Henry Wentworth Acland first suggested licensure for nurses in England.
1892	American Society of Superintendents of Training Schools for Nurses organized and supported licensure in the United States.
1901	First nursing licensure in the world: New Zealand.
1903	First nursing licensure in the United States: North Carolina, New Jersey, New York, and Virginia (in that order).
1915	ANA drafted its first model nurse practice act.
1919	First nursing licensure in England.
1923	All 48 states had enacted nursing licensure laws.
1935	First mandatory licensure act in the United States: New York (effective 1947).
1946	Ten states had definitions of nursing in the licensing act.
1950	First year the same examination used in all jurisdictions of the United States and its territories: State Board Test Pool Examination.
1965	Twenty-one states had definitions of nursing in the licensing act.
1971	First state to recognize expanded practice in the nursing practice act: Idaho.
1976	First mandatory continuing education for relicensure: California.
1982	Change to nursing process format examination: National Council Licensure Examination for Registered Nurses (NCLEX-RN).
1986	First state to require baccalaureate degree for initial registered nurse licensure and associate degree for licensed practical nurse licensure: North Dakota (effective 1987).
1994	Computer-adapted testing initiated nationwide.
1998	Mutual Recognition Nurse Licensure Compact finalized. Utah is the first state to become part of the Compact.

included graduating from a school that satisfied certain standards and passing a comprehensive examination. Only those who had met these standards could use the title "registered nurse." An employer or a member of the public then could differentiate between a registered nurse and an individual who used the title "nurse," but had not met the standards required to be registered. Under this system no one was required to have a license to practice nursing.

The community benefited from these standards because an established credential attested to a registered nurse's level of competence. The individual licensed as a registered nurse profited by better job availability and salary when employers differentiated between those with licenses and those without licenses.

North Carolina passed the first law providing for permissive licensure in 1903. By 1923, all the existing 48 states had permissive licensure laws. Alaska and Hawaii passed licensure laws while they were still territories, and continued to recognize these laws when they became states. The set of laws regulating the practice of nursing is termed the Nurse Practice Act.

Mandatory Licensure for Nursing

After permissive licensure laws came into being, nurses' activity regarding licensure became less intense because most individuals graduating from nursing schools sought and received licenses to practice. However, there was still concern that some persons were practicing nursing without having demonstrated skill and knowledge. The majority of those functioning without licenses were nursing school graduates who had failed the licensing examinations; they were referred to as graduate nurses, rather than registered nurses. Other nurses who practiced without licenses included individuals who had been educated as nurses in foreign countries.

To end this situation and provide greater protection to the public, many nurses began to call for mandatory licensure. Mandatory nursing licensure requires that all persons who wish to practice nursing meet established standards for education, pass standardized examinations, and secure a license to practice in the state, province, or territory in which they wish to work.

The first mandatory licensure law took effect in New York in 1947. Today, mandatory licensure is the standard in the United States and Canada, and in most other countries. Therefore, if you wish to work as a nurse in any state, territory, province, or other country, you must obtain a license that is valid there before you begin working. Even though you are licensed to practice in one place, that does not allow you to practice elsewhere without seeking a new license in that jurisdiction (Fig 7-2).

Although the terms "registered nurse" and "licensed practical nurse" (or licensed vocational nurse, as used in Texas and California) were protected in law, the more gen-

FIGURE 7–2 A standard credential makes hiring easier.

eral term "nurse" has not been protected historically. Many individuals describe themselves as nurses when their roles in health care are assistive. Their employers also may refer to them as "nurses" to support their status. Some states have made "nurse" a protected term. In these states only registered nurses or practical (vocational) nurses may use the title "nurse." Others, such as certified nurses' aides/assistants and medical assistants, may use only their specific title.

CURRENT NURSING LICENSURE LAWS

The authority for establishing a licensure law lies with the legislature of each jurisdiction. However, new legislation regarding nursing licensure most often is initiated through the nurses' association or through the State Board of Nursing. The group initiating the action may spend months preparing and planning the content of the bill and gaining the support of legislators for its passage.

A proposed change in the law enters the legislative process through an elected member of the legislature who has been persuaded that the change is in the best interest of the public. The proposal must go through the entire legislative committee review, a public hearing, and a legislative voting procedure before it can become a law. When finally passed by the legislature, the legislation becomes part of the licensure law.

During the legislative process, individuals and organizations may affect the content of the proposed legislation by influencing the legislators. In 1974, for example, a bill was introduced in New York that would have changed the educational requirements for entry into nursing practice; the bill established that the minimum requirement for practice would be a baccalaureate degree. During the legislative process a great deal of lobbying occurred, and changes were made in the bill. Even those who had initiated the bill dropped their support of the new language. The result was the defeat of the bill; the proposed change in educational requirements was not enacted.

Rules and Regulations

Each state has its own set of administrative rules and regulations to carry out the provisions of laws regulating nursing. These rules and regulations are established by an administrative body, usually the *State Board of Nursing*, that is given responsibility for administering the Nurse Practice Act. This responsibility is authorized in the Nurse Practice Act itself. (See the section later in this chapter on the Role of the Board of Nursing.) Most states require that public hearings be held in regard to proposed rules and regulations, but the board has the authority to make the final decision. The rules and regulations must be within the scope outlined by the legislation that was passed. Those that are accepted by the appropriate board have the force of law unless they are challenged in court and are found not to be in accord with the legislature's intent. These rules are termed the administrative law.

In some states, the Nurse Practice Act is detailed and specifies most of the critical provisions regarding licensure and practice. In other states, the practice act is broad, and the administrative body is given a great deal of power to make decisions through rules and regulations.

The difference between what is contained in the enacted law and what is contained in rules and regulations is illustrated by the educational requirements for licensure in each state. In some states the enacted law specifies that a diploma, an associate degree, or a baccalaureate degree is acceptable preparation for registered nursing. In those states, the enacted law would have to change in order for the educational requirements to change. In other states, educational requirements are not in the enacted law—they are established by the Board of Nursing through rules and regulations. In North Dakota, for example, the educational requirement for the registered nurse license was changed to the baccalaureate degree through state regulations. Thus, both the Nurse Practice Act and state rules and regulations govern nursing in your state.

Nursing Licensure Law Content

In the early 1900s, the ANA, assuming its leadership role in nursing licensure, formulated a model nurse practice act to be used by state associations when planning legislation (Snyder & LaBar, 1984). The most recent revision of this model was in 1990 by the ANA Congress for Nursing Practice (ANA, 1990). The National Council of State Boards of Nursing (NCSBN) also developed a model nurse practice act (NCSBN, 1982). The NCSBN continues to update its model act as part of its role in supporting the state boards of nursing, with the most recent revision being published by the National Council in 1994 (NCSBN, 1994c). In addition, the NCSBN has written the Model Nursing Administrative Rules, which was also updated in 1994 (NCSBN, 1994d). Currently the ANA is working cooperatively with the NCSBN to develop a single model nurse practice act (ANA, 1999).

We recommended that you carefully read the Nurse Practice Act for the state in which you will practice. A copy of the act may be obtained from the State Board of Nursing (see Appendix A for addresses). In some states, one act includes both practical nursing and registered nursing; other states have two separate, but similar, acts. Historically, the role of the nursing assistant was not outlined in nursing laws. As federal legislation mandating classes and certification for nursing assistants in long-term care took effect, some states are modifying laws, and rules and regulations, to address the role of the nursing assistant. In other states regulations governing nursing assistants rest within a different department of the state government.

The following general topics usually are covered in state licensure laws for nursing.

PURPOSE

The purpose of regulating the practice of nursing is twofold: regulations protect the public and make individual practitioners accountable for their actions. Note that the protection of the status of the licensed individual is not the reason for licensure. With this in mind, you can better understand the inclusion of some other topics in the act.

Definitions

All of the significant terms in the act are defined for the purpose of carrying out the law. This is where the legal definition of nursing and the scope of practice are spelled out.

The NCSBN has given the following definition: "the 'practice of nursing' means assisting individuals or groups to maintain or attain optimal health, implementing a strategy of care to accomplish defined goals, and evaluating responses to care and treatment. This practice includes, but is not limited to, initiating and maintaining comfort measures, promoting and supporting human functions and responses, establishing an environment conducive to wellbeing, providing health counseling and teaching, and collaborating on certain aspects of the health regimen. This practice is based on understanding the human condition across the lifespan and the relationship of the individual within the environment" (NCSBN, 1994, p. 3). The National Council document then proceeds to distinguish between registered nurse practice and licensed practical/vocational nurse practice.

No state adopts the exact wording of any recommended definition, but most states include references to performing services for compensation, the necessity for a specialized knowledge base, the use of the nursing process (although steps may be named differently), and components of nursing practice. Several states include some reference to treating human responses to actual or potential health problems; this was first addressed in New York State's license law and was later incorporated in the ANA's "Nursing: A Social Policy Statement" (1980). Most states refer to the execution of the medical regimen, and many include a general statement about additional acts that recognize that nursing practice is evolving and that the nurse's area of responsibility can be expected to broaden.

Definitions of practical (vocational) nursing are more restrictive, and usually state that the individual must function under the direction of a registered nurse or physician, in areas demanding less judgment and knowledge than is required of the registered nurse; in the NCSBN model act, this is referred to as "a directed scope of nursing practice" (NCSBN, 1994, p. 4). Practical nurse standards usually focus on the assessment and intervention portions of the nursing process. There has been much discussion about the role of the licensed practical/vocational nurse in the analysis of data and planning for care. States differ in the independence permitted for practical nurses. Some states provide a list of specific functions appropriate to the practical nurse, or list specific functions not permitted.

A variety of nursing assistants are employed in health care facilities; they may have titles such as mental health technician, nursing assistant, or medication technician. The preparation for and scope of practice for these individuals is a matter of serious concern to the public. With the current pressure to contain costs, these individuals may be assigned tasks and responsibilities requiring more than their educational preparation and competence. Laws regarding educational requirements and legal definitions of scope of practice have been used to control nursing assistant practice. For example, through the OBRA 1987 regulations for long-term care facilities, a nationwide standard was established for the training and certification of nursing assistants employed in these facilities. Each state administers the regulations and is free to raise the standards, but may not lower them.

QUALIFICATIONS FOR LICENSURE APPLICANTS

The qualifications for licensure may be described in detail in the law, or only general guidelines may be given, leaving the details up to the State Board of Nursing. The most common basic requirements are graduation from an approved educational program and proficiency in the English language. Some states make the educational requirements more specific—requiring, for example, high school graduation and either an associate or baccalaureate degree, or a diploma in nursing, for the registered nurse applicant.

All states require a passing score on a comprehensive examination, but do not specify which examination in the law; the current licensing examinations are discussed later in this chapter. Many states require that an applicant be of "good moral character." There is usually a requirement for disclosure of criminal convictions, some of which are a barrier to licensure. Some require "good physical and mental health," but more commonly there is a requirement for disclosure of any illness or medication use that might affect practice.

TITLING

This section of the law specifies the titles to be used for those who have met the licensure requirements. In some states, only the titles registered nurse and licensed practical nurse are regulated. Many states also regulate the use of titles for advanced practice, such as nurse practitioner and nurse midwife. Titles used in these expanded roles vary from state to state. Some current titles are advanced practice nurse (APN), advanced registered nurse (ARN), specialized registered nurse (SRN), nurse practitioner (NP), independent nurse practitioner (INP), advanced nurse practitioner (ANP), advanced registered nurse practitioner (ARNP), and certified registered nurse (CRN). In some states, the specialized nurse uses the title of a specific certification, such as family nurse practitioner (FNP) and pediatric nurse practitioner (PNP). As legal regulation of advanced practice expands, titles are likely to be systematized through the NCSBN.

GRANDFATHERING

Whenever a new law is written, it usually contains a statement specifying that anyone currently holding a license may continue to hold that license if and when requirements for the license change. Without this provision, the enactment of a new law would require individuals who are currently licensed to reapply and to show that they meet the new standards.

However, not all changes in the law are grandfathered. When new requirements are instituted that the legislature believes are important for the safety of the public, all currently licensed individuals may be required to meet the new standards within a given period. For example, in 1987 the legislature in Washington State passed a bill requiring all licensed health professionals to have 7 hours of education regarding certain topics related to the acquired immunodeficiency syndrome (AIDS). New applicants had to provide evidence of meeting this requirement before their licenses were granted; current license holders had to meet this requirement before their licenses were renewed. Individuals seeking licensure by endorsement also were required to verify that they had completed the equivalent of 7 hours of AIDS education. For additional discussion of grandfathering, please refer to Chapter 6.

LICENSE RENEWAL AND CONTINUING EDUCATION REQUIREMENTS

The length of time for which a license is valid and any requirements for its renewal are specified in the law. In some states, license renewal requires only the payment of a fee. Many jurisdictions require evidence of continuing education for renewal. The documentation of continuing education may be the submission of records, or it may be attested to by signing a form. For example, California requires that the person seeking to renew an RN license list all continuing education courses taken, along with the number of continuing education units earned and the provider number of the agency offering the courses. In many states where the applicant is not required to submit records at the time of renewal, a procedure for random checking ensures compliance with the law. Continuing education requirements vary greatly, from as few as 15 hours every 2 years to as many as 24 hours every year.

FINANCIAL CONCERNS

Although the nurse practice act itself usually does not specify the fees to be charged for obtaining or renewing a license, general restrictions on the method of calculating fees and on how the fees may be used are often included in the act. The act may specify how the expenses of the Board of Nursing are to be met and who has legal authority to make decisions regarding the use of funds.

All states charge a fee for processing an application for licensure. At initial licensure there are also fees for taking a licensing examination, and a fee must be paid to the company that prepares and scores an examination. The total cost for an initial examination and license is usually close to $200. In addition, there is a fee each time a license is renewed. For specific information on current licensure fees, temporary permits, and continuing education requirements, contact the Board of Nursing in the state in which you will practice.

NURSING EDUCATION PROGRAMS

Some state laws describe the requirements of nursing education programs in only the most general terms, leaving the details up to the Board of Nursing; in other states, the laws are specific. The law may specify the number of years of education required, the courses or content that must be included, and the approval process for particular programs. If the law is general, then the board sets more specific standards. All nursing education programs in a state must fulfill the requirements of the state law.

DISCIPLINARY ACTION

Disciplinary action refers to all penalties that may be imposed against an individual who has violated provisions of a licensing law. Disciplinary actions include restrictions on practice (such as working only under supervision), suspension of a license for a specified period, or revocation of a license. Disciplinary action can only be taken based on criteria stated in the law (Fig 7-3). In the past, most state acts contained general

FIGURE 7–3   A nursing license may be revoked by the State Board of Nursing.

rules about such matters as immoral and unprofessional conduct. Because of their vagueness, however, these general rules proved difficult to enforce in court. In addition, most courts have supported revocation of a license only when the offense was related in some way to practice issues that affected the public. Thus, most modern laws contain specific concerns such as the following:

- Fraud in obtaining a license
- Conviction of a felony
- Substance abuse
- Harming the public

Some states now have clauses that call for license revocation for individuals who default on government-sponsored educational loans or on agreements regarding service in return for scholarship aid (New Legislation, 1996).

VIOLATIONS AND PENALTIES

Specific power is provided to the nursing board to prosecute those who violate the provisions of the law. The board may be authorized to ask a court to halt a specific practice that it believes is contrary to the law until a full hearing can be held. This is called "injunctive relief." This term refers to the court order called an injunction that requires an individual or organization to stop a particular activity.

EXCEPTIONS

Certain provisions may allow those who are not licensed to act as nurses in specific situations. Performing as a student while in an educational program is usually the primary exception. Those who are caring for family members or friends without pay are also exempted from license regulations. Those who are practicing nursing in a federal agency, such as a military hospital, are exempted from the local state law as long as they maintain a current license in another state. Some states are adopting exceptions for self-directed care by the disabled. In these situations, a paid care provider may perform certain care that is usually considered nursing when directed to do so by the mentally competent, physically disabled client. This includes administering medications in the home and carrying out specific care procedures, such as catheterization.

ADMINISTRATIVE PROVISIONS

Each law requires administrative specifications detailing when the law will become effective and when a previous act will no longer be in force. Such provisions are of particular interest to nurses when a law is first passed, because nurses want to know when changes affecting them will take place.

Advanced Practice Nurses

Advanced practice nurses include nurse practitioners, nurse anesthetists, and nurse midwives. Licensure requirements for advanced practice vary from state to state. Many, but not all, require the master's degree in nursing. Gradually states are moving toward the master's degree as the standard. None of the states administers a state licensing examination for advanced practice nursing.

Often the law requires that a person be certified for advanced practice by the ANCC or a nursing specialty organization (see section on certification later in the chapter) to receive a license as an advanced practice nurse. This certification includes testing. The requirements and methods for obtaining certification remain with the organization granting the certification, but the nurse receives a license from the state to practice in the expanded role. This is true of certified nurse anesthetists, who are all certified through the Council on Certification of Nurse Anesthetists, but who receive legal status to practice in anesthesia by the appropriate authority in their state. Some states do not specifically mention advanced practice nurses, but the Board of Nursing approves specialty practice based on the provisions in the basic act. In still other states, advanced practice nurses are governed under the medical practice act. Contact the Board of Nursing in the state in which you are interested for information about advanced practice.

The NCSBN has adopted the position that the testing and licensing of nurses in advanced practice is the responsibility of the legal jurisdiction. Therefore, the NCSBN is developing a testing program for advanced nursing practice. In 1996, the NCSBN began a study process that could lead to a state-run testing program. Another of the goals of this study was the standardization of other licensing requirements for advanced nursing practice across the country.

Those who now certify advanced practice nurses have voiced opposition to this plan (Boards will weigh, 1996). The ANA does not believe that regulating advanced practice through the law and state-administered testing is the best method of ensuring safety in expanded practice. Some of the laws regulating advanced practice have provided for physician review of nursing's scope of practice. The ANA is concerned that these laws will take autonomy away from nursing and allow medicine to control some aspects of the nursing profession. The ANA also is concerned about the rigidity of these laws, which may not allow for evolving nursing roles. The ANA holds the position that the licensure law should regulate minimum safe practice, and that the profession should regulate advanced practice. This is the procedure in medicine, in which there is only basic licensure because a physician in specialty practice is regulated by specialty boards in the profession.

The Role of the Board of Nursing

The Board of Nursing (or its equivalent) is legally empowered to carry out the provisions of the law. The membership of the board, the procedures for appointment and removal, and the qualifications of board members are determined by the Nurse Practice Act. The board has the power to write the rules and regulations used in daily operations.

The governor of the state usually appoints the members of the State Board of Nursing. The law specifies the occupational background of the candidates; nominations may be made by nurses' organizations and other interested parties. North Carolina is the only state in which the registered nurse members of the state board are elected by the registered nurses in the state.

Boards of nursing range in size from 7 to 17 members. Prerequisites regarding the educational background of nurses who serve as board members vary from state to state. Some states require that the board include nurses from different occupational areas, such as education and nursing service. Most states have at least one public member of the board. A few have at least one physician on the nursing board.

Most states have a single board for registered nurses and licensed practical nurses. In some states, two separate boards exist. Each state board has a paid staff that usually is headed by a registered nurse who is employed as the executive director of the State Board of Nursing. The executive director is responsible for administering the work of the board and seeing that rules and regulations are followed. Some duties related to professional licensure may be performed by a centralized state agency acting in that capacity for all licensed occupations. The responsibilities of these centralized agencies may range from administrative matters (such as collecting fees, managing routine license renewals, and providing secretarial services) to decision making, relegating individual boards like the Board of Nursing to an advisory status.

Each state board must operate within the framework of its own state law regarding the practice of nursing, but all cooperate with one another through the NCSBN. For example, state boards acting together through the NCSBN contract with the company that prepares the licensing examinations for registered nurses and practical nurses that are used throughout the United States. They also cooperate with the ANA and the National League for Nursing (NLN) in some matters, but maintain the separation that is required of a governmental body.

The Board of Nursing typically must perform the following functions:

1. Establish standards for licensure
2. Examine and license applicants
3. Provide for interstate endorsement
4. Renew licenses, grant temporary licenses, and provide for inactive status for those already licensed who request it
5. Enforce disciplinary codes
6. Provide rules for revocation of license
7. Regulate specialty practice
8. Establish standards and curricula for nursing programs
9. Approve nursing education programs

OBTAINING A NURSING LICENSE

There are two different procedures for obtaining a nursing license; one is used for obtaining an initial license and the other for obtaining a license when the nurse is already licensed in another jurisdiction. The initial licensure process is called *licensure by examination*. Obtaining a license in a second jurisdiction is called *licensure by endorsement*. In both instances, the applicant for licensure must meet all provisions of the law (such as educational preparation, language proficiency, and legal residency status) in the state where he or she is seeking licensure. In the initial licensure process, the applicant must take and pass the standard licensing examination (NCLEX). When seeking licensure by endorsement, the applicant is not required to take another examination; the licensing examination results from the initial state are accepted as proof of minimum safe practice, but other requirements must be met. This process is discussed later in the chapter.

Licensure by Examination

The establishment of a licensing examination was an important part of early efforts to achieve a professional standard for the registered nurse. When each state adopted a licensing law, it also established a mechanism for examining license applicants. A major achievement in the history of licensure was the formation of the Bureau of State Boards of Nurse Examiners, which eventually led to the use of an identical examination in all states in 1950. The original examination, called the State Board Test Pool Examination, was prepared by the testing department of the NLN, under a contract with the state boards. Although each state initially determined its own passing score, most states agreed on an acceptable test score; eventually all states adopted a common passing score for the State Board Test Pool Examination. The current examination, called the NCLEX-RN for registered nursing and the NCLEX-PN for practical nursing, is used in all states and territories of the United States. It is prepared and administered by the Educational Testing Service of Princeton, New Jersey, under a contract with National Council of State Boards of Nursing. Beginning in October 2002, a new testing company, National Computer Systems of Edin Prairie, Minnesota, will prepare and administer the examination.

Critical Thinking Activity

A student about to graduate from a registered nursing program in New York wishes to practice nursing in New Jersey. Investigate the steps she should take to ensure that she may legally practice nursing in New Jersey as soon after graduation as possible.

CONTENT OF THE EXAMINATION

Historically, the content of the nursing examination was divided into the categories of medical, surgical, obstetric, pediatric, and psychiatric nursing. Because nursing had changed in nature and these categories no longer adequately reflected nursing practice, the NCSBN adopted a different examination plan, which was implemented in July 1982. For this new examination, the National Council supported a research study, called the "RN Job Analysis," that identified nursing behaviors critical to maintaining a safe and effective standard of care (Display 7-2). This research has been repeated periodically to ensure that the test plan remains relevant to current nursing practice.

In all of these studies, newly licensed, practicing registered nurses are studied to determine both the frequency and the criticality of various behaviors. *Frequency* refers to how often the behaviors are required of the newly practicing registered nurse. *Criticality* refers to those actions that, if performed incorrectly or omitted, could cause serious harm to the client. These studies are reflected in the "Test Plan for the National Council Licensure Examination" (NCSBN, 1998).

The NCLEX-RN examination questions are organized into categories based on the interaction of client needs and the steps of the nursing process. The four client needs with their subcategories are noted in Table 7-1 (NCSBN, 1998). The nursing process is divided into five steps. These two sets of concepts form a matrix in which each question tests a step of the nursing process and one subcategory of client need. Another set of broad concepts is integrated into the test. These are also listed in Table 7-1. The multiple choice questions in the examination typically are based on situations that require a nursing response. They are designed to test judgment and decision making, not simply knowledge of facts. Setting priorities may be one aspect of that judgment (NCSBN, 1998).

Within these categories, safe practice behaviors are tested. For example, one question might determine an applicant's ability to assess in relationship to infection control, while another question might determine whether an applicant would implement the correct action to maintain infection control. In the category of physiologic integrity, a question might focus on the appropriate planning for a client to minimize the risk of a complication and another might focus on evaluating the outcomes of pharmacologic intervention. In this way, questions address two aspects of the matrix plan (Fig. 7-4).

Display 7–2
CRITICAL REQUIREMENTS FOR PRACTICE

I. Exercises Professional Prerogatives Based on Clinical Judgment
   A. Adapts care to individual patient needs
   B. Fulfills responsibility to patient and others despite difficulty
   C. Challenges inappropriate orders and decisions by medical and other professional staff
   D. Acts as patient advocate in obtaining appropriate medical, psychiatric, or other help
   E. Recognizes own limitations and errors
   F. Analyzes and adjusts own or staff reactions to maintain therapeutic relationship with patient
II. Promotes Patient's Ability to Cope with Immediate, Long-range, or Potential Health-related Change
   A. Provides health care instruction or information to patient, family, or significant others
   B. Encourages patient or family to make decision about accepting care or adhering to treatment regimen
   C. Helps patient recognize and deal with psychological stress
   D. Avoids creating or increasing anxiety or stress
   E. Conveys and invites acceptance, respect, and trust
   F. Facilitates relationship of family, staff, or significant others with patient
   G. Stimulates, remotivates patient, or enables patient to achieve self-care independence
III. Helps Maintain Patient Comfort and Normal Body Functions
   A. Keeps patient clean and comfortable
   B. Helps patient maintain or regain normal body functions
IV. Takes Precautionary and Preventive Measures in Giving Patient Care
   A. Prevents infection
   B. Protects skin and mucous membranes from injurious materials
   C. Uses positioning or exercise to prevent injury or the complications of immobility
   D. Avoids using injurious techniques in administering and managing intrusive or other potentially traumatic treatments
   E. Protects patient from falls or other contact injuries
   F. Maintains surveillance of patient's activities
   G. Reduces or removes environmental hazards
V. Checks, Compares, Verifies, Monitors, and Follows up Medication and Treatment Processes
   A. Checks correctness, condition, and safety of medication being prepared
   B. Ensures that correct medication is given to the right patient and that patient takes or receives it
   C. Adheres to schedule in giving medication, treatment, or test
   D. Administers medication by correct route, rate, or mode
   E. Checks patient's readiness for medication, treatment, surgery, or other care
   F. Checks to ensure that tests or measurements are done correctly

(continues)

Display 7–2
CRITICAL REQUIREMENTS FOR PRACTICE *(Continued)*

    G. Monitors ongoing infusions and inhalations
    H. Checks for and interprets effect of medication, treatment, or care, and takes corrective action if necessary
VI. Interprets Symptom Complex and Intervenes Appropriately
    A. Checks patient's condition or status
    B. Remains objective, further investigates, or verifies patient's complaint or problem
    C. Uses alarms and signals on automatic equipment as adjunct to personal assessment
    D. Observes and correctly assesses signs of anxiety or behavioral stress
    E. Observes and correctly assesses physical signs, symptoms, or findings, and intervenes appropriately
    F. Correctly assesses severity or priority of patient's condition, and gives or obtains necessary care
VII. Responds to Emergency
    A. Anticipates need for crisis care
    B. Takes instant, correct action in emergency situations
    C. Maintains calm and efficient approach under pressure
    D. Assumes leadership role in crisis situation when necessary
VIII. Obtains, Records, and Exchanges Information on Behalf of the Patient
    A. Checks data sources for order and other information about patient
    B. Obtains information from patient and family
    C. Transcribes or records information on chart, Kardex, or other information system
    D. Exchanges information with nursing staff and other departments
    E. Exchanges information with medical staff
IX. Utilizes Patient Care Planning
    A. Develops and modifies patient care plan
    B. Implements patient care plan
X. Teaches and Supervises Other Staff
    A. Teaches correct principles, procedures, and techniques of patient care
    B. Supervises and checks the work of staff for whom she or he is responsible

The NCLEX-PN has a similar construction pattern. A "PN Job Analysis" study is conducted and then the test plan is developed. The most recent PN Job Analysis was completed in 1997; the newest test plan for the PN was approved in 1998 and implemented in April 1999. The practical nurse is expected to assume a more dependent role in assessment; therefore, the category is titled data collection. Analysis is not part of the test plan. Whereas the RN examination includes management of care, the PN examination focuses on coordinated care. Even when topics are the same, the level of judgment expected of the PN differs from that expected of the RN. The newest test recognizes that many licensed practical nurses are employed in long-term care settings,

TABLE 7–1. NCLEX-RN Test Plan

Concepts	Percentage of Test Questions
Client Needs	
• Safe, effective care environment	
Management of Care	7–13
Safety and Infection Control	5–11
• Health promotion–health maintenance	
Growth and Development Through the Life-Span	7–13
Prevention and Early Detection of Disease	5–11
• Psychosocial integrity	
Coping and Adaptation	5–11
Psychosocial Adaptation	5–11
• Physiologic integrity	
Basic Care and Comfort	7–13
Pharmacological and Parenteral Therapies	5–11
Reduction of Risk Potential	12–18
Physiologic Adaptation	12–18

Steps of the Nursing Process	**Integrated Concepts**
• Assessing	• Caring
• Analyzing	• Communication
• Planning	• Cultural Awareness
• Implementing	• Documentation
• Evaluating	• Self-care
	• Teaching/learning

with clients older than 65 years of age, through a life span focus that emphasizes the older population. The percentages of questions in each category of the NCLEX-PN are shown in Table 7-2 (NCLEX-PN, 1999).

PREPARING AND ADMINISTERING THE EXAMINATION

Preparing questions for the examination is a complex process. Individuals who teach in nursing programs across the country are brought together as item writers. Together they write questions based on the test plan. Questions then are reviewed by content experts, who are nurses currently working with new graduates. Another panel of individuals reviews the questions for bias. Each question then is verified for accuracy by using current nursing references; test construction experts also review the structure of all of the questions. The final versions of all questions are tested by inclusion in a non-graded part of the license examinations being given to new graduates; the questions are evaluated for their level of difficulty and appropriate use as part of a future scored examination.

In addition to assuming responsibility for test preparation, the testing service administers the computerized tests through contracted testing centers, scores the examinations, and reports scores to the state boards. The testing service is authorized to sell

FIGURE 7–4   Questions on the NCLEX exam are designed to test ability to function safely as a nurse. Setting correct priorities is one aspect of safe practice.

statistical information related to the examinations to the states and to individual schools.

COMPUTERIZED ADAPTIVE TESTING

All NCLEX examinations (both RN and PN) are now administered through computerized adaptive testing (CAT). The CAT consists of a bank of examination questions administered through a computerized system. CAT had its first field trials in 1990, was tested across the country in 1993, and was adopted for all testing beginning in April 1994.

In this computerized test, the multiple choice questions are on a computer screen. The computer contains a large bank of questions; different individuals may be presented with different questions. The development of questions and the design of the computer program ensures that all tests are equivalent even when not identical. The computer program evaluates each response, and then selects an appropriate question to present next, choosing a slightly harder question if the previous question was answered correctly, or an easier question if the response was incorrect. The computer program ensures that all essential aspects of the test matrix plan are part of every examination. On the NCLEX-RN the minimum number of questions that might be

TABLE 7–2.   NCLEX-PN Test Plan

Concepts	Percentage of Test Questions
Client Needs	
• Safe, effective care environment	
Coordinated Care	6–12
Safety and Infection Control	7–13
• Health promotion–health maintenance	
Growth and Development Through the Life-Span	4–10
Prevention and Early Detection of Disease	4–10
• Psychosocial integrity	
Coping and Adaptation	6–12
Psychosocial Adaptation	4–10
• Physiologic integrity	
Basic Care and Comfort	10–16
Pharmacological Therapies	5–11
Reduction of Risk Potential	11–17
Physiologic Adaptation	13–19

Steps of the Nursing Process	*Integrated Concepts*
• Data Collection	• Caring
• Planning	• Communication
• Implementation	• Cultural Awareness
• Evaluation	• Documentation
	• Self-care
	• Teaching/learning

administered is 75 and the maximum is 265. The maximum length of time for the examination is 5 hours, but a candidate performing either especially well or very poorly might complete the exam in just 1 hour. One break is required after 2 hours of testing, and others may be taken at the discretion of the applicant. Testing ends when the scoring analysis clearly indicates a pass, clearly indicates a fail, the maximum number of questions have been answered, or the maximum time has been completed.

Each candidate for licensure makes an individual appointment at a testing site. At the testing site, the computers are located in a quiet room without distractions. Pencil and paper are provided for notes or calculations (calculators are not permitted). Security is tightly monitored.

Each question, along with its possible answers, is presented on a separate screen; if there is a brief situation, it appears on the same screen as the question and answers. Only two keys are used throughout the examination: the space bar moves between the alternative answers, and the "enter" key must be pressed twice to make a selection. A selection must be made to move to the next question. It is not possible to go back to a question previously answered. Some practice questions are provided to assure that the individual understands the process. When the individual has completed enough questions for the computer program to determine either a "pass" or a "fail," the testing session is ended.

SCORING THE EXAMINATION

The computer calculates the score as the applicant answers questions. Based on the computation made as the applicant progresses, additional questions are presented to clearly determine whether the applicant meets the standards for safe, effective practice in all areas of the test plan. The score used to determine a pass or a failure is not a raw score (ie, the number correct), but is derived from a complex statistical process that takes into consideration both the difficulty of a question and whether the response was correct. As soon as the statistical computation provides a clear prediction of "pass" or "fail," the test is terminated. If the computerized score has not provided a clear prediction of pass or fail by the end of the examination (either time is up or maximum questions are answered), the performance on the last 60 questions becomes key to determining pass or fail. The test was not designed for the purpose of differentiating levels of excellence, only for demonstrating basic safe practice, and this is what the pass or fail communicates.

Although the computer immediately determines a score (upon the completion of the examination), the individual is not notified of the result at that time. The scoring information is communicated to the Educational Testing Service, which then notifies the appropriate board. The Board of Nursing then notifies the individual whether they received a "pass" or "fail."

Every three years, the National Council of State Boards considers the appropriateness of the passing standards for both the PN and RN examinations. In October 1997 the decision was made to increase the passing standard for the NCLEX-RN beginning in 1998 based on the increased expectations placed upon nurses in their work environments (NCSBN, 1997). In 1998 the NCSBN approved a change in the passing standard for the PN examination. This increased standard took place in April 1999, coincident with the implementation of the NCLEX-PN Test Plan (NCSBN, 1998).

PREPARING FOR THE NCLEX

Each individual must determine how best to prepare for the licensure examination. This is determined based on background and preferred study style. A review of the knowledge basic to nursing is important for most individuals. This may be done using course notes and texts. Those who become anxious in testing situations may want to focus on exercises to decrease anxiety during the examination. Those who find the process of test taking difficult can gain greater self-confidence by practicing test-taking techniques. This can be done through printed tests in books or computerized test preparation programs.

For both the NCLEX-RN and the NCLEX-PN, many commercial study aids are available. To prepare applicants to take the examination, the NCSBN has authorized the preparation of a study book that explains the examination, how it was written, and the scoring system, and that provides sample questions to familiarize applicants with the way the test is written. The NCSBN also provides an on-line NCLEX-RN study program available by subscription. Many companies also prepare NCLEX-RN and NCLEX-PN review books, sample examination questions, audiotapes, and computerized practice examinations that are used to prepare for the licensing examinations. Manuals that outline standard nursing practice relative to many different health care problems may be useful for reviewing nursing content. Live and videotaped review courses, both by individual schools of nursing and by commercial publishers, are available to those who want assistance with preparation.

FUTURE TRENDS IN EXAMINATION

The NCSBN spent many years examining the potential for computerized Clinical Simulation Testing (CST), a more complex form of computerized testing of nursing licensure applicants (Bersky & Yocom, 1994). In this type of test, a client situation is presented on the computer screen. The applicant is asked to determine the appropriate action and type the answer into the keyboard. The applicant receives points for correct actions, and for the order or priority in which actions are chosen. Points are subtracted for inappropriate actions. Special note is made of actions that might harm a client. This type of testing is much more expensive to develop and administer than a multiple-choice question examination. CST was first field tested in 1991 (Overview, 1996). Further testing in schools of nursing was completed during the 1997–1998 academic year. When the analysis of this testing was presented in 1999, the Delegate Assembly of the NCSBN decided that the CST will not become a part of the licensing examination. The complexity of scoring and the high cost make it impractical for that purpose. Whether it might be used for any other purpose remains to be seen.

Licensure By Endorsement

The process of obtaining a nursing license in a new state (when already licensed in another state) is called licensure by endorsement. Sometimes people incorrectly assume *reciprocity* exists among states for nursing licenses. Technically, reciprocity is the type of recognition provided for such items as a driver's license; you can drive in any state as long as your license from your home state is valid. A similar type of recognition has been developed between some states (see Multistate Licensure, below), but is not the universal pattern.

In licensure by endorsement, each case is considered independently, based on the rules and regulations of the state. However, owing to the uniformity of licensing laws throughout most of the United States and its territories, nurses have enjoyed easy mobility between geographical areas.

Because the same licensure examination and same passing standard are used nationwide, no state requires that the examination be retaken. Basic educational and legal requirements of the individual state where a license is sought must be met. Sometimes a nurse moving to a new state must meet the current criteria for new licensure. In other states, a nurse must fulfill only the requirements that were in effect at the time of the original licensure. A state may require a nurse to meet other criteria, such as those for continuing education, before granting licensure by endorsement. In all cases, appropriate paperwork must be completed, necessary fees paid, and a license obtained before a nurse may begin employment.

A temporary license, which allows the applicant for licensure by endorsement to be employed while credentials are being verified and processed, is available in some states. Other states require that a permanent license be obtained before any employment is legal in those jurisdictions.

If a nurse wishes to maintain licensure in more than one state, this may be done by paying the renewal fees and meeting other requirements for continued licensure, such as continuing education, in each state. Some nurses hold licenses in several different states in order to be able to work as a traveling nurse or to choose work in different locations. Nurses working close to state lines may need more than one license to be employed by an agency that operates in more than one state. This might be true of a nursing education program that has clinical sites in two adjacent cities or a home care agency with clients in two states.

At present, North Dakota does not offer straightforward licensure by endorsement to all nurses licensed in other states. In North Dakota, an associate degree is required for initial licensure as a practical nurse, and a baccalaureate degree is required for initial licensure as a registered nurse. All nurses registered in North Dakota were grandfathered into their licenses when this change in licensure regulations occurred. A registered nurse or licensed practical nurse from another state, who does not have the required degree and who seeks licensure by endorsement in North Dakota, must meet specific conditions and standards identified by the North Dakota Board; the conditions may include enrollment in an educational program to obtain the required degree. Based on individual evaluation, a temporary license may be granted while the individual fulfills the conditions specified for a regular license. North Dakota represents an exception to the general pattern of easy mobility for all registered nurses.

 Critical Thinking Activity

A registered nurse who has been working in Indianapolis, Indiana, for 10 years decides to relocate to Orlando, Florida. What are the steps that the nurse should take to ensure that she is able to work as a registered nurse in Florida?

MULTISTATE LICENSURE

Multistate licensure involves an individual receiving a registered nurse license in one state and being legally permitted to practice in additional states without obtaining additional licenses for those states. Originally two approaches to multistate licensure were explored by the NCSBN: rapid endorsement and mutual recognition. The NCSBN finally endorsed a mutual recognition compact that requires states to share disciplinary information and basic licensure information (National Council Begins, 1996). Other states remain interested in exploring the rapid endorsement process.

A computerized databank titled NURSYS is scheduled for completion in 2000. This data bank will contain disciplinary information from every state and will be used in the Multistate Compact states to track disciplinary concerns (Majek, 1996; Ventura, 1999). It also may prove useful in any moves toward rapid endorsement.

The Multistate Licensure Compact

The Multistate Licensure Compact is the agreed upon standard for mutual recognition of registered nursing licensure that was adopted by the NCSBN. Those states that have entered into the NCSBN Multistate Licensure Compact have all passed legislation adopting the terms of the compact into their licensure laws (NCSBN, 1998). This law applies only to basic registered nursing licensure and does not apply to any form of advanced practice nursing.

All of the states that have signed the compact are referred to as *party states*. A person's *home state* is the state in which an individual resides and in which that individual has a registered nursing license. An individual maintains only one license, the license granted in the home state, but is legally permitted to practice in any party state. When renewing a license, the individual renews in the home state. The individual nurse cannot hold a license in two party states at the same time. When an individual changes residence to a new party state, he or she would apply for a new home state license based on residency. If an individual wished to practice in a non-party state, that person would still need to apply for a license in the non-party state before practicing nursing.

A *remote state* is a place other than the nurse's home state where the patient or recipient of nursing practice is located. For purposes of this law, nursing care is located where the patient is, not where the nurse is. The individual nurse must comply with the state laws regulating nursing practice in the state in which the client is located. Any party state where nursing care occurs (whether the home state or the remote state) may institute disciplinary action based on appropriate procedures. The home state is notified of the action being taken in the remote state through a coordinated information system. When a remote state institutes disciplinary action, they may revoke the privilege to practice in that state only. Only the home state may revoke the license itself. If an individual has been assigned to some type of alternative program (such as drug treatment and monitoring) as part of the disciplinary process by any party state, the conditions of the disciplinary process must prohibit the individual from practicing in other states in the compact until the problem is resolved.

As you can see, the registered nurse who is licensed in a Multistate Licensure Compact state, who chooses to work outside the home state, must follow the directives contained in the compact and become familiar with the nursing practice act in any state in which clients are located. The State Board of any state participating in the compact will provide complete information on the specific requirements to be met.

States Involved

Some states have already entered into the multistate licensure agreement. These include Arkansas, Iowa, Maryland, Mississippi, Nebraska, North Carolina, South Dakota, Texas, Utah, and Wisconsin. Others are considering the potential. Still other states have decided that at this time it would not be in their best interests to join such a pact.

States currently in the Multistate Licensure Compact share disciplinary information and basic licensure information.

Reasons Nurses Seek Multistate Licensure

Under standard licensing laws, the nurse who practices in more than one state must hold multiple nursing licenses. This is both costly and complex. As the health care system grows more diverse, it is not uncommon for a health care-providing organization to operate across state boundaries. *Telenursing* includes the use of telecommunications technology (eg, telephone, fax, computers, teleconferencing, interactive television, and video phone) to provide nursing services to individuals and groups. A telenurse may be in one state, with a client in a distant state, thus raising questions regarding licensure requirements for a nurse who serves clients in more than one state. Does the nurse who provides telephone monitoring and advice for the client in another state need to be licensed in that client's state? Another area of concern is the nurse who works for an agency that serves clients across state borders. This nurse needs to visit clients in more than one state. The nursing case manager may follow clients in several states. All of these create situations in which both health care agencies and individual nurses would like a simpler system for licensing.

Concerns Regarding Multistate Licensure

Not all nurses have supported multistate licensure. The ANA has identified that nurses could be practicing side-by-side who have differing requirements for relicensure; for example, one home state requires continuing education and another does not. Some state attorneys general have given opinions that it would be unconstitutional to allow another state to control the requirements for practice in their own state. Privacy concerns regarding the data stored in the NURSYS system are another area of concern. The multistate licensure system may save money for the nurse who practices in multiple states because only one license would be purchased. However, if fewer nurses are licensed in the state, but the same number practice in the state, one would expect that disciplinary costs would remain even. The cost of licenses for all nurses, therefore, would have to rise to assure adequate funds to support disciplinary costs (Ventura, 1999).

A major concern is the disciplinary process. Although the board of nursing can investigate nursing practice and enforce its own standards in the state, it cannot change the licensure status of the person whose licensure is in a different state; this fact is troubling to some boards of nursing. They are concerned that they would be unable to protect the public adequately. A person disciplined in a remote state still would possess what would appear to be a valid home state license, but perhaps would not legally be able to practice in the remote state. For the individual nurse, the differences in licensure regulations could result in the same behavior being the cause of disciplinary action in one state but not in others; however, if the license were removed, then it would be invalid in all states. Simpson (1999) suggests that technology can solve most of these concerns if it is applied effectively. The ANA has expressed concern that multistate licensure would facilitate bringing in out-of-state nurses for "union busting" and thus interfere with valid collective bargaining. (See Chapter 12 for a further discussion of collective bargaining.)

The future holds many exciting possibilities for nursing but also poses many potential pitfalls. This is a complex issue, because state licensing agencies are charged with protecting the public and have legitimate concerns regarding such areas as disciplinary action.

REVOCATION OR LIMITATION OF A LICENSE

A license to practice any occupation becomes a property right of the individual once the state has awarded it. As long as the individual renews a license by paying the appropriate fees and meeting any requirements, such as continuing education, a license cannot be revoked without cause. The possible reasons for revoking or limiting a license are spelled out in the law. (The common reasons were listed earlier, in the discussion of disciplinary action.)

The procedure for revoking a license includes a fact-finding process and a hearing, which functions in many ways like a court proceeding. The state board or a specially designated hearing board is responsible for conducting the hearing and making a decision. The board may provide a license with conditions, suspend a license until certain conditions are met, or revoke a license completely. For example, a nurse faced with charges of chemical dependency might be directed to enter a treatment program, to refuse employment involving direct responsibility for clients or access to drugs, and to be monitored for compliance. If these conditions are met, the individual may be allowed to work in a restricted environment and then be reinstated to full rights and privileges of licensure when treatment is completed. The board's decision may be appealed in a court of law in most states. The individual being investigated for any violation of the nursing practice act or who is in the hearing process should have an attorney for legal counsel throughout the proceeding. A license to practice nursing is valuable to the individual nurse and should be protected. The nurses association can often provide referrals of attorneys who are familiar with the disciplinary process. If a board of nursing finds that the individual's actions constitute a felony, the board is obligated to report that to the criminal authorities for prosecution.

As a licensed professional, you should be aware that you are responsible to your clients and to the state for your practice. You can act to protect your license through maintaining current knowledge and appropriate standards of practice. You should also understand and abide by the scope of practice as described in your individual nurse practice act (Green and others, 1995).

Critical Thinking Activity

A nurse in your state receives a notification from the Board of Nursing that a complaint has been lodged with the board in regard to her practice. Find out what the process would be in your state for this nurse to respond to the complaint. What resources will this nurse need? What are the possible consequences if the complaint is sustained?

SUNSET LAWS

Most laws remain in effect until the legislature votes to rescind or replace them. Because this has resulted in archaic laws remaining in effect for many years, some states have passed what are known as "sunset laws." Sunset laws provide that any regulatory act, such as the Nurse Practice Act, will automatically be rescinded if not reauthorized. In states with sunset laws, nurses cannot wait for an opportune time to support changes in the Nurse Practice Act. Instead, they must identify when sunsetting will occur and work in advance to sustain the current law or make changes. The advantage of sunset laws is that they guarantee that the legislature will review and evaluate agencies and programs.

LICENSURE OF GRADUATES OF FOREIGN NURSING SCHOOLS

Many nurses from foreign countries have immigrated to the United States and sought licensure to be able to work in their new home. Some nurses have come to the United States for additional education and need a license to engage in clinical practice associated with that education. Still others are attracted by the better salaries and living conditions for nurses in the United States. During the nursing shortage of the early 1980s, employers in the United States actively recruited foreign nurses, sometimes providing support for travel and relocation expenses.

All graduates of foreign nursing schools who want to practice nursing in the United States must provide verification that their foreign education meets state requirements, and they must take the appropriate NCLEX examination. In the past, institutions would sometimes hire foreign nurses into lower paying positions until they obtained a license. When many did not pass the examination, they felt exploited by the system.

The U.S. Department of Labor, the Department of Health and Human Services (formerly known as the Department of Health, Education, and Welfare), the Immigration and Naturalization Service, the ANA, and the NLN were different agencies and organizations concerned about the safety of the public and about the well-being of the foreign-educated nurse. To address these problems, these organizations and governmental agencies collaborated in the development of an independent organization called the Commission on Graduates of Foreign Nursing Schools (CGFNS). This organization reviews foreign educational credentials, assures English language proficiency by evaluating scores on the TOEFL (Test of English as a Foreign Language), and administers a nursing proficiency examination to foreign-educated nurses. Based on these data, the CGFNS provides certification to Boards of Nursing, educational institutions, and the Immigration and Naturalization Service of the nursing education status of the individual seeking to go to school or work in the United States. Nurses may take the CGFNS examination in 40 sites around the world before undertaking expensive relocation. Up to 85% of foreign-educated nurses who have obtained CGFNS certification pass the licensing examination. This contrasts to the 5% to 10% who passed the licensing examination without CGFNS screening. Because many foreign-educated nurses still come to the United States without having taken the CGFNS examination, it also is offered in selected cities in the United States. Some states make CGFNS certification a requirement for graduates of foreign nursing schools who wish to take the NCLEX-RN.

During the nursing shortage of the 1980s in the United States, recruitment of foreign-educated nurses was prevalent. A special regulation allowed these nurses to obtain the H-1A nonimmigrant preference visa from the U.S. Immigration and Naturalization Service, or a work permit from the U.S. Labor Department. The foreign-educated nurse had to obtain CGFNS certification to get this visa. Because the special regulation was not renewed, it was automatically rescinded, or "sunsetted" in September 1995 (see section on Sunset Laws earlier in this chapter). The H-1B nonimmigrant visas remained available for foreign-educated nurses with a bachelor's degree and experience.

As a new shortage of registered nurses begins in the United States, permission for recruitment of foreign-educated nurses has been sought again. In 1999, the "Nursing Relief For Disadvantaged Areas Act" was signed into law. This law provides for a special H-1C visa for foreign-educated nurses who work in areas of documented nursing shortage. The visa is good for 3 years and is not renewable. This legislation will sunset in 2003.

INTERNATIONAL NURSING LICENSURE

Nursing education and nursing licensure differ greatly throughout the world. In Australia, nursing education has been moved into university settings, and future applicants for licensure in that country will be required to have a university education. In Italy, nursing education is now consolidated under broad, multisite programs administered by university nursing departments. The nations of Eastern Europe face many drastic changes in their health care systems as they change internally and form different relationships with the West. Nursing education was restricted during Soviet domination and many nurses had limited nursing educational opportunities, with basic nursing education sometimes occurring at the high school level. These nurses are now seeking ways to broaden nursing education in their own countries and to interface with the international nursing community.

Because of these great differences, nursing credentials are not easily transferred internationally. The International Congress of Nurses (ICN) has supported the development of effective licensure legislation worldwide. In 1988, the ICN launched a project called "Nursing Regulation: Moving Ahead," which was funded by the W. K. Kellogg Foundation. This ongoing project involved nurses and officials from 77 countries in seminars and studies. To date, nursing licensure laws in the United States have not been affected by this study, but it has supported the development of more restrictive licensure laws in some parts of the world.

Individuals who are interested in international nursing need to consider their language proficiency and educational backgrounds. Not all countries welcome nurses educated elsewhere. They may have a surplus of nurses and wish to avoid displacing local nurses. Others are concerned that nurses educated in affluent societies such as the United States and Canada may understand little about the health care needs and nursing practices in a developing country. Organizations actively working in the international health field usually will provide information on opportunities and licensure requirements in various countries. The ICN in Geneva can provide addresses of appropriate governmental authorities to contact regarding licensure in certain countries.

CERTIFICATION IN NURSING

Certification in nursing is primarily a professional, and not a legal, credential. The definition of certification adopted by the Interdivisional Council on Certification of the ANA (1978) states: "Certification is the documented validation of specific qualifications demonstrated by the individual registered nurse in the provision of professional nursing care in a defined area of practice." Certification is available from many professional nursing and health care organizations (Fig. 7-5).

ANCC Certification

In 1988, the ANA established a credentialing center called the American Nurses' Credentialing Center (ANCC), which assumed all of the ANA credentialing activities. The ANA invited all other organizations providing credentialing for nurses to join; some joined, but many retained their individual programs.

FIGURE 7–5 Certification acknowledges an expert level of nursing practice.

ANCC certification is a method of recognizing nurses who have special expertise. Applicants must demonstrate current practice and knowledge beyond that required for licensure as a registered nurse. Effective in 1998, as approved by the House of Delegates in 1991, individuals seeking certification as generalists in all specialties are required to have a baccalaureate in nursing; those seeking certification as specialists or advanced practice nurses need a master's degree in nursing. After submitting evidence of completing all requirements, a nurse may take the national examination for a specific certification. Certification is granted for a period of 5 years, after which a nurse may renew the certification by submitting new evidence of current practice and ability. Display 7-3 lists the various certification credentials available from the ANCC.

In addition to certifying specialty practice, the ANCC provides an accreditation mechanism for institutions or organizations desiring to be an "approver" or a "provider" of nursing continuing education programs. State nurses associations and specialty organizations often seek accreditation as approvers of programs. Accreditation as a provider assures the nurse consumer that the continuing education offering meets appropriate standards (Consultation services, 1999).

Display 7–3
NURSING CERTIFICATION AVAILABLE THROUGH THE AMERICAN NURSES' CREDENTIALING CENTER

Generalists (bachelor's degree required)*
Cardiac Rehabilitation
CE/Staff Development
College Health
Community Health
General Nursing
Gerontological
Home Health
Medical-Surgical
Pediatric
Perinatal
Psychiatric and Mental Health
School Nurse

Nurse Practitioners (master's degree required)
Acute Care
Family
Pediatric
Adult
Gerontological
School

Clinical Specialists (master's degree required)
Community Health
Home Health
Gerontological
Medical-Surgical
Adult Psychiatric and Mental Health
Child/Adolescent Psychiatric and Mental Health

Nursing Administrators
Nursing Administration
Nursing Administration, Advanced (master's degree required)

Modular (specialty certification or additional test required)
Nursing Case Management
Ambulatory Care

*A new plan that includes "board certified" for BSN preparation and "certified" for diploma and associate degree education was announced in 2000.

American Board of Nursing Specialties

In 1991, eight national nursing certification programs joined to establish the American Board of Nursing Specialties. These organizations were the American Nurses' Credentialing Center of the ANA, the American Board for Occupational Health Nursing, the American Board of Neuroscience Nursing, the Association of Rehabilitation Nurses, the Council on Certification of Nurse Anesthetists, the National Board of Nutritional Support Certification, the Nephrology Nursing Certification Board, and the Orthopaedic Nurses Certification Board. According to their report, in 1991 these eight organizations represented more than 65% of the total number of registered nurses certified in specialty practice (Specialty Certification, 1991). The goals of this board are to ensure quality in specialty nursing, to improve the public's perception of specialty nurses, and to provide specialty nurses who bring a consistent standard of education and experience to their practice. This is a major breakthrough in the entire certification process for nursing. This Board has established a peer review process for certification organizations that provides evaluation and recognition of the certification granted (Display 7-4).

Other Certification Programs

Other specialty organizations in nursing also have certification programs (Table 7-3). Most are administered by a separately titled and funded certification organization that

Display 7–4
NURSING CERTIFICATION AVAILABLE THROUGH THE SPECIALTY NURSING ORGANIZATIONS*

Addictions Nursing	Neonatal Nurse Practitioner
Childbirth Educator	Nephrology Nursing
Critical Care Nursing	Neuroscience Nursing
Diabetes Educator	Nurse Anesthetist
Emergency Nursing	Nurse Midwife
Gastroenterology	Occupational Health Nursing
Healthcare Quality	Oncology Nursing
Holistic Nursing	Ophthalmic Nursing
Hospice Nurse	Orthopedic Nursing
Inpatient Obstetric Nurse	Pain Management
Intravenous Nursing	Plastic and Reconstructive Surgical
Lactation Consultant	Nursing
Legal Nurse Consultant	School Nurse
Low Risk Neonatal Nurse	Urology Nursing
Maternal Newborn Nurse	Women's Health Nursing
Neonatal Intensive Care Nurse	

*Educational requirements vary.

TABLE 7–3. Certification Available Through Specialty Organizations*

Certification	Organization
Addictions Nursing (CARN)	CARN Certification, National League for Nursing
Critical Care Nursing (CCRN)	American Association of Critical Care Nurses Certification Corporation
Diabetes Educator (CDE)	National Certification Board for Diabetes Educators
Emergency Nursing (CEN)	Board of Certification for Emergency Nursing
Flight Nursing (CFRN)	
Enterostomal Therapy (CETN)	Enterostomal Therapy Nursing Certification Board
Gastroenterology (CGC)	Certifying Board of Gastroenterology Nurses and Associates
Hemodialysis Nurse (CHN)	Board of Nephrology Examiners Nursing and Technology
Peritoneal Dialysis Nurse (CPDN)	
Infection Control (CIC)	Certification Board of Infection Control
Intravenous Nursing (CRNI)	Intravenous Nurses Certification Corporation
Lactation Consultant (IBCLC)	International Board of Lactation Consultants Examiners
Maternal/Child Specialties	National Certification Corporation for the Obstetric, Gynecologic, and Neonatal Nursing Specialties
Ambulatory Women's Health Care Nurses (RN,C)	
High-Risk Obstetric Nurse (RN,C)	
Inpatient Obstetric Nurse (RN,C)	
Low-Risk Neonatal Nurse (RN,C)	
Maternal Newborn Nurse (RN,C)	
Neonatal Intensive Care Nurse (RN,C)	
OB/GYN Nurse Practitioner (RN,C)	
Reproductive Endocrinology/Infertility Nurse (RN,C)	
Neuroscience Nurse (CNRN)	American Board of Neuroscience Nursing Professional Examination Service
Nurse Administrator—Long-Term Care (RN,C)	Center for Credentialing Services NADONA/LTC Professional Exam Review System
Nurse Anesthetist (CRNA)	Council on Certification of Nurse Anesthetists
Nurse Midwife (CNM)	Association of Certified Nurse Midwives Certification Council
Nutrition Support Nurse (CNSN)	National Board of Nutrition Support Certification
Occupational Health Nursing (COHN)	American Board for Occupational Health Nurses
Oncology Nursing (OCN)	Oncology Nursing Certification Corporation
Ophthalmic Nursing (CRNO)	National Certifying Board for Ophthalmic Registered Nurses
Orthopedic Nursing (ONC)	Orthopaedic Nurse Certification Board
Pain Management (CNOR)	American Academy of Pain Management
Pediatric Specialties	National Certification Board of Pediatric Nurse Practitioners & Nurses
General Pediatric Nurse (CPN)	
Pediatric Nurse Practitioner (CPNP)	
Perioperative Nurse (CNOR)	National Certification Board of Perioperative Nursing
Plastic and Reconstructive Surgical Nurse (CPSN)	Plastic Surgical Nursing Certification Board
Post-Anesthesia Nurse (CPAN)	American Board of Post-Anesthesia Nursing Certification Professional Examination Service
Rehabilitation Nurse (CRRN)	Rehabilitation Nursing Certification Board
School Nurse (CSN)	National Board for Certification of School Nurses
Urology Nurse (CURN)	American Board of Urologic Allied Health Professionals

*See Appendix B for addresses of organizations.

is closely related to the specialty organization. This administrative structure is set up to protect the sponsoring organization from economic liability, to preserve tax-exempt status, and to provide a more objective approach to the credentialing process. Information on any of these specialty certification programs can be obtained by writing directly to the organization (see Appendix B). Some of these organizations require a BSN for certification, but others certify based on the RN license, role-specific education and practice, and an examination. The Oncology Nurses Society adopted the BSN as a requirement, but in December 1999 announced the requirements were changing to admit any registered nurse meeting other requirements. Their rationale for the change was that they were unable to demonstrate any practice differences between those prepared with various basic nursing credentials once they had the required specialty education and practice. This illustrates the constant changes that are occurring in the field of nursing.

The National Association of Pediatric Nurse Associates/Practitioners (NAPNAP) supports an independent certification for the pediatric nurse practitioner. This has resulted in certificates being awarded in the same area by two organizations. NAPNAP and the ANCC have had joint conferences regarding certification, with the hope of developing one jointly sponsored certification; however, fundamental differences still exist between the two organizations on how authority for determining standards should be established.

The Association for Women's Health, Obstetric, and Neonatal Nursing (AWHONN), formerly called the Nurses' Association of the American College of Obstetricians and Gynecologists (NAACOG), sponsors certification for nurses working in women's health care, obstetrics, and neonatal nursing.

The American Association of Critical Care Nurses (AACCN) sponsors certification of nurses in the critical care arena. Their certification confers the title Critical Care Registered Nurse (CCRN). Although this certification is not required to work in critical care, it attests to ongoing practice in critical care, along with continuing education directly related to the critical care field and a passing score on a critical care examination.

The American College of Nurse Midwives sponsors a certification program for nurses specializing in nurse midwifery. Nurses graduating from approved midwifery programs apply for certification through this organization. Approved programs may be at a basic level or at a master's degree level.

Some organizations of health care workers offer credentialing to individuals in specific occupations that may include nurses. For example, the Society of Gastroenterostomal Assistants offers certification to individuals employed in gastroenterology laboratories. This certification is available to both registered nurses and licensed practical nurses. The Association for Practitioners in Infection Control certifies individuals who are professionals in infection control, including physicians, public health officers, and nurses.

Critical Thinking Activity

A registered nurse with 5 years of general medical-surgical acute care experience is interested in working in the critical care unit of a hospital in your community. Seek information regarding how this nurse could obtain a critical care position in your community. Compare that process with what would be required of you as a new graduate to move into such a position.

Certification for Licensed Practical Nurses

Certification for LPNs (LVNs) is available for those practicing in long-term care. The National Association of Practical Nurse Education and Service (NAPNES) determined that many LPNs have responsible positions in long-term care and that recognition of their abilities through certification would be appropriate. They contracted with the National Council of State Boards of Nursing to develop and administer a certification examination. Those taking this examination use the title CLTC (Certified in Long-Term Care). This is the only nursing certification available to LPNs. LPNs may be eligible for certification programs that are not specifically nursing.

THE FUTURE OF CREDENTIALING IN HEALTH CARE

Because credentialing in nursing involves so many different aspects of education, licensure, and certification, it has confused the public, nurses, and other health care professionals. The ideal credential clearly communicates qualifications and competence; therefore, it is important for nursing to have a credentialing system that can be understood by others. Current changes are moving nursing closer to an effective credentialing system.

Institutional Control of Credentials

Many new health care occupations related to new procedures and processes in medical care are being developed as new technology develops. Those who believe the state should take positive action to protect the public continue to exert pressure to license additional health care providers. Those who oppose credentialing of additional individual groups of health care workers believe that modern-day employers are able to assess workers and to differentiate among them on the basis of competence. Some who oppose credentialing of individual health occupations believe that licensing the institution that hires the employees would be an adequate safeguard for the public.

Another approach to credentialing in health care is certifying specific competencies rather than an entire field of practice. Those advocating this approach believe that it would facilitate the development of individuals with a broad range of competencies suited to a particular setting. For example, in a rural area one individual might be certified as competent to perform certain basic x-ray examinations (such as for simple fractures), basic laboratory studies (such as complete blood count and urinalysis), and some basic client care procedures (such as bathing, toileting, feeding, and positioning). Because more complex procedures are sent to a larger center and there is no need for a full-time person in any of these positions, basic care would be made available in a convenient and low-cost manner. Certification of specific competencies by the employing agency is sometimes referred to as *site-based examination* and *site-based certification*. One concern about this method of certifying competencies is the focus on technical skills, without adequate recognition of the knowledge base needed for decision making and judgment. Other concerns are the complexity of keeping track of the many specific competencies, and the difficulty with job mobility when competencies are not standardized.

Pew Report

A comprehensive reform of all health care workforce regulation was proposed by the Center for the Health Professions (Finocchio et al., 1995). Based on a study supported by the Pew Charitable Trust, the report titled "Reforming Health Care Workforce Regulation" (commonly referred to as one of the "Pew Reports on Health Care Workforce Regulation"), made ten recommendations for changes in regulations. These are found in Display 7-5. These recommendations are based on what is termed a SAFE focus: *S*tandardized where appropriate, *A*ccountable to the public, *F*lexible to support optimal access, and *E*ffective and *E*fficient in protecting and promoting the public's health, safety, and welfare. Many of the recommendations, such as educating the public about health professional regulation and collecting data on the health professions, are supported by almost everyone. Others, such as developing, implementing, and evaluating continuing competency requirements, raise many questions in the minds of both health professionals and regulatory boards.

The National Council of State Boards of Nursing provided leadership in a national meeting in December of 1995 to discuss the Center for Health Professions' recommendations and their implications for nursing regulation. The response of those in

Display 7–5
RECOMMENDATIONS FOR REFORMING HEALTH CARE WORKFORCE REGULATION

1. Standardize regulatory terms
2. Standardize entry-to-practice requirements
3. Remove barriers to the full use of competent health professionals
4. Redesign health professional board structures and functions
5. Educate the public
6. Collect data on the health professions
7. Develop, implement, and evaluate continuing competency requirements
8. Reform the professional disciplinary process
9. Develop tools to evaluate regulatory effectiveness
10. Understand the organizational context of health professions regulation; develop partnerships to streamline regulatory structures and processes

The Center for the Health Professions. "What's the fuss?" Front & Center, San Francisco: University of California, Summer, 1996.

attendance was that nursing has supported the broad goals of the recommendations and has achieved goals in many areas. However, there was concern that the stated goals are unfocused and go beyond what can be accomplished through regulation alone. Although some of the policy suggestions in the report are controversial, there appeared to be a willingness to engage in constructive dialogue and encourage the participation of legislators, consumers, and health professionals in decision making. In August 1996 the NCSBN published a detailed response to the Pew Report as a special section in its Issues Newsletter. For each recommendation, a discussion and specific policy option were provided (Lund et al., 1996).

Continued Competency

Once an individual receives a license to practice as a health professional, a serious event (or series of serious events) must occur for that license to be removed. Even in states that require continuing education, the question has been asked "How can anyone be sure that an individual who was judged competent through an examination at one time is still competent years later?" The National Council of State Boards of Nursing has defined competence as "the application of knowledge and the interpersonal, decision-making, and psychomotor skills expected for the nurse's practice role, within the context of public health, welfare, and safety." The NCSBN has further indicated that the nurse should be expected to perform as necessary for the particular situation or restrict practice if the RN cannot safely perform (Green & Ogden, 1999).

In 1996 the Center for the Health Professions provided grants for the State Initiatives Program to Reform the Healthcare Workplace. Some states established specific programs to examine competency issues. Focusing on the concern regarding continued competency, state boards of nursing, nurses associations, and others have worked together. The states of Kentucky, Oklahoma, Texas, and Nebraska are addressing the issue of continued competence (Green & Ogden, 1999; Burback & Exstrom, 1999).

One concern that has emerged is the difference between identifying beginning competence as a generalist in all areas of nursing, and the expectation of higher level competence in a special sphere of nursing that is needed by the experienced nurse. There are clear differences in roles of nurses between urban and rural settings, between acute care and long-term care, between ambulatory care and inpatient care. The role of the employer in assessing the nurse's competency is another area of discussion. The Joint Commission on the Accreditation of Healthcare Organizations requires that accredited organizations have a program in place to evaluate competency of all employees.

The expectation for personal self-assessment and growth also must have a place in the search for continued competence. What responsibility should nurses take in identifying their own learning needs, seeking appropriate professional development opportunities, and monitoring their own learning from those opportunities? Should nurses be required to establish professional goals? To keep portfolios documenting self-assessment and professional development? To take advanced examinations? Chapter 9 offers suggestions for a personal self-evaluation plan. Whatever the rules and regulations, nurses do have a professional, ethical obligation to maintain their own competence.

KEY CONCEPTS

- Credentials are written proof of qualifications and may include diplomas conferred by educational programs, certification or registration by professional groups, and legal licenses conferred by governmental agencies.
- Permissive licensure allows for those meeting certain standards to be licensed, whereas mandatory licensure requires that all individuals who wish to practice in the field be licensed to practice.
- Nursing leaders began efforts to obtain legal licensure in 1896. The first permissive licensure law was passed in 1903 by North Carolina, and the first mandatory licensure law was passed in New York in 1947.
- Legal rules governing nursing practice are found in the licensure law passed by a legislative body. Further provisions governing nursing are found in the rules and regulations established by the administrative agency in which the legislation vests authority.
- The nursing practice act usually contains a definition of nursing, and addresses qualifications for licensure applicants, use of titles, renewal and continuing education requirements, grandfathering, financial concerns, nursing education programs, disciplinary action, violations and penalties, administrative provisions, and expanded nursing roles.
- The Board of Nursing (or its equivalent) is the administrative agency with the authority to carry out the provisions of the Nurse Practice Act.
- A license to practice nursing must be obtained from the state or province in which you wish to work. An initial license is termed licensure by examination, and subsequent licenses may be obtained in other jurisdictions through licensure by endorsement.
- Advanced practice nurses are regulated by each state. Most require professional certification in an advanced practice nursing specialty to be licensed in that role.
- Multistate licensure involves a compact between certain states that allows nurses who are licensed in those states to work freely among all the compact states without the need for obtaining additional licenses.
- The NCLEX-RN examination is administered through a computerized plan that covers the five steps of the nursing process and four areas of client needs, and that identifies competence for entry-level safe nursing care.
- Graduates of foreign nursing schools must have their credentials reviewed and may be required to take the CGFNS examination, which reviews both nursing content and English language ability, before being admitted to take the NCLEX examination.
- A license may be revoked by the State Board of Nursing, a designated disciplinary board, or a court of law based on specific reasons stated in the Nurse Practice Act.
- Certification provides evidence of specialized clinical knowledge and ability beyond the basic level. Certification as a nurse practitioner may be used as a basis for legal approval to practice in an expanded role.
- Concerns about the future of health care worker credentialing include issues of public accountability and continued competence.

REFERENCES

American Nurses Association. Nursing's Agenda for Healthcare Reform. Washington, DC: American Nurses Publishing Co., 1991

American Nurses Association Congress for Nursing Practice. Suggested State Legislation: Nursing Practice Act, Disciplinary Diversion Act, Prescriptive Authority Act. Kansas City, MO: American Nurses Association, 1990

American Nurses Association. Nursing: A Social Policy Statement. Kansas City, MO: American Nurses Association, 1980

American Nurses Association. The Study of Credentialing in Nursing: A New Approach, vol 1. The Report of the Committee. Kansas City, MO: American Nurses Association, 1978

Bersky A, Brady D. A new generation of competence assessment in nursing: Computerized clinical simulation testing (CST). Issues 14(1):1–8, 1993

Bersky AK, Yocom CJ. Computerized clinical simulation testing: Its use for competence assessment in nursing. Nurs Health Care 15(3):120–127, 1994

Boards will weigh plan to test NPs. Am J Nurs 96(6):69, 73, 1996

Boards call for work to continue on a multistate license for nurses. Am J Nurs 96(10):78, 18, 1996

Burback V, Exstrom S. Continued Competency in Nebraska: Process and Progress. Issues 20(2): 1, 5–11, 1999

Consultation services now available for ANCC magnet and accreditation programs. American Nurse 31(5):11, 1999

Finocchio LJ, Dower CM, McMahon T, Gragnola CM, and the Taskforce of Health Care Workforce Regulation. Reforming Health Care Workforce Regulation: Policy Considerations for the 21st Century. San Francisco: Pew Health Professions Commission, 1995

Foreign RNs' fate unclear as visa program ends. Am J Nurs 95(10):77, 80–81, 1995

Green A, Crismon C, Waddill L, Fitzpatrick O. Are you at risk for disciplinary action? Am J Nurs 95(7):36–42, 1995

Green A, Ogden BS. Three state nursing boards examine continued competency. Available at: *www.nursingworld.org/tan/99marapr/competen.htm*. Accessed June 26, 2000.

Lund E, Bouchard J, Graves C, Osman C, VanWingerden C, Bosma J, Creal D, Hutcherson C, Sheets V. National Council of State Boards of Nursing's Response to the Pew Taskforce on Health Care Workforce Regulation. Issues 17(3):Special Section 1–6, 1996

Majek M. Licensure verification process under construction by Boards of Nursing. Issues 17(3):5, 1996

National Council of State Boards of Nursing. Model Nursing Practice Act (revision) Chicago: National Council of State Boards of Nursing, 1994c

National Council of State Boards of Nursing. Model Nursing Administrative Rules. Chicago: National Council of State Boards of Nursing, 1994d

National Council of State Boards of Nursing. National Council begins revising models for nursing regulation. Issues 17(3):3, 1996

National Council of State Boards of Nursing. New Test Plan for PN Approved. Issues 19(3), 1998

National Council of State Boards of Nursing. New Test Plan for RN Approved. Issues 18(4), 1997

National Council of State Boards of Nursing, Nurse Licensure Compact: Final Version, November 6, 1998. Available at: *www.ncsbn.org*. Accessed January 4, 2000.

National Council of State Boards of Nursing. Test Plan for the National Council Licensure Examination for Registered Nurses. Chicago: National Council of State Boards of Nursing, 1992b

New Legislation. The Nursing Commission Newsletter 2(1):2. Olympia, WA: Washington State Department of Health, 1996

Overview of the computerized clinical simulation test (CST) project. Issues 17(1):7–9, 1996

Parkman CA. Health care workforce regulation reform. Nursing Management, 28(9):34–37, 1997

Schaefer B. International credentials review: Crucial and complex. Nurs Health Care 11(8):431–432, 1990

Simpson RL. State regulation in a world of "boundary-less" technology. Nursing Management 28(2):22, 1997

Simpson, RL. Tech talk on multistate licensure. Nursing Management 30(1):12–13, 1999

Snyder ME, LaBar C. Issues in Professional Practice, vol 1. Nursing: Legal Authority for Practice. Washington, DC: American Nurses Publishing Co., 1984

Specialty certification groups form organization. Am Nurse 23(4):20, 1991

Ventura MJ. The great multistate licensure debate. RN 62(5):58-63, 1999

FURTHER READING

American Association of Colleges of Nursing. Position statement: Certification and regulation of advanced practice nurses. Washington, DC: AACN, 1994

Bruce D: State Rights, Nursing Futures and Regulation Conference: Summary Report, Online Journal of Issues in Nursing. Appendix A: Summary of presentations. Available at: *www.nursingworld.org/ojin/tpc3/tpc3_3.htm, November 6, 1997.* Accessed January 14, 2000.

Cronenwett LR. Molding the future of advanced practice nursing. Nurs Outlook 43(3):112–118, 1995

Donaho B: Health Care Systems, Nursing Futures and Regulation Conference: Summary Report, Online Journal of Issues in Nursing. Appendix A: Summary of presentations. Available at: *www.nursingworld.org/ojin/tpc3/tpc3_3.htm. November 6, 1997.* Accessed January 14, 2000.

Fiesta J. Why nurses lose their licenses, Part I. Nurs Management 24(10):12, 14, 1993

Fiesta J. Why nurses lose their licenses, Part II. Nurs Management 24(11):14–15, 1993

Fiesta J. Why nurses lose their licenses, Part III. Nurs Management 24(12):16, 1993

Henry PF. Your due process rights in a disciplinary action. Nurse Pract Forum 2(4):210–211, 1991

Hutchenson C: Crossing Borders, Nursing Futures and Regulation Conference: Summary Report, Online Journal of Issues in Nursing. Appendix A: Summary of presentations. Available at: *www.nursing world.org/ojin/tpc3_3.htm. November 6, 1997.* Accessed January 14, 2000.

Parker J. Development of the American Board of Nursing Specialties. Nurs Management 25(1):33–35, 1994

Spencer-Cisek P, Sveningson L. Regulation of advanced nursing practice: Part two—certification. Oncology Nursing Forum 22(8):39–42, 1995

State Legislative Trends and Analysis: Special Report to the 1998 House of Delegates. Available at: *www.nursingworld.org/gova/hod98/, June 1999.* Accessed June 26, 2000.

Stuckey, CD, Nursing practice across fiber optics. Nurs Management 29(7):24–25, 1998

Relevant web sites

Certification information
Lippincott/AJN Web site *www.nursingcenter.com/career/certification.cfm*
American Nurses Association *www.nursingworld.org*
Licensure information
National Council of State Boards of Nursing *www.ncsbn.org*
Lippincott/AJN Web site *www.nursingcenter.com/career/licensure.cfm*
Commission on Graduates of Foreign Nursing Schools *www.cgfns.org*

8

Legal Responsibilities for Practice

As the legal profession becomes increasingly aware of the education and experience of the professional nurse, as well as the unique role a nurse plays in the health care delivery system, it is anticipated that nurses will become more legally accountable for their actions.

(Fiesta, 1988)

OBJECTIVES

After completing this chapter, you should be able to:

1. Identify two general sources of law and describe their differences.

2. Explain the role of institutional policies and protocols in legal decision making.

3. Describe some situations in which nurses may be involved in criminal law.

4. Define liability, identifying situations in which liability is shared by employers or supervisors.

5. State points to be considered in the purchase of professional liability insurance.

6. Explain the most commonly recurring legal issues in nursing.

7. Explain how informed consent, advance directives, and the Patient Self-Determination Act support the patient's rights.

8. Discuss the nurse's responsibility in the specific issues that can constitute malpractice.

9. Identify factors that contribute to a suit being instituted against a health care professional, and explain how an individual nurse might prevent legal suits.

10. Explain the various aspects of a legal action.

11. Outline the role of the nurse when testifying for a legal proceeding.

KEY TERMS

Administrative law	Durable power of attorney	Negligence
Advance directive	Durable power of attorney for health care	Patient Self-Determination Act
Assault	Expert witness	Plaintiff
Battery	False imprisonment	Privileged communication
Case law	Felony	Prudent person
Claims-brought insurance	Fraud	Prudent professional
Claims-occurred insurance	Guardian	Regulatory law
Common law	Informed consent	Res ipsa loquitor
Constitutional law	Judicial law	Standards of practice
Court	Liability	Statutory law
Criminal law	Liability insurance	Suit
Decisional law	Malpractice	Testimony
Defendant	Minor	Tort
Deposition	Misdemeanor	Voluntary consent
Discovery		Witness to fact

Every newspaper contains reports of sensational cases being decided in our courts. Concerns about lawsuits and liability are voiced in every business. Health care remains at the forefront of professions where legal issues constitute a major area of concern. Nurses express concern about their responsibilities and whether they might be vulnerable to lawsuits. A wise nurse considers legal issues before a crisis arises and uses sound information to help guide action in situations where questions arise.

Legal issues are those that are decided by law. *Law* includes those rules of conduct or action recognized as binding, or enforced by a controlling authority such as the local, state, or national government. *Ethics* are the principles of conduct governing one's relationships with others—basic beliefs about right and wrong. Legal and ethical issues are often discussed together because they go hand in hand, with one supporting the other. Ethics also may address questions that are entirely different from those addressed by the law. Hall (1996, p. 49) states, "Law is the minimum ethic, written down and enforced; behavior that is not merely desired but mandated." In this chapter we focus on how the law affects nursing practice. Ethics are introduced here in Chapter 8 and are discussed in more detail in Chapter 9.

Examples and situations relating to legal issues discussed throughout this chapter are given to help you understand the application of the specific concepts. Many more factors would be considered in arriving at an actual legal decision than can be presented in a paragraph or two. It is the interaction of multiple factors that makes it impossible to provide absolute predictions regarding legal outcomes in specific situations. Specific factual data may contribute to contradictory decisions in cases that appear similar on the surface. Different judges and juries may also interpret facts and law in various ways, resulting in dissimilar outcomes for cases that appear to be alike.

If you have a question about a specific personal situation, you would be well advised to consult an attorney who is experienced in medicolegal matters. The facility where you are employed may have a legal counselor who is available to you. Another source of legal aid is your nurses' association attorney. If you desire private counsel, suitable names may be recommended by the nurses' association in your state or the local bar association. And, of course, you may always identify and seek the services of an attorney in your community who works in the area of law about which you are concerned.

SOURCES OF LAW

If nurses know the source of law, then they know how it can be challenged and changed, and how powerful it can be. There are two general sources of law: statutory law and common law (Fig. 8-1). Both are relevant to nursing practice.

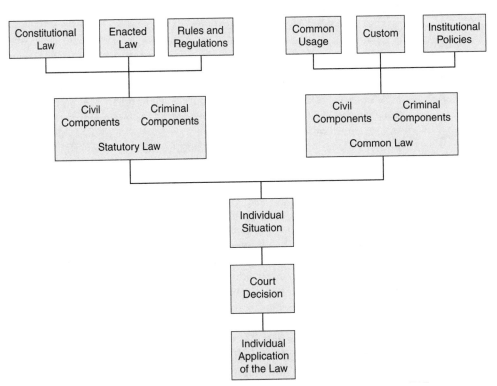

FIGURE 8–1   Civil law and criminal law both may affect a nursing situation.

Statutory Law

A *statute* is a rule or formal regulation, established by governmental authority, that appears in writing. A violation of a statute is legally punishable. Statutory law is published in codes. A key aspect of all statutory law is that it is written down as specific rules. In the United States, statutory law includes constitutional law, enacted law, and regulatory law. These laws are in a hierarchy of authority, with constitutional law having the greatest authority, enacted law the next, and regulatory law the last. The US Constitution always has precedence over any other law.

CONSTITUTIONAL LAW

The highest law of the United States is *constitutional law*. It is the law established by the federal government and based on the US Constitution. The Constitution was developed and passed by the Continental Congress and then ratified by all of the states. The Constitution establishes the general organization of the federal government, and specifies the federal power and limitations to that power. The powers not specifically given to the federal government in the Constitution are retained by the states. Amendments to the US Constitution require similar passage and ratification by the states. The first amendments were contained in the Bill of Rights, which was passed a few years after the Constitution was established. Each state has its own constitution that acts as the highest law for that individual state. Many other nations, such as Great Britain, do not have a constitution or equivalent document.

ENACTED LAW

Enacted law includes all bills passed by legislative bodies, whether at the local, state or province, or national level. Enacted laws of the US federal government all carry the designation "US" in their official title. Enacted laws of states or other governing bodies carry a similar designation. The federal Social Security Act is an example of federally enacted law. Nurse practice acts in the various states are examples of enacted law at the state level.

REGULATORY LAW

Regulatory law (also referred to as executive or administrative law) includes the rules and regulations established by governmental agencies to carry out enacted law. At the federal level, the Health Care Finance Administration (HCFA) writes regulations governing the payment of Medicaid and Medicare funds that were authorized through legislation. At the state level, the State Board of Nursing is authorized through enacted laws to establish rules and regulations that govern the practice of nursing in that particular state. The rules and regulations they establish identify the requirements of nursing program curricula, educational requirements for licensure, continuing education requirements, and so forth (See Chapter 7). They are established and enforced to protect the safety of the public. Rules and regulations of administrative bodies can be enforced in court.

Common Law

Common law derives from common usage, custom, and judicial law (judicial decisions or court rulings). It is based in the English common law. Common law is less clear and exact than statutory law because it is composed of many actions and documents that are not specific written rules that apply to everyone. Common law is fluid and changes over time. In general, statutory law carries more weight in court than does common law.

COMMON USAGE AND CUSTOM

As the term seems to imply, courts are empowered through the concept of common law to examine the common usage and custom in a community for patterns that reflect the community's standards for behavior. Common usage and custom are not usually written down and specific. However, written documents can be used to support common usage and custom in specific cases. For example, when examining standards of professional practice in a court case, the court may examine documents that specify standards of professional practice as reflecting common usage. These documents may be changed by the organization and thus are not fixed.

The issue of abandonment of a patient illustrates how common usage applies to nursing. No statutory laws dictate that a nurse cannot leave a seriously ill patient without ensuring that someone else will provide care, but common practice and custom (which could be supported through the testimony of nurses and other health care workers) require that nurses do not abandon their patients. Failure to meet this standard might be deemed a violation of common law.

JUDICIAL LAW

Judicial law (also referred to as decisional, or case law) is derived from decrees or judgments from the courts. Judicial decisions or rulings in court cases apply statutory and common law to specific situations. These decisions then become precedents for interpretations of both statutory and common law in other cases. Court rulings are binding within the jurisdiction of the particular court that determines them, but are used in a more general way (as guidelines) in other jurisdictions. In any specific situation, the final determination of the application of all types of law is the court decision in that case. While the decision may be appealed to higher courts, the final application of law is always the authority of a court of law.

OTHER FACTORS AFFECTING LEGAL DECISIONS

In addition to the sources of law discussed above, several other factors can affect how laws are interpreted and enforced. These factors also play an important role in our legal system.

Rulings

A *ruling* or *advisory opinion* made by a state board or by an attorney general is an attempt to provide a guideline based on an interpretation of the enacted and regulatory law relative to a specific situation, and is not a final legal decision. Different boards and attorneys general might vary in their opinions. The validity of an opinion only stands until the issue is brought before a court and the court rules on the situation. The final decision in any legal issue rests with a court.

Rights and Responsibilities in Health Care

Rights and responsibilities have both legal and ethical aspects. In the United States, basic rights are specified in the first fourteen amendments to the Constitution (see above); this section of the Constitution is called the Bill of Rights and is an example of one of the limitations placed on the federal government. These rights protect the individual from governmental interference in basic areas of life. From these primary rights, other rights are deduced. For example, although the right to privacy of medical records is not specifically discussed in the Bill of Rights, the right to be secure in one's own home against unreasonable search and seizure is guaranteed. This basic right has led to court decisions supporting the right to privacy regarding one's own affairs, including medical records.

In the United States, because the Constitution is supreme over any other source of law, no statutory or regulatory law may interfere with the rights enumerated in the Bill of Rights. In other countries, rights may be more limited, or may be part of the statutory law enacted by a legislative body. These laws may carry less weight than the US Constitution. Some countries have no counterpart to the rights found in the United States.

Some of the rights of which we speak are not legally supported, but are based on ethical beliefs. For example, we often speak of a "right to health care." There is no legal basis for this right in the United States, but many people believe there is an ethical basis for this right. In some countries, such as Canada and Great Britain, health care is a right supported by the law. In these countries, health care for all has been established through legislation and administrative rules and regulations.

During 1999 several different forms of a Health Care Consumer's Bill of Rights were submitted to the US Congress. The focus and provisions of each were slightly different, but the major thrust of all concerned privacy of records, access to information about health care options, and a guarantee of due process for appeals of health care coverage. The American Nurses Association (ANA) has strongly supported this effort. Concerns about the way managed care organizations were responding to individuals prompted these efforts. There is an expectation that a patient's bill of rights will be passed by both houses of the federal legislature in the year 2000.

Responsibilities often accompany rights. If a right is guaranteed, the government and designated others have legally mandated responsibilities to ensure that the right is upheld. In the matter of the right to privacy of medical records, for example, all health care workers have legally mandated responsibilities to ensure that privacy is upheld.

The individual who holds a right also may have responsibilities. These responsibilities are sometimes a matter of ethics, rather than mandated by law. An individual with a right to health care may have the responsibility to use that resource wisely and to cooperate effectively in achieving the desired health outcomes.

Institutional Policies and Protocols

Institutional policies provide guidance in the proper actions to be taken in specific situations, and identify the individuals responsible for taking action. Established agency policies may be considered the *standard of practice* for that agency and, therefore, common usage (common law) by the court, and may become important as a basis for legal decisions. Policies may protect the institution itself and the employees of an institution from legal difficulties if they are based on current practice and sound legal advice.

Members of the hospital staff who have expertise in the practice area under consideration usually develop the specific policy. An attorney also may be consulted to ensure that policies conform to legal requirements. Final approval of policies often rests with the board of trustees, directors, or commissioners, who have ultimate responsibility for the financial and legal management of the organization.

Institutional policies are changed in response to new situations and new expectations in society. Usually there is an established institutional route for the change or expansion of a hospital policy. Nurses may be in a position to recognize the need for such a change as they use a policy and compare it with the latest professional information.

A *protocol* or *procedure* provides specific guidelines on performing a task. The purpose of protocols and procedures is to ensure that there is consistent, sound practice in an institution. Just as policies must be updated, so should protocols and procedures (see Chapter 12).

CLASSIFICATION OF LAWS

Law is divided into civil and criminal components. Both statutory law and common law may be subdivided in this way.

Criminal Law

Criminal law addresses the general welfare of the public. A violation of criminal law is called a *crime* and is prosecuted by the government. On conviction, a crime may be punished by imprisonment, parole conditions, a loss of privilege (such as a license), a fine, or any combination of these. The punishment is intended to deter others from committing the crime and to punish the violator. Crimes may be classified as either *misdemeanors* or as *felonies*. A misdemeanor is a lesser infraction of the law and is punished by a fine or an imprisonment of less than a year. A felony represents a more serious violation of the law, and carries heavier fines and longer periods of imprisonment, perhaps even death.

Civil Law

Civil law regulates conduct between private individuals or businesses, and is enforced through the courts as damages or money compensation. A *tort* is a violation of a civil law in which another person is wronged. Private individuals or groups may bring a legal action (a lawsuit) to court for breach (or breaking) of civil law. The judgment of the court results in a plan to correct the wrong and may include a monetary payment to the wronged party. Nurses may find themselves involved with both civil and criminal laws, either separately or within the same situation.

CRIMINAL LAW AND NURSING

Because a violation of any law governing the practice of any licensed profession may be a crime, you must be aware of the extent of the Nurse Practice Act of the state in which you are practicing. Where the Nurse Practice Act requires that actions (such as administering drugs) be performed only under the direction of a physician, that explicit authorization must exist. Standing orders that refer to specific situations, as well as the usual orders written for an individual patient, may be adequate authorization. However, custom or usual practice will not substitute for the specific authorization required by law. A violation of a professional practice act may be prosecuted as a crime even if no actual harm occurred to the patient.

It is costly to the state to undertake criminal prosecution; therefore, even when they are discovered, some violations of criminal law are not prosecuted in court. Knowing this, some nurses make the error of believing that "minor" violations are acceptable. Even when not prosecuted in court, criminal action could result in the loss of a job and in the loss of a license to practice nursing.

S I T U A T I O N   **Violation of a Practice Act**

A registered nurse working nights in a nursing home has an elderly resident who wakes and states he has indigestion. The nurse assesses the resident carefully and determines that this, indeed, appears to be simple indigestion and heartburn. After checking the medication record, the nurse determines that there is no prn order for any type of antacid or other medication that might relieve the resident's distress. She notes that the physician is one who dislikes being called at night and that, further, this physician is considered a very approachable individual when she visits residents. The nurse decides to give a dose of an antacid and ask the day nurse to call the physician and request a telephone order for the medication.

The Nurse Practice Act does not give the nurse the authority to diagnose disease and prescribe medication, regardless of the situation. The Medical Practice Act and the Nurse Practice Act on Advanced Nursing Practice contain this authorization. This, then, is a violation of the law and is a crime, even though the resident was not harmed.

Violation of laws related to the care and distribution of controlled substances is also a crime.

SITUATION   **Violation of Narcotic Laws**

In making the routine check of the narcotic record before going off duty, the night nurse notes that the record does not match the actual count of morphine in the supply. She is tired and does not wish to spend the time searching the record and correcting the mistake. Instead, she makes a false entry for a patient who did not receive a narcotic so that the record appears correct.

Because the laws regulating controlled substances are rigid, this would be a violation of the law. In this situation, the presumably innocent action by one nurse actually may serve to obscure the fact that someone else is diverting narcotics for personal use. As a nurse, you need to look beyond temporary convenience to the potential consequences of your action.

Nurses also have been charged by states with committing crimes while in the role of caregiver. These legal actions may be based upon such charges as reckless endangerment or criminal negligence. Errors resulting in the serious injury or death of a patient are investigated and may be prosecuted and tried by the criminal courts. A license to practice nursing may be temporarily withdrawn while such charges are investigated and tried. If the individual is found innocent, the license then may be restored. If the individual is convicted of the crime, the nursing license may be revoked in addition to sentencing and other penalties.

In the state of Colorado, criminal charges were brought against three nurses for negligent actions that resulted in the death of an infant. Through a series of actions by the nurses, the infant was given a ten-fold overdose of intravenous penicillin. This case clearly shows that the state has the power to prosecute as a crime professional conduct that results in serious harm or death (Fiesta, 1999). Many nurses are distressed by the actions of the prosecutor in the Colorado case because the facts as currently known do not seem to indicate a criminal level of negligence (Curtin, 1997).

Nurses who commit felonies such as theft, abuse, or deliberate harm to a patient are always charged under both criminal laws and the laws regulating nursing practice. Nurses who commit felonies outside of the care setting can be prosecuted under criminal law and under the law regulating nursing practice if the felony reflects on their fitness to practice nursing. For example, an individual who was prosecuted for selling narcotics usually would have action taken under the nurse practice act as well.

CIVIL LAW AND NURSING

Civil law relates to legal disputes between private parties. Malpractice actions brought in health care situations involve civil law.

Torts

Torts are civil wrongs committed by one person against another (Bernzweig, 1996). The wrong may be physical harm, psychological harm, or harm to reputation, livelihood, or some other less tangible value. The action that causes a civil wrong may be either intentional or unintentional. An intentional tort is one in which the outcome was planned, although the person involved may not have believed that the intended outcome would be harmful to the other person.

SITUATION   **Intentional Tort**

An elderly, somewhat forgetful, but competent resident in a long-term care facility decides not to take an ordered antidepressant medication, although he clearly shows signs of depression. The nurse believes that the patient needs the medication. Therefore, she dissolves it in juice and does not tell the resident. She later informs the resident's son of her action, thinking it will be praised. She is surprised to find the son very angry, and he threatens legal action.

The nurse purposely made the resident take the medication, even though he had refused it. This was her planned intent. Even though she thought it was in the resident's best interests, the resident was wronged in losing his right to informed consent. A court would generally agree that loss of informed consent is a wrong. If legal action is taken, the nurse may be found to have committed an intentional tort (that is, a planned wrong to another person).

An unintentional tort is a wrong committed against another person or property that was not intended to happen. The most common cause of an unintentional tort is negligence.

Negligence

Negligence is a general term that refers to conduct that does not show due care (Guido, 1997). If harm is caused by negligence, it is termed an *unintentional tort*, and damages may be recovered. *Negligence* is a broad term that has many applications in society. All negligence has the following four essential characteristics (Fiesta, 1994):

1. Harm must have occurred to an individual.
2. The negligent person must have been in a situation where he or she had a duty toward the person harmed.
3. The person must be found to have failed to fulfill his or her duty. This is called "breach of duty." This might include either doing what should not have been done (commission of an inappropriate action) or failing to do what should have been done (omission of a necessary or appropriate action).
4. The harm must be shown to have been caused by the breach of duty.

SITUATION   **Negligence**

A homeowner fails to repair a broken step at the entrance to his home. He fails to warn a guest of the broken step, and the guest trips on the broken step in the dark and is injured.

Negligence could be charged: the injury is the harm; the homeowner had a duty toward the guest to safeguard that guest from foreseeable harm; a reasonably *prudent person* would have repaired the step or at least warned the guest; and the injury can be shown to be a direct result of the homeowner's failure to act prudently.

Malpractice

Malpractice is a term used for a specific type of negligence. It refers to the negligence of a specially trained or educated person in the performance of his or her job. Therefore, *malpractice* is the term used to describe negligence by nurses in the performance of their duties.

The definition of malpractice is almost the same as the definition of negligence, but looks at the professional standard of care as well as the professional status of the caregiver (Guido, 1997). The professional person must have had a *professional duty* toward the person injured. For example, the nurse was acting as a nurse for the person injured (in either a paid or volunteer capacity). Additionally, the harm that occurred to the injured person or to the property must be based on a failure to act as a reasonably *prudent professional* would have acted in the situation. This is a higher standard than is required of the general public (Bernzweig, 1996) (see Display 8-1).

Just as all parts of the situation are clear in some general negligence situations and not in others, the professional duty is similarly clear in some instances and not in others. The nurse who is assigned to care for a patient in a hospital clearly has a duty to that patient. In some situations, duties overlap and more than one nurse might have a duty toward the same patient; whether a supervisor, another nurse on the unit, or a nurse visitor has a professional duty to a patient might be in dispute. Again, the court would decide whether a duty was present.

 ### Critical Thinking Activity

> You have taken a new position as a home health nurse. One of your patients is an elderly woman with a long history of diabetes who has a leg ulcer. Your role is to assess the patient in relationship to her diabetic management and wound care, and teach as needed. While you are in the home, her husband tells you that he has been having pain in his knee and asks if you would examine it and tell him whether it is all right to use a heating pad on it, and whether he should take ibuprofen or some Tylenol. Do you have a duty to help him? Why or why not? What will your response be? What legal issues are involved in this situation? If you advise him and your advice turns out to be incorrect, what legal action could he take?

A breach of duty, as mentioned earlier, is a failure to act as a prudent professional, that is, according to the *standard of care* for the profession in a particular situation (Fiesta, 1994). Standards of nursing care are determined in variety of ways (Guido, 1997). State boards of nursing set some standards; accrediting agencies such as the Joint Commission and professional nursing organizations set others. Standards of care

Display 8–1

ESSENTIAL ELEMENTS OF MALPRACTICE

- Harm to an individual
- Duty of a professional toward an individual
- Breach of duty by the professional
- Breach of duty as the cause of harm

also appear in policies, protocols, and procedures of the institution. Current nursing references, educational material, and articles may contribute to an understanding of an appropriate and current standard of care. Still other standards of care are determined by seeking the input of an expert professional. To determine that a breach of duty was present in a particular case, a court will officially determine what constitutes a professional standard of care for that situation. This is the application of both statutory law and common law, as previously discussed.

The final question becomes one of identifying the cause of the harm that occurred. Malpractice is present only if a breach of duty was the cause of the harm. The presence of harm is often clear. For example, if a person fractured a hip, no one would dispute that this was harm. However, the cause of a fractured hip might be the person's own responsibility, not the responsibility of someone else. When the harm is so clear, and the responsibility for the harm so straightforward, that anyone would agree on it, the expression *res ipsa loquitur* is used. This is Latin for "the thing speaks for itself." In this case the harm and responsibility do not need to be "proved" to the court, because all would agree that harm occurred.

SITUATION   *Res Ipsa Loquitor*

An individual was undergoing surgery. During the surgery, an emergency occurred that demanded a great deal of attention by all of the care providers. During this emergency situation, the failure to complete a count of the sponges used in the open abdomen was overlooked. The wound was closed and the patient was transferred to post-anesthesia recovery, and from there to a unit. The wound did not begin to heal but rather showed signs of infection. When this was not corrected with treatment, an x-ray of the abdomen was performed and the radiopaque thread in the sponge revealed its position. The patient was returned to surgery and the sponge was removed. If this case were taken to court, the court might well determine that the doctrine of *res ipsa loquitor* applied. There was a sponge in the abdomen; it was the cause of infection; the sponge could not have gotten in the abdomen except during surgery; and the surgical team was responsible in the operating room for all that occurred to the patient while there. The thing quite literally would speak for itself.

Remember that, as discussed earlier in the chapter, a breach of duty may be either the omission of a correct action or the commission of an incorrect action (Fig. 8-2). The following two situations illustrate this.

FIGURE 8–2   A reasonably prudent nurse uses common sense as well as nursing theory.

SITUATION   **Omission of Correct Action**

An elderly, disoriented person is admitted to an acute care facility. The nurse fails to establish a plan for monitoring and maintaining safety for this person. The patient falls out of bed during the night, sustaining a fractured hip.

This could be found to be malpractice. The nurse was working in a professional capacity and had a duty to this patient. The patient can be shown to have sustained an injury. Through testimony by nurses and reference to standard nursing texts, it can be demonstrated that a reasonably prudent registered nurse would have been expected to take action to protect this patient from falls. It was the nurse's failure to act that caused the fall and fracture. This failure to act could constitute malpractice.

SITUATION   **Commission of Inappropriate Action**

A postoperative patient has an order to ambulate. The nurse assigned to this patient finds that the patient's condition has changed drastically since the order was written. The patient has fever and a rapid pulse and is complaining of severe abdominal pain. The nurse proceeds to have the patient ambulate. The patient faints, sustaining a head injury in the fall. This necessitates additional hospitalization, x-ray films, and diagnostic procedures.

Again, this could be found to be malpractice. The nurse was working as a professional with a duty to this patient. The patient can be shown to have sustained an injury. It may be demonstrated that a reasonably prudent nurse would have recognized that the change in the patient's condition called for altering the plan of care and not ambulating at this time. This was the breach of duty. Ambulating the patient in that condition was the cause of the fall and the head injury. Therefore, malpractice could be found, owing to inappropriate action on the part of the nurse.

LIABILITY

A *liability* is an obligation or debt that can be enforced by law. In the case of malpractice, a person found guilty of any tort (whether intentional or unintentional) is considered legally *liable*, or legally responsible, for the outcome. The person legally liable usually is required to pay for damages to the other person. These may include actual costs of care, legal services, loss of earnings (present and future), and compensation for emotional and physical stress suffered. Although liability is legally determined by a court, an individual who believes that he or she would be held legally liable if a court were consulted, may agree to pay damages (or that individual's insurance company may agree to pay) without actually going to court. This may be done even when the person denies true negligence or malpractice, but chooses to settle the issue because a court case would be more costly than the damages to be paid.

LIABILITY INSURANCE

Liability insurance transfers from the individual to a large group the legal costs and any settlement related to a suit. The expectation is that most individuals will not be sued, and that the pool of premiums therefore will adequately cover the costs of those who are sued, the administrative costs of managing the policies, and the profit for the insurance company. Individuals benefit by transferring risk from themselves to the insurance company for the cost of the insurance policy.

A liability insurance crisis exists in the United States. The cost of liability insurance for primary health care providers (such as physicians and nurse practitioners) has escalated at an extraordinary rate. Some of the factors that have caused this to happen are the large judgments that have been made, the number of suits that have been brought, the large fees that attorneys receive, and the high profits of insurance companies. Nurses in independent advanced practice have been especially affected by the increase in premiums, because their incomes have traditionally been moderate and they cannot charge fees sufficient to cover insurance costs that may equal those of physicians. Nurses who are employed in more traditional roles are able to obtain malpractice insurance for a modest cost.

The American Nurses Association (ANA) has initiated a data bank related to legal claims against nurses. The organization is asking all registered nurses to provide information to it regarding legal action in which they have been named as a defendant. The ANA's purpose is to have adequate records to support its contention that the low level of suits against nurses in all areas of practice should translate into low-cost liability insurance.

Some states have initiated legislation that allows for awards to cover actual losses and costs of care, while limiting awards for pain and suffering and other nontangible factors. Sometimes this legislation has been accompanied by restrictions on insurance company rates. Some laws are also being amended to restrict the monetary liability of any party according to the percentage of responsibility. For example, if damages were set at $10,000 and each of two defendants were determined to be responsible for 50% of the problem, one party could not be made to pay more than $5,000, even if the other party had no assets and could not pay. Liability laws continue to be a major concern for nurses because nurses are being named in an increasing number of suits.

Institutional and Individual Insurance

Many hospitals and other institutional employers carry liability insurance that covers both the institution and its employees. Some hospitals may limit the coverage that their policies provide for individual employees in an effort to hold down costs. Kihm (1999) pointed out that when health care institutions merge, are bought out, or go bankrupt, liability insurance coverages may be called into question. Some institutions have chosen to self insure part of their liability requirements. If such an institution goes bankrupt, there are no funds left to pay liability claims and pending claims may revert to individuals named in the suits. Tammello (1997) identified several reasons to carry your own liability insurance, including the limitations in institutional policies, the existence of charitable immunity laws, and the need for ongoing personal protection in many settings.

In some states, nonprofit hospitals have *charitable immunity*. This means that the nonprofit hospital cannot be held legally liable for harm done to a patient by its employees. The employees of that nonprofit hospital are still legally liable for their own actions. When the institution does not bear any of the financial responsibility in a lawsuit, the individual employee is more exposed to financial risk. In Massachusetts, a nonprofit hospital that was protected by the State's charitable immunity laws was involved in a liability suit. Because the hospital was protected, the entire judgment fell on the individual nurse (Kihm, 1999). The trend in legislation is toward the repeal of laws providing for charitable immunity. Those active in the consumer movement have argued that no institution should be relieved of responsibility in such a blanket fashion. If you are employed by a nonprofit or governmental institution, you should learn whether the law in your state provides charitable immunity for the institution.

Even if an employer carries liability insurance, it is often advisable for the individual professional to carry an independent policy. An independent policy may cover the person in voluntary activities and on the job. It also will follow the person who moves from one employer to another. If a legal action is instituted against the professional, the individual liability insurance policy may provide independent legal counsel.

Some nurses state that they do not carry insurance because it might encourage people to bring suit against them. They mistakenly assume that people will not sue if it means financial hardship for the person being sued; most individuals who sue do not know whether a nurse carries individual insurance. In addition, insurance is not the only source of payment for a judgment. Judgments may be levied against most tangible assets, including houses, cars, and savings; judgments also may be levied against future earnings. Married nurses who reside in community property states should realize that one half of the assets of a family may be vulnerable to a judgment. Community property states at this time include Arizona, California, Idaho, Louisiana, Nevada, New Mexico, Texas, and Washington. These factors combine to support the need for the individual professional to carry liability insurance that will provide legal counsel and protection in the case of any judgment.

Analyzing Insurance Coverage

Individual liability insurance for registered nurses is available from a variety of insurance companies (directly through their agents) and through professional organizations that offer coverage as a service to members. When investigating individual liability insurance, ask the agent or company the questions in Display 8-2.

Asking these questions can help you to compare policies from different insurance carriers. When coverage appears equal, you might ask how long a company has been in business and how long it has been providing nursing liability insurance. You want to be insured with a reliable, stable company.

The nurse employee should investigate just as carefully liability insurance coverage that is carried by the hospital. Questions 1 through 4 in Display 8-2 apply to institutional insurance policies as well as to individual insurance policies. In addition, you should ask the questions in Display 8-3 about any institutional policy.

Insurance Cost and Coverage

The ANA has a group policy providing $500,000 per claim and $1 million total in 1 year as basic coverage for the registered nurse. Optional higher limits are available.

Display 8–2
QUESTIONS TO ASK REGARDING INDIVIDUAL LIABILITY INSURANCE

1. In what situations would I, as an individual, be covered?
2. In what situations would I not be covered?
3. How is my coverage affected by my actions? For example, if I failed to follow hospital policy, would I still be covered?
4. What are the monetary limits of the policy?
5. Does the policy provide me with an attorney?
6. Is the policy renewable at my option? What factors affect renewability?
7. Does the insurance cover incidents that occurred while the policy was in force, regardless of when the claim is brought (claims-occurred insurance coverage), or does it cover incidents only if I am currently insured (claims-brought insurance coverage)?
8. What is the cost compared with other policies?

Display 8–3

ADDITIONAL QUESTIONS REGARDING AN INSTITUTIONAL LIABILITY POLICY

1. Does the policy provide me with a personal attorney, or will the same attorney be working for the hospital?
2. At what point would the hospital no longer be responsible and would I become personally responsible?
3. How would my job be affected if a lawsuit were filed or payment awarded based on an action against me? (Check institutional policy as well as the insurance company policy.)
4. Does the insurance company have the right to seek restitution from me if it pays a claim based on my actions?

(It is important that you have accurate answers to these questions so that you can make an informed decision regarding your need for an individual policy.)

The cost for basic coverage in 1999 was approximately $90 per year. Inflation can be expected to increase this cost. Since the 1970s, the cost of the basic coverage provided by the ANA policy rose from approximately $12 per year to its current amount. Several commercial companies and other nursing organizations offer liability insurance policies with comparable rates. These are often advertised in nursing journals.

As previously stated, liability insurance coverage for specialty practice as a nurse practitioner, nurse anesthetist, or nurse midwife is much more expensive. Group policies are available for some of these practitioners through professional organizations. Some individuals are covered by institutional policies and do not try to maintain individual policies. This is especially true of those who work part time and find that insurance premiums are comparable whether working full time or part time.

Critical Thinking Activity

You are accepting a position in a clinic. When might you ask about professional liability insurance coverage? Formulate specific questions. Identify the person who would be the best source of this information. How will you proceed if this person does not have the information you seek? If the interviewer tells you that the clinic is very well covered by liability insurance, will you purchase personal malpractice insurance? Why or why not?

NATIONAL DATA BANK

In the United States, the federal government maintains a "National Data Bank" on licensed health care providers. This is separate from and has a purpose different from the data collected by the ANA or the NCSBN. By law, all judgments, settlements paid, or convictions for malpractice, and all situations in which a health care provider's privileges to practice are curtailed or withdrawn, must be reported to this data bank. All institutions must consult this data bank for information before giving any health care provider privilege to practice in the institution. The purpose of the National Data Bank is to protect the public from incompetent professionals who continue to practice by moving from one place to another.

LEGAL ISSUES COMMON IN NURSING

Some legal issues recur frequently in nursing practice. It is wise for the nurse to understand these particular issues as they relate to individual practice.

Personal Liability

As an educated professional, you are always legally responsible or liable for your actions (Bernzweig, 1995). Thus, if a physician or supervisor asks you to do something that is contrary to your best professional judgment and says, "I'll take responsibility," that person is acting unwisely. The physician or supervisor giving the directions may be liable if harm results, but that would not remove your personal liability.

SITUATION   Personal Liability

The registered nurse giving medications on a large medical unit notes that an order for digoxin (a heart medication) is considerably larger than the usual dose. She looks up the medication in a reference book and finds that she is correct about the dosage. The ordered dose is several times the usual dose. The nurse then calls the supervisor and explains the situation.

The supervisor double checks the order with the registered nurse and then states: "Dr. Jones is an outstanding physician. I am sure he has a good reason for ordering this dose. Go ahead and give the medication as ordered. I'll take responsibility." The nurse then gives the medication, and the patient suffers a toxic reaction.

The registered nurse could be held liable for giving the incorrect amount of medication. She had the knowledge and judgment to recognize that the dose was much larger than usual, and she failed to check with the physician. A statement by the supervisor does not remove the nurse's personal responsibility for her own actions. Because even a competent physician might make an error, the nurse had a responsibility to clarify the order. The supervisor and the physician could be held liable in addition to the nurse, but not instead of her.

Although each person is legally responsible for his or her own actions, the example above illustrates that there are also situations in which a person or organization may be held liable for actions taken by others.

Employer Liability

The most common situation in which a person or organization is held responsible for the actions of another is in the employer-employee relationship. In many instances, an employer can be held responsible for torts committed by an employee. This is called the doctrine of *respondeat superior* (let the master respond). The law holds the employer responsible for hiring qualified persons, for establishing an appropriate environment for correct functioning, and for providing supervision or direction as needed to avoid errors or harm. Therefore, if a nurse, as an employee of a hospital, is guilty of malpractice, the hospital also may be named in the suit. The employer's liability may exist even if the employer appears to have taken precautions to prevent error.

It is important to understand that this doctrine does not remove any responsibility from the individual nurse, but it extends responsibility to the employer in addition to the nurse. If, for example, a hospital has a procedure that does not conform to good nursing practice as you know it, and you follow that procedure, you will still be liable for any resulting harm. You are expected to use your education and experience to make sound judgments regarding your work.

SITUATION   **Employer Responsibility for a Staff Nurse**

A nurse working in a long-term care facility is responsible for planning and coordinating the care of a severely debilitated resident. This elderly man is totally dependent for all activities of daily living due to a recent stroke. He is not eating and drinking adequately. He faints and is discovered to have very low blood pressure and a rapid weak pulse. He is sent to the local hospital, where he is admitted for dehydration secondary to inadequate fluid intake. Investigation reveals that no assessment of his fluid or nutritional status has been recorded, nor was there any plan to ensure that nutritional and fluid needs were met.

Both the nurse and the long-term care facility in this situation might be found liable for harm that resulted. The nurse had a personal, professional responsibility to accurately assess the resident and to institute care to meet his basic needs. The facility also had a responsibility to make sure that policies, procedures, and protocols were in place to ensure appropriate assessment and care, and that employees followed through on them.

Supervisory Liability

In the role of charge nurse, head nurse, supervisor, or any other role that involves delegation, supervision, or direction of other people, the nurse is potentially liable for the actions of others. The supervising nurse is responsible for exercising good judgment in a supervisory role. This includes making appropriate decisions about assignments and delegation of tasks. If an error occurs and the supervising nurse is shown to have exercised sound judgment in all decisions made in that capacity, the supervising nurse may not be held liable for the error of a subordinate. If poor judgment was used in assigning an inadequately prepared person to an important task or oversight was inadequate, the supervisory nurse might be liable for resulting harm. The extent of the subordinate's responsibility would depend on his or her level of education and training. People with limited education or training might not be liable for some errors; the more education subordinates have, the more likely they will be liable. (See Chapter 12 for more discussion of delegation.)

SITUATION   **Supervisory Responsibility for an Educated Staff Member**

Two sudden admissions to the coronary care unit create a situation in which additional help is needed to care for the patients in the unit. A "float" nurse is sent to the CCU to assist. The charge nurse does not ask the temporary float nurse whether she has education or experience in coronary care, nor does the temporary float nurse volunteer this information. The temporary float nurse, however, has no background or experience in coronary care.

The temporary nurse is assigned by the charge nurse to the complete care of two patients. Because of the float nurse's inability to accurately interpret the monitors, a potentially life-threatening problem is not identified until the patient "arrests." Resuscitation efforts are successful, but the patient suffers some brain damage.

Both the charge nurse who assigned the inadequately prepared nurse to total care, and the temporary nurse, could be found liable: the charge nurse for incorrectly assigning the nurse, and the temporary nurse for not recognizing her own limitations. The educational preparation of the temporary nurse gave her the background to understand that expertise was needed in this situation, and that she did not possess that expertise. If the situation were changed so that the temporary nurse was reviewed for expertise in coronary care and found to have that expertise, then the charge nurse might not be liable for the error of the temporary nurse. The supervisory function of ascertaining level of preparation and ability to meet the standards of the job would have been carried out.

SITUATION   **Supervisory Responsibility for Staff Member With Limited Education**

The registered nurse is working on a unit that assigns a nursing assistant to work with each RN. One evening, the regular nursing assistant is absent due to illness. A new nursing assistant is assigned to work with the RN. During the evening, the RN asks the nursing assistant to monitor the new postoperative patient. The RN lists for the nursing assistant the items that are to be checked: vital signs, hourly urine output, pain, and condition of the dressing. Each hour, the RN stops the nursing assistant, asks if the patient is doing okay, and receives an affirmative reply. When the RN stops to chart, he reviews the last 4 hours of flow sheet information listed by the nursing assistant. He sees that the urine output has been only 15 mL/hr for the last 4 hours. When he questions the nursing assistant, he learns that the nursing assistant had no idea what information needed to be reported immediately. The RN completes an assessment and calls the physician. The patient is found to have developed renal failure.

The RN might be found negligent in this case for assigning the nursing assistant to monitor a critical postoperative patient without proper direction or supervision. The nursing assistant might not be found negligent because she had no basis for recognizing the seriousness of the situation or for recognizing her own lack of ability to meet the responsibilities involved in this assessment. She could carry out the tasks assigned and had done those correctly.

Duty to Report or Seek Medical Care for a Patient

A nurse who is caring for a patient has a legal duty to ensure that the patient receives safe and competent care. This duty requires that the nurse maintain an appropriate standard of care and that the nurse take action to obtain an appropriate standard of care from other professionals when that is necessary. For example, if a nurse identifies that a patient needs the attention of a physician, and fails to make every effort to obtain that attention, the nurse has breached a duty to the patient.

S I T U A T I O N   Failure to Seek Medical Care for Patient

The registered nurse is caring for a postoperative patient during the night. The patient's blood pressure begins to drop and the pulse begins to rise. The nurse's assessment indicates that the patient may be bleeding internally. The nurse institutes a plan for close nursing monitoring and calls the surgeon to describe the situation. The surgeon gives a telephone order to increase the intravenous fluid rate and states that he will see the patient in the morning. The patient's condition continues to deteriorate, but the nurse does nothing further to ensure that a physician examines the patient.

If the outcome is unfavorable, the nurse can be found to have breached a duty to the patient. The patient relies on the nurse to provide appropriate care and to identify when a physician is needed. The nurse could have made more telephone calls to the surgeon and failing the success of that, could have followed the facility's procedure for asking another physician (such as the emergency department physician) to see the patient.

The nurse has a duty to continue all efforts to obtain appropriate medical care for the patient. If the nurse had followed all procedures, sought another physician, and continued efforts when initial attempts were unsuccessful, the nurse would not have breached a duty. The nurse cannot guarantee a physician's care, but can guarantee that the patient will not be left without an advocate.

Additionally, the nurse has a responsibility to examine critically medical orders that are written for a patient. Although the nurse is not responsible for the medical order itself, the nurse's education provides a background to identify obvious discrepancies or problems. In one reported case (Anonymous, Nursing 97), two doctors left conflicting orders, which the charge nurse then transcribed. The court ruled that the nurse had a duty to understand the patient's plan of care and to communicate with the doctors who had written the conflicting orders.

Confidentiality and Right to Privacy

Confidentiality and the right to privacy with respect to one's personal life are basic concerns in our society. All information regarding a patient belongs to that patient. This right has been inferred from interpretation of the federal constitution, but is explicitly stated in some state laws.

In theory, this right should protect a patient's privacy. However, third party payers (such as insurance companies and HMOs) will not reimburse for care if they do not receive the records they request. The result is that patients must often sign statements giving blanket approval for all information to be sent to the third party payer. They may be unaware of exactly what information is sent or who may see it.

When computerized records are transmitted to insurance companies, they no longer contain only a brief statement of diagnosis and treatment; they may contain detailed accounts of interactions between a patient and a mental health professional, health information of a sensitive nature, and genetic information that could be used inappropriately. Because increased use of computerized records can result in easier retrieval and cross-referencing of records from many sources, the general public, health care providers, and government officials are becoming more concerned about potential invasions of privacy.

A nurse who gives out information without authorization from the patient or from the legally responsible guardian can be held liable for harm that results. If you have any question about who the legally responsible guardian of a patient is, be sure to consult with your administrative authority. There may be a court-appointed legal guardian, or the situation may be governed by specific state laws regarding who becomes the responsible guardian when the person is unable to give personal consent. The hospital administration should be able to ascertain the correct guardian.

Only those professional persons involved in the patient's care who have a need to know about the patient can be allowed routine access to the record. A physician who is not involved in the patient's care or who does not have an administrative responsibility relative to that care is not allowed routine access. Persons not involved in care can be allowed access to the record only by specific written authorization or by court order. You should be cautious about what information you share verbally and with whom.

A directory information policy has been adopted by many acute care hospitals. This policy gives specific guidelines regarding what may be revealed according to freedom of information laws, and does not violate confidentiality; usually a patient's name and sex, and a general statement of condition (satisfactory, serious, and so on) may be revealed. This is a wise standard for general hospitals and nursing homes with no written policy to follow. In some instances, especially those involving treatment for alcoholism, drug abuse, and AIDS, even revealing the information that an individual is hospitalized is considered a legal violation of confidentiality.

Medical records professionals state that it is not uncommon for attorneys, family members, media representatives, or law enforcement officials to request access to patient records or specific patient information without having express consent of the patient or a legal court order to view the records or be given information. Those unfamiliar with laws regarding privacy sometimes reveal information inappropriately. If you are ever approached for patient information by someone who purports to have authority, your best course of action is to refer that individual to appropriate administrative personnel who can determine the validity of the request.

SITUATION   Breach of Confidentiality

A nurse in a small community hospital discusses with a friend the admission of a woman community member for treatment of cancer. The nurse's friend then talks to others, who talk to still others, until there is widespread knowledge of the patient's cancer in the community. The woman's daughter hears about her mother's cancer diagnosis at school and is very upset.

The nurse could be held liable for revealing this information in a suit charging breach of privacy and confidentiality. The harm is the emotional distress to the woman and her family. If the breach of confidentiality could be traced to the nurse's conversation, the nurse's action would be considered the direct cause of harm.

A newer concern is that more health care agencies are using fax machines to send patient information to one another and even between departments within an institution. Faxes have a legitimate purpose in that continuity of care is enhanced when information is shared. When you send a document by fax machine, however, you cannot assure that confidentiality is maintained. Some facilities have a policy requiring that you call ahead and designate a specific person who is to be present to receive the fax. The cover page often states that this is confidential material and should not be read by anyone other than the designated recipient. If your facility or agency has no policy regarding the safeguarding of faxed information, you would be wise to raise the concern.

Other new areas of concern are the Internet and e-mail. Through these avenues, a health care provider may consult with other professionals to provide the best diagnostic and treatment services to the patient. However, online computer communications are not private. Those with the necessary skill may intercept and read any e-mail or Internet message. Therefore, the identity of patients must be protected in any such communication.

Defamation of Character

Any time that shared information is detrimental to a person's reputation, the person sharing the information may be liable for defamation of character. Written defamation is called libel. Oral defamation is called slander. Defamation of character involves communication that is malicious and false. Sometimes such comments are made in the heat of anger. Occasionally statements written in a patient's chart are libelous. Severely critical opinions may be stated as fact. An example of such a statement might be "The patient is lying," or "The patient is rude and domineering." Patients may charge that comments in the chart adversely affected their care by prejudicing other staff against them. The prudent nurse will chart only objective information regarding patients and give opinion in professional terms, well documented with fact. A chart might read:

"The patient states . . . Observation reveals . . ."; this provides factual information for the reader without making potentially libelous accusations. In conversations, the prudent nurse avoids discussing patients.

SITUATION   Slander

Two registered nurses are leaving the floor for their coffee break. They are discussing the patients in their care as they wait for the elevator. They enter the elevator with several other people and continue their conversation. The first nurse says: "That Mrs. Johnson in room 201. I don't know whether I can take another day of her! She's impossible!" The other nurse replies: "I know just what you mean. I had her a couple of days ago and she was just on the bell all the time. If you ask me, there's nothing wrong with her that a good swift kick wouldn't cure!" First nurse: "Do you really think she's faking?" Second nurse: "I'm sure of it. Have you ever watched her when her husband comes to visit?"

A relative of the patient is one of the people in the elevator and overhears the conversation. The relative reports the conversation to the patient.

If the patient brings suit, the nurses involved might be found guilty of slander. The nurses were discussing the patient in a place where others could hear the conversation. The comments clearly identified the patient, reflected opinions that were not supported with fact, and potentially could jeopardize the patient's reputation and standing in the community.

Defamation of character also may be charged by a health care provider who believes that statements made by another professional are false, malicious, and have caused harm. There are accepted mechanisms for confidentially reporting inappropriate care or errors; these should be used, and critical statements to uninvolved third parties should not be made. In many states, licensed professionals are required to report poor practice or illegal acts on the part of other professionals. Criticism reported without malice and in good faith, through the appropriate channels, is protected from legal action for defamation.

Privileged Communication

Privileged communication refers to information shared by an individual with certain professionals that does not need to be revealed even in a court of law. All states consider certain types of communication (between client and attorney, between patient and doctor, or between an individual and a member of the clergy) privileged. Not all states recognize the nurse-patient relationship as one in which privileged communication takes place; even those states that recognize nurse-patient communication as potentially privileged do not consider *all* communication between patients and nurses privileged. It is important that you understand that privilege is a limited concept. Only a court can determine if privilege exists in any specific case (Fig. 8-3). If a court does not determine information to be privileged, then you are legally obligated to testify about the communication.

FIGURE 8–3 Privileged communication is a very narrow concept under the law. A judge must determine whether communication between a nurse and a client is privileged.

Informed Consent

Every person has the right to either *consent* (agree) to or refuse health care treatment. The law requires that a person give voluntary and informed consent. *Voluntary* means that no coercion exists. *Informed* means that a person clearly understands the choices being offered.

CONSENT FOR MEDICAL TREATMENT

Consent for medical treatment is the responsibility of the medical provider (eg, physician, dentist, nurse practitioner). Included in the discussion must be the alternatives for treatment, the risks of any treatment proposed, the relative value of any treatment proposed, and the risks of not having treatment. This consent may be either verbal or written. Written consent usually is preferred in health care to ensure that a record of consent exists, although a signature alone does not prove that the consent was informed. A blanket consent for "any procedures deemed necessary" is not usually considered adequate consent for specific procedures. The form should state the specific proposed medical procedure or test.

The patient's medical condition usually is not accepted by the courts as a valid reason for not giving the patient complete and accurate information. Currently, there are no clear guidelines as to what constitutes complete information. What constitutes adequate information about various alternative approaches to treatment is often unclear. Is it always necessary to discuss a treatment the physician does not believe is a good choice? Courts have generally supported the idea that usual risks need to be disclosed, but that rare or unexpected risks do not have to be discussed.

The law places the responsibility for obtaining consent for medical treatment on the physician. It is the physician's responsibility to provide appropriate information, and he or she is liable if the patient charges that appropriate information was not given. A nurse may present a form for a patient to sign, and the nurse may sign the form as a witness to the signature. This does not transfer the legal responsibility for informed consent for medical care to the nurse. If the patient does not seem well informed, the nurse should notify the physician so that further information can be provided to the patient. Although the nurse would not legally be liable for the lack of informed consent, the nurse has ethical obligations to assist the patient in exercising his or her rights and to assist the physician in providing appropriate care (see Chapter 9 for discussion of the ethical obligations regarding informed consent).

CONSENT FOR NURSING MEASURES

Nurses must obtain a patient's consent for nursing measures undertaken. This does not mean that exhaustive explanations need to be given in each situation, because courts have held that patients can be expected to have some understanding of usual care. Consent for nursing measures may be verbal or implied. The nurse may ask, "Are you ready to ambulate now?" The patient answers, "Certainly," providing verbal consent. Alternatively, the nurse may state, "I have the injection the doctor ordered for you. Will you please turn over?" If the patient turns over, this is implied consent.

The nurse should remember that the patient is free to refuse any aspect of care offered. Like the physician, the nurse is responsible for making sure that the patient is informed before making a decision. Good nursing care requires that you use all means at your disposal to help the patient comprehend the value of proposed care. For example, the postoperative patient needs to understand that getting into a chair is part of the plan of care, not a convenience for the nurse or simply a change to prevent boredom. Thus, a patient's refusal of care is accepted only after the patient has been given complete information. The nurse would then carefully document this situation.

ADVANCE DIRECTIVES

Advance directives are legal documents attesting to the wishes of an individual regarding health care in situations in which he or she is no longer capable of giving personal informed consent. They are completed in "advance" of the situation in which they might be needed, and "direct" the actions of others. There are several types of advance directives. A living will provides information on general preferences regarding end-of-life issues.

A *durable power of attorney for health care* is a document that legally designates a decision-maker should the person be incapacitated. This document also may contain specific advance directives such as whether tube feedings, intravenous fluids and nutrition, ventilator support, and other such treatments should be instituted if the individual is found to be terminally ill or in a persistent vegetative state.

In 1990, the Patient Self-Determination Act (PSDA) was passed by the US Congress. It took effect in 1992, and required that on admission to any health care service (hospital, long-term care center, or home care agency) patients be given an opportunity to determine what lifesaving or life-prolonging actions they want to be carried out. The agency must provide adequate information for the individual to make an informed decision regarding these important matters. As a result of this legislation, agencies reviewed and revised policies and protocols regarding consent. In many agencies, a nurse has the responsibility to provide the education and obtain a signature on a document indicating preferences.

Information regarding the results of the PSDA is being analyzed by several government agencies to determine whether there has been a change in practice. Some have suggested that the manner in which self-determination and the possible alternatives are explained greatly influences patient choices; one suggestion has been that these matters first be discussed in the health care provider's office, before admission. When this is possible, it allows for more time to consider alternatives and consult significant others. The final decision is then made away from the pressure of the health care environment. (See Chapter 10 for a further discussion of planning for end-of-life issues.)

COMPETENCE TO GIVE CONSENT

A person's ability to make judgments based on rational understanding is termed *competence*. Dementia, developmental disabilities, head injuries, strokes, and illnesses creating loss of consciousness are common causes of an inability to make judgments. Determining competence is a complex issue. The patient's illness, age, or condition alone does not determine competence. Legal competence is ultimately determined by the court. The general tendency of the courts has been to encourage whatever decision making an individual is capable of and to restrict personal decision making as little as possible.

When a person is determined legally to be incompetent, a legal guardian is appointed and consent is obtained from the legal guardian. A legal guardian is constrained from making some types of decisions. For example, if the health care action could be identified as injurious to the individual involved, a court may need to be consulted regarding consent for that specific action. An example would be the decision about discontinuation of dialysis for an incompetent individual. When such an individual leaves no clear advance directive regarding personal wishes, the health care providers might insist on getting a court decision before accepting the consent of the guardian to terminate the dialysis.

Health care providers often encounter those for whom no legal determination of competence has been made, but who do not seem able to make an informed decision; examples include the very confused elderly person, the inebriated person, and the unconscious person. The law in each state specifies who is allowed to give consent in such situations. Frequently, this is the spouse, the parent, the children, or the siblings. There are also guidelines to follow in determining that a person cannot give his or her own consent. Your facility policy should contain directions to guide you in obtaining legal consent; if it does not, you should consult an administrative person for a decision. In situations where there are several persons in the category, such as children of an elderly person, agreement regarding decisions is needed before proceeding. Determining who is able to give legal consent in such a situation is not a nurse's responsibility.

Competence may change from day to day, as a person's physical illness changes. The person who has had a major surgery and is receiving large doses of narcotics for pain may not be able to reason clearly. Forty-eight hours later this same individual may be perfectly alert and capable of considering complex issues. An individual may be competent to make some decisions, such as "I don't like rice and I won't eat it!" but incompetent to make others, for example, decisions regarding financial matters. These differences in competence require care providers to adjust their own planning to incorporate patient self-determination whenever possible, even when the person is legally incompetent. If a person truly is not capable of making decisions, the nurse should attempt to present necessary nursing actions in a way that elicits cooperation and avoids confrontation over decisions.

WITHDRAWING CONSENT

Consent may be withdrawn after it is given. People have the right to change their minds. Therefore, if after one intravenous infusion a patient decides not to have a second one started, that is his or her right. As a nurse, you have an obligation to notify the physician if the patient refuses a medical procedure or treatment.

CONSENT AND MINORS

The consent of a minor usually is given by a parent or legal guardian. You also should obtain the minor's consent when he or she is able to give it. Increasingly, courts are emphasizing that minors be allowed a voice when it concerns matters that they are capable of understanding. This is especially true for the adolescent, but this consideration should be given to any child who is 7 years of age or older. When a minor refuses care and the legal guardian has authorized that care, you should not proceed until legal clarification is given. Your nursing supervisor should be consulted.

Minors who live apart from their parents and are financially independent, or who are married, are termed *emancipated minors*. In most (but not all) states an emancipated minor can give consent to his or her own treatment. Some states have specific laws relating to the *mature minor*, allowing a sexually active minor to give personal consent (without also obtaining parental consent) for treatment of sexually transmitted disease, or for obtaining birth control information and supplies (see Chapter 10). You should be sure of the law in your own state if you practice in an area where this is a concern. Most institutions have developed policies to guide employees in making correct decisions in this and other areas dealing with consent.

Emergency Care

Care in emergencies has many legal repercussions, therefore, the judgment that an emergency exists is important. Certain actions may be legal in emergencies and not legal in nonemergency situations. In emergencies, the standard procedures for obtaining consent may be impossible to follow. Further, in emergencies, personnel must sometimes take on responsibilities that they would not undertake in a nonemergency situation. Critical thinking on the part of all health care professionals is essential when differentiating an emergency from a nonemergency.

Most facilities that provide emergency care have policies and procedures designed to ensure adequate support for claiming that an emergency exists. Thus, the policy will often state that at least two physicians in the emergency department must examine the patient and concur that the emergency requires immediate action, without waiting for consent. This ensures maximum legal protection for the physician and the institution.

CONSENT IN EMERGENCIES

If a true emergency exists, consent for care is considered to be implied. The law holds that if a reasonable person were aware that the situation was life threatening, he or she would give consent for care. An exception to this is made if the person has explicitly rejected such care in advance; an example is a Jehovah's Witness carrying a card stating his personal religion, and that he does not wish to receive blood or blood products. This is one reason emergency department nurses should check a patient's wallet for identification and information related to care. Checking a patient's wallet should be done with another person, and a careful inventory of contents made and signed by both. There should be little concern about liability in taking emergency action if this is completed.

STANDARDS OF PRACTICE AND EMERGENCIES

Standards of practice in emergencies also differ from those in nonemergency situations. In hospital emergencies, the nurse sometimes may be in the position of identifying an emergency and whether a needed action is one that only a physician usually performs. The hospital is expected to have a policy and procedure, which the nurse would follow, to verify and document the situation fully. This usually involves consultation with a supervisory nurse and verification of the emergency situation, as well as attempts to obtain medical assistance. Again, critical thinking by the nurse is essential to determine whether a true emergency exists.

When "life or limb" is truly in danger, the courts have held that a nurse can do those things immediately necessary, even if they usually are considered medical functions, provided the nurse has the essential expertise to perform the actions safely and correctly. The matter of having essential expertise is crucial; this is why all members of an emergency response team must learn all aspects of the "code" procedure. If, for any reason, the physician were unable to respond to the code, a nurse who was prepared with this essential expertise would assume the role of the leader.

S I T U A T I O N   **Nursing Action in a Hospital Emergency**

In an orthopedic unit, it is common to care for patients with new casts. A young man with a newly applied long-leg cast is admitted through the emergency department at 6 PM. The nurse assigned to this patient's care carefully makes all the appropriate observations throughout the evening and documents his findings. The nurse notes that the leg is beginning to swell and that the edges of the cast are beginning to cut into the skin. At that time, the nurse notifies the supervisor that a problem is developing, and that he thinks the physician should be notified. The supervisor agrees and the nurse begins trying to contact the physician. The nurse continues to make observations, noting increasing swelling, color changes in the exposed toes, and loss of sensation. The physician cannot be reached and no other physician is immediately available.

The nurse follows the hospital procedure for seeking medical attention and for determining when an emergency exists. After consultation with the supervisor, the nurse decides that an emergency exists and that the cast needs to be cut open to relieve the pressure. Cutting a cast open is considered a medical procedure in this hospital.

The nurse has been taught how to use a cast cutter in emergency situations. Thus, the nurse possesses the essential expertise. The nurse, with the supervisor's approval, cuts open the cast and secures it in place with an elastic bandage. All observations made, consultations carried out, attempts to notify the physician, and the final action taken are documented carefully in the patient's record. Hospital policy was followed throughout the situation to ensure that all necessary steps had been taken.

Although this action went beyond usual nursing practice, it would not be considered a violation of either the nursing or the medical practice acts, because an emergency existed and the results of inaction would have been serious. Additionally, the nurse had the expertise and was prepared to carry out the necessary action safely. This emergency care usually is limited to specific technical procedures that the nurse has learned. It does not include diagnosing disease or prescribing medication, unless there are specific standing orders relative to the situation.

NONINSTITUTIONAL EMERGENCY CARE

Emergencies encountered outside the health care environment present other problems. Anyone rendering aid in an emergency is expected to behave as a reasonably prudent person would in such a situation. The nurse rendering aid in an emergency must behave as a reasonably prudent nurse in that situation. Thus, the standard is higher than for the nonprofessional person, although the nurse is not expected to perform as if he or she were operating in a health care setting. The physical situation and the psychological situation are both considered when determining what is reasonably prudent nursing action.

All states and Canadian provinces have "Good Samaritan" statutes that excuse negligence on the part of rescuers in an emergency; the term refers to a person who voluntarily helps another in need (Hall, 1996). These laws are of interest to health care professionals who are concerned about law suits. The first of these statutes was enacted in California in 1959 (Bernzweig, 1995). These statutes vary in content and comprehensiveness, but relieve a professional of some liability when reasonable care is used. These laws often make people feel more secure when rendering aid.

Each nurse must make an individual decision about rendering emergency aid in a specific situation. The decision involves ethical as well as legal considerations. If the profession of nursing is a public trust and nurses are truly involved in the business of caring, then failure to aid an individual who is in serious danger is an ethical violation of that trust. To date, there has been no instance of a nurse being sued for coming to the aid of someone in an emergency situation (Bernzweig, 1995; Fiesta, 1994). Professional liability insurance does provide coverage when the nurse assists in this way, which may make you feel more comfortable about rendering emergency aid. Statutes in Vermont, Minnesota, Wisconsin, Wyoming, and Quebec mandate that *anyone* assist persons in danger but may not be enforceable (Hall, 1996).

In many states, emergency personnel must render all possible aid, including all resuscitative measures, when they are called to an emergency situation. This has sometimes resulted in the resuscitation of a terminally ill person who had previously stated that resuscitation was not desired; as more individuals receive terminal care in their homes, this will become an increasing concern.

Legislation allowing for patient self-determination regarding emergency responders has now been passed in some states. The law usually stipulates the precise circumstances under which an individual may provide an advance directive in regard to emergency procedures, and how that directive must be documented so that emergency personnel can honor it. All emergency responders must be aware of their responsibilities in regard to advance directives.

Fraud

Fraud is deliberate deception for the purpose of personal gain and is usually prosecuted as a crime. However, it may also serve as the basis of a civil suit. Situations of fraud in nursing are not common. One example would be trying to obtain a better position by giving incorrect information to a prospective employer. By deliberately stating (falsely) that you had completed a nurse practitioner program to obtain a position for which you would otherwise be ineligible, you are defrauding the employer. This may be prosecuted as a crime, because you are also placing members of the community in danger of receiving substandard care. You may also commit fraud by trying to cover up a nursing error to avoid legal action. Courts tend to be more harsh in decisions regarding fraud than in cases involving simple malpractice, because fraud represents a deliberate attempt to mislead others for your own gain and could result in harm to those assigned to your care.

SITUATION   **Fraud**

A registered nurse is giving medications to the patients to whom she is assigned. When she presents a patient with his pills, he states that he was sure the doctor had discontinued the red pill because he had had a reaction to it the evening before. The nurse states that she is sure these are the correct medications. The patient takes the pills and the nurse charts the medications. The patient subsequently has a reaction. The nurse becomes frightened, goes back, and alters the medication record to make it appear that the medication was not given.

This situation could be considered fraud. The deception was the changing of the record, and the personal gain was freedom from responsibility for the error.

Assault and Battery

Assault is saying or doing something to make a person genuinely afraid that he or she will be touched without consent. *Battery* involves touching a person when that individual has not consented to the action. Neither of these terms implies that harm was done; harm may or may not occur. For an assault to occur, the person must be afraid of what might happen because the individual appears to have the power to carry out the threat. "If you don't take this medication, I will have to put you in restraints" is an example of an assault. For battery to occur, the touching must occur without consent. Remember that consent may be implied rather than specifically stated. Therefore, if the patient extends an arm for an injection, he cannot later charge battery, saying that he was not asked. But if the patient agreed because of a threat (assault), the touching still would be considered battery because the consent was not freely given.

Assault and battery are crimes under the law. However, most of these cases in health care are instituted as civil suits by the injured party, rather than as criminal cases by the governmental authorities. An example of a case that is most likely to be prosecuted as a civil case is given in the following situation.

SITUATION   Assault and Battery

A patient who was voluntarily admitted to a psychiatric hospital refused to take any antipsychotic medications. The staff decided that her need for the medications was great; therefore, they planned to restrain her and give her injectable antipsychotic medications.

A court might consider this to be assault and battery. Although the patient was mentally ill, there is no indication that a court ever found her incompetent to make her own decisions or ordered her to be treated against her will. Mental illness alone does not constitute incompetence and this woman had the right to refuse treatment.

Assault and battery are most commonly treated as criminal cases when they involve suspected abuse of a patient. Most of us in health care are shocked and dismayed to learn of instances where care providers were abusive. Individuals who have difficulty with impulse control and anger may become frustrated with a patient and threaten, push, shove, or otherwise harm the individual. Most jurisdictions have laws requiring that anyone who knows of abuse to a dependent patient, whether a child, a developmentally delayed adult, or an elderly person, report that abuse to the proper authorities. Within an institution, there should be policies and procedures for this type of reporting. Appropriate authorities must conduct a careful investigation to ensure protection of the rights of the person accused.

Critical Thinking Activity

You have taken a position as a night nurse in a long-term care facility. One of the nursing assistants speaks of residents in very negative terms. You have observed her assisting a resident to the bathroom, and she seemed abrupt and somewhat rough with the resident. Another resident says to you, "You have to be really nice to her [gesturing toward the door where the nursing assistant just exited] or she'll take it out on you next time." What should be your response to the resident? What action, if any, should you take? What is your legal liability if you do nothing? What is your legal liability if you initiate action against this nursing assistant?

False Imprisonment

Making a person stay in a place against his wishes is *false imprisonment*. The person may be forced to stay either by physical or verbal means. It is easy to understand why restraining a patient or confining a patient to a locked room could constitute false imprisonment, if proper procedures were not first carried out. Again, false imprisonment is a crime, but when it occurs in health care it is most often the basis of a civil suit rather than a criminal case (Fig. 8-4).

FIGURE 8–4 The improper use of restraints may constitute "false imprisonment."

The law is less clear about keeping a patient confined by nonphysical means. If you remove a patient's clothes for the express purpose of preventing his leaving, you could be liable for false imprisonment. Threatening to keep a person confined with statements such as, "If you don't stay in your bed, I'll sedate you," can also constitute false imprisonment. If a person needs to be confined for his or her own safety or well-being, it is best to help the person understand and agree to that course of action.

Any time a patient poses a danger to self or others, the law requires that the least restrictive means available be used to protect the patient and others. Health care providers are obligated to document the behavior of concern, problem solve alternative actions, and then try those alternative actions before resorting to any type of restraint. Documentation of this entire process is essential. Nurses who determine the need for restraints must obtain a physician's order as soon as possible. Be sure to follow the policies of the facility.

In a conventional care setting you cannot restrain or confine responsible adults against their wishes. All persons have the right to make decisions for themselves, regardless of the consequences. The patient with a severe heart condition who defies orders and walks to the bathroom has that right. You protect yourself by recording your efforts to teach the patient the need for restrictions and by reporting the patient's behavior to your supervisor and the physician.

In the same context, the patient cannot be forced to remain in a hospital. If a patient wants to leave against medical advice, that is the patient's right. Again, you document your efforts in the record and follow applicable policies to protect the facility, the physician, and yourself from liability. The example of an intentional tort given earlier in this chapter involved false imprisonment.

A hospital may not detain a patient for nonpayment of a bill. The hospital is free to take legal action against the person who does not pay, but refusing discharge also constitutes false imprisonment.

False imprisonment suits are a special concern in the care of the psychiatric patient. Particular laws relate to this situation. In the psychiatric setting, you may have patients who have voluntarily sought admission. The same restrictions on restraint or confinement that apply to patients in the general care setting apply to these patients. Other patients in the psychiatric setting may have been committed involuntarily according to the laws of the state. Specific measures may be used to confine the involuntarily committed patient. Law in terms of situation, type of restraint allowed, and the length of time restraining may be used usually defines these measures. If you work in a psychiatric setting, you should review specific policies regarding restraint to protect patients and to assist staff in functioning within the legal limits.

Medication Errors

Medication errors are one of the most common causes of adverse outcomes for hospitalized patients. The incidence of errors related to medications ranges from 4% to 17% of all people being admitted to hospital (Bates et al, 1993, 1995; Lesar et al, 1990). In these studies antibiotics, analgesics, and cardiovascular drugs most frequently were associated with errors. Errors had many different sources, including inappropriate medication for the condition being treated; incorrect dosage or frequency of administration of medication; wrong route of administration; failure to recognize drug interactions; lack of monitoring for drug side effects; and inadequate communication among members of the health care team, and the patient.

Many different health care team members were responsible for the errors and many different team members can prevent errors. Although individuals must exercise extraordinary care and follow procedures carefully, systems for medication administration also need to be carefully scrutinized. Some errors result from drugs with similar names; look-alike medication containers contribute to other errors; still other errors are created by poor systems for communication in which handwriting problems may contribute to lack of clarity. Verbal orders have such a potential for error that most systems are set up to avoid them as much as possible.

When medication errors do occur, the health care professionals involved should institute corrective action immediately and communicate with the patient and family. Fiesta (1998) points out that if health care professionals are not straightforward with patients and families, fraud or intentional concealment may be charged and may contribute to the awarding of punitive damages as well as ordinary damages. Most malpractice insurance will not cover punitive damages.

FACTORS THAT CONTRIBUTE TO MALPRACTICE CLAIMS

A suit usually does not follow the poor results or harm that occur in the course of nursing practice. However, an understanding of the factors that enter into whether a suit is instituted may be helpful to you.

Social Factors

Much is being written about changes in the public's attitudes toward health care personnel. Health care is big business, and patients complain increasingly of not being accepted and respected as individuals. Patients are more willing to bring suit against someone who is part of a large, impersonal system.

Health costs are high, and some people think hospitals and physicians have the ability to pay large settlements, whether directly or through insurance. If a patient's own income is lessened or disrupted by an illness, he or she might bring suit as a solution to economic difficulties. Increased public awareness of the size of monetary judgments that have been awarded may also be an economic incentive to initiating a suit.

 Critical Thinking Activity

A good neighbor and friend experiences an unfortunate episode of extremely poor care in a local hospital where you are employed. She discusses this with you and asks your advice about initiating a suit. What are your obligations in this situation, both as a friend and as a professional? What are your obligations as an employee of the institution? If you need help reaching a decision, to whom can you turn?

Suit-Prone Patients

Some people are more likely to bring suit, for real or imagined errors. If these people are recognized as being suit-prone patients, it is possible for you to protect yourself through increased vigilance in regard to care and thorough record-keeping. Although we would warn you to guard against stereotyping, the following general descriptions may help you to avoid problems. Suit-prone patients usually are identified by overt behavior in which they are persistent fault finders and critics of personnel and of all aspects of care. They may be uncooperative in following a plan of care and sensitive to any perceived slight.

Persons who exhibit hostile attitudes may extend their hostile feelings to the nurses and other health care persons with whom they have contact. The nurse who becomes defensive when faced with hostility only widens the breach in the nurse-patient relationship. It is necessary to pay careful attention to those principles of care learned in psychosocial nursing that deal with how to help the hostile patient. Assisting patients in solving their own problems and offering support are the best forms of protection for the nurse.

Another type of patient who appears more suit-prone is the very dependent person who uses projection to deal with anxiety and fear. These individuals tend to ascribe fault or blame for all events to others and are unable to accept personal responsibility for their own welfare. Again, meeting these patients' needs with a carefully considered plan of care is the answer.

A common error is to withdraw and become defensive when confronting a suit-prone patient; this reaction occurs partly because a situation is unpleasant and partly because a staff member feels personally threatened by the patient's behavior. This reaction increases the likelihood of a suit if a poor result occurs.

Another incorrect nursing response to the suit-prone patient is to become more directive and authoritarian. This tends to increase the patient's feeling of separation and distance from the staff and again increases the likelihood of a suit.

When the staff is helped to view the patient as a troubled person who manifests his or her problems in this manner, sometimes they find it easier to be objective. The patient is in need of all the skill that the prepared nurse can bring to the emotional problems. The suit-prone patient does not always end up suing; much depends on the response of health care personnel.

Suit-Prone Nurses

Nurses may also be suit-prone. Nurses who are insensitive to the patient's complaints, who do not identify and meet the patient's emotional needs, or who fail to identify the limits of their own practice may contribute to suits instituted not only against the nurse but also against the employer and the physician. The nurse's self-awareness is critical in preventing suits (Fig. 8-5).

Staff members may contribute to a patient's distrust of care through complaining about working conditions, telling patients about problems occurring on the unit, and disparaging other health care providers. There is a distinction between informing a patient that you must meet someone else's needs, and therefore will not return for a specified period of time, and giving the patient the impression that you do not have time to attend to his or her needs.

FIGURE 8–5 Certain things can be done to prevent malpractice suits.

PREVENTING MALPRACTICE CLAIMS

The most significant thing you can do to prevent malpractice claims is to maintain a high standard of care. To do this, you may work at improving your own nursing practice and also the general climate for nursing practice where you work. You can do this in many ways.

Self-Awareness

Identify your own strengths and weaknesses in practice. When you have identified a weakness, seek a means of growth. This may include education, directed experience, or discussion with colleagues.

Be ready to acknowledge areas of weakness to supervisors, and do not accept responsibilities for which you are not prepared. For example, the nurse who has not worked in pediatrics for 10 years and accepts an assignment to a pediatric unit without orientation and education is setting the stage for an error to occur. Lack of current familiarity with the area is not a defense against liability. As a professional you should not accept a position if you cannot meet the criterion of being a reasonably prudent nurse in that setting. In instances of true emergency (eg, disaster, flood), courts may be more lenient, but "we need you here today" is not an emergency.

Adapting Proposed Assignments

As discussed previously, nurses may find themselves assigned to units where they have little or no experience with the types of patient problems they will encounter. It is reasonable to be assigned to assist an overworked nurse in a special area if you can assume duties that are within your own competence, and allow the specialized nurse to assume the specialized duties. It is not reasonable or safe for you to be expected to assume the specialized duties. Thus, if you were not prepared for coronary care, you might go to that unit, monitor the intravenous lines, take vital signs, and make observations to report to the experienced coronary care nurse; the experienced nurse then would be able to check the monitors, administer the specialized medications, and make decisions. Note that this does fragment the patient's care, and would not be appropriate as a permanent solution, but could alleviate a temporary problem in a safe manner.

Following Policies and Procedures

It is your responsibility to be aware of the policies and procedures of the institution that employs you. If they are sound, they can be an adequate defense against a claim, providing they were carefully followed.

For example, the medication procedure may involve checking all medications against a central medication Kardex; if you do this and there is an error in the Kardex, you might not be liable for the resulting medication error because you followed all appropriate procedures and acted responsibly. The liability would rest with the person who made the error in transcribing the medication from the physician's orders to the Kardex. If, however, you had not followed procedure in checking, you might also be liable because you did not do your part in preventing error. As discussed previously, policies are often designed to provide legal direction.

Changing Policies and Procedures

As nursing evolves, changes are needed in policies, procedures, and protocols. Part of your responsibility as a professional is to work toward keeping these up to date. Are there written policies to deal with emergency situations? Statements such as, "Oh, we've always done it this way" are not adequate substitutes for clearly written, officially accepted policies. Often facilities that are reluctant to make changes based on the suggestions of individual nurses are much more receptive to new ideas when the legal implications of outmoded practice are noted. References such as the guidelines produced by the Agency for Health Care Policy and Research (AHCPR) may provide strong support for needed changes in practice.

Documentation

Nurses' records are unique in the health care setting. They cover the entire period of hospitalization, 24 hours a day, in a sequential pattern. Your record can be the crucial factor in avoiding litigation. Documentation in the record of observations made, decisions reached, actions taken, and the evaluation of the patient's response are considered much more solid evidence than verbal testimony, which depends on one's memory.

Because each case is determined by the facts as well as by the applicable law, clear documentation of all relevant data is important. For legal purposes, observations and actions that are not recorded may be assumed not to have occurred. Documentation needs to be factual, legible, and clearly understandable. Only approved abbreviations should be used. Narrative notes should have clear statements, and errors should be corrected according to the policy of the facility. Liquid erasing fluid, erasures, and heavy crossing out may be interpreted as attempted fraud in record keeping. You should avoid any statement that implies negligence on the part of any health care provider. Although primarily focusing on physician's records, Kightlinger provides examples of how poorly kept health care records actually may contribute to the likelihood of a successful suit (Kightlinger, 1999). Nurses should be aware that their notes protect not only themselves, but often other members of the health care team and the facility.

Properly kept records also may protect you from becoming liable for the error of another, by demonstrating that you did everything in your power to prevent harm, including consulting with others. These records might include a complete log of telephone calls to a physician, and consultation with any relevant supervisor. Documentation should support that you followed all relevant policies and procedures when an emergency occurred. Although it is easy to become impatient with the time required by "paper work," complete and clear documentation is often the basis of a successful defense against a claim of malpractice.

One concern about problem-oriented records and charting "by exception" is that these formats may provide less detailed information and may be less helpful in defense against litigation. This does not have to be the case. You can use any system of charting and record-keeping to provide appropriate and adequate documentation of care. If you identify something that needs to be recorded and cannot find a provision within your system to make that recording, you can be sure that others have experienced the same difficulty. You might begin inquiries toward establishing a clear mechanism for the record-keeping that concerns you. When nurses serve on committees to review and plan charting procedures, it is wise for them to seek consultation with the attorney for the facility; this helps to ensure that the plan for record-keeping is legally sound as well as professionally useful.

ELEMENTS OF A LEGAL ACTION

Any legal action begins with the process of *discovery* and then may be dropped, settled out-of-court, or go to trial for settlement.

Discovery

In a civil lawsuit (one between parties for the recovery of damages) a lengthy discovery process leads up to the trial. *Discovery* involves gathering information through documents (such as previous medical records and results of mental and physical examinations), interrogatories (written questions answered under oath), and depositions. A *deposition* is a formal proceeding in which each attorney has an opportunity to question a witness outside of court, and a sworn verbatim record is made by a court reporter (Guido, 1997). Depositions are often held in attorneys' offices or in a health care facility for the convenience of the health care providers. Sometimes depositions are taken to preserve the testimony of a witness for trial and are used in place of live testimony at trial. Most depositions in which you would participate, however, would be depositions for discovery purposes.

Settlement Out of Court

Often cases are settled before trial because of information obtained in the discovery process. The person bringing suit may be persuaded that no malpractice occurred or that it cannot be proved, and may drop the suit. On the other hand, the persons or institutions being sued (or their insurance companies) may determine that it is in their best interests to avoid a trial and agree to pay damages; this is often done without admitting that malpractice occurred. A settlement may require that no party to the settlement reveal its terms to others. Often the cost in time and money to defend a malpractice case exceeds the cost of a settlement. However, any settlement must be reported to the National Practitioner Data Bank. This has made many health care professionals reluctant to settle a legal action for reasons of finances and convenience.

Trials

A *trial* is a legal proceeding that takes place in a courtroom and is presided over by a judge. Some trials are settled before the judge (or panel of judges) alone, and others also have a jury present. In most instances a trial is a public hearing and anyone can attend and listen to the proceedings. The various witnesses may appear in person or, when agreed to by both sides, a deposition may be accepted in place of in-person testimony. The judge has full authority over all that takes place in the courtroom. The *plaintiff* is the individual bringing suit. The *defendants* are all those being named in the suit. Each side presents its witnesses who are examined (questioned) by the attorney. The attorney for the other side then is able to cross-examine (question) that witness about any of the information presented. The final decision is made by a vote of the jury meeting in private or by the judge who considers all the information and makes a ruling. Monetary awards may be made at the time of the decision or may be established by further deliberation.

THE NURSE AS WITNESS

In the course of your practice as a registered nurse, a time may come when you are asked to serve as a witness in a legal proceeding. Several kinds of cases may involve the nurse as a witness to fact or as an expert witness. When you become involved in any legal action, you should be sure that you understand both your rights and your obligations in regard to legal action.

As a witness, you will be required to swear or affirm to tell the entire truth. Failure to tell the entire truth is perjury. You are expected to answer the questions asked of you to the best of your ability; however, you do not have to provide an answer that would incriminate yourself, nor do you have to answer a question for which you do not remember or know the answer. It is perfectly permissible to state "I do not remember" or "I do not know" if you do not.

It is helpful to use words and terms that can be understood by those who are not familiar with medical terminology, or to explain medical terminology when its use is essential. If hypothetical situations or cases are presented for your response, be sure to note the differences between the hypothetical case and the one currently under consideration before you respond.

Be brief and direct when answering questions. Do not volunteer additional information that has not been asked for by the attorney. You may open up entire areas of inquiry that would not be considered without your comments. It is the attorney's job to ask the question to bring out the facts to which he or she wants you to testify. The opposing attorney will have an opportunity during cross-examination to ask you additional questions that the attorney believes are necessary for the facts of the case. However, be cautious about simply answering "yes" or "no." In some instances an explanation is essential; a simple answer may sound as if you did not perform appropriately (Aiken, 1994).

Witness to Fact

A *witness to fact* is an individual who has firsthand knowledge of the specific situation that is the basis of the legal action. As a witness to fact, you will be testifying to the exact situation and circumstances of the event or events in question. You should always consult an attorney before talking to anyone about a matter in which you have been asked to testify, especially a malpractice action (Display 8-4).

For example, a nurse might be asked to testify as a witness to fact when a person has been injured (for example, in an automobile accident) and you or your organization were involved in the care of that person. Your testimony in such a case might be on behalf of the injured person, to help describe the injuries and the care received for those injuries. For example, you may be asked to testify regarding the care given in a burn center to a victim of an electrical accident who received considerable nursing care during the recovery period.

Another situation involving the nurse as a witness to fact is one in which a patient brings a lawsuit against persons or organizations who have provided health care that the patient believes was below the standard of the community. Medical malpractice is alleged in such a situation. The nurse may be included among those who are charged with malpractice. For example, the nurse may have to give evidence regarding medical record notes, or care given to the patient in the days before the alleged malpractice occurred.

In both of these situations, the nurse's concern is with the specific factual details of a particular case. The nurse will be testifying only to what he or she has observed or done, not to hearsay. When nurses are asked to testify as to the facts of a situation, they sometimes believe that because they have done nothing wrong they do not need legal counsel. The law is complex, and you could jeopardize the position of an institution for which you work, or even jeopardize yourself and your professional future, with unwise statements. The person who is bringing suit may alter or amend the orig-

Display 8–4
GUIDELINES FOR TESTIFYING

- Answer only the questions asked.
- Do not volunteer additional information.
- Admit if you do not remember.
- Refer to your written documentation to support your answers.
- Be brief and direct.
- Do not use medical or technical terminology unless essential—then explain your terms.
- Explain when a simple yes or no would be misleading.
- Note differences between hypothetical cases presented and the one under consideration.

inal complaint to involve new defendants, including you. If you have liability insurance, you should advise your insurance company of your role as a witness, and an attorney will be assigned to talk with you. If you are covered by an employer's policy, you should consult with the appropriate administrative representative immediately to obtain legal counsel. This attorney should assist you in understanding the questions in the case, your role, and how you can protect yourself in the situation (Fig. 8-6).

Critical Thinking Activity

> You have been called as a witness of fact to testify in a malpractice case against a local orthopedic surgeon regarding a patient for whom you cared. You are anxious about testifying. How can you best prepare for this? From whom should you seek assistance and guidance?

Expert Witness

A nurse also may be involved in a lawsuit as an expert witness. An *expert witness*, under Rule 702 of the Federal Rules of Evidence, accepted in the federal courts and many state courts, is defined as "a witness qualified as an expert by knowledge, skill, experience, training, or education" who may testify in the form of an opinion or otherwise. The purpose of testimony as an expert witness is to provide information and opinion that can be used by the court in making a decision. When you appear as an expert nursing witness, your testimony provides an opinion that will assist the judge or jury to understand complex areas of nursing care. You provide a professional opinion, related to your area of expertise, on the appropriate care for a given situation. For example, if you are an operating room nurse, you may be given medical records from another hospital and asked to render an opinion, on the basis of your expertise, as to whether the standard of nursing care given at the first hospital was within the standards of the community. Your role as an expert may not be accepted without question in a legal action. You may have to state clearly the qualifications, including your edu-

FIGURE 8–6 When testifying in court you should answer only the questions asked. Do not introduce other information.

cation and experience, that enable you to make a judgment. Nurses serving as expert witnesses usually have many years of experience, specialty education, and perhaps certification in their area of specialty.

The attorney who asks you to testify as an expert witness should be able to provide you with the information you need about your testimony. Feel free to ask that attorney what your role is in the case, and in which areas you are expected to testify. The attorney is likely to discuss in detail what questions will be asked of you and to ask what your answer would be to those questions.

KEY CONCEPTS

- Law includes those rules of conduct or action recognized as binding or enforced by government.
- Statutory law includes all written laws and governmental codes.
- Constitutional law, which has the greatest authority in any jurisdiction, is found in the US Constitution and in state constitutions.
- Enacted law includes those laws passed by legislative bodies.
- Regulatory law, also referred to as administrative or executive law, includes those rules and regulations established by administrative bodies within the government.

- Common law includes judicial law, also referred to as case law, and common usage or custom.
- Civil law encompasses those laws regulating private conduct between individuals.
- Criminal law regulates actions having to do with the safety of the community as a whole.
- Violations of criminal law are considered crimes, whereas violations of civil law are considered torts.
- Legal rights are derived from constitutional guarantees, and carry with them responsibilities. Other rights are ethically determined, and while not supportable by law, do govern the behavior of health care professionals.
- Malpractice actions brought against health care workers involve civil law. Nurses may be involved in cases related to intentional torts, negligence, or malpractice.
- The individual who is negligent or has committed malpractice is legally liable for the effects of that action. This means there is an obligation to the individual wronged.
- Liability may be focused on the individual, the supervisor, or the employer.
- Liability insurance may be purchased that transfers the cost of being sued and the cost of any settlement from the individual to a large group.
- A number of legal issues recur in nursing. Among these are the duty to report or seek medical care for a patient, protection of the patient's confidentiality and right to privacy, defamation of character, privileged information, issues related to informed consent, medication administration, and issues related to different types of emergency care.
- Nurses also can be involved in criminal cases related to fraud, assault and battery, and false imprisonment. In some cases, however, a civil suit may be brought against a nurse, in which case the nurse may not be prosecuted for criminal behavior.
- Many factors contribute to malpractice claims. These include social factors, characteristics of suit-prone patients, and characteristics of suit-prone nurses.
- A nurse can do many things to prevent malpractice claims. Being aware of your own practice, accepting only those assignments for which you are prepared, following policies and procedures, and properly documenting care are among the most important.
- A legal action may include a process of discovery, dropping the action, settlement out of court, or a trial.
- Nurses may be called as witnesses in trials because of their expertise in a particular area, or because of personal knowledge of the case. You must understand both your rights and your obligations in regard to legal action before giving a deposition or testimony.

REFERENCES

Aiken TD. Legal, Ethical, and Political Issues in Nursing. Philadelphia: FA Davis, 1994

Anonymous. Court case: A failure to communicate. Nursing 97 27(2):32, 1997

Bates DW, Cullen DJ, Laird N, et al. Incidence of adverse drug events and potential adverse drug events: Implications for prevention. JAMA 274:29–34, 1995

Bates DW, Leape LL, Petrycki S. Incidence and preventability of adverse drug events in hospitalized adults. J Gen Intern Med 8:289–294, 1993

Bernzweig EP. The Nurse's Liability for Malpractice, 6th ed. St. Louis: Mosby-Year Book, 1996

Curtin L. When negligence becomes homicide. Nursing Management 28(7):7–8, 1997

Fiesta J. The Law and Liability, 2nd ed. New York: John Wiley & Sons, 1994

Fiesta, J. Law for the nurse manager: Legal aspects of medication administration. Nursing Management 29(1):22–23, 1998

Fiesta J. Do no harm: When caregivers violate our golden rule, part 2. Nursing Management 30(9):10, 1999

Guido GW. Legal Issues in Nursing. Norwalk, CT: Appleton-Lange, 1997

Hall JK. Nursing Ethics and Law. Philadelphia: WB Saunders, 1996

Kightlinger, R. Sloppy records: The kiss of death for a malpractice defense. Medical Economics 76(8):109–113, 1999

Kihm NC. My hospital will cover me. The Washington Nurse. 29(4):32–33, 1999

Lesar TS, Briceland LL, Delcoure K, Parmalee JC, Masta-Gornic V, Pohl H. Medication prescribing errors in a teaching hospital. JAMA 263:2329–2334, 1990

Neufeldt V (ed). Webster's New World Dictionary, 3rd ed. New York: Macmillan, 1996

Tammelleo AD. Malpractice insurance: For your protection. RN 60(10):73–77, 1997.

FURTHER READING

Aiken TD. Depositions: What you need to know. J Legal Nurs Consult 6(4):9–10, 1995

Bates DW, Leape LL, Petrycki S. Incidence and preventability of adverse drug events in hospitalized adults. J Gen Intern Med 8:289–294, 1993

Carson W. Nursing and professional boundaries: Legal barriers to practice. Am Nurse 25(2):24, 1993

Eskreis, TR. Seven common legal pitfalls in nursing. Am J Nurs 98(4): 34–40, 1998

Fiesta J. Law for the nurse manager: Legal issues in long-term care, Part I. Nurs Manage 27(1):18–19, 1996; Part II. Nurs Manage 27(2):18–19, 1996

Grant AE, Ashman AA. Legal issues: Fax machines can land you in court. Regist Nurs J 8(1):16, 1996

How to read and understand your professional liability insurance policy. Am Nurse 27(8):24–25, 1995

The legal side. Am J Nurs (regular feature)

The legal side: Bedside computers and confidentiality. Am J Nurs 95(10):75–76, 1995

Regan Reports on Hospital Law. Providence: Medica Press (quarterly publication)

Regan Reports on Medical Law. Providence: Medica Press (quarterly publication)

Regan Reports on Nursing Law. Providence: Medica Press (quarterly publication)

Regan WA. OR nursing law. AORN J (regular column)

Schirm V, Gray M, Peoples M. Nursing personnel's perceptions of physical restraint use in long term care. Clin Nurs Res 2(1):98–110, 1993

Sullivan GH. Legally speaking. RN (regular column)

Tammelleo AD. Court upholds nurse's refusal to float. Case in point: Winkleman v. Beloit Memorial Hospital (483 N.W. 2d 211, WI;ob1992;cb). Regan Reports on Nursing Law 33(2):2, 1992

Weiler K. Patient self-determination: Is anyone really listening? J Gerontol Nurs 19(10):42, 1993

Relevant Web Sites

Board of Nursing web sites (see Appendix A or links from *www.ncsbn.org*) may contain information on advisory opinions regarding nursing practice in that state

Health Care Practice *www.healthcarepractice.com*

Medical-Legal Consulting Institute *www.legalnurse.com/cer/cer_1.html*

Official state web sites with statutes are available in some jurisdictions

9

Ethical Concerns in Nursing Practice

Only an ethics which is grounded in the breadth of being, not merely in the singularity or oddness of man, can have significance in the scheme of things.

(Salk, *The Phenomena of Life*, 1982)

KEY TERMS

Authoritarian	Codes of ethics	Ethical dilemma
Autonomy	Cultural relativism	Ethics
Beneficence	Deontology	Fidelity
Boundary violations	Distributive justice	Ideal observer theory
Chemical dependency	Duty	Justice

Morality	Social equity	Values
Mores	Teleology	Values clarification
Natural law	Theory of obligation	Values conflict
Nonmaleficence	Utilitarianism	Veracity
Paternalistic		

Morality refers to the rightness or wrongness of an action and is based largely upon a society's mores or customs. Ethics is the study of morality. Decisions that must be made regarding ethical and moral issues are primarily concerned with what is "right" or "good" for an individual. In nursing today it is impossible to escape situations that call for judgments requiring serious consideration of what is right or best for our clients, their families, and the community. Although some of these decisions can be based on the clinical knowledge that you have been developing, many will require additional expertise in the realm of ethical and moral decision making.

You have already had exposure to some of these decisions, such as the decision not to resuscitate a patient, or the decision to withdraw treatment. You already understand that these decisions are not made easily. Fortunately there are guiding principles to assist us in the process. And as you work at the process of applying critical thinking to your nursing decisions, you have learned to look seriously at the assumptions that have been made. Assumptions are often based on ethical and moral values. All of these are good reasons why, as nurses, we need knowledge of ethics, morality, and the process of ethical decision making.

It is not possible in this text to explore the topic of ethics in depth; however, we provide an overview of the topic in this chapter. To assist you in understanding some of the terminology used in the discussion of ethics (and as a point of reference), we have provided a list of definitions in Table 9-1 that are not more fully explained in the text of this chapter. We discuss some of the approaches to ethical decision making, and give examples of its application in health care. We also provide some direct application to your performance as a nurse and to personal decision making. As you read about ethical issues and conflicts, and discuss them in your classroom or with a classmate, we urge you to respect others by listening carefully to them and honestly attempting to understand their positions and their accompanying values and beliefs. Only by considering all aspects of an issue can we seek and find understanding for ourselves.

UNDERSTANDING THE CONCEPT OF ETHICS

In the formal sense, ethics is a branch of *philosophy* (the study of beliefs and assumptions) referred to as moral philosophy. The word *ethics* is derived from the Greek term *ethos*, which means customs, habitual usage, conduct, and character. DeGeorge (1993) defines ethics as a "systematic attempt to make sense of our individual and social

TABLE 9–1. Some Terminology Related to Ethics

Term	Definition
Absolutism	The view that there is only one correct moral principle or code for which there are no exceptions
Altruism	Behavior motivated by concern for the well-being of others and which is intended to benefit others
Amoral	The state or quality of being indifferent to morality
Categorical imperative	From Immanuel Kant's ethics, the view that for an act to be moral, it must be able to be applied to everyone
Cultural relativism	The view that there is enormous variety in the mores and morals of people in different cultures and times and no single cultural position is correct
Descriptive ethics	Focuses on what people actually do in given situations
Ethics	A specific area of study of morality, which concentrates on human conduct and human values (from the Greek *ethos*, meaning character, habitual uses, customs)
Ethical/Moral egoism	When one considers only his or her own good or self-interest
Ethical/Moral nihilism	The view that there are no valid moral principles; nothing is morally right or wrong
Ethical/Moral objectivism	The view that universally valid or true moral principles exist
Ethical/Moral relativism	The view that no universally valid or true moral principles exist but rather that all moral principles are valid relative to culture or individual choice
Ethical/Moral skepticism	The view that we cannot know whether there are universally valid moral principles
Hedonism	A view that good can be defined as that which is pleasurable
Meta-ethics	Deals with the extent to which moral judgments are reasonable or justifiable
Moral	Generally accepted as dealing with what is good and what is bad, what is right and what is wrong
Moral agent	A person capable of making distinctions between what is right and what is wrong
Moral philosophy	The branch of philosophy that examines beliefs and assumptions about the nature of certain human values
Moral thought	Individual cognitive evaluation of right and wrong, good and bad
Naturalism	A view of moral judgment that regards ethics as dependent on human nature and psychology
Normative ethics	Examines individual rights and obligations as well as common good
Philosophy	The intense and critical examination of beliefs and assumptions (from the Greek words *philia*, meaning love or friendship, and *sophia*, meaning wisdom)
Situationism (Situational ethics)	The view that one's actions are governed entirely by the situation rather than by principles or rules
Subjectivism	The view that moral principles are applicable to the agent alone, that what is right for one might not be right for another

moral experience, in such a way as to determine the rules that ought to govern human conduct, the values worth pursuing, and the character traits deserving development in life." Since the time of Socrates and the Golden Age of Greece, philosophers have attempted to provide a logical approach to the questions of human conduct that arise in our lives. Some divide this discipline into three areas: *meta-ethics*, which deals with the extent to which moral judgments are reasonable or justifiable; *normative ethics*, which examines individual rights and obligations as well as the common good; and *descriptive ethics*, which focuses on what people actually do in given situations (Davis & Aroskar, 1991).

Closely associated with the concept of ethics is that of *morals*. This word, derived from the Latin *mores*, means custom or habit. Morals are the basic standards for what we consider right and wrong. Morals or standards are usually based on religious beliefs and, to some extent, social influence and group norms. Together, the two words ethics and morals form constructs related to conduct, character, and motives for action. We typically describe the behavior we observe as good, right, desirable, honorable, fitting, or proper; or, we might describe the behavior as bad, wrong, improper, irresponsible, or evil. Quickly you will realize that such perceptions are based on *values*, and that each of us (and each society) has a differing set of values. Values are most commonly derived from societal norms, religion, and family orientation and provide the framework for making decisions about the actions we take every day (Aiken, 1996). For example, if you were raised to believe in and support the teachings of the Roman Catholic Church, you value human life as beginning at the time of conception. Therefore, you probably would have difficulty accepting abortion as an alternative to unwanted pregnancy. We all have been in a situation in which we experienced a *values conflict*. This occurs when we must choose between two things, both of which are important to us. For example, if you are a new mother you probably would like to spend all of your time with your child; however, if you also must help provide support for the family, and that requires leaving the child to go to work, you have a values conflict.

Most of the time we don't think about our values—we just accept them. We are most apt to think about them when we have a difficult decision to make, when something goes wrong, or when we find ourselves in a conflict because of differing values. In nursing we work with a diverse patient population and therefore are exposed to a variety of values and ethical standards. The need to give conscientious care to all patients often forces us to examine our own values. The process that fosters the identification of significant values is known as *values clarification* (Steele & Harmon, 1979). We examine what we believe is good, bad, beautiful, worthy, meaningful, and so forth, and explore the process of determining our personal values. The process of values clarification assists us in making choices and facilitates decision making, because we have a better understanding of our own value systems and, therefore, a better understanding of ourselves.

At times you will be faced with an ethical dilemma and will be much better prepared to work with the situation if you have a good understanding of yourself. An *ethical dilemma* occurs when an individual must choose between two equally unfavorable alternatives. For example, assisted suicide provides an ethical dilemma for many. Although they are certainly opposed to seeing a loved one spend the last months of life in great pain and suffering, they are equally opposed to assisting with an earlier death. Ethical dilemmas usually have no perfect solution, and those making decisions may find themselves in the position of having to defend their decisions. Although there are times when a difference in values and decisions can be accepted, at other times differences put people into direct conflict. Should you experience such a situation, we urge you to be constructive (rather than destructive) in the methods you choose to work toward resolving the differences.

Critical Thinking Activity

> Identify situations you might confront in nursing in which your personal religious or philosophical values would be involved. What would be the consequences of following the dictates of your value system? Do conflicts exist between your value system and actions required by the situation? If so, how will you recognize the differences and how will you deal with them? Are there any other alternatives? What might they be?

BASIC ETHICAL CONCEPTS

Various authors and theorists identify different concepts as basic to ethics. Those concepts that are most frequently addressed include rights, autonomy, beneficence, non-maleficence, justice, fidelity, veracity, and the standard of best interest. Identifying how they apply to a particular situation and balancing their competing claims often present a challenge.

Rights

Typically we think of a *right* as a just claim or entitlement, or as something that is owed to an individual on a legal, moral, or ethical basis. In common usage this is often extended to include privileges, concessions, and freedoms. Rights form the basis of most professional codes and legal judgments. (See Chapter 8 for more discussion of rights as used in the legal sense.) The discussion of the other ethical concepts is founded on the belief that people are entitled to certain rights. We deal with the issue of "rights" any time we are talking about the right of a person to self-determination. If a patient is admitted to a hospital and refuses treatment, and there is a strong indication that the patient could recover, should the physicians and nurses respect the patient's right to self-determination? The problems that occur when one individual's rights come in conflict with the values of another provide us with many challenges and dilemmas.

SELF-DETERMINATION RIGHTS

Federal legislation has been passed to ensure that individual rights are respected. The Patient Self-Determination Act, also known as the Danforth amendment, requires that agencies receiving Medicare money ask patients if they have advance directives, inform patients of their right to refuse treatment under state law, and educate staff and the community about those rights. This act was created because of our society's fundamental belief in the individual's right to decide. However, this act does little to recognize cultural diversity and sensibility to groups such as Chinese-Americans, who have a unique but different set of values and well-defined role relationships (Fung, 1994).

RIGHTS AND CULTURAL RELATIVISM

Although the concept of rights is almost taken for granted in our Western culture, there are some who suggest that there are no human rights and that we cannot talk about rights, the violation of rights, or moral judgments, because the validity of all moral judgments is culturally relative. In other words, all rights and judgments must be able to be applied to all cultures. This concept is known as *cultural relativism*. Carried to the fullest extent, the concept of cultural relativism would limit us to determining when rights are being violated in our culture (Buchanan, 1996). Cultural relativism embraces the notion that groups and individuals hold different sets of values that must be respected. If the same values are not held by all cultures, then they are not considered valid and should not be applied in any situation. This is an interesting concept to consider in relationship to health care practices with which we, in the Western culture, have great difficulty, such as female circumcision. Although it is appalling to us, in some non-Western cultures concerns about virginity, marriageability, the husband's sexual pleasure, and religious beliefs dictate that female children be circumcised. Members of these cultures do not view this practice as mutilation; rather, it is thought to result in the improved appearance of female genitalia and to be referred to as uncircumcised is a terrible insult (Lane & Rubinstein, 1996). As our world becomes smaller, we need to learn how to deal with such differences.

RIGHTS OF THE UNBORN

There are many times when we grapple with whose rights should be respected. The most obvious example of this situation occurs when we consider the rights of the unborn to life versus the right of the mother to make choices regarding her own body. This issue is one that has continued to divide members of our society and is often an issue brought forth when candidates are running for election. The concern becomes even more contradictory, paradoxical, and convoluted when we consider that some states will permit a late-term abortion; however, in that same state, if an automobile accident occurs in which a pregnant women is killed (thus also killing the fetus she is carrying), the offending driver can be charged with two cases of manslaughter—both the mother and the unborn child.

RIGHTS OF PRIVACY AND CONFIDENTIALITY

An area receiving much attention today is that of the rights of the patient to privacy and the confidentiality of medical information. This has surfaced as a major concern because sensitive health records are now computerized and can be e-mailed, telecommunicated, faxed, or copied to various individuals or groups who may have an interest in the information. In 1996, Congress passed legislation in the Health Insurance Portability and Accountability Act that required that steps be taken or legislation be passed to ensure the privacy of individually identifiable health information. Badzek

(1999, p 52) defines privacy as the "right to be left alone and free from intrusion, including the right to choose care based on personal beliefs, feelings, or attitudes . . . and the right to control when and how sensitive information is shared."

Confidentiality deals with not sharing this information. People are concerned that exposure to personal health information, especially that related to genetic tests, could result in loss of or denial of health insurance, or could result in embarrassment or discrimination in the work environment. The information technology on which we have come to rely for prompt communications creates problems in this area even with the best efforts to remain confidential. Materials that are faxed often arrive at a central location where individuals who should not have access to it could see the information. An employee in an organization could log on to a computer in which patient-sensitive information is stored.

The American Nurses Association (ANA) has been concerned about this issue for some time. In 1995, the House of Delegates of the organization approved a policy called "Privacy and Confidentiality Related to Access to Electronic Data." In 1998, the Board of Directors endorsed the "Core Principles of Telehealth" intended to regulate telecommunication technologies used to provide long-distance care, education, and patient data. The organization continues to work with other national groups on the issue of privacy and confidentiality. As a student and as a nurse of the future, you will want to remain ever mindful of your responsibility to maintain patient privacy and confidentiality in all matters.

Autonomy

Autonomy involves the right of self-determination, independence, and freedom (Aiken, 1994). It comes from the Latin *auto* meaning "self" and *nomy*, which means "control." Some refer to autonomy as respect for the individual and include the expectation that each individual will be treated as unique and as an equal to every other individual (Davis, Aroskar, Liaschenko, & Drought, 1997). Writers may refer to it as the Principle of Individual Freedom (Thiroux, 1998). Other words often associated with autonomy include dignity, inherent worth, self-reliance, and individualism.

When we consider an individual's autonomy, the way we approach a problem may result in the decision-making process becoming more time consuming. It is closely tied to *informed consent* (see Chapter 8), which requires that clients be provided clear and sufficient information about their situation to make a rational decision for themselves. Giving consideration to an individual's autonomy also requires that justification be provided for why the patient is not participating in decision making, if in fact the patient is not. In today's health care delivery system, it is important to respect patients' rights to make decisions about and for themselves, even when we do not agree with those decisions. For example, you may have difficulty supporting the decision of a new mother, who is a Jehovah's Witness and whose life is in danger because of blood loss, to refuse to have a blood transfusion.

As with most other rights, there may be restrictions on the right to choose—autonomy does not mean that individuals can do anything they want. When one person's autonomy interferes with another individual's rights, health, or well-being, limitations may be imposed. Does a patient's right to self-determination allow that individual to choose a certain expensive treatment if that choice would unjustly deny money to another person for another treatment? What if a patient demands a bone marrow transplant that wipes out the health department's entire budget for immunizations? Does the autonomy of a patient with a highly communicable disease take precedence over the right of the community not to be exposed to the disease? If there are to be limitations, what should those limitations be? In what instances should the legal system interfere with personal decision making?

For some individuals, autonomy may be less important than values related to the family. Is this acceptable? Who decides how much autonomy is "enough"? Once again, we must consider the idea that autonomy is predominantly a Western value. For example, tribal life occurs under more strenuous circumstances than we normally encounter; it requires more cooperation, less variation from the norm. The individual's freedom to do things is far more limited because it is directed toward the common good of the community.

Beneficence and Nonmaleficence

Beneficence refers to the obligation to do good, not harm, to other people. It also maintains that we ought to prevent evil or harm (Burkhardt & Nathaniel, 1998). Thus, the concept of beneficence extends from promoting good to *nonmaleficence* (the prohibition of intentional harm). As far back as Hippocrates, physicians were entreated to do no harm. Florence Nightingale stated that the patient should be no worse for having been nursed. The *Code for Nurses with Interpretive Statements* (1985) addresses this issue when it very clearly delineates the steps to be taken to remove harm or evil. Some examples include reporting unethical practice of a colleague to appropriate authorities or expressing concern to the individual who is engaged in practices that result in substandard practice.

In health care we recognize that sometimes we unintentionally do harm to individuals. Nosocomial infections, adverse drug reactions, and the side effects of such treatments as irradiation and chemotherapy for cancer are certainly harmful to the individuals who experience them. In some cases, given the alternatives, a patient will opt not to have the treatment (eg, irradiation). The ethical mandate is that we refrain from intentionally inflicting harm. Sometimes it is difficult to accept that a side effect of a particular treatment might result in harm to a patient.

Good is a general term of approval or commendation, and may be defined as that which produces favorable results, is beneficial, effective, honorable, worthy, respectable, proper, valid, desirable, pleasant, or healthy (Webster's New World College Dictionary, 1996, p. 581). Thus, we tend to think of it as that which promotes life, development, and fulfillment. We view it as "good" when a friend makes a quick recovery from surgery, when a child graduates from high school or college, or when aging parents are able to take that long-awaited trip they have been planning for years.

It is sometimes difficult to decide who will determine what is good for a specific person in a specific situation. In most instances, we expect that people will make their own decisions about what is good for them. But who decides for the infant with regard to procedures such as immunizations that inflict some degree of pain, but have long-lasting and positive benefits? Who decides for the individual who is unconscious or is mentally incompetent?

Another problem centers on what is good. Is all life good, or are there situations in which not living is better than life? Is it better to sustain life in the face of disability, or is it better to allow a person to die and have suffering end? If giving good care to one patient means that lesser care will be given to another (a situation encountered more and more frequently in today's health care environment), how can we defend such an action? What if giving good care means violating good nursing economics (cost containment)? There are no simple answers, and the answers are not the same for everyone.

The issue of sanctity of life is of major concern in the health care arena. Some would argue that all life is good. Others would adamantly assert that life is not good when the quality of life is poor; this latter belief has led to serious discussions regarding euthanasia, supported the establishment of such groups as the Hemlock Society, and has resulted in at least three states initiating legislation supporting assisted suicide. Many people, particularly physicians, believe that the principles of respect for the patient and relief from suffering fail to do justice to the internal values, professional integrity, and norms of medicine (Miller & Brody, 1995). Another example of a situation in which quality-of-life issues also emerge can be seen in an instance in which parents are advised that a fetus has a life-compromising condition such as meningomyelocele. The parents must weigh the quality of the life against the complications inherent in the meningomyelocele if the pregnancy is allowed to go to term. Surrounding all issues dealing with the sanctity of life are religious views and values, particularly those maintaining that all life is sacred. Certainly arguments regarding the "right to life" play a major role in discussions regarding abortion, whether supported by religious beliefs or personal value systems. The "right to life" also affects our personal beliefs about capital punishment.

Thus it can be said that although the topics of medical futility and the sanctity of life are widely discussed, there exists little consensus about them. As a nurse you will often encounter difficult situations in the care of your patients in which opposing values play against one another. Understanding your own values, which may change over time, is important in these situations.

Critical Thinking Activity

Identify ways in which the concept of beneficence has shaped medical and nursing care provided to patients. Do you believe this is a concept that will have the same impact in years to come? What assumptions are you making? Are your data accurate? What are the implications for the future?

Justice

Justice refers to the obligation to be fair to all people. It looks at the concepts of fairness, just deserts, and entitlements (Edge & Groves, 1999). We must ask, "How is fairness defined?" Does fairness mean that people should be treated the same? In terms of access to health care, is it just for one person to receive more resources than another receives? If so, what makes it "just," and how does that relate to the distribution of scarce medical resources? Does age make a difference in what we consider just? Should it? Does justice imply that the government should provide the resources or services individuals are unable to provide for themselves? Can we measure fairness in any objective sense? What should occur when one person's rights interfere with the rights of another? These issues will be discussed in greater detail in Chapter 10.

DISTRIBUTIVE JUSTICE

The concept of *distributive justice* requires the fair distribution of burdens and benefits (Davis, Aroskar, Liaschenko, & Drought, 1997). It requires that all individuals have an equal opportunity to access scarce resources and requires health care organizations and health plans to provide to individual recipients the care and service each is due. This would include the frail elderly, poor, and disabled. Providers, managers, and policy-makers struggle with complicated and complex rules that fail to provide guidance in difficult or ambiguous situations (Maddox, 1998).

Armstrong and Whitlock (1998) cite six criteria that inform the just distribution of limited resources: need, equity, contribution, ability to pay, effort, and merit. Need involves known medical need, not elective procedures. Equity addresses trying to distribute equally to all, although no one would give a certain proportion to healthy individuals just to assure equity. Contribution considers what an individual might be expected to give to society at a future date. Ability to pay is self-explanatory, but to deny needed health services because an individual cannot pay contradicts the concepts of charitableness that exist in our society. Patient effort deals with a patient's compliance or noncompliance with medical advice. Merit addresses the potential that exists for benefit from the additional investment of limited health resources. These six criteria have not always provided a strong basis for decision making, and the ethical issues related to allocation of scarce resources promise to become more complex in the coming years.

ETHICS AND FINANCIAL COMPENSATION

Another issue receiving attention, discussion, and review is the practice of rewarding physicians monetarily or nonmonetarily for limiting care. This process was first seen in the advent of diagnosis-related groups (DRGs) under Medicare that established limits for payment for services (Silva, 1998). Recently, health maintenance organizations (HMOs) have come under fire for rewarding physicians who maintain lower costs of care or for penalizing those who do not. What impact might this have on nurses who are involved in the care of clients who the nurse believes are not receiving adequate treatment? How does this affect the nurse's obligation to serve as an advocate for the patient? These and similar issues are yet to be played out in the health care environment, but certainly point to the need for all nurses to understand ethics and ethical principles.

Fidelity

Fidelity refers to the obligation to be faithful to the agreements, commitments, and responsibilities that one has made to oneself and others. Interestingly, it is one of the ethical concepts not addressed specifically in some textbooks of nursing ethics. Fidelity is the foundation of the concept of accountability that we hear about so often in nursing today. What are the responsibilities of health care personnel to individuals, employers, the government, society, and self? When these responsibilities conflict, which should take priority? In reality, which do take priority? Are nurses obligated to provide care to all patients? Under what circumstances, if any, might this be challenged? What are the nurse's promises to society? Would it also cover areas such as competence? Abiding by institutional policies? Operating within the profession's Code of Ethics?

A situation that often challenges us in health care is that of confidentiality. Is maintaining confidentiality one of the promises that nurses make to clients? Is maintaining confidentiality a moral/ethical issue as well as a legal issue? Are there any instances when it is acceptable to violate the principle of confidentiality? If you are working with an impaired colleague, is it appropriate and ethical to violate a confidential situation in the interest of patient well-being? We discuss this issue in detail later in this chapter.

Veracity

Veracity refers to telling the truth or not intentionally deceiving or misleading patients. From childhood, we are all admonished to tell the truth and to avoid lying. When we are children, this seems straightforward. As we become adults, we see more and more instances where the choices are less clear. For example, do you tell the truth when you know the truth will cause harm to an individual (nonmaleficence)? Do you tell a lie when it would make someone less anxious and afraid? You might see this as beneficence (doing good), but then you have abandoned the principle of veracity. Edge and Grove (1999) refer to the lack of truth telling as leading to a slippery slope, because when we conceal the truth to a patient, it teaches all others involved (eg, family members, friends, housekeeping staff) that health practitioners lie. This deception is later remembered and the concept that one cannot rely on health professionals pervades. In her writing, Bok (1978) emphasized that lying is detrimental both to the person doing the lying and to the person being told the lie. She suggests that it diminishes the person's dignity and integrity, and therefore lying should be seen as an unusual step that requires serious consideration of alternatives (Fig. 9-1).

The Standard of Best Interest

When a decision must be made about a patient's health care and the patient is unable to make an informed decision, it is done in the *standard of best interest*. As the name implies, it is based on what the health care providers or family believe is best for that individual, taking into account tangible factors such as how the patient may be harmed, how the patient may benefit, and physical and fiscal risks. Such decisions are based on the individual's expressed wishes or on documents such as living wills. Health care professionals strive to avoid unilateral decisions made by a health care provider. Unilateral decisions often imply that the decision-maker knows what is best for the patient. When this occurs, it is referred to as *paternalism*, or the deliberate limiting of the patient's autonomy. In instances where parents have denied their children lifesaving care, the courts have, on occasion, overturned the parent's decision on the best-interest standard (Edge & Groves, 1999).

THERE, THERE DEAR... YOU'LL SOON BE JUST FINE!

FIGURE 9–1 Statements that may seem to allay a patient's fear and anxiety actually result in abandonment of the principle of veracity.

ETHICAL THEORIES

It is not our intent to delve with any depth into the writings of early philosophers. However, because ethical theories are mentioned frequently in the literature that deals with bioethical issues, some background seems appropriate.

An ethical theory is a moral principle or a set of moral principles that can be used to assess what is morally right or morally wrong in a given situation. Over the years we have called on the theories of philosophers to guide us in our decision making.

The most widely used theories are presented in Table 9-2. You are encouraged to consider various ethical approaches and discuss with your classmates when each might be used appropriately. For example, an application of utilitarianism (or consequential-ism) as seen in the health care industry would be the justification of capitation in the managed care organization (MCO). Because the MCO pays a certain amount of money per member per month to a contracted provider, the MCO would argue that it has provided the greatest good for the greatest number of members (Stahl, 1996). An example of deontology might be applied to the situation in which all persons involved in a research study have a complete understanding (informed consent) of the study and its purposes. The participant is not simply a means to an end. In applying Rawls' the-

TABLE 9–2.   Major Ethical Theories and Theorists

Title of Theory (Other Names)	Theorist Associated With Work	Basic Principles of Theory
Natural Law (Objectivism)	St. Thomas Aquinas (1225–1274)	Actions are morally right when they are in accord with our nature and end as human beings. Good should be promoted, evil avoided, and ethics is grounded in our concern for human good.
Deontology (formalistic system, the principal system of ethics, or duty-based ethics)	Immanuel Kant (1724–1804)	Ethical decision making is based on moral rules and unchanging principles (or motivations that are derived from universal values) considered separately from the consequences. The fundamental principle is called the categorical imperative, unconditional commands that must be applied similarly in all situations without exception.
Utilitarianism (often referred to as teleology, consequentialism or situation ethics, although there are some differences)	Jeremy Bentham (1748–1832) and John Stuart Mill (1806–1873)	An act is right when it is useful in bringing about a desirable or good end. A second principle allows the end to justify the means. Fits well into Western society's values regarding work ethic and the behavioristic approach to education, philosophy, and life. Applicable to research.
Social Equity and Justice	John Rawls (1921–)	Addresses two fundamental principles of justice developed in 1971. The second principle allows social and economic positions to be to everyone's advantage and open to all. Introduces a "veil of ignorance" whereby persons making choices would not have any specific information regarding those involved, thus choosing the alternative that supported the most disadvantaged person. Supports justice and equal rights for everyone.
Ideal Observer	Raymond W. Firth (1901–)	Requires that decisions be made from a dispassionate, disinterested, and consistent viewpoint with full information about the situation and the consequences available (difficult criteria to fulfill).

ory of social justice, we could not ethically justify using income inequalities or the ability to pay to determine a patient's eligibility for access to health care.

 ## Critical Thinking Activity

> Of the ethical theories provided in this chapter, select the one that most appeals to you and describe the aspects of the theory that make it most attractive. Examine factors that bring you to this point of view. What are the consequences of support of this ethical theory on your professional practice?

FACTORS THAT INFLUENCE ETHICAL DECISION MAKING

Ethical decisions are not made in a vacuum. Many factors exert pressure and demand response as we search for appropriate answers to the dilemmas that we face. All facets of today's world are experiencing change, and nursing is no exception. The realities and new problems confronting us today are challenging the truths of yesterday.

All people must determine their own bases for making ethical decisions. Some individuals rely on formal philosophical or religious beliefs that define matters in relation to what is believed to be the truth or good or evil. Others make decisions based on personal life experiences or on the experiences of those close to them. Still others rely on professional codes of ethics to give guidance on ethical issues. In reality, ethical decision making often involves a combination of all of these factors.

In studying ethical issues it is important for you to understand the many forces that are operating simultaneously in our society. These forces are not independent or mutually exclusive, but act and react with one another in a constantly changing milieu, causing evolutionary changes in all segments of society (Fig. 9-2). The following is a dis-

FIGURE 9–2 Decisions made in relation to one aspect of an ethical situation will affect all other aspects of the problem.

cussion of some of the factors that affect ethical decision making in the health care environment.

Codes for Nurses

Through their professional organizations, nurses have developed some common guidelines to use in making ethical decisions. They are contained in the American Nurses Association's (ANA) Code for Nurses and the International Council of Nurses' Code for Nurses. Each attempts to outline the nurse's responsibilities to the patient and to the profession of nursing.

The ANA code is unique among professional codes because it addresses fairly specific issues and does not confine itself to matters of etiquette or broad general statements. Warren T. Reich, editor-in-chief of the *Encyclopedia of Bioethics*, was quoted as stating, "This is probably the most interesting and responsive code I have ever read" (New encyclopedia, 1977, p. 8). Nurses presented tentative codes in the 1920s, the 1930s, and the 1940s. Finally, in 1950, a code of ethics was adopted. It has been revised several times since then (Table 9-3). Early versions stated that a nurse had an obligation to carry out a physician's orders; later versions, however, stress the nurse's obligation to the patient. This includes protecting the patient from incompetent, unethical, or illegal practice. An ad hoc committee of the ANA also developed interpretive statements, which enlarge upon and explain the code in detail. The interpretive statements were last revised in 1985. The Code for Nurses is presented in Display 9-1. However, this Code is currently being revised. You may check out the progress on this revision through the ANA web site: *www.nursingworld.org*.

The International Council of Nurses' Code was revised in 1973 and again in 2000. The introductory section of this code addresses the general responsibilities of the nursing profession. Four sections follow, dealing with the more specific concerns of people, practice, the profession, and coworkers. In addition, the International Council of Nurses has written a Pledge for Nurses, which is a statement of affirmation and acceptance of the personal and ethical responsibilities of being a member of the nursing profession. Both of these documents can serve as guidelines for ethical conduct. The International Council of Nurses' Code is presented in Display 9-2.

The Patient's Rights

The patient's rights are another consideration in decision making. Ideally, we have always recognized them in some way. As early as 1959, the National League for Nursing formulated a statement regarding patient's rights. For many years, however, health care professionals assumed that they knew what was best for patients and made many decisions without consulting or considering the rights of the patient. For example, a patient with a specific disease was not offered information about possible treatment alternatives, even when valid alternatives did exist. The patient's physician decided which treatment method was preferable, and that was the only one presented to the patient. This is another example of paternalism, discussed earlier in this chapter.

As the health consumer movement became more active, greater attention was paid to the rights of the patient (see earlier discussion of rights). Today patients may expect

TABLE 9-3. Chronology of the Development of Code for Nurses and Distinguishing Characteristics	
Date	**Characteristics**
1896	The Nurses' Association Alumnae of the United States and Canada identify their purposes—the first is to establish and maintain a code of ethics
1921	The National League for Nursing Education appoints an advisory Committee on Ethical Standards. Development of a statement recommended
1923	Task of developing a Code of Ethics shifted to the American Nurses Association (ANA)
1926	"A Suggested Code" published in August issue of AJN to solicit input. Rhetorical and effusive in style; never formally adopted; discussed moral duties of the nurse and ideal of service.
1940	"A Tentative Code" published, expressing more overt concern for the profession of nursing; input sought from AJN readers.
1950	The Code for Professional Nurses unanimously adopted at ANA House of Delegates. The Code had a preamble and listed 17 provisions; several related to personal ethics of the nurse. Response solicited.
1960	Code revised to reflect social context of increasing assertiveness of nurses and increasing sense of nurses participation in the care of patients (as opposed to subordination).
1968	Code revised. Preamble deleted and provisions reduced to 10. Omits, for the first time, any reference to the private behavior of the nurse.
1976	Code revised with greater emphasis on patients participating in their care. Published with Interpretive Statements. Changed the word "patient" to "client."
1985	Code remained basically the same but Interpretive Statements revised to reflect concerns of the day—bioethics, legal language, societal discrimination, effects on the person of technologic advances in medicine.
1996	ANA convened a task force to examine the Code. Task force recommended revision of both the Code and the Interpretive Statements.
1998	Revised draft of code presented to the ANA House of Delegates. Task Force asked to provide rationale for changes and to present a complete document (preamble, provisions, and interpretive statements). Changes primarily addressed content related to whom nurses serve, nurses' duty to themselves, the ethical obligations of all nurses, work conditions, patients rights, and efforts to meet public health needs.

Material for this table primarily compiled from article written by Martha Fowler.

to be informed of all alternatives for treatment and often want to participate in choosing a type of treatment, weighing the possible benefits and risks of the treatment methods presented. The law also has supported the right to informed decision making. Despite these efforts, a recent study done to characterize the nature and completeness of informed decision making in routine office visits of both primary care physicians and surgeons found that informed decision making was often incomplete. The study involved a total of 1057 audiotaped encounters among 59 primary care physicians and 65 general and orthopedic surgeons (Braddock, et al, 1999).

In 1973, the American Hospital Association published *A Patient's Bill of Rights* (AHA, 1992), which outlines the rights of the hospital patient and serves as a basis for making decisions about hospitalized patients. Some have criticized this document, saying that it is rather innocuous because it simply reminds patients of their rights (such as privacy, confidentiality, and informed consent) but says nothing of hospitals that fail to act in accordance with these rights. The AHA revised this document in 1992. In the introduction, hospitals are encouraged to modify and adapt the AHA document to their individual situations and communities. The revised document speaks more force-

Display 9–1
AMERICAN NURSES ASSOCIATION CODE FOR NURSES

Preamble

The Code for Nurses is based on belief about the nature of individuals, nursing, health, and society. Recipients and providers of nursing services are viewed as individuals and groups who possess basic rights and responsibilities, and whose values and circumstances command respect at all times. Nursing encompasses the promotion and restoration of health, the prevention of illness, and the alleviation of suffering. The statements of the Code and their interpretation provide guidance of conduct and relationships in carrying out nursing responsibilities consistent with the ethical obligations of the profession and quality in nursing care.

1. The nurse provides services with respect for human dignity and the uniqueness of the client unrestricted by considerations of social or economic status, personal attributes, or the nature of health problems.
2. The nurse safeguards the client's right to privacy by judiciously protecting information of a confidential nature.
3. The nurse acts to safeguard the client and the public when health care and safety are affected by the incompetent, unethical, or illegal practice of any person.
4. The nurse assumes responsibility and accountability for individual nursing judgments and actions.
5. The nurse maintains competence in nursing.
6. The nurse exercises informed judgment and uses individual competence and qualifications as criteria in seeking consultation, accepting responsibilities, and delegating nursing activities to others.
7. The nurse participates in activities that contribute to the ongoing development of the profession's body of knowledge.
8. The nurse participates in the profession's efforts to implement and improve standards of nursing.
9. The nurse participates in the profession's efforts to establish and maintain conditions of employment conducive to high quality nursing care.
10. The nurse participates in the profession's effort to protect the public from misinformation and misrepresentation and to maintain the integrity of nursing.
11. The nurse collaborates with members of the health professions and other citizens in promoting community and national efforts to meet the health needs of the public.

Source: Code for Nurses with Interpretive Statements. *Reprinted with permission of the American Nurses Association.*

fully of the hospital's responsibility for providing medically indicated care and services. In addition, it emphasizes the collaborative nature of health maintenance, which requires patient as well as provider responsibility. The *Patient's Bill of Rights* is presented in Display 9-3.

Some groups, nurses' associations among them, also have formulated statements regarding the rights of the health care consumer. In some states, the rights of the health care consumer are being formalized into legal statements.

INTERNATIONAL COUNCIL OF NURSES CODE FOR NURSES ETHICAL CONCEPTS APPLIED TO NURSING (2000)

Nurses have four fundamental responsibilities: to promote health, to prevent illness, to restore health and to alleviate suffering. The need for nursing is universal.

Inherent in nursing is respect for human rights, including the right to life, to dignity and to be treated with respect. Nursing care is unrestricted by considerations of age, colour, creed, culture, disability or illness, gender, nationality, politics, race or social status.

Nurses render health services to the individual, the family and the community and coordinate their services with those of related groups.

Nurses and People

The nurse's primary responsibility is to people requiring nursing care.

In providing care, the nurse promotes an environment in which the human rights, values, customs and spiritual beliefs of the individual, family and community are respected.

The nurse ensures that the individual receives sufficient information on which to base consent for care and related treatment.

The nurse holds in confidence personal information and uses judgment in sharing this information.

The nurse shares with society the responsibility for initiating and supporting action to meet the health and social needs of the public, in particular those of vulnerable populations.

The nurse also shares responsibility to sustain and protect the natural environment from depletion, pollution, degradation and destruction.

Nurses and Practice

The nurse carries personal responsibility and accountability for nursing practice and for maintaining competence by continual learning.

The nurse maintains a standard of personal health such that the ability to provide care is not compromised.

The nurse uses judgment regarding individual competence when accepting and delegating responsibilities.

The nurse at all times maintains standards of personal conduct which reflect well on the profession and enhance public confidence.

The nurse, in providing care, ensures that use of technology and scientific advances are compatible with the safety, dignity and rights of people.

Nurses and the Profession

The nurse assumes the major role in determining and implementing acceptable standards of clinical nursing practice, management, research and education.

The nurse is active in developing a core of research-based professional knowledge.

The nurse, acting through the professional organisation, participates in creating and maintaining equitable social and economic working conditions in nursing.

Nurses and Co-workers

The nurse sustains a cooperative relationship with co-workers in nursing and other fields.

The nurse takes appropriate action to safeguard individuals when their care is endangered by a co-worker or any other person.

Source: Reprinted with permission of the International Council of Nurses.

Display 9–3
THE PATIENT'S BILL OF RIGHTS

Introduction

Effective health care requires collaboration between patients and physicians and other health care professionals. Open and honest communication, respect for personal and professional values, and sensitivity to differences are integral to optimal patient care. As the setting for the provision of health services, hospitals must provide a foundation for understanding and respecting the rights and responsibilities of patients, their families, physicians, and other caregivers. Hospitals must ensure a health care ethic that respects the role of patients in decision making about treatment choices and other aspects of their care. Hospitals must be sensitive to cultural, racial, linguistic, religious, age, gender, and other differences as well as the needs of persons with disabilities.

The American Hospital Association presents *A Patient's Bill of Rights* with the expectation that it will contribute to more effective patient care and be supported by the hospital on behalf of the institution, its medical staff, employees, and patients. The American Hospital Association encourages health care institutions to tailor this bill of rights to their patient community by translating and/or simplifying the language of this bill of rights as may be necessary to ensure that patients and their families understand their rights and responsibilities.

Bill of Rights*

1. The patient has the right to considerate and respectful care.
2. The patient has the right to and is encouraged to obtain from physicians and other direct caregivers relevant, current, and understandable information concerning diagnosis, treatment, and prognosis.

   Except in emergencies when the patient lacks decision-making capacity and the need for treatment is urgent, the patient is entitled to the opportunity to discuss and request information related to the specific procedures and/or treatments, the risks involved, the possible length of recuperation, and the medically reasonable alternatives and their accompanying risks and benefits.

   Patients have the right to know the identity of physicians, nurses, and others involved in their care, as well as when those involved are students, residents, or other trainees. The patient also has the right to know the immediate and long-term financial implications of treatment choices, insofar as they are known.

3. The patient has the right to make decisions about the plan of care prior to and during the course of treatment and to refuse a recommended treatment or plan of care to the extent permitted by law and hospital policy and to be informed of the medical consequences of this action. In case of such refusal, the patient is entitled to other appropriate care and services that the hospital provides or transfer to another hospital. The hospital should notify patients of any policy that might affect patient choice within the institution.

4. The patient has the right to have an advance directive (such as a living will, health care proxy, or durable power of attorney for health care) concerning treatment or designating a surrogate decision maker with the expectation that the hospital will honor the intent of that directive to the extent permitted by law and hospital policy.

(continued)

Display 9–3
THE PATIENT'S BILL OF RIGHTS *(continued)*

Health care institutions must advise patients of their rights under state law and hospital policy to make informed medical choices, ask if the patient has an advance directive, and include that information in patient records. The patient has the right to timely information about hospital policy that may limit its ability to implement fully a legally valid advance directive.

5. The patient has the right to every consideration of privacy. Case discussion, consultation, examination, and treatment should be conducted so as to protect each patient's privacy.

6. The patient has the right to expect that all communications and records pertaining to his/her care will be treated as confidential by the hospital, except in cases such as suspected abuse and public health hazards when reporting is permitted or required by law. The patient has the right to expect that the hospital will emphasize the confidentiality of this information when it releases it to any other parties entitled to review information in these records.

7. The patient has the right to review the records pertaining to his/her medical care and to have the information explained or interpreted as necessary, except when restricted by law.

8. The patient has the right to expect that, within its capacity and policies, a hospital will make reasonable response to the request of a patient for appropriate and medically indicated care and services. The hospital must provide evaluation, service, and/or referral as indicated by the urgency of the case. When medically appropriate and legally permissible, or when a patient has so requested, a patient may be transferred to another facility. The institution to which the patient is to be transferred must first have accepted the patient for transfer. The patient must also have the benefit of complete information and explanation concerning the need for, risks, benefits, and alternatives to such a transfer.

9. The patient has the right to ask and be informed of the existence of business relationships among the hospital, educational institutions, other health care providers, or payers that many influence the patient's treatment and care.

10. The patient has the right to consent to or decline to participate in proposed research studies or human experimentation affecting care and treatment or requiring direct patient involvement, and to have those studies fully explained prior to consent. A patient who declines to participate in research or experimentation is entitled to the most effective care that the hospital can otherwise provide.

11. The patient has the right to expect reasonable continuity of care when appropriate and to be informed by physicians and other caregivers of available and realistic patient care options when hospital care is no longer appropriate.

12. The patient has the right to be informed of hospital policies and practices that relate to patient care, treatment, and responsibilities. The patient has the right to be informed of available resources for resolving disputes, grievances, and conflicts, such as ethics committees, patient representatives, or other mechanisms available in the institution. The patient has the right to be informed of the hospital's charges for services and available payment methods.

(continued)

Display 9–3
THE PATIENT'S BILL OF RIGHTS *(continued)*

The collaborative nature of health care requires that patients, or their families/surrogates, participate in their care. The effectiveness of care and patient satisfaction with the course of treatment depend, in part, on the patient fulfilling certain responsibilities. Patients are responsible for providing information about past illnesses, hospitalizations, medication, and other matters related to health status. To participate effectively in decision making, patients must be encouraged to take responsibility for requesting additional information and instructions. Patients are also responsible for ensuring that the health care institution has a copy of their written advance directive if they have one. Patients are responsible for informing their physicians and other caregivers if they anticipate problems in following prescribed treatment.

Patients should also be aware of the hospital's obligation to be reasonably efficient and equitable in providing care to other patients and the community. The hospital's rules and regulations are designed to help the hospital meet this obligation. Patients and their families are responsible for making reasonable accommodations to the needs of the hospital, other patients, medical staff, and hospital employees. Patients are responsible for providing necessary information for insurance claims and for working with the hospital to make payment arrangements, when necessary.

A person's health depends on much more than health care services. Patients are responsible for recognizing the impact of their life-style on their personal health.

Conclusion

Hospitals have many functions to perform, including the enhancement of health status, health promotion, and the prevention and treatment of injury and disease; the immediate and ongoing care and rehabilitation of patients; the education of health professionals, patients, and the community; and research. All these activities must be conducted with an overriding concern for the values and dignity of patients.

*These rights can be exercised on the patient's behalf by a designated surrogate or proxy decision maker if the patient lacks decision-making capacity, is legally incompetent, or is a minor.

A patient's Bill of Rights was first adopted by the American Hospital Association in 1973. This revision was approved by the AHA Board of Trustees on October 21, 1992.

© 1992 by the American Hospital Association, 840 North Lake Shore Drive, Chicago, Illinois 60611. Printed in the U.S.A. All rights reserved. Catalog no. 157759.

Social and Cultural Attitudes

Changes in the attitudes of society as a whole profoundly influence each of its segments. For example, the changing roles of women, the shifting attitudes toward marriage and the family, and the changing status of minorities have all required nurses to reexamine their personal feelings and alter their way of providing nursing care.

Ethical concerns are the by-products of many factors at work in our society today, including the role of the individual and the family. In the health care field this is most pointedly illustrated by the use of the terminology "health care" as opposed to "medical care." Health care suggests much greater involvement of others and places the patient in the center of the activity, whereas medical care places the physician in the key role. We see similar language being applied to "telehealth" as opposed to "telemedicine." The meaning of "consumer unit" is shifting from an individual to a whole family or even a whole community. The focus of care also has changed from one that was primarily disease oriented to one that focuses on prevention and wellness.

The size of the group being affected by ethical decisions has a bearing on the decision-making process. The smaller the group, organization, or society involved in or affected by the decision making, the easier the process of arriving at an acceptable alternative. For example, the Oregon Medicaid system limits care for HIV-infected people based on the reasoning that their average life expectancy is short (Hall, 1996). It is unlikely that this decision could have been made if the state had a large population of people who were HIV-infected. The larger the group affected by a decision, the more complex it becomes. Many of our ethical considerations now involve our society as a whole or, in some cases, the world; therefore, solutions are difficult.

The value a society places on the individual or the family directly influences the standard of care (Fig. 9-3). In Western society, we believe in each person's right to exercise choice based on individual beliefs and conscience. We also place high value on preserving individual life; therefore, we often use tremendous resources to try to achieve additional years, months, or even days of life. A society that placed greater emphasis on the community good than on the individual might not choose to use resources in

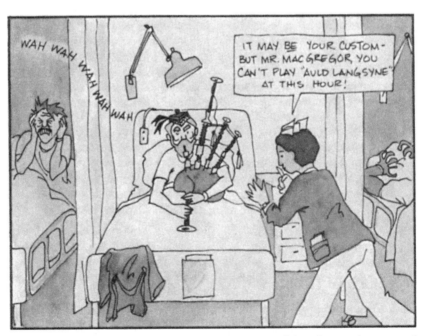

FIGURE 9–3 In providing care, the nurse respects the beliefs, values, and customs of the individual.

that way. The standard of care might aim for comfort without the use of expensive treatment modalities.

A culture's religious values and belief in an afterlife directly affect ethical issues. The Hindu belief in rebirth after death and the immutability of fate affects decisions about using health care resources. Those who believe that an outcome is predetermined by fate will not choose to commit major resources and efforts toward altering that outcome.

The population, or, more accurately, the overpopulation of a country relative to its resources also may have a direct bearing on the value placed on life. The material resources to provide many health services may not be available. Decisions may be made to eliminate certain costly health care procedures even though they are known to be effective and desired by individuals.

 ## Critical Thinking Activity

> Identify two sociocultural factors with which you have had personal experience that could impact ethical decision making. How is your view of this different than it might have been 5 years ago? In what ways have your views remained the same? Why do you think your views have changed or remained the same? What implications does this have for the way you will view things in the future?

Science and Technology

Scientific advancement and technology have left us wrestling with concerns that would have been considered science fiction 50 years ago. Before the development of kidney dialysis, we accepted the fact that people with nonfunctioning kidneys would soon die. After machines that could filter body wastes became available, a genuine dilemma arose over who would have dialysis and who would not; the number of people needing treatment far exceeded the personnel, time, and equipment available to treat them. As the technology became available, the ethical questions refocused on decisions to end treatment rather than on issues related to initiating treatment.

Other technology has had similar effects. The advent of machines that could artificially breathe for someone challenged the medical and legal professions to examine their definitions of life, and brought into focus problems of whether and when to turn off a ventilator. Heart and lung machines that could adequately perfuse the body while the heart was stopped for surgical procedures enabled operations to be performed that were unheard of 50 years ago. Fetal monitors, which can be attached to women in labor, provide a continuous readout of the status of the fetus. Such monitoring has resulted in a greater number of infants delivered by cesarean section. The transplantation of organs from one individual to another has created untold ethical dilemmas. Individuals with AIDS have a limited life expectancy even with the best of health care. Should they be encouraged to participate in research that is sometimes risky in order to advance scientific knowledge and the possibility of future benefit to others? How far should experimentation go? Should it include the transfusion of bone marrow from a baboon? Thus, scientific and technologic advances continue to present some ethical questions for which no answers are readily apparent.

Legislation

Social change and legislation are constantly interacting. Legislation may follow changes in society's attitudes, converting new ideas into law. For example, a greater acceptance of infants born to single mothers has resulted in legislation that changed the wording of birth certificates, and dropped the word "illegitimate." Similarly, attitudes are being challenged regarding parenting by lesbian and gay couples, either through artificial insemination or adoption.

When social change is desired, legislation may be actively sought to require people to behave in new ways. This was true for civil rights legislation. A change in society was desired, and supporters of civil rights sought legislation as one step toward change. Recent legislative action that addresses the needs and opportunities available to the disabled has brought about changes in public policies, procedures, and even architecture.

Judicial Decisions

The judicial system provides a major avenue for debating and trying to solve ethical problems. More issues are being taken to court, and judicial decisions are used more often as the basis for determining appropriate action. As you continue to study this topic, note that we have often cited a landmark decision in regard to an ethical issue. The process does not stop there, however. Some people may disagree with a judicial decision and continue to oppose it. Higher courts also may overturn judicial decisions. Meanwhile, the questions regarding the individual person's role in carrying out a judicial decision remain. For example, although the law in the past forbade abortions, some physicians believed strongly in the right of the individual to have the procedure done. These physicians were upset by the results of abortions performed by individuals who lacked the necessary education and skill to do it safely, and therefore were willing to perform abortions despite the law prohibiting the procedure. These physicians were, of course, liable to prosecution if it was discovered they were performing illegal abortions, and some were prosecuted. The issues of abortion and government funding of the procedure are still controversial. It is not likely that these issues will be resolved in a way that is satisfactory to everyone.

Funding

The financing of health care represents a major area of conflict that has ethical dimensions. The government has become more involved in providing funds for health care. Some people are asking how much time, money, and energy we should allocate to health care, and how those resources should be divided. How obligated are we as a society to make some form of health care available to all? What is it that health care can and cannot provide? Which is more important, prevention or cure?

Health care includes controversial procedures, such as abortion, sterilization, and transplantation; some taxpayers do not ethically sanction these procedures and do not want their tax dollars used to fund them. Thus, decisions about funding challenge basic values.

Personal Religious and Philosophical Viewpoints

Your personal viewpoint certainly will be a major factor influencing your ethical decision making. Achieving self-understanding in values is a lifelong learning task, and undoubtedly your position on various issues will change as you move through life. Values are the product of our life experiences and are influenced by family, friends, religion, culture, environment, education, and many other factors. Because of this our values may change.

RELIGIOUS BELIEFS AND ETHICAL DECISION MAKING

Religious beliefs form the basis for ethical decision making for some people; however, a person who is a member of a particular religious group may not ascribe to all of the beliefs of that group. Some individuals make their own decisions with regard to each situation, which in some cases may not parallel the doctrines of their religious group. For example, some Muslims maintain that women should be completely separated from men, and wear veils when in the presence of men. They would find any health care setting that did not respect this belief to be in conflict with their basic values. Other Muslims do not adhere to this strict interpretation of Islamic law, and women wear modest clothing but need not wear veils. They would be more comfortable in most Western health care settings because they would not feel a conflict with their personal values.

RECOGNIZING THE IMPACT OF PERSONAL VALUES

You will want to consider your personal values when seeking a nursing position after graduation. Nursing offers a variety of job opportunities to the new graduate. In choosing a job, you certainly cannot expect to avoid all conflict or problem situations, but you will want to avoid working in an area in which conflict is constant. Before you accept a position, you may want to consider whether it has the potential to conflict with your basic beliefs. For example, if you were ethically opposed to abortion, it would be wise to avoid employment on an obstetric unit or in a community clinic where therapeutic abortions are performed routinely. In this situation, making your views known and refusing certain assignments after you begin employment might result in termination because the employer may justifiably assert that you agreed to fulfill all the responsibilities of the position when you accepted employment.

Similarly, you might choose to work in an area that supports your personal value system or strong ethical commitment. For example, religious groups who saw value in the life of the dying person began the hospices for the dying in England. Their religious beliefs were and have continued to be part of their approach to care. If you strongly value your own ethnic or cultural approach to health care, you might choose to work in a health care setting where that approach is part of the philosophy.

FACTORS IN THE WORK ENVIRONMENT THAT AFFECT ETHICAL DECISION MAKING

By virtue of the positions they hold in the health care system, nurses have special pressures influencing them as they try to make decisions. An awareness of these factors may help you as you struggle with personal problems in decision making.

Status as an Employee

Most nurses are not in independent practice, but are employed by hospitals, nursing homes, community agencies, or outpatient facilities. Pressures divide the nurse's loyalty among patient, employer, and self. You will notice that codes do not speak of responsibilities to the employer, yet, from an ethical standpoint, you have certain loyalties and obligations to the employer who pays your salary and makes decisions regarding your work. It is not unusual for an ethical decision to involve conflict between the best interests of the employer and the patient.

When discussing ethical decisions in the abstract, most people say that, of course, the patient's best interest should be the only priority. In real situations, however, the issues often are not so clearly defined. If a nurse's decision affects the employer adversely, the result may be job loss, poor references, and a severely curtailed economic and career future. For example, one physician was known to routinely require his patients to sign blank surgical permits on admission to the hospital; a staff nurse became upset with this procedure after learning that the patients often did not understand what was being planned. Eventually, she discussed the matter with the physician, pointing out that she did not believe it was ethical to require the patients to sign the blank documents, especially because they were not informed of alternative methods of treatment. The physician became angry and complained to the hospital administration, threatening to take his surgeries elsewhere. This might have created a considerable economic loss for the hospital and, depending on the action of the administrator, the nurse might have been labeled a troublemaker, and even discharged to placate the physician.

Collective Bargaining Contracts

Collective bargaining contracts can protect nurses in making ethical decisions. By formalizing reasons and procedures for termination of employment, and outlining grievance measures to provide a mechanism by which the individual nurse can be protected, a contract may provide greater freedom. (See Chapter 12 for more discussion of collective bargaining and grievance measures.)

Some people believe that contracts hamper individual freedom. The supervisor who believes that an employee does not deliver optimal care may feel unable to do anything about the situation, because the correction and termination processes under a contract are so complex or time consuming. Often many steps related to notifying the employee of unsatisfactory work and providing assistance for improvement are required before an employee can be discharged.

Collegial Relationships

An excellent climate for ethical decision making can be provided when nurses who work together support one another, share in decision making, and present a unified approach to others. All too often such relationships are lacking in health care institutions. Nurses feel alone and are not experienced in seeking and providing support to one another. Greater effort on the part of all nurses in this area might be rewarding and is certainly long overdue.

Authoritarian and Paternalistic Backgrounds

The historically authoritarian and paternalistic attitudes of physicians and hospitals often have relegated nurses, most of whom are women, to dependent and subservient roles. These role differentiations have discouraged nurses from taking independent stands on issues, and they continue to affect relationships in the health care field. In some settings, ethical decisions are made without the participation of nurses, yet nurses are expected to implement the decisions.

More nurses are speaking out against an approach that leaves them out of the decision-making process. Nurses today might expect a physician to discuss the possibly futile treatment of a critically ill patient with the patient, with the family, and with the nursing staff. The patient would be encouraged to express personal needs, the family's views would be included, and the nurses' input would be part of the decision-making process regarding the medical plan of care.

If a nurse makes an ethical decision on the basis of the patient's best interest, but contrary to the physician's or hospital's interest, public support may be forthcoming. The public increasingly sees health care as big business, and tends to support those who champion consumer interests that conflict with the institution's interests. This support may be short lived, and therefore should not be relied on for protection against the adverse consequences of an ethical decision.

Ethics Committees in Health Care

Many hospitals have had ethics committees for years. Such committees traditionally were composed of physicians and existed for the purpose of monitoring the behavior of physicians. They acted when a physician's inappropriate behavior, such as arriving at the hospital intoxicated, was reported to them. Today the scope of ethics committees has enlarged considerably. Membership has grown, and representatives of the hospital administration, the community, and a variety of health care disciplines are being included. An ethicist may serve as a consultant or as a member of the committee. If nurses participate, a formal mechanism allows them to share in ethical decision making.

With their expertise and experience, the members of ethics committees help individuals who must make ethical decisions to identify whether they have all the relevant information, to determine other options they have not considered, and to compare the situation with basic ethical principles and theories. Often the committee acts in an advisory capacity to medical staff members and families struggling with difficult decision making. Ethics committees may also help institutions establish policies in regard to ethical concerns that tend to recur in that setting.

Consumer Involvement in Health Care

With consumers involved in decision making, nurses again may face situations in which they are expected to take action based on the conclusions of others. Many nurses may find this problematic. For example, an elderly diabetic who has gangrene of the foot may refuse amputation, saying, "If I'm going to die, I'm going to die whole." The nurse, recognizing the lifesaving benefit of the amputation, may have difficulty maintaining effective communication and rapport with the patient and family, because of her own convictions that an amputation is the best treatment. Mental health is another area in health care in which nurses may struggle. Patients may refuse to comply with the recommended treatment and as a result live in a homeless, psychiatrically unhealthy situation. This also is very difficult for family members.

A FRAMEWORK FOR ETHICAL DECISION MAKING

When faced with ethical decisions, most of us hope to find the "right" answers. Unfortunately, a right answer may not exist for everyone or every situation; such is the nature of dilemmas. However, you can proceed from a basic framework that encourages you to look beyond your first thoughts or feelings to basic issues. A great deal has been written about the decision-making process in the last two decades—more in recent years than before. Along with this, several models have been developed to assist us with ethical decision making (Curtin, 1978; Thompson & Thompson, 1981; Jameton, 1984; Milner, 1993). The steps identified below, gleaned from various approaches, offers a process you can use to guide you in this task. In studying it, you will realize it is not much different than the nursing process with which you are already familiar.

Identify and Clarify the Ethical Problem

To define the ethical concern with which you are struggling, you need to review the situation and gain as clear a perception of the problem as possible. Is there something wrong? How deep does the issue go? Are there legal or institutional concerns? What is the decision to be made? You need to clarify information about which you are not certain. Consider what ethical principles might be involved. Are those principles in conflict? Who are the relevant parties to this decision? What are their values? Ask yourself what your role and relationship to the problem is. Is this really someone else's decision, which you should not assume, or is it one in which a collaborative decision must be made? What are the time boundaries for making this decision? What other factors influence the decision?

Gather Data

It is important to have as much information about the unique situation as possible. The facts of the situation make a difference in what options are possible. Remember that there is no magic pattern or formula to facts in most situations; they are screened through each person's background and experience. What clearly appears to be a "true fact" to one person may seem to be "opinion" to another. Therefore, seeking other viewpoints may help you to see the situation more clearly. You need to identify the relevant people in the situation and understand their concerns and perspectives as much as possible. Consider whether legal cases might affect decision making in this case.

Identify Options

Most ethical problems have more than one possible solution. If only one solution existed, there would be no ethical dilemma, because there would be no choice. In some cases more than one solution may be satisfactory; in others, none of the options will seem satisfactory. The more options you can identify, the more likely you are to find one you can support. What is the range of actions that could be taken? What would be the anticipated outcome of those actions? For each option, consider its impact on each person involved. Also think about the impact on society as a whole if this option were chosen. Consider the ethical theories presented and explore how each option compares with the basic principles of each theory. In this way, you might determine that one option is basically a utilitarian approach (seeking the greatest good for the greatest number), whereas another is clearly supporting a deontological position of doing one's duty. Which option does the greatest good while at the same time doing the least harm? Which option respects the rights and dignity of all persons involved? Is one approach more appropriate than another in this situation? Is this approach in keeping with your own moral and ethical position?

Make a Decision

At some point, you have to make a decision. This is often difficult and in some instances painful. However, refusing to make a decision that is yours is not a responsible position and, in fact, doing nothing is indeed making a decision. There will never be enough time, enough data, or enough alternatives in some situations. No matter how thorough your analysis or how carefully you weigh all competing claims, you may still be left with uncomfortable feelings. When dealing with these feelings, you might think ahead to the action you plan to take. If you explained to someone you respect why you chose this option, what would that individual say?

Act and Assess

Once you have chosen a course of action, you must carry out your decision. This may involve working with others or personally carrying out plans. Assess the outcomes as you proceed. Unforeseen outcomes are common in ethical situations. Share your thoughts and concerns with others as you proceed, and continue to seek new insights into the situation. As you assess the outcome in this particular situation, consider its relevance for a wider range of situations and concerns. Use this situation as a foundation from which to grow and develop. Ask yourself, "What have I learned from this experience that will be useful in the future?" "What would I do in another situation?" "What would I change?"

SPECIFIC ETHICAL ISSUES RELATED TO THE PROFESSION OF NURSING

Some ethical issues of concern to nurses relate specifically to the nursing profession; others relate to bioethical issues confronting all of society. In this section we discuss the issues facing nurses through commitment to the patient, commitment to personal excellence, and commitment to the nursing profession as a whole. Bioethical issues that relate to the whole society are discussed in Chapter 10. We present a definite viewpoint regarding ethics in the nursing profession. We feel strongly about the individual nurse's responsibility for nursing practice and place high value on personal integrity in professional relationships.

Commitment to the Patient

Nursing has a strong history of being committed to the well-being of patients who need care. Both the ANA Code for Nurses and the International Code for Nurses, presented earlier in this chapter, clearly point out the nurse's obligation to fulfill this commitment. This obligation has been used to try to persuade nurses that they must not be concerned for themselves, their working conditions, their salaries, or other aspects of their employment. This is not realistic, and may even be counterproductive to the development of effective, autonomous nurses. However, rejection of the handmaiden philosophy does not require rejection of a basic philosophy that nursing is focused on providing patients and their families with support for growth toward maximum health and well-being. Patients can never become objects for nursing, but must be approached as unique individuals who deserve concern, respect, and the best we have to offer.

Recommending a Care Provider

Patients and acquaintances may ask you to recommend a physician or other care provider because they believe that, as a nurse, you have special knowledge and insight in such matters. In the past, nurses were admonished not to express opinions about care providers and were encouraged to direct patients to the yellow pages, directories, or hospitals that referred patients to staff physicians on a rotating basis. If you have no personal knowledge about the requested information, then this would be a reasonable approach, or you might honestly tell an individual requesting information that you have no personal or professional knowledge regarding a particular care provider. But if you do have knowledge, it seems inappropriate to sidestep the issue. You could recommend several competent persons, pointing out characteristics of each that might be factors in personal choice. For example, if you were asked to recommend an obstetrician, you might recommend three. You then could state further that Drs. A, B, and C are all board-certified specialists in obstetrics. You might add some information about their practices: Dr. A is an older physician with a more traditional approach to childbirth; Dr. B is a young and innovative physician who strongly advocates father participation and the Lamaze natural childbirth method; Dr. C is new in the community but appears to allow patients a great deal of choice in their approach to childbirth. The patient can further research these physicians and make a personal choice.

If you are asked specifically about a physician whose care you believe to be less than satisfactory, you are faced with a different dilemma. Making severely critical statements might leave you open to a legal charge of slander by the physician (see Chapter 8). However, saying nothing is ethically a problem because you are not acting to protect the patient. A safe approach is to state, "I personally would not choose Dr. X as my physician. Instead I would prefer to see Dr. N or Dr. O." If pressed to give reasons, you are legally more secure if you say that you would prefer not to discuss specifics.

You need to be careful that any recommendations are not based on hearsay or gossip. If you do not have solid information on which to base a referral, do not be drawn into making one. Being a nurse does not obligate you to be an expert on all health care questions.

Confronting Substandard Care

The day has passed when nurses could be expected to provide unwavering support of all members of the health care team, whatever their actions and whatever the outcome for the patient. Concern for the welfare of patients requires that nurses acknowledge the existence of substandard care and work toward change. We see the issue in terms of the form and extent the involvement should take, rather than whether the nurse should become involved.

This issue is complicated by many factors. First of all, you need to consider whose care you are criticizing. If it is the care of another nurse, or a care provider with less educational preparation than you possess, the situation is more straightforward. If you have questions about medical care delivered or the action of a physician, it becomes more difficult, especially if you are concerned about the medical actions taken. Many would suggest that as a registered nurse you do not have the necessary knowledge to challenge medical practice. You want to be careful about how you proceed, referring to hospital policy manuals, trusted colleagues, and your supervisor for advice before proceeding.

When you observe a colleague practicing what you think is poor patient care, such as poor sterile technique, it is not as difficult. Various avenues of action are available to you. What you choose to do depends on the seriousness of the situation you have observed.

Usually the simplest and most effective solution to any problem is to go directly to the person involved and to state: "I observed this specific incident, and it seemed to me that it was not in the best interest of the patient because . . . What is your perception of the situation?" With this response, you are not making accusations of poor nursing and it allows the nurse to give a rationale for the action taken. When you understand the situation more fully, you may have a different point of view. If you disagree with your colleague and the situation is not critical, you might want to state simply that you do disagree. Sometimes just calling an incident to the attention of the person will result in a change in behavior, even if there is no open agreement that a change is needed.

If you observe poor care a second time, you might again approach the person. State what you have seen, and note that it is the second time. If the person still disagrees that a problem exists, state that you feel obligated to discuss this with your immediate superior, because it is not in the best interest of the patient. You should then follow through on this.

If you have a reputation on the unit for maintaining a focus that enhances the welfare of patients, and you have been quick to praise the good care provided by others, your action in response to poor care will be more readily accepted. Remember that your attitude when approaching another nurse is crucial. Facial expressions and tone of voice, as well as words, need to be considered. If you are perceived as friendly and caring, your comments probably will be accepted in a far different manner than if you are seen as being negative and critical.

However, you cannot always count on this reaction. Many nurses feel threatened by the idea of evaluation, or have had bad experiences in which evaluation only involved pointing out deficiencies. These nurses may be angry and upset with any colleague who considers evaluation part of the colleague role. There is a great deal of pressure in these situations to close your eyes to what is happening around you and concentrate only on your own care. The following is a suggested plan for action in such situations.

A BASIC PATTERN FOR ACTION

The first step in any situation in which you believe substandard care exists is to collect adequate, valid information. It is most desirable if you have personally observed the behavior that you believe to be substandard. Do not make decisions based on gossip, hearsay, or a single isolated instance. If you do, you may create problems for yourself rather than solving problems for the patient. Sometimes a single incident is serious enough that you want to act, but before taking action be sure of your facts.

Your second step is to be certain you understand both the official and the unofficial systems of authority and responsibility within your facility—the formal and the informal operations of the organization and the laws of the state in which you are practicing. In some states, laws exist requiring that poor practice be reported directly to the relevant licensing board. You need to know which people have the authority to make decisions and changes, what the official prescribed route of change is, and what the hidden priorities of the institution might be. For example, the official lines of authority may provide the physician who has been elected chief of staff with authority within the medical group. Your knowledge of the informal system may reveal that a certain respected physician who does not have an official position actually is able to exert more influence for change. Within the nursing chain of responsibility, you may be aware that the head nurse of your unit, although officially having authority, in reality refers all decision making to the supervisor. The head nurse's role may actually be one of information gatherer and sharer.

It is most commonly recommended that once you are certain of your data and know how the system works in your organization, you take concerns to your immediate supervisor. Many people believe that reporting to a supervisor fulfills your ethical responsibility as well as your legal responsibility. If the system always worked effectively, your supervisor would forward the concern until it reached the individual or committee with the authority and duty to act.

When you approach a supervisor, you need to give specific information that includes the dates, situations, and the action you took. You should not indulge in generalities or sweeping statements, but should stick to specific observed instances by simply describing what you saw. Let the supervisor know that you have talked with the person under discussion and have informed the person that you would speak with the supervisor. It is important to specify the action you would like to see occur. You might ask the supervisor to discuss the matter with both of you to clarify the correct nursing procedure. Or you might ask the supervisor to discuss the matter with the other nurse or observe the nurse. A vague declaration of "You need to do something about this!" is not helpful. It is also important to remember that once you have initiated this action, you may be involved in some follow-up.

If you observe an incident that has the potential to cause a patient danger (eg, an unreported medication error) or one that has legal ramifications (eg, the falsifying of narcotic records), you have a legal as well as an ethical responsibility to go immediately to a supervisor with your information. In a situation that has the potential for legal involvement, it is prudent to keep an exact personal record of your observations and actions. Your record should include times and dates of incidents and of your reporting efforts (see Chapter 8).

ALTERNATIVE APPROACHES FOR ACTION

At times, the system does not always work as expected. Your concern regarding what you perceive as poor practice may be dropped or ignored at any one of many points. You may never learn what was done, even when positive action was taken, because of the constraints of confidentiality for the affected employee. Occasionally, results emerge only much later, when a change in procedure and policy occurs.

Often there are good reasons for this. Perhaps the persons in authority want to collect more specific data about a situation, with as little general discussion as possible. Sometimes there are aspects of a legal contract or a collective bargaining contract of which you are unaware that must be considered in the actions that are taken. Other times, professional confidentiality may make it seem that nothing is being done when, in fact, steps have been taken to correct a situation. It is easy as a newcomer to the health care scene to see only part of a picture.

However, there are times when an alternative initial approach is more appropriate. There are several ways you can bring about change. You may volunteer to serve on committees that deal with peer review. If there are no such committees, you may work to have them established, perhaps through a bargaining unit. This route of action will require a considerable investment of your own time and effort. The cry of "Why doesn't somebody do something?" may often be answered "Because nobody takes the time." This is a real constraint on action.

Another initial approach is to use the informal system within the facility. You may discuss your concern with a trusted person (or mentor) who has influence within the system. You may learn that you are not alone in your concerns, that efforts toward change are being made, and that your input of data is welcomed. Another approach would be to seek the assistance of another individual with power within the organization. However, we must caution you about using informal systems; informal systems can backfire. If your immediate superior learns that you went over his or her head with your concerns, he or she may direct anger at you. Additionally, the person with whom you choose to share your concern may recognize that you have "skipped a step" in the reporting process and send you back to your supervisor. Therefore, we suggest that you use these alternative approaches only when the ones suggested earlier have failed to bring about the desired results.

If your initial approach is not effective, a formal route for seeking further change would lead you through the official lines of authority within your facility. After discussing your concern with your immediate supervisor and receiving no satisfactory response, you would tell the supervisor formally that you intend to carry your concern to the next higher authority. Technically you could proceed in this manner until you reached the administrator or even the board of directors. Informing your supervisor of your plans should help to avoid the problems mentioned above, but you should be prepared to listen to some words of warning from the supervisor or efforts to discourage you from taking action. There are reasons this individual has chosen not to pursue the issue.

Another formal route for seeking further change is through designated committees or procedures within your facility. As hospitals move into models of shared governance, this may be your best alternative. Discussing or sharing a problem with a particular committee might require a carefully written and documented report explaining your concern. You then might be called to answer questions that the committee believes it is important to ask.

A final alternative to a problem in your work setting is to offer your resignation if a change is not made. Continuing to work in an environment in which poor practice exists may place you in conflict with your ethical standards and values. If you find it necessary to do this, be careful that you do not jeopardize your own future with angry letters or intemperate remarks. The old saying, "Don't burn your bridges behind you" is relevant in such a situation. Render your resignation in a polite and professional manner even when expressing dissatisfaction with the system.

Reporting directly to a state licensing board or professional organization's disciplinary committee is an avenue of action outside of the employment setting. The licensing board exists to assure the public of safe practice; therefore, these organizations and agencies usually deal with serious problems that represent a breach of the public trust or serious harm. They may not have the capacity or desire to pursue minor (though still important) problems. The same constraints apply when reporting to these organizations. Remember that their investigation and decisions may be done in a judicial or legal manner. This may involve the requirement that you provide legal testimony in regard to your complaints.

PERSONAL RISKS IN REPORTING

If you decide to pursue any of these routes, you need to be fully aware of the possible consequences. You may be labeled a troublemaker, or worse. You may lose the opportunity to be promoted because you are seen as being antagonistic to the system. It is even possible that you could lose your job for creating too many waves. Officially this should not happen, but in reality it can and does. In 1996, a nurse working in a New England hospital became increasingly concerned about the quality, safety, and dignity of patient care and took action to see the situation corrected. He was eventually fired from his job but sued and won his case (Fletcher, Sorrel, & Silva, 1998). The hospital appealed and lost the case. However, litigation is expensive, both financially and emotionally. We do not mean to be unduly discouraging, but we want to warn you that the role of change agent is not easy, and you should be aware of and weigh the consequences before you decide to act. And above all, be certain that your perceptions are correct and that your concerns are well grounded.

Commitment to Personal Excellence

To meet the commitment to a patient, each individual nurse must be committed to personal excellence. Basic to moving toward personal excellence is a willingness to engage in self-evaluation and assume responsibility in the work setting. It is critical that you assume the responsibility for maintaining competence. (For more discussion of this topic, see the discussion on competency in Chapter 7.)

SELF-EVALUATION

Self-evaluation is discussed throughout this text in relationship to personal career goals, legal concerns, and continuing education. The health care professional also has a strong ethical responsibility to practice self-evaluation. You are the one who is best able to identify your weaknesses and practice deficits as well as your strengths. Your careful self-evaluation is the patient's best protection against poor or inadequate care.

Self-evaluation is not always an easy or pleasant task. If we are truly honest with ourselves, we will be likely to uncover areas we wish were not there. Remember, done informally, these do not have to be shared with anyone; that is one of the beauties of self-evaluation. On the other hand, do not hesitate to ask for assistance if you think you need it. One is seldom criticized for trying to do a better job. Many institutions are now including self-evaluation and the establishment of personal goals in the formal evaluation of employees. If this is the case, you may be asked to prepare a written self-evaluation that will be shared with at least your immediate supervisor.

One approach to self-evaluation is the use of the nursing process format. Begin with a thorough personal assessment. To do this you need to gather data about your own performance. This requires a level of objectivity that is not easy. You might outline areas in which you want to gather data and actually keep notes on yourself.

After data have been collected, you need to give yourself time to reflect on it and analyze it thoroughly. The self-assessment outline includes questions you should ask yourself; however, the criteria that you use to determine whether your answers reflect the quality of performance you want to attain are not included. Those specific criteria must be individualized to the setting in which you work and the nature of your role in that setting. The breadth of data that represent excellent practice for the nurse in the emergency department differs from what would represent excellence for the nurse working in a rehabilitation setting. The amount of decision making in which the patient participates differs between the post-anesthesia recovery room and the outpatient clinic. Thus, criteria specific to your work situation are needed.

Your analysis can reveal strengths, weaknesses, and areas for growth or improvement. Congratulate yourself on the strengths identified and then clearly delineate those areas in which you want to change or to improve. As in nursing care planning, clearly identifying and stating the problems or growth needed helps you to plan more effectively.

After you have identified your problems or areas for growth, it is appropriate to establish a plan of action. The plan is more helpful to you if it contains clearly defined goals. What is a realistic expectation? How long should it take to reach that expectation? As part of realizing these goals, you might find it helpful to establish criteria to identify your progress. Once the goals are set, you are better able to plan appropriate action to meet them. You might consider such things as requesting in-service education, taking continuing education courses, consulting with colleagues, and doing independent reading and study. Some plans need to include specific things to do in your daily nursing care for improvement. To do this you may want to request assignments that provide opportunities for practice of skills. Perhaps you are interested in transferring to a specialty area of care. This will involve communication with your immediate supervisor and may involve enrolling in some special classes.

All this planning should not go to waste. Implementing this plan will require you to remain focused on what you are trying to accomplish. Keeping records on your progress is often helpful. It also provides positive reinforcement when you realize that some of your goals have been met.

Periodic evaluation of your progress is necessary so that you do not become discouraged. Any records you have kept are valuable for this purpose. Sometimes it is hard to identify gradual change. You might even plan rewards for yourself for improvement that occurs. Try not to become discouraged if you do not see the improvement you desire. Remember that just as a reassessment and a new plan are often necessary in patient care planning, a revised plan may be needed in the self-evaluation process. Keep in mind that your overall goal is personal excellence in nursing practice. Display 9-4 suggests questions that can be asked in a self-evaluation plan.

RESPONSIBILITY FOR SUPPLIES

Pilfering includes stealing in small amounts or stealing objects of little value. Many people who are scrupulously honest in other aspects of their lives do not recognize that taking small items from a place of employment is indeed theft. Employees often take home adhesive bandage strips, pens, and other such objects so routinely that they do not even consider whether this is right or wrong. With the large number of employees in modern agencies, this constant petty theft may total thousands of dollars. The cost of this must be passed on to those who pay the bills—the patients. As a leader in the

Display 9–4
SELF-EVALUATION PLAN

Assessment of Patients
- Do I gather enough data about patients and families, including both strengths and deficits?
- Is there sufficient depth and breadth in the data I gather?
- Do I listen closely to the patient and attend to what is being said?
- Do I regularly use all available sources for information about my patients (eg, patient, family, other staff, chart, Kardex)?
- Have I recognized problems quickly so that they did not become worse through inattention?
- Do I recognize physiologic, social, and psychologic problems?
- Is my assessment free of personal biases and viewpoints?
- Do I separate relevant from irrelevant data?

Planning for Patient Care
- Do I routinely seek more information on which to base decisions about patient care?
- Are my assumptions correct?
- Do I include the patient in decision making whenever possible?
- Do I consult with others on the health care team when planning?
- Are my written plans clear, concise, and reasonable to carry out?
- Do I take into account the realities of the situation when planning care?
- Are my plans for care sound and appropriate to the individual patient?
- Do I employ principles from the biologic and social sciences in planning?
- Have I considered all alternatives?

Intervention
- Is my work organized and finished on time?
- Do I maintain optimum safe working habits?
- Do I perform technical skills in an efficient and safe manner?
- Do I communicate clearly and effectively with patients, family, and staff?
- Do I use therapeutic communication techniques appropriately and effectively?
- Do I use teaching approaches appropriate to the individual patient and family?
- Do I keep accurate and complete written records?
- Do I understand and perform any administrative tasks that are my responsibility (eg, ordering supplies, planning for laboratory tests)?
- Do I make the effort to learn about new techniques and procedures?
- Do I function as a team player?
- Do I incorporate critical thinking into all of my activities?

Evaluation
- Do I routinely evaluate the effectiveness of the nursing care I give?
- Do I effectively assist in evaluation of the patient's response to medical care and to ordered therapies?
- Do I encourage the patient to participate in evaluating both the process and the outcome of care?
- Have I evaluated all aspects of care fair mindedly?

(continued)

Display 9-4
SELF-EVALUATION PLAN *(continued)*

Personal Growth and Relationships
- Have I established a sound trust and working relationship with coworkers?
- Do I support and assist my coworkers when possible?
- Do I communicate effectively with others on the health care team?
- Do I seek answers to questions for which I have no answer?
- Have I sought opportunities for learning and personal growth?
- Is my attitude helpful and productive?
- Do I have sound working habits (eg, appearing on time, limiting coffee and lunch breaks to the correct time)?
- Is my appearance appropriate to the working environment?
- Do I use appropriate channels of communication within the institution?
- Do I handle criticism constructively?
- Do personal biases interfere with the care that I provide or my relationship with colleagues?
- Am I doing my share in overall professional activities (eg, serving on committees, assisting with development projects)?
- Am I honest with myself, being neither too harsh nor too easy on myself?
- Do I have personal values and beliefs that interfere with providing quality nursing care?

care setting, the registered nurse is often in a position to communicate clearly to all employees that pilfering is unacceptable. The nurse can set an example of careful stewardship of the hospital supplies.

Sometimes removing supplies is an oversight rather than a planned action (Fig. 9-4). To make efficient use of time, nurses commonly place many small items such as alcohol wipes, extra needles, and pens in their pockets. One hospital unit found that their yearly supply budget for black pens was almost exhausted in the first 6 months of the year. The simple action of placing a basket in the lounge into which nurses dropped everything from their pockets before leaving cut the pen costs dramatically. Perhaps you can be equally creative in helping to solve such problems in your work setting.

Commitment to the Nursing Profession

Commitment to the nursing profession requires that each individual nurse be concerned not only about personal performance, but also about how nursing is practiced. This involves participation in formal and informal evaluation of nursing care, dealing with poor care, and identifying the impaired nurse. Nurses always have evaluated one another in both formal and informal ways. Some people think that evaluation implies noting error or deficiency. Good evaluation is much broader than this. The main purpose of peer evaluation is to maintain consistent high-quality nursing care. This is an ethical, professional obligation.

FIGURE 9–4   Many people who are otherwise scrupulously honest do not recognize that taking small items from a place of employment is theft.

FORMAL EVALUATION

Formal evaluation of nursing care is occurring in most settings under the title of quality assurance and quality improvement. Quality assurance is a planned program of evaluation that includes ongoing monitoring of the care given and of outcomes of care. It includes a mechanism for instituting change when problems or opportunities for improvement are identified. Quality assurance programs are required by the Joint Commission on the Accreditation of Healthcare Organizations and by Medicare. Special nursing projects such as the work done on nursing outcomes (see Chapter 6) have a focus on the quality of care provided.

All types of evaluation first call for establishing specific criteria to be used in the evaluation. These criteria may refer to process, to outcome, or to both. The creation of the criteria is a professional nursing responsibility.

The first aspect of nursing care that is usually evaluated is whether nursing actions taken are complete and appropriate. Criteria developed to evaluate this aspect are called process criteria. One basis for developing process criteria is the "Standards of Clinical Nursing Practice" developed by the ANA (American Nurses Association, 1991). General standards refer to all settings, and more specific ones exist for gerontologic, maternal-child, community health, psychiatric-mental health, and other specialty areas of nursing. Some specialty organizations, such as the Intravenous Nurses' Society, also have published standards that refer to their specialty.

Another basis for formal evaluation is the use of outcome criteria for patient care. Outcome criteria are specific, observable patient behaviors or clinical manifestations that are the desired results of care. The criteria usually are established by nurses who work in groups to develop them. Nursing literature is consulted so the appropriate criteria are established (see Chapter 6).

Several methods have been used to evaluate both the process and the outcomes of nursing care. Conferences designed to discuss the matter to be evaluated are personal and flexible but may lack objectivity. Simple interviews with either patients or staff also lack objectivity, although valuable insight and direction may be gained from them. Direct observation of patients provides an excellent means of evaluation if specific criteria are set up before the observation, but it is time consuming. The method that is gaining wider acceptance in nursing is the audit based on review of the patient's record. If information does not appear in the record (other than situations in which "charting by exception" are employed) then, for the purposes of the audit, the appropriate observations were not made or the actions were not taken. This may come as a shock to nurses who reply, "But we always do that!"

The chart review involves comparing the patient record with the criteria. Often the evaluation is completed by medical records personnel. The accuracy of the review depends on the adequacy of the charting. This is just one of the reasons why you must recognize the importance of your charting and make sure that you maintain a high standard in written records. If audits are being done at your institution, you should become familiar with the criteria being used. These criteria can serve as guidelines in evaluating your own care and record-keeping.

The chart review has raised serious concerns that have resulted in greater attention to documentation, and even revision of record systems. Once the information has been gathered, nurses again take the initiative in determining the meaning of the data and what the next step should be. Because the goal is improvement of patient care, it is hoped that the audit will result in plans to enhance patient well-being. Changes in policies and procedures and in-service education classes are some approaches that have been used. Once remedial action has been taken, reevaluation is done to determine its effectiveness. Formal evaluation of nursing care is successful only if all nurses recognize their individual responsibility and accountability for practice and are willing to learn and grow to enhance patient care.

INFORMAL EVALUATION

An important day-to-day evaluation of patient care occurs informally as peers observe the performance of others. Often coworkers are the ones who are best able to observe a nurse's performance. Watching other nurses also helps you to grow in your own practice. When you observe coworkers, you need to strive for objectivity. A common mistake is to let personal feelings, likes, and dislikes influence our observations so that we see only what we want to see. We may view a close friend only in a positive light, whereas we see only the negative aspects of a nurse with whom we have a poor personal relationship.

Another important aspect of evaluation is examining results or outcomes of care. Two nurses may use different approaches or techniques in similar situations, but both may achieve positive results.

This type of observation and evaluation provides an excellent opportunity for ongoing learning. As you observe behavior and outcomes in nursing practice, you most often will see good nursing care. Do not hesitate to commend others and share your positive feelings. Everyone benefits from positive reinforcement of skill; it helps nurses to create a good climate for personal growth and sharing.

The Chemically Impaired Professional

The *chemically impaired professional* is a term used to describe that person whose practice has deteriorated because of chemical abuse, specifically, the use of alcohol and drugs. There is a strong possibility that each of you, if you remain active in the profession, at some time will find yourself working with a chemically impaired colleague; perhaps you already have.

One would like to believe that nurses, who have studied the physiologic effects of alcohol and drugs on the system, would avoid such abuse. This is not the case, however. Statistics on chemical dependency in nurses are flawed, owing to the social stigma and the subsequent efforts to protect the individuals involved (Sullivan, Bissell, & Williams, 1988). From September 1980 to August 1981, the National Council of State Boards of Nursing collected data on disciplinary actions from its member state boards. Of the cases reported during that period, it was determined that 67% of the disciplinary proceedings involving nurses were related to some form of chemical abuse (Sullivan, Bissell, & Williams, 1988). The state boards have not published data since then. Several studies of alcoholic physicians and nurses have revealed that only a small percentage were ever reported to their respective state boards (Bissell & Haberman, 1984; Bissell & Skorina, 1987). In their discussion of chemical dependency in nursing, Sullivan and colleagues (1988) estimated the number of chemically dependent nurses based on statistics for the general population and the number of nurses in treatment. Although both physicians and nurses are overrepresented among those in chemical dependency treatment programs, it may be that they are more predisposed to enter treatment than the population at large. Sullivan and colleagues conclude that the percentage of chemically dependent nurses is at least as great as the percentage of chemically dependent people in the general population, and it may be that there is a greater percentage in the nursing population based on accessibility of drugs.

Recently, studies have assessed probable alcoholism among nursing students. Marion and colleagues (1996) reported that the use of alcohol by nursing students paralleled the alcohol consumption of other college students, an age group recognized as demonstrating high usage. Their findings indicate significant drinking problems among the students sampled. Campbell and Polk (1992) also have expressed concern about substance abuse among students, and have encouraged nurse educators to identify students suspected of abuse and to educate students about the problem. Sullivan, Bissell, and Leffler (1990) reported that the addiction process was starting earlier, sometimes even before nursing school, and that younger nurses were more likely to use narcotics, resulting in serious problems in job performance.

Why are nurses affected by this problem? Factors that lead to chemical dependency include the stress of the nursing profession, particularly in intensive care units and emergency departments. Frequent shift changes and staffing shortages add to the situation. Unrealistic personal expectations, frustration, powerlessness, anxiety, and depression contribute to the problem. Once the problem exists, denial is a big part of the disease.

Jefferson and Ensor (1982) provide the following information about addiction:

> Addiction is an insidious process that occurs as the result of a) prolonged intake of a chemical, b) processes going on within the individual (including genetic, psychological, and chemical), and c) processes external to the individual (that is, the actions and reactions of family, friends, co-workers, supervisors, and society). . . . Addiction is present any time a chemical interferes with any aspect of a person's life and that person keeps using the chemical.

All areas of the profession are affected by the problem of chemical dependency in nursing. A significant financial impact is realized by institutions that employ nurses with dependency problems in the forms of sickness, absenteeism, tardiness, accidents, errors, decreased productivity, and staff turnover. Early recognition and treatment have been recommended to help offset this problem (LaGodna & Hendrix, 1989). Nurse managers who are confronted with the problem of impaired practitioners may begin to question the efficacy of treatment (Hendrix, Sabritt, McDaniel, & Field, 1987).

In 1981, the ANA appointed a Nursing Task Force on Addiction and Psychological Disturbance to develop guidelines for the treatment and assistance of nurses whose practice was impaired by alcoholism, drug abuse, or psychologic dysfunction. The guidelines were designed for use by state nurses' associations. These guidelines served as a basis for state associations to approach chemical dependency in nursing from a treatment and rehabilitation viewpoint rather than from a punishment viewpoint. In 1990, the ANA developed suggested state legislation to respond to the problems of chemical dependency and drug diversion in nurses (American Nurses Association, 1990). The emphasis in this recommendation was on a voluntary treatment and monitoring program for nurses with problems rather than traditional legal proceedings.

The concerns about the chemically impaired nurse are twofold. The first is a personal concern for the nurse who is afflicted: the illness may go undetected and untreated for years. The second concern is for the patient, whose care is jeopardized by the nurse whose judgment and skills are weakened.

Because nurses, by virtue of their education, are socialized into caring roles, they have not always dealt with the problem in a straightforward fashion. The impaired nurse was often protected, transferred, ignored, and, in some instances, promoted. None of these actions helped solve the problem.

What are some of the behaviors you will notice in a chemically impaired colleague? The following characteristics are commonly seen in alcoholic nurses:

- More irritable with patients and colleagues; withdrawn; mood swings
- Illogical and sloppy charting
- Excessive errors
- Unkempt appearance
- Social isolation; wants to work nights, lunches alone, avoids informal staff gatherings

- Elaborate excuses for behavior such as being late for work
- Blackouts: complete memory loss for events, conversations, phone calls to colleagues; euphoric or "glossed over" recall of events on floor (ie, arguments or unpleasant events)
- Frequent use of breath purifiers, drinks high volume of "sodas"
- Flushed face, red or bleary eyes, unsteady gait, slurred speech
- Signs of withdrawal; tremors, restlessness, diaphoresis (Washington State Nurses Association, 1992, p. 10)

A drug-addicted nurse commonly exhibits the following behaviors:

- Extreme and rapid mood swings, irritable with patients, and then calm again (after taking drugs)
- Wears long sleeves all the time
- Suspicious behavior concerning controlled drugs
- Consistently signs out more controlled drugs than anyone else
- Frequently breaks and spills drugs
- Purposely waits until alone to open narcotics cabinet
- Constantly volunteers to be the medications nurse
- Disappears into bathroom directly after being in narcotics cabinet
- Vials/medications appear altered
- Incorrect narcotic count
- Discrepancies between his or her patient reports and others' patient reports on effect of medications
- Patient complaints that pain medications dispensed by this individual are ineffective
- Defensive when questioned about medication errors
- Abnormal number of syringes being used or missing
- Frequent use of restroom by the nurse; evidence of broken syringes, bloody pieces of cotton in bathroom (Washington Health Professional Services, 1992)

Problems related to drug abuse are complicated by the fact that the nurse usually is obtaining drugs from the supply available on the hospital unit and is therefore in violation of the Controlled Substances Act.

In addition to personal behavior changes, job performance changes also occur in those with drug and alcohol problems. These job performance changes include:

- Doing the minimum necessary
- Difficulty meeting schedules and deadlines
- Illogical and sloppy charting
- Excessive medication errors
- Excessive incidence of controlled drugs broken or spilled
- Increasing absences without adequate explanation (Washington State Nurses Association, 1992, p. 11)

As a registered nurse, what should you do if you suspect that a colleague has a chemical dependency problem? First of all, you need to know what the law in your state requires of you. In many states every professional is legally obligated to report a chemically dependent health care professional. This reporting most commonly is done through channels at the place of employment, but also may be done directly to the State Board of Nursing. If you do not know the requirements, you should immediately learn what they are. In some states, failure to report can result in disciplinary action toward you.

When planning to report you do not have to be sure beyond any doubt that a problem exists. You need to have enough data to represent a reasonable concern. The investigation to clearly establish the problem is the responsibility of the employing agency or the state board.

To establish reasonable concern, collect data and document it, including objective facts, dates, and times that support your concern. Do not confront or accuse the person whom you suspect. For several good reasons, you should not confront the person whom you suspect at this time.

First, the person may become more secretive about the behavior because of the danger of being caught. This will make collection of data more difficult, if not impossible. Personal defenses and denial may become stronger. The suspected person may ask for a transfer to another shift or to a different part of the facility, or, if truly threatened, may seek employment in another facility.

Second, the person may feel attacked and rejected. To ensure that it not end in a disaster, a confrontation needs the support of a knowledgeable professional. With the support of the appropriate health care person, the individual may be guided to appropriate choices for treatment and rehabilitation.

We have already alluded to another reason you should not confront the suspected person at this time. You are still collecting data and documenting it. You cannot be sure from a single observation that a problem exists. There are often reasons why things are not the way that we initially perceived them to be. If the person is someone you know well, who confides in you regarding personal problems, you might use those occasions to refer the individual to appropriate resources for personal assistance and counseling.

Once you feel you have data to support a realistic concern, you should report it to a supervisor to validate your observations. Usually, once you have notified your supervisor, he or she will assume responsibility for the problem, but may ask for your continued assistance with data collection or with confrontation (see earlier discussion on reporting to your supervisor).

Once adequate information has been gathered, agency administrative personnel will notify the State Board of Nursing. In addition, they usually must notify the State Board of Pharmacy if drugs are involved. More investigation will be carried out; records will be examined. If a problem exists, actions appropriate to the situation will be taken. These usually include a carefully planned confrontation by an intervention team, a requirement that treatment be sought, and a presentation of the consequences of not seeking treatment.

The worst thing you can do if you suspect a problem is to ignore it or help a colleague "cover" for inadequacies. The problem will not get better if it is not recognized and treated. The longer the delay, the greater the chance that an innocent patient will be placed in jeopardy.

Fortunately, help and rehabilitation are being made available to those who need it. Many states now have programs to provide treatment of health care professionals with chemical dependency. These programs usually provide a specific contractual agreement in regard to professional practice during the treatment and monitoring period. This is often done without formal disciplinary proceedings. The goal of this process is restoration of the individual to effective functioning. At the present time, 16 states have special programs for chemically dependent nurses that serve as alternatives to standard disciplinary action (Smith & Hughes, 1996).

In some states the licensing boards may institute formal disciplinary proceedings to suspend a license or issue a license with limitations on practice, and to provide monitoring and supervision while the individual seeks treatment. When treatment is completed, the board may reinstate the license with temporary limitations and continued monitoring and support. The goal is the eventual full rehabilitation of the health care professional to the service of the community. Baldwin and Smith (1994) reported a much higher treatment success rate in nurses than in the general population. These researchers further identified that successful recovery was most likely in those nurses who retained their employment during treatment. Therefore, reporting a chemically dependent colleague may be the most caring action you can take.

If, as a nursing student, you suspect that a fellow classmate (or worse yet, an instructor) has a problem with chemical abuse, you would be wise to discuss your concerns with your instructor or with the director of the program. Because such problems typically get worse with time, the earlier they are addressed and corrected, the better it is for everyone. Again, it is important that you have accurate information to report, along with times, dates, and examples of the behavior that caused your concern.

Critical Thinking Activity

Assume that you have serious concerns that a colleague is delivering poor patient care because of problems with chemical dependency. Where would you begin? What is your personal responsibility? What is your responsibility to your colleague? What is your responsibility to the patients? What steps should you take? Do you have a personal liability in the situation?

Boundary Violations

The term *boundary violations* is used to refer to situations in which nurses move beyond a professional relationship and become personally involved with patients and the patient's life. Professional sexual misconduct has been defined as "any expression by a nurse or other health care provider of erotic or romantic thoughts, feelings, or gestures that are sexual or may be reasonably construed by the patient as sexual" (Smith, Taylor, Keys, & Gornto, 1997). At present, there is no official reporting of the violation of sexual boundaries; however, it is the topic of focus groups and workshops conducted by the National Council of State Boards of Nursing. It is of particular concern because it represents a violation of the trust relationship that exists between the patient and the nurse. Between the patient and the nurse, the nurse necessarily holds power, creating a vulnerable situation for the patient. The nurse also has access to confidential and privileged information about patients and their families. The trust relationship must be maintained (Fig. 9-5).

Although sexual misconduct is the major focus of this concern, it expands into other areas of conduct, such as overidentifying with a particular family member or moving into pseudofamily relationships with the patient's family. If this happens, the family may question the nurse's motives, wondering if she is looking for a bequest in a will or other tangible benefit. Such overinvolvement will interfere with the nurse's personal life and even could result in legal actions on the part of the family.

Some early indications that boundaries are beginning to break down include situations in which the nurse spends extended time with a patient beyond assigned duties or visits the patient when not on duty. Showing favoritism or possessiveness of a patient, meeting patients in isolated areas not required in direct patient care, or personal disclosure by the care provider are other indicators that boundaries are being violated (Ellis & Hartley, 2000).

It is important that you are able to recognize situations in which a colleague may cross sexual boundaries. If you believe sexual misconduct is occurring on the unit where you are employed, the steps you would follow are similar to those you learned

FIGURE 9–5 Everyone benefits when boundaries are clearly established and maintained.

to use in dealing with chemical abuse. Documenting the behavior carefully, noting dates, times, and the names of individuals involved is extremely important. Keep your documentation focused on factual information and objective data. You would then share this information with your immediate supervisor.

KEY CONCEPTS

- Ethics is a branch of philosophy referred to as moral philosophy. It seeks to provide answers to some of the questions of human conduct that arise in our life, and attempts to determine what is "right" or "good."
- Inherent in the study of ethics is an appreciation of individual values that are derived from societal norms, religious, and family orientation. We can get in better touch with our own value system through the process of values clarification.
- The basic ethical concepts of beneficence, nonmaleficence, autonomy, justice, fidelity, veracity, and the standard of best interest underlie ethical decision making and may be in conflict in an individual situation.
- The ethical theories of utilitarianism, deontology, natural law, and social equity and justice may be used to examine the implications of ethical decisions.
- The concept of justice has been expanded to include distributive justice that is applied in situations requiring the allocation of scarce resources. The problems associated with the allocation of scarce resources are expected to increase in the near future.
- Ethical decision making may be based on personal religious and philosophical viewpoints, but must always be grounded in professional standards seen in the Codes for Nurses and the statements of patient rights.
- A variety of social and cultural factors including attitudes, science and technology, legislation, judicial decisions, and funding all influence ethical decision making.
- The nurse's status as an employee, collective bargaining contracts, collegial relationships, the authoritarian and paternalistic backgrounds of health care, deliberations of ethics committees, and consumer involvement create pressures in regard to ethical decision making.
- A basic framework for ethical decision making emphasizes identifying and clarifying the problem, gathering data, identifying options, making a decision, acting, and assessing.
- Nurses have ethical obligations to the patient, and must maintain an objective stance in regard to other health care providers, and when confronting substandard care. Commitment to personal excellence and to the profession of nursing also characterizes the excellent nurse.
- The chemically impaired nurse is a concern to the profession and a danger to patients. All nurses have an obligation to report those who demonstrate chemical impairment and to assist impaired colleagues in finding treatment and rehabilitation.
- Boundary violations, a situation in which the nurse moves beyond a professional relationship and becomes involved with patients and their families, has become a concern in nursing. Educational programs to increase understanding of this problem and help avoid its occurrence are being conducted.

REFERENCES

Aiken TD, Catalono JT. Legal, Ethical, and Political Issues in Nursing. Philadelphia: F.A. Davis, 1994

American Hospital Association. A Patient's Bill of Rights. Chicago, IL: AHA, 1992

American Nurses Association. Standards of Clinical Nursing Practice. Washington, DC: American Nurses Association, 1991

American Nurses Association. Suggested State Legislation: Nursing Practice Act, Nursing Disciplinary Diversion Act, Prescriptive Authority Act (Publ. No. NP-78). Washington, DC: American Nurses Association, 1990

Armstrong CR, Whitlock R. The cost of care: Two troublesome cases in health care ethics. The Physician Executive 24(6):32–35, 1998.

Baldwin L, Smith V. Relapse in chemically dependent nurses: Relevance and contributing factors. Issues 15(1):1, 4–5, 1994

Bissell L, Haberman PW. Alcoholism in the Professions. New York: Oxford University Press, 1984

Bissell L, Skorina J. 100 alcoholic women in medicine. JAMA 257:2939–2944, 1987

Bok S. Lying: Moral choice in public and private life. New York: Random House, 1978

Braddock CH, Edwards KA, Hasenberg NM, Laidley TL, Levinson W. Informed decision making in outpatient practice: Time to get back to the basics. JAMA 282(24):2313–2320, 1999

Buchanan A. Judging the past: The care of the human radiation experiments. Hasting Center Report 2(13):25–30, 1996

Campbell AR, Polk E. Legal and ethical issues of alcohol and other substance abuse in nursing education. Atlanta, GA: Southern Council on Collegiate Education for Nursing, 1992

Cohen MM, Cohen EN, Thomasma DC. Making treatment decisions for permanently unconscious patients. In Monagle JF, Thomasma DC: Medical Ethics: A Guide for Health Professionals. Rockville, MD: Aspen, 1988

Curtin L. A proposed model for critical ethical analysis. Nursing Forum 17(1):12–17, 1978

Davis AJ, Aroskar MA, Liaschenko J, Drought TS. Ethical Dilemmas & Nursing Practice, 4th ed. Stamford, CT: Appleton & Lange, 1997

DeGeorge RT. Business Ethics. Englewood Cliffs, NJ: Prentice-Hall, 1993

Detmer DE, Steen EB. Shoring up protection of personal health data. Issues in Science and Technology XII(4):73–78, 1996

Edge RS, Groves JR. Ethics of Health Care: A Guide for Clinical Practice, 2nd ed. Albany, NY: Delmar, 1999

Ellis JR, Hartley CL. Managing and Coordinating Nursing Care, 3rd ed. Philadelphia: Lippincott Williams & Wilkins, 2000

Firth R. Ethical absolutism and the ideal observer. In Sellars W, Hospers J: Readings in Ethical Theory. Englewood Cliffs, NJ: Prentice-Hall, 1970

Fletcher JJ, Sorrell JM, Silva MC. Whistleblowing as a failure of organizational ethics. Available at *www.nursingworld.org/ojin/topic8/topic8_3.htm*. Accessed January 8, 2000

Fowler M. Nursing ethics. In Davis AJ, Aroskar MA, Liaschenko J, Drought TS: Ethical Dilemmas & Nursing Practice, 4th ed. Stamford, CT: Appleton & Lange, 1997:17–34

Fung L. Implementing the Patient Self-Determination Act (PSDA): How to effectively engage Chinese-American persons in the decision of advance directives. Journal of Gerontological Social Work 22(1-2):161–174, 1994

Hall JK. Nursing Ethics and Law. Philadelphia: WB Saunders, 1996

Hendrix M, Sabritt D, McDaniel A, Field B. Perceptions and attitudes toward nursing impairment. Research in Nursing and Health 10:323–333, 1987

Jameton A. Nursing Practice: The Ethical Issues. Englewood Cliffs, NJ: Prentice-Hall, 1984

Jefferson LV, Ensor BE. Confronting a chemically impaired colleague. Am J Nurs 82(4):574, 1982

LaGodna G, Hendrix M. Impaired nurses: A cost analysis. J Nurs Admin 19(9):13–18, 1989

Lane SD, Rubinstein RA. Judging the other: Responding to traditional female genital surgeries. Hastings Center Report 26(3):31–40, 1996

Maddox PJ. Administrative ethics and the allocation of scarce resources. Online Journal of Issues in Nursing. Available at *www.nursingworld.org/ojin/topic8/topic8_5.htm* Accessed December 7, 1999.

Marion LN, Fuller SG, Johnson NP, Michels PJ, Diniz C. Drinking problems of nursing students. J Nurs Educ 35(5):196–203, 1996

Miller FG, Brody H. Professional integrity and physician-assisted death. Hastings Center Report 25(3):8–17, 1995

Milner S. An ethical nursing practice model. J Nurs Admin 23(3):22–25, 1993

Neufedt V, Guralnik DN. Webster's New World Collegiate Dictionary, 3rd ed. New York: Macmillan, 1996:581

New encyclopedia of bioethics includes A.N.A. code. Am J Nurs 77(8):872, 1977

Rawls J. A Theory of Justice. Cambridge MA: Harvard University Press, 1971

Salk J. Phenomena of Life. Chicago: University of Chicago Press, 1982 as cited in Hasting Center Report 25(7): inside back cover

Silva MC. Financial compensation and ethical issues in health care. Online Journal of Issues in Nursing. Available at *www.nursingworld.org/ojin/tpc6/tpc6_4.htm* Accessed October 4, 1999.

Smith LL, Hughes TL. Re-entry: When a chemically dependent colleague returns to work. Am J Nurs 96(2):32–37, 1996

Stahl DA. Ethics in subacute care—Part I. Nurs Management 27(9):29–30, 1996

Steele SM, Harmon VM. Values Clarification in Nursing. New York: Appleton-Century-Crofts, 1979

Sullivan E, Bissell L, Leffler D. Drug use and disciplinary actions among 300 nurses. International Journal of the Addictions 25(4):375–391, 1990

Sullivan E, Bissell L, Williams E. Chemical Dependency in Nursing: The Deadly Diversion. Menlo Park, CA: Addison-Wesley, 1988

Thompson J, Thompson H. Ethics in Nursing. New York: Macmillan, 1981

Washington Health Professional Services. A Guide for Assisting Colleagues Who Demonstrate Impairment in the Workplace. Olympia, WA: Washington State Department of Health, 1992

Washington State Nurses Association. Handbook for Working With the Chemically Dependent Nurse. Seattle: Washington State Nurses Association, 1992

FURTHER READING

Bagwood T. Substance abuse and obligations to colleagues. Nurs Management 21(8):40–41, 1990

Badzek LA, Mitchell K, Marra SE, Bower MM. Administrative Ethics and Confidentiality Privacy Issues. Online Journal of Issues in Nursing. Available at *www.nursingworld.org/ojin/topic8/topic8_2.htm.* Accessed December 7, 1999.

Beckel J. Resolving ethical problems in long-term care. J Gerontol Nurs 22(1): 20–26, 1996

Bosek MSD. Nursing ethics. Optimizing ethical decision making: The decision analysis model. Med-Surg Nurs 4(6):486–488, 1995

Bowden PL. The ethics of nursing care and "the ethic of care." Nursing Inquiry 2(1):10–21, 1995

Browne A. A conceptual clarification of respect. Journal of Advanced Nursing 18(2):211–217, 1993

Browne AJ. The meaning of respect: A First Nations perspective. Canadian Journal of Nursing Research 27(4):95–109, 1995

Buchanan A. Judging the past: The care of the human radiation experiments. Hasting Center Report 26(3): 25–30, 1996

Capron AM. Constitutionalizing death. Hastings Center Report 25(6):23–24, 1995

Conlon C. Developing ethical competence. Am Nurs 26(3):1, 11, 1994

Cunningham ME. Afrocentrism and self-concept. Journal of National Black Nurses' Association 7(1):15–24, 1994

Czerwinski BS. An autopsy of an ethical dilemma. J Nurs Admin 20(6):25–29, 1990

Erlen JA. Managed care and the nurse's ethical obligations to patients. Orthopaedic Nursing 14(6):42–45, 1995

Esterhuizen P. Is the professional code still the cornerstone of clinical nursing practice? J Adv Nurs 23(1):25–31, 1996

Evans LK. Knowing the patient: The route to individualized care. J Gerontol Nurs 22(3):15–19, 47–53, 1996

Farquhar M. Definitions of quality of life: A taxonomy. J Adv Nurs 22(3):502–508, 1995

Fealy GM. Professional caring: The moral dimension. J Adv Nurs 22(6):1135–1140, 1995

Freedman B. Respectful service and reverent obedience: A Jewish view on making decisions for incompetent parents. Hasting Center Report 26(4):31–37, 1996

Gilfand G, Long P, McGill D, Sheerin C. Prevention of chemically impaired nursing practice. Nurs Management 21(7):76–78, 1990

Gobis IJ. Computerized patient records: Start preparing now. J Nurs Admin 24(9):15–16, 60, 1994

Greipp ME. Culture and ethics: A tool for analyzing the effects of biases on the nurse-patient relationship. Nursing Ethics: An International Journal for Health Care Professionals 2(3):211–221, 1995

Grossman D. Cultural dimensions in home health nursing. Am J Nurs 96(7):33–36, 1996

Hendin H. Selling death and dignity. Hasting Center Report 25(3):19–23, 1995

Hughes TL, Smith LL. Is your colleague chemically dependent? Am J Nurs 94(9):30–35, 1994

Johnson E. Cultural diversity: Considerations for ethical and culturally sensitive practice. Md Nurs 14(1):6, 1995

Katims I. The contrary ideals of individualism and nursing value of care. Scholarly Inquiry for Nursing Practice 9(3):231–244, 1995

Kikuchi JF. Multicultural ethics in nursing education: A potential threat to responsible practice. J Prof Nurs 12(3):159–165, 1996

Kroeger-Mappes EJ. Ethical dilemmas for nurses: Physicians' orders versus patient's rights. In Mappes TA, Zembaty JS: Biomedical Ethics, 2nd ed. New York: McGraw-Hill, 1986:127

Laffey J. Bioethical principles and care-based ethics in medical futility. Cancer Practice 4(1):41–46, 1996

Laischenko J. Artificial personhood: Nursing ethics in a medical world. Nursing Ethics 2(3):185–196, 1996

Lippman H. Addicted nurses: Tolerated, tormented, or treated? RN 55(4):36–41, 1992

McAlpine H. Critical reflections about professional ethical stances: Have we lost sight of the major objectives? J Nurs Educ 35(3):119–126, 1996

McGee P. The concept of respect in nursing. British Journal of Nursing 3(13):681, 683–684, 1994

McGrath P. It's ok to say no! A discussion of ethical issues arising from informed consent to chemotherapy. Cancer Nursing 18(2):97–103, 1995

Merrell J, Williams A. Beneficence, respect for autonomy, and justice: Principles in practice. Nurse Researcher 3(1):24–34, 1995

Milner S. An ethical practice model in the age of empowerment. Miss RN 57(5):16, 1995

Morrissey J. Data Security. Modern Healthcare 26(40):32–40, 1996

Morrissey J. Patient privacy requires cultural revolution. Modern Healthcare 26(40):36, 1996

Parmee R. Patient education: Compliance or emancipation? Nursing Praxis in New Zealand 10(2):13–23, 1995

Riley JM, Fry ST. Nurses reflect widespread ethical conflicts. Reflections on Nursing Leadership. Vol 26(2):35–36, 2000

Schneiderman LJ, Jecker NS. Wrong Medicine. Baltimore, MD: Johns Hopkins University Press, 1995

Sherry D. Autonomy vs. beneficence. Home Healthcare Nurse 8(6):13–15, 1990

Smith G. Attitudes of nurse managers and assistant nurse managers toward chemically impaired colleagues. Image 24(4):295–300, 1992

Smith KV. Ethical decision-making in nursing: Implications for continuing education. Journal of Continuing Education in Nursing 27(1):42–45, 1996

Spindel PG, Suarez SH. Informed consent and home birth. Journal of Nurse-Midwifery 40(6):541–554, 1995

Sugirtharjah S. The notion of respect in Asian traditions. British Journal of Nursing 3(14):739–741, 1994

Tallon RW. Computer-based patient records: Hype versus reality. Nurs Management 27(3):53–56, 1996

Taylor C. Medical futility and nursing. Image: Journal of Nursing Scholarship 27(4):301–306, 1995

Taylor SL. Quandary at the crossroads: Paternalism versus advocacy surrounding end-of-treatment decisions. Am J Hosp Palliat Care 12(4):43–46, 1995

Wennerstrom PA, Rooda LA. Attitudes and perceptions of nursing students toward chemically impaired nurses: Implications for nursing education. J Nurs Educ 35(5):237–239, 1996

Whitbeck C. Ethics as design: Doing justice to moral problems. Hastings Center Report. 26(3):9–16, 1996

Relevant Web Sites

The American Nurses Organization *www.nursingworld.org/* (Click on Ethics and Human Rights)

Hastings Center *www.hastingscenter.org/*

John Hopkins University Center *www.med.jhu.edu/bioethics_institute*

Midwest Center *www.midbio.org/*

National Catholic Bioethics Center *www.ncbcenter.org/*

National Reference Center for Bioethics Literature *www.georgetown.edu/research/nrcbl/*

Nursing Ethics Network *www/bc.edu/nursing/ethics*

Poynter Center *www.indiana.ceu/~poynter/index.html*

University of British Columbia Center *www.ethics.ubc.ca/*

10

Bioethical Issues in Health Care

Ironically, while the desire for progress leads to greater knowledge and innovation, it also raises the general level of discontent with the status quo, which tends to be seen as inadequate in light of the future possibilities.

(Callahan, 1997)

OBJECTIVES

After completing this chapter, you should be able to:

1. Analyze why bioethical issues are a concern to nurses and to nursing.

2. Examine the controversy surrounding the Human Genome Project, identifying the potentials for both positive and negative outcomes resulting from this information.

3. Outline the history of family planning in the United States and discuss how various value systems and beliefs have affected it.

4. List some of the ethical and legal problems associated with artificial insemination, surrogate motherhood, and in vitro fertilization.

5. Discuss the problems associated with determining when death has occurred.

6. Analyze the multiple factors in right-to-die issues, including the difference between active and passive euthanasia.

7. Analyze the various arguments related to withholding and withdrawing treatment.

8. Discuss the ethics that establishes the foundation for providing clients with informed consent and involving them in decisions regarding treatment.

9. Identify the major concerns associated with organ transplantation.

10. Discuss the multiple concerns that affect decisions regarding the treatment of the mentally ill.

11. Outline concerns related to the rationing of health care.

K E Y   T E R M S

Abortion (spontaneous, therapeutic, elective)

Advance directives

Age of consent

Amniocentesis

Artificial insemination

Assisted death

Behavior control

Bioethics

Death

Durable power of attorney for health care

Emancipation of a minor

Eugenics

Euthanasia

Gene therapy

Genetic mother

Genetic screening

Genetics

Gestational mother

Family planning

Futile treatment

Informed consent

In vitro fertilization

Living will

Mature minor

Negative euthanasia

Negative right simpliciter

Organ procurement

Organ transplantation

Patient self-determination (PSD)

Positive euthanasia

Property rights

Rationing

Right to die

Scarce medical resources

Spare-the-mother syndrome

Surrogate mother

Withdrawing/withholding treatment

Wrongful birth

Xenografts/ xenotransplantation

ioethics is the study of ethical issues that result from technologic and scientific advances, especially as they are used in biology and medicine. This area of study is also called biomedical ethics because of its association with medical practices. It is a subdiscipline within the larger discipline of ethics, which (as discussed in Chapter 9) is the philosophical study of morality, or what is right and what is wrong. Today more than ever, nurses and their patients need to keep pace with the technologic changes occurring in health care. The choices that must be made by patients and caregivers are the result of changes that were not a part of our decision making in earlier times.

This chapter discusses some of the choices with which nurses and their clients must grapple. It should be read, studied, and discussed within the framework of the information concerning ethical decision making that was provided earlier. The content of the chapter should provide a basis with which you can look at judicial rulings, legal mandates, and social standards, and how they can be used to assist in resolving concerns with which we are faced in health care delivery. You have had some experience in looking at what is right or wrong with regard to your personal professional practice. This chapter examines more specifically the issues that apply to the bioethics of patient care.

MAJOR AREAS WHERE BIOETHICS ARE APPLIED

The bioethical issues surrounding the delivery of health care grow in number each year. They are always in the process of changing and taking on new scope and proportions.

At an earlier time, most of the truly serious debates related to birth, death, or the processes that bring a person to either point. Today, issues related to birth and death represent just the "tip of the iceberg." Of equal or greater concern are such matters as universal access to health care and insurance for all, rationing of health care, cost containment and quality of care, where and how federal dollars should be spent with regard to the nation's health, and the obligation of others to assist the homeless.

It is estimated that our society currently spends 13.7% of the gross domestic product (GDP) on health care—more than a trillion dollars each year. This amount was calculated to increase to $1.7 trillion by the year 2000, when it will equal approximately 18.1% of the GDP (Edge & Groves, 1999). As a nation, our population is getting older and living longer, with the health needs of the elderly placing an even greater burden on an already stressed system. Because of lifestyle changes and medical breakthroughs, today many persons live to reach old age. Life expectancy has increased a year or two in each recent decade; in the United States, the life expectancy for females born today is 79.1 years and for males, 72.3, compared with 47 years at the beginning of the 20th century. Diseases such as Alzheimer's and AIDS, for which no cures exist at this time, have increased in prevalence. New technologies have led to treatments that were not available 15 years ago; rather than decreasing health care needs, they have had the result of increasing needs because these specialized services are available today. Many treatments require use of technologies so expensive that they are priced beyond what an individual or family can afford without help from third-party payers. Finding new and better ways to treat life-threatening conditions challenges medical researchers, and the treatments that become available often invite debate among *bioethicists*. For example, the use of *xenografts* (animal-organ transplants) has been suggested to meet the increasing demand for healthy organs to transplant, but many people question this practice and, to date, it has not developed.

Some would indicate that the "birth of bioethics" occurred with the publication of an article in Life Magazine titled "They Decide Who Lives, Who Dies" (November 9, 1962). This article told the story of a group of individuals in Seattle whose duty it was to select patients for a recently opened hemodialysis program in the city. Many more patients needed treatment than could be accommodated; those not selected would likely die. This event was followed several years later by an article about the ethics of medical research that provided impetus for examining these issues. When Christiaan Barnard performed the first heart transplant in 1967, the world again responded with awe and concern. Who was the donor? Where did he come from? Was he truly dead (Jonsen, 1993)?

Centers for research in bioethics emerged, most notably the Institute of Society, Ethics, and the Life Sciences, located in Hastings-on-Hudson, New York (often called The Hastings Center), and the Kennedy Institute of Ethics, located at Georgetown University in Washington, DC. The Kennedy Institute of Ethics, founded in 1971 by Joseph and Rose Kennedy, is a teaching and research center that provides ethical perspectives on major policy issues. It boasts the largest university-based faculty in the world devoted to research and teaching biomedical ethics. Journals such as the *Hastings Center Report* and the *Journal of Medicine and Philosophy* have come into being, and an encyclopedia, *The Encyclopedia of Bioethics*, has been published. Web sites devoted to the topic of bioethics are so numerous that they cannot be listed in the confines of this textbook. Today bioethicists are included in many important task forces and special committees.

Entire textbooks have been devoted to bioethical considerations. Initially most of these were written for medical students, but now just as many are written for nursing students. Some nursing programs include a course in ethics and bioethics in the curriculum. This chapter can only introduce the topic and, we hope, broaden your perspective and deepen your interest. You are encouraged to read about and study these issues further as they affect your nursing practice.

As we mentioned earlier, most of the bioethical issues with which we wrestle were not a concern 20 or even 10 years ago. They have evolved as a product of the technologic advances that have occurred in medical practice and research. Table 10-1 lists some of the significant medical milestones that have occurred since 1920, some of which we have come to take for granted (eg, antibiotics and DNA). You readily can see that in 1960 there was no quest for human organs or critical decisions with regard to the life status of a possible donor. We were not able to fertilize ova outside the human body and reimplant fertilized eggs in a woman's uterus until 1978. Certain life-saving machines (eg, ventilators) and miracle drugs (eg, some of the chemotherapeutic agents used today) were not available to offer extension of life. Technologies such as magnetic resonance imaging (MRI), which gives us information about the structure of tissues and allows for early diagnosis and treatment, were not available. Concerns that related to the quality of life were often more clear-cut. As advances occur in medical practice, we must challenge ourselves to think through our own beliefs and feelings about these practices.

It is our intent in this short section to share with you some of the major bioethical issues confronting the new graduate today. You will have an opportunity to gain information, explore philosophical and religious issues, and integrate your own beliefs into your role as a nurse (see Table 10-1).

THE HUMAN GENOME PROJECT

A *genome* may be defined as all the DNA in an organism, including the genes that carry information for making the proteins required by all organisms. You will remember from your biology classes that the human genome consists of 46 chromosomes: 22 pairs of autosomes and a pair of sex chromosomes. Genomes have been studied for many reasons, including disease prevention, determination of the effects of radiation and chemicals on living species, and more recently, genetic therapy.

The Human Genome Project (HGP) was first proposed by Nobel prize-winning virologist Renato Dulbecco in 1986. The international project (at least 18 countries have established human genome research projects) officially started in October 1990. It was planned to last for 15 years, but the completion date has been accelerated to 2003 because of rapid technologic advances. Its cost is estimated at $3 billion. The project has two goals: to discover all the approximately 100,000 human genes (the human genome), make them accessible for further biologic study, and determine the order (sequence) of the individual nucleotides in the DNA of the 3 billion DNA subunits (bases). An additional part of the HGP includes parallel studies being carried out

TABLE 10–1. Some Medical Milestones of the 1900s

When	Who	What
1928	Alexander Fleming	This British bacteriologist noticed that one of his culture plates had grown a fungus and the colonies of staphylococci around the edge of the mold had been destroyed. Because this fungus was a member of the *Penicillium* group he named it penicillin.
1938	Howard Florey & Ernst Chain	These two pathologists took up the work of Fleming and demonstrated the efficacy of penicillin in treating infection. In 1945 the three were jointly awarded the Nobel Prize for Physiology of Medicine.
1951	Forrest Bird	The first Bird breathing device was developed (Bird Mark 7) and breathing treatment machines were introduced. Inhalation (respiratory) therapy rapidly developed as a health profession (Pilbeam, 1992).
1953	James Watson & Francis Crick	These two geneticists deciphered DNA's double-helix structure. Researchers began to focus on the internal functioning of the cell and molecular biology developed as a specialty.
1954	Physicians in Boston	Transplanted the kidney from one twin to the other, thus moving kidney transplantation from the experimental stage it had occupied since 1902. Kidney transplantations have been the most successful of transplantations (Miller-Keane, 1992).
1955	Jonas Salk	Public health officials began immunizing children against polio with Dr. Salk's vaccine, which contained dead virus.
1957	Albert Sabin	A polio vaccine was developed, which was based on weakened live virus, that could be administered orally.
1967	Christiaan Barnard	This South African surgeon performed the first human-heart transplant.
1972	British engineers	The computed tomography (CT) scanner, which assembles thousands of x-ray images into a highly detailed picture of the brain, was developed in England. It was later expanded to provide scans of the entire body.
1978	English physicians	The process of in vitro fertilization was developed. Louise Brown became the first person to be conceived in a test tube, then implanted into the mother's uterus.
1979	World Health Organization	This group declared that smallpox had been eradicated 2 years after the last known case was identified. This occurred because of world-wide immunization against the disease.
1981	Physicians in San Francisco and New York	Doctors from these two cities reported the first cases of what would later become known as acquired immunodeficiency syndrome (AIDS). To date, no cure exists.
1982	The U.S. Food and Drug Administration	The first drug developed with recombinant-DNA was approved by this group. It was a form of human insulin; its availability saves thousands of lives.
1995	Duke University surgeons	Hearts from genetically altered pigs were transplanted into baboons, proving that cross-species transplantations can be done. Transmission of animal viruses to humans emerges as a serious concern.
1998	Scientists from University of Wisconsin—Madison	Culture embryonic stem cells (cells that are the parent cells of all body tissues) from donated human blastocysts, opening the door to potential repair or replacement of diseased tissues or organs (UW Madison, Stem Cell, 1998).

Much of the material for this table was gathered from an article by Sherwin B. Nuland, *Time Special Issue*, Fall 1996.

on selected model organisms such as the *Escherichia coli* bacterium (Genome FAQs File, 1999).

This research is inspired by the discovery that an estimated 4,000 disease genes reside within the human genome. Identification and isolation of defective genes, and their replacement with functional genes (*gene therapy*), could result in the elimination of diseases that have plagued society for generations. Several significant conditions currently under study are cystic fibrosis, Huntington's disease, myotonic dystrophy, gout, and adult polycystic kidney disease.

Gene therapy can be divided into two categories. The first kind is an alteration in germ cells (sperm or ova) that results in a permanent genetic change in a whole organism and subsequent generations. For ethical reasons, this is not currently being considered for humans. The second is called "somatic cell gene therapy," and is similar to an organ transplant. Several cases of somatic cell gene therapy have been initiated, most relating to treatment of cancers and blood disorders (Rossiter & Caskey, 1993).

The Human Genome Project brings the promise of improved diagnosis and possible treatments for many inherited diseases (Fig. 10-1). It also raises other questions. Once this technology has been developed, where does it end? Who among health care providers will provide access to patients? Will the responsibility fall to the family practitioner, who will most likely be the first contact for those with a genetic disor-

FIGURE 10–1 Another interesting issue involves the creation of life or, more correctly, the circumstances under which it may occur.

der? How prepared are family practitioners for this type of care delivery? In a study of family physicians' perspectives on genetics and the Human Genome Project conducted in the midwestern United States, many family physicians indicated that they felt educational opportunities to learn about genetics have been inadequate, and some indicated reluctance to gain the additional education that would be required (Fetters, Doukas, & Phan, 1999). Will we see the advent of a new medical specialty in structural genomics? Will molecular medicine teams be developed in our society (Trent, 1999)? Will new and expensive technology result, such as a program of high-throughput X-ray crystallography aimed at developing a comprehensive mechanistic understanding of normal and abnormal human and microbial physiology (Burley, et al 1999)?

Initially, people were excited at the possibility of preventing such diseases as diabetes or cystic fibrosis. Then they began to think about other ramifications. Once identified, how is this information handled with regard to issues of privacy and confidentiality? What is the impact if third-party payers gain access to the information? What might be the advantages and disadvantages of knowing the diseases to which you are susceptible? With whom should that information be shared? Employers? Insurance companies? The government? What would be the effects of manipulating stature, intelligence, or sex? Do we run the risk of creating "superbabies?" Does this project represent eugenics revisited? The following are some of the ethical, legal, and social issues identified by those working with the HGP:

- Fairness in the use of genetic information by insurers, employers, courts, schools, law enforcement, and other social agencies
- Privacy and confidentiality of genetic information: who owns and controls it?
- Psychologic impact and stigmatization because of an individual's genetic differences
- Issues surrounding genetic testing due to family history: should it be done when no treatment is available? Are tests reliable?
- Reproductive issues, including informed consent and use of information in decision making: do health care personnel provide proper counseling?
- Gene therapy that someday may be used to treat, cure, and prevent genetic disorders
- Genetic enhancement, which involves using gene therapy to supply certain desired characteristics, such as height
- Fairness in the use of genetic technologies: access and who will pay
- Clinical issues, including education of health care providers, the public, and patients
- Commercialization of products, including property rights: who owns the genes?
- Conceptual and philosophical implications regarding human responsibility as related to genes and behavior (Human Genome Project Information, 1999)

You can see that the HGP poses many controversial bioethical challenges, with many questions yet to be answered. Students interested in having more extensive knowledge of this project are encouraged to do research in their school or local library, and on the Internet, which is replete with information.

Critical Thinking Activity

> Identify as many positive outcomes of the Human Genome Project as you
> can. Then identify as many disadvantages as you can that society might
> experience as a result of the Human Genome Project. Compare and contrast
> the value of these when weighed one against another.

BIOETHICAL ISSUES CONCERNING THE BEGINNING OF LIFE

Many bioethical issues with which we wrestle are focused on the process by which
conception occurs, the products of conception, and the beginning of life, including
whether it should occur. Much of the early debate related to family planning and
conception.

Family Planning

The modern population control movement probably can trace its beginnings to the
writings of a minister in the Church of England. In 1798, Thomas Malthus, in an essay
titled "On Population," expressed deep concern about a population that was growing
faster than were the resources to support it. To offset this problem, he advocated late
marriage, no marriage, or sexual abstinence in marriage. No forms of contraception as
we know them today were available, although women sometimes developed home-
made devices in an effort to prevent pregnancy. Most commonly these devices were
sponges dipped in various herbs and other substances that, when inserted in the vagina,
soaked up or inactivated semen.

In the United States, another approach was taken that undoubtedly led to some of
the controversy related to the issue of birth control. In 1873, Congress passed the
Comstock Act, prohibiting the sale, mailing, or importing of any drug or article that
prevented conception. This resulted in the illegal importation and distribution of contraceptive devices. You may have read about Margaret Sanger (1883–1966), a nurse
who championed for contraceptive practices at a time when such activities and viewpoints were extremely unpopular and illegal. Although charged and sentenced for disseminating information on birth control, she went on to establish the National Committee on Federal Legislation for Birth Control, the forerunner of the Planned
Parenthood Federation.

It was not until 1965 that a clear, legal concept of planned parenthood was developed, when the Supreme Court of the United States established the right of the individual to obtain medical contraceptive advice and counseling in the case of *Griswold
and Buxton v. the State of Connecticut* (Hayt, 1977).

Additional controversy over birth control is related to the theological teachings of
some religious groups, who believe interference with procreative powers is wrong.
Through encyclicals from the popes, the Roman Catholic Church strongly has advo-

cated the natural use of reproductive powers to ensure the propagation of the human race; anything that impedes attainment of the purpose for which these organs were created (ie, reproduction) is considered immoral. We see high birth rates in countries that are predominantly Roman Catholic. Orthodox Judaism has specific rules about when sexual intercourse may or may not occur; these rules are geared toward increasing the Jewish population. The Orthodox Jewish population is so small, in proportion to other groups, that the impact is not significant. The members of the Church of Jesus Christ of Latter Day Saints (Mormons), although less adamant in their teachings, also discourage the use of artificial birth control under normal circumstances. Some conservative Protestant Christians and conservative Muslims also advocate allowing God to plan families and do not use birth control methods.

When caring for individuals whose personal beliefs prohibit the use of artificial birth control, you must be knowledgeable about natural methods of family spacing, such as fertility awareness methods, that will meet the patient's needs. If your personal views regarding contraception differ, your views must be set aside as you focus on assisting the patient in selecting a method that is compatible with the patient's personal values and beliefs.

Among the methods of birth control available to those who have no religious sanction against their use, not all methods are acceptable to all people. For example, some find the intrauterine device unacceptable because they believe that interfering with a fertilized egg should be viewed as abortion (researchers are not entirely sure how the intrauterine device works, but some suggest that it prevents the fertilized egg from implanting in the wall of the uterus). Those who find abortion an acceptable method of coping with an unwanted pregnancy represent the other extreme. During your career as a nurse, you will care for patients who represent many differing viewpoints.

Central to all discussions of contraception is the issue of freedom to control one's body. This immediately raises a second question: who has that right? Is it the woman's right because it is her body? Avid feminists would answer with a resounding "yes." What if the partners disagree about family planning practices? Does one have more say than the other? What if one partner wants to have a family and the other does not? It is not within the scope of this chapter to explore the ramifications of all these concerns, but nurses working in this area need to be aware of the many issues that are present.

Largely because of personal values, there is disagreement over how contraception should be practiced, by whom, and at what age. In general, it is assumed that adults are capable of giving free and informed consent. The ability to procreate precedes what is generally considered legal age, however, and we find ourselves grappling with problems related to age of consent, its definition, and the role of the parents and the family.

Problems of Consent and Family Planning

In legal terms, the *age of consent* is "the age at which one is capable of giving deliberate and voluntary agreement, especially to marriage or to unlawful sexual intercourse" (Thomas, 1993). This implies physical and mental ability and the freedom to act and make decisions. The age of consent is established state by state and varies from age 14 in Hawaii and Pennsylvania to age 18 in fourteen other states. Most states have established age 16 as the age of consent (&TOTSE, 1999). Until children reach the age of consent, parents are required to give consent for the care of their children. Implicit in this is the assumption that the parents have the best interests of the child at heart and that they are better qualified than the child to make decisions in the child's best interest. (Do you see how this generates the concept of "paternalism" that has been discussed in other parts of the book?) The authority to give consent goes along with the understanding that the parents are responsible for the care (including medical costs) and education of the minor. However, today's trends cloud the issue, and legislators and concerned citizens continue to struggle with legislating "rights" through arbitrary criteria such as age. In former times, the age of 7 was considered an appropriate age at which to give consent, because by age 7 children were expected to know right from wrong and to have reached the age of reason. Although few of us would think that this is an age at which a child should be responsible for consenting to medical treatment, guidelines of the Department of Health and Human Services have allowed that this age is sufficient for refusing consent, despite parental opinion (Hellegers, 1975).

The trend recently has been toward the concept of the "emancipated minor." An *emancipated minor* is a child legally under the age of majority who is recognized as having the legal capacity of an adult under circumstances prescribed by state law. Generally, minors are deemed emancipated when they are self supporting or not living at home; married; pregnant or a parent; in the military; or declared to be emancipated by a court. Emancipated minors may give consent for medical treatment regardless of their parent's or legal guardian's knowledge or agreement (Kelley, 1994). Most states recognize some form of emancipation of minors.

Another term we often hear is *mature minor*, a relatively new concept. This term is applied to "youths who are sufficiently mature and intelligent to understand the nature and consequences of a treatment that is for their benefit" (Mancini, 1978, p. 126). Under this definition, a minor who wants birth control devices because he or she is sexually active demonstrates the ability to make a mature decision, although the parents may not agree with the decision. The mature minor also may consent to therapy for sexually transmitted disease, drug abuse, and pregnancy care. Health care workers have no legal obligation to inform parents of any such treatment. The most liberal legislation applies to the treatment of sexually transmitted disease and is endorsed by most states. Minors of any age can consent to diagnosis and care for sexually transmitted disease. The following illustrates the problems that can occur in this situation.

An 11-year-old girl sought treatment for gonorrhea. At her insistence, the physician promised to honor her legal right to confidential health care and not to inform her parents. Later, a public health nurse who was working with the girl learned that the child was being repeatedly sexually assaulted after school by a 16-year-old neighbor while her parents were still at work. The nurse also felt bound to a pledge of confidentiality but was able, with encouragement, to get the child to discuss this with her parents and enlist their support. In this instance the statute that protected the "rights" of the child may have led health care professionals to become involved in activities that did not serve the best interests of the child.

In 1976, the American Academy of Pediatrics (AAP) published a policy statement on the legal concept of informed consent in pediatric practice. This statement recommended that minors be allowed to give consent for health services when they are pregnant or afflicted with reportable communicable disease (including venereal diseases) or drug or substance abuse (including alcohol and nicotine). It is generally accepted that the age of the patient is not to be considered for some treatments, but that parental consent is automatically required for other treatments (when the patient is younger than 18). In 1995 the Committee on Bioethics of the AAP provided an updated statement that analyzed the issues surrounding informed consent, parental permission, and child assent. It emphasized the ethical obligation physicians have to obtain parental permission to undertake recommended medical interventions. It also encouraged physicians to seek patient assent when developmentally appropriate, and supported informed consent obtained directly from patients when working with emancipated or mature minors with adequate decision-making capacity (Committee, 1995).

Certainly, there are times when physicians' ethical and moral convictions prevent them from complying with adolescents' requests for care. This occurs most commonly in response to requests for contraceptive pills and abortions. In such cases, physicians often discuss their beliefs with the adolescent, and frequently refer the patient to a medical colleague for assistance.

A major controversy exists around the role of the school in the sex education of high school students and the dispensing of contraceptives through high school health clinics. The advent of emergency contraception in the form of birth control pills taken in high dose for a limited time after intercourse has added another dimension to these ethical issues about birth control and minors. In some states, emergency contraception is available directly from a pharmacy without a physician's prescription. The pharmacist, therefore, is drawn into the decision-making web.

Those who are concerned about the high incidence of teenage pregnancies and sexually transmitted diseases argue that the information must be disseminated, regardless of who does it. Conservatives think that this promotes erosion of the role of the family, and worry that the indiscriminate dispensing of contraceptives encourages promiscuity among teenagers. Concern about the spread of AIDS has done much to alter thinking, particularly in regard to the dispensing of condoms.

Abortion

What has been said about contraception becomes an even greater issue when related to abortion. In medical terms, abortion is the termination of pregnancy before the viability of the fetus—that is, any time before the end of the sixth month of gestation. An abortion may occur spontaneously as a result of natural causes (*spontaneous abortion*). A pregnancy may be interrupted deliberately for medical reasons (*therapeutic abortion*), or for personal reasons (*elective abortion*). It is the last two classifications (especially the latter) that induce bioethical debate. Ethically, the entire debate revolves around the definition of human life and when the fetus should be considered a human being. There are two major schools of thought about the nature of the fetus: one supports the belief that new life occurs at the moment of conception; the other contends that human life does not exist until the fetus is sufficiently developed biologically to sustain itself outside the uterus.

The legal aspects of abortion were clarified on January 22, 1973, when the US Supreme Court ruled that any state laws that prohibited or restricted a woman's right to obtain an abortion during the first 3 months of pregnancy were unconstitutional. The following excerpt details the case of *Roe v. Wade*, in which the Supreme Court recognized that, during the first trimester of pregnancy, a privacy right exists that allows an individual woman to make the final decision with regard to what happens to her own body (*Roe v. Wade*, 1973).

"Jane Roe" was the fictitious name Norma McCorvey used when two young attorneys, both women, filed her lawsuit. A pregnant, divorced waitress, and a victim of a gang rape and beating, Jane Roe sued the State of Texas because she could not obtain a legal abortion in that state and was too poor to travel to New York or California, where abortion was legal. Without access to abortion, she had the baby, whom she placed for adoption. Four years later, the Supreme Court struck down the laws that prevented her seeking abortion. Certain time limitations as to when an abortion can be performed were determined to be necessary, because of the state's interest in protecting potential life. At the period of viability, the state's interest took precedence over the mother's desire for an abortion. Supreme Court Justice Blackmun, in writing an opinion that met with agreement from six other justices, decided that a woman's decision to terminate a pregnancy was encompassed by the right to privacy, up to a certain point in the development of the fetus (Blackmun, 1981); it was established that this lasted until the end of the first trimester. Thus, the courts ruled that the state could not prevent abortions during the first trimester, but could regulate abortions in the second and third trimesters of pregnancy, at which point the interests of the fetus took precedence over those of the mother.

The basic principles of the 1973 decision were reaffirmed by the Court in 1992. Despite these rulings, the issue of abortion versus right to life continues to surface, with new legislation and rulings being considered each year and the issue debated each presidential election. In 1977, Congress barred the use of Medicaid funds for abortion with the exception of those done for therapeutic reasons and in other specific circumstances. However, the legal positions do little to help us deal with bioethical concerns. Many people view termination of life at any point after conception as murder. The Roman Catholic Church firmly upholds its traditional position on abortion. Many conservative Protestant Christian groups are also active in opposing abortion.

Some believe that although abortion is not desirable, under certain circumstances it would be justifiable—for example, in cases of rape or incest, or in instances where amniocentesis indicates that a fetus would be born retarded or genetically defective. Others think that early termination of a pregnancy might be acceptable, but that termination after the fourth month would not be appropriate.

Those who support abortion without restriction usually do so because they believe that women should have control over their own bodies. They further argue that the quality of life of an "unwanted" child, or a child born with a deformity or genetic defect, may be minimal. Interesting and challenging cases have emerged with respect to this concept. These are generally known as *wrongful birth* cases, and are based on the principle that it is wrong to give birth to children (such as those with birth defects or limitations that can be diagnosed or anticipated before birth) who will not have the same quality of life as other children.

As a nurse, these issues present some difficult questions you will need to answer. To what extent do you believe you can personally participate in the abortion procedure? You may find it easier to assist with an abortion performed as a dilation and curettage at 10 weeks' gestation, in a doctor's office or clinic, than to assist with a saline abortion carried out at 5 months' gestation in a hospital labor room. The products of conception aborted at 10 weeks have little that is lifelike in their appearance. The fetus aborted at 5 months appears much like a premature infant. Certainly, as a nurse, you have the right to refuse to be involved in abortion procedures or the care of patients seeking abortion. Employment in certain areas (eg, labor and delivery rooms) however, may rest on the nurse's willingness and ability to assist with abortions and to give conscientious care to the patient who has had an abortion. Some religiously affiliated hospitals have elected to close their labor and delivery suites rather than perform abortions.

Although textbooks traditionally have defined the age of viability (the earliest age at which fetuses could survive if they were born at that time) as 20 to 24 weeks' gestation, technology has increased the ability to enable very low birth weight and premature babies to survive. The age of viability is less clear than it once seemed. Attention has been focused on incidents in which an abortion was attempted toward the end of the fifth or sixth month of gestation, and the fetus was born showing signs of life. Is the doctor or nurse obligated to try to keep the infant alive? Is the doctor or nurse guilty of malpractice, or even murder, if he or she does anything to hasten the infant's death? Should this infant be considered a human being? Does the infant have "rights"? Does the mother have legal possession of and responsibility for the child if, in fact, she attempted to abort the fetus? This issue, like so many others, probably will be settled in a court of law while we continue to debate it ethically.

The abortion issue also is complicated by consent problems. Many states have recognized the special problems related to parental consent for teenagers and to health care involving pregnancy and have legislated special exceptions.

In the last few years, the abortion issue has been made more complex by research that would use the fetal tissue resulting from an abortion for therapeutic purposes. Research has suggested that fetal brain tissue (recovered at the time of abortion), if implanted in the brain of the patient with Parkinson's disease, may help in the treatment of the disease. The ramifications of this type of research and treatment are so great that a special committee has been appointed to develop guidelines to govern future research and treatment activities requiring the use of fetal tissue.

As a society, it seems likely that we will continue to debate the issue of abortion. Ultimately, the decision rests with the individual who must make the choice. Certainly the legal entanglements become more complex with each court ruling, and will be limited only by our willingness to challenge other aspects of the question.

Critical Thinking Activity

Select one of the positions taken regarding abortion. Defend your position, providing a strong rationale for your thinking. Examine your thinking for biases. Why did you develop those biases? Discuss the topic of abortion with a classmate who holds a different position, remembering that all persons are entitled to their own viewpoints.

Prenatal Testing

The ability to identify birth defects and genetic disorders of the fetus has created a different dimension in the abortion debates. A major breakthrough in our ability to detect genetic abnormalities in the fetus occurred in the 1970s with the development of techniques to carry out *amniocentesis*. An amniocentesis is performed between 14 and 20 weeks after the woman's last menstrual period. This test is performed after identifying the placental site and locating a pocket of amniotic fluid using an ultrasound scan; a 22-gauge needle is then inserted through the pregnant woman's abdomen and uterus, and 15 to 20 mL of fluid is removed and analyzed. From these cells, many genetic problems can be diagnosed prenatally, including such conditions as Down syndrome (which accounts for about one third of the cases of mental retardation in western countries), hemophilia, Duchenne's muscular dystrophy, Tay-Sachs disease, and problems related to the brain and spinal column (eg, anencephaly and spina bifida).

Down syndrome, a condition occurring with higher frequency in mothers in their early 40s and older, is the most common reason for seeking amniocentesis. When genetic screening reveals a genetic disease, a woman will often choose to have an abortion. Rothstein (1990, p. 39) reports that "termination rates for muscular dystrophy, cystic fibrosis, and alpha and beta thalassemia are nearly 100%; they are 60% for hemophilia; and 50% for sickle cell anemia." Some couples request amniocentesis if they are in an "at-risk" group, but state that they would not abort the fetus under any circumstances; instead they believe that an additional 5 months will give them time to adjust to the presence of a disease before the baby is born. Usually doctors are reluctant to do an amniocentesis under these circumstances, because the risk of performing the procedure, although small, does not seem justified.

Some people are concerned about this procedure because of where it might lead. Is mass genetic screening a possibility? Ethicists have expressed concern about the possibility of the government making diagnostic amniocentesis and abortion of all defective fetuses mandatory. Others argue against genetic counseling and amniocentesis because of the stress it places on a marriage, and because of the guilt placed on the partner carrying the defective gene (when that can be determined). They argue that there are some things we are better off not knowing. Genetic screening also may result in at least one of the partners (often the carrier) seeking voluntary sterilization to prevent pregnancies with less than favorable outcomes. Despite concerns, amniocentesis has become a fairly common test offered to mothers who are in an "at risk" group.

Chorionic villus sampling (CVS) involves securing a sample of chorionic villi from the developing placenta. Using a fine needle inserted through the abdomen or a thin plastic cathether inserted through the cervix, these cells are collected and then analyzed in a laboratory. Like amniocentesis, these tests can predict birth defects and certain diseases. CVS can be performed earlier than an amniocentesis, usually in the 10th or 11th week of pregnancy.

The advent of amniocentesis and CVS heralded the development of yet another medical specialty: prenatal surgery. Although the specialty is still new, some corrective surgery is being performed on infants while they are in their intrauterine environment.

As a nurse, you may care for clients with varying viewpoints regarding prenatal screening and abortion, and you will also have your own values to consider. Will your values conflict with those of your clients? Are you obligated to advocate for a client when the client's request is squarely in opposition to what you believe to be right? Should you try to sway a woman who is indecisive toward either decision?

Sterilization

For years, surgical operations resulting in permanent sterilization have been performed for therapeutic purposes. Examples of this include the removal of reproductive organs to halt the spread of cancer or other pathologic processes. Although problems may arise for the patient and family as a result of such surgeries, usually they are resolved without serious ethical debate (depending on the family's religious values, the patient's body concept, family plans, and personal values).

With increasing frequency, voluntary sterilization has been requested by couples to terminate reproductive ability. For all intents and purposes, these surgical procedures, whether performed on men or women, should be considered permanent and irreversible. Sterilization may pose few problems for those who are satisfied with the size of their family. In most cases, full and informed consent is obtained from both partners before the surgery is performed. Some people question whether a man or woman is free to make an independent decision regarding sterilization without consulting the partner. Although many people see it as the prerogative of a couple, others find any type of sterilization in conflict with their religious and moral beliefs. A few states still have laws forbidding voluntary sterilization for contraceptive purposes, but these laws may not be enforced. However, surgical sterilization under any other circumstances than those described above is controversial.

Eugenics

Eugenics is the study of methods to improve inherited human characteristics. The practice of eugenics is not new. The idea of improving the quality of the human race is at least as old as Plato, who wrote on the topic in his *Republic*. The philosophical beliefs of certain 18th century thinkers about the notion of human perfectibility were central to the eugenics movement, which is thought to have started in the 19th century. Charles Darwin's theory of evolution was advanced by his cousin Francis Galton, who created the term *eugenics*. When Mendel's law provided a framework for explaining the transmission and distribution of traits from one generation to another, the eugenics movement took hold. Organizations focusing on eugenics were created around the world.

The center of the eugenics movement in the United States was the Eugenics Record Office in Cold Spring Harbor, New York, and its leader was geneticist Charles Davenport. Until the early 1930s, the eugenics movement grew. Eugenicists presented a two-part policy. Negative eugenics advocated the elimination of unwanted characteristics from the nation by discouraging "unworthy" parents. This included a variety of approaches such as marriage restriction, sterilization, and permanent custody of "defectives." Many eugenicists were actively involved in other issues of the day, including prohibition, birth control, and legislation that would outlaw miscegenation (ie, marriage between two persons of different races, especially between white and black people in the United States). During this time, states passed compulsory sterilization bills affecting certain developmentally disabled groups. By 1929, California, for example, had sterilized approximately 6,250 people, almost twice as many as all other states combined (Kevles, 1993). The Immigration Restriction Act of 1924 also was passed at this time, dramatically limiting the immigration of people from southern and eastern Europe on the grounds that they were "biologically inferior."

Positive eugenics encouraged increasing the desirable traits in the population by urging "worthy" parents. "Superior" couples were encouraged to have more children.

The eugenics movement also grew in Germany. In 1933, Hitler sanctioned the Hereditary Health Law, or the Eugenic Sterilization Law, which ensured that the "less worthy" members of the Third Reich did not pass on their genes. It resulted in the sterilization of several hundred thousand people and helped lead to the death camps.

By the late 1930s, eugenics in the United States began a tremendous decline. Americans became concerned about the concept of a "master race." At the same time, psychologists and anthropologists were conducting research that indicated that culture and environment also had great influence over human development.

When the eugenic movement was rekindled in the 1960s, it had a different focus—one related to genetic counseling and genetic research. Today, a couple giving birth to a child with a congenital anomaly (or who realize that one of them is carrying a genetic trait that could cause a child to have a congenital anomaly) might voluntarily seek genetic counseling, and possibly opt for the sterilization of one of the partners. Again, this approach offends the religious and moral values of some, but generally it is viewed as the couple's prerogative.

Problems are created when the concept of eugenics is applied to minors or to institutionalized persons. Problems also arise in the language of laws in certain states that would include "epileptics, habitual criminals, and moral degenerates" among those eligible for compulsory sterilization. Some states extended compulsory sterilization to include those who might become wards of the state (Hayt, 1977). In the case of epilepsy, modern medical advances have changed our understanding of the role of heredity in the disease and our attitudes toward people who are affected. The trend in recent years has been for states to modify, repeal, or ignore their eugenic sterilization laws.

In states that still permit compulsory eugenic sterilization, questions can be raised about who may request sterilization, who may sign the consent, and who must fund the procedure. As the result of a court decision, federal dollars may not be used for this purpose (Hellegers, 1975). However, the taxpayer contributes to the cost of institutionalizing people who are not capable of living independently in today's society, and caring for those with severe illnesses and disabilities. The question also must be raised regarding the ability of two individuals who are mentally retarded to care for children they may parent. Therefore, it is not only a personal concern, but also society's concern.

The sterilization of sex offenders also has been discussed recently. In some instances, sterilization has been recommended for individuals convicted of repeated sexual offenses, particularly those against children. Because sex crimes are related to power and aggression, and not just to sex drive, this remains a controversial issue.

In Vitro Fertilization

In 1978 in England, much attention focused on the birth of the first child who was conceived in a test tube, a process we refer to as *in vitro fertilization* (IVF). Owing to a blockage in the mother's fallopian tubes, conception in her tubes was impossible. The ovum was removed from the mother, united with the father's sperm in a laboratory setting, and then implanted in the mother's uterus, where it grew to term and was delivered by cesarean section. Today, IVF and similar procedures (Table 10-2) help many infertile couples (approximately 26,000 so far) to become parents. An additional 40,000 couples have found the procedure to be unsuccessful (Grady, 1996).

Many herald this as one of medical science's great advances. For others, it raises many concerns. Several fertilized ova are usually returned to the uterus to assure that at least one will survive. If more than one implant successfully, it is possible for the mother to have multiple births. Multiple births seldom go full term, resulting in financial and emotional costs. When the number of implanted embryos is too great, consideration is given to aborting several of them to improve the chances of full development for the remaining ones; this creates additional ethical dilemmas for the family.

What should be done with fertilized ova that are not returned to the uterus? Should they be thrown away? Given to a donor? Used for research? Should tax dollars be used to fund this type of research? If frozen, how long should they remain frozen? What should be done with them at the end of that time? In England in 1996, 3,300 embryos were allowed to defrost and die because of a 1990 law that limits storage time to 5 years unless donor couples seek an extension (English cardinal, 1996).

Despite the objections raised against IVF, it is now recognized as a viable alternative for many couples who otherwise would be childless (at least as far as natural parenting is concerned). Reproductive problems often stem from blocked fallopian tubes. By harvesting the eggs, fertilizing them in a laboratory, and implanting them in the woman's uterus, this problem can be bypassed.

Other offshoots of in vitro fertilization allow people who are carrying a severe genetic disease to be assured that their children will not be affected by the condition or carry the defective gene. Fertilized ova are examined for possible disease before being implanted in the uterus; those that are diseased would not be implanted.

TABLE 10–2.   Types of Assisted Reproductive Techniques

Name	Initials	Description	First Used With Humans
Artificial Insemination: Homologous	AIH	Husband's semen is collected and then deposited at the cervical os or in the wife's uterus by mechanical means.	United States, 1884
Artificial Insemination: Donor	AID	Donor's semen is collected and deposited at the the cervical os or in the woman's uterus by mechanical means.	United States, 1884
In Vitro Fertilization	IVF	After heavily medicating the woman with hormones to trigger ovulation, eggs are harvested and fertilized with father's sperm in a laboratory. Several of the resulting embryos are implanted in the mother's uterus.	England, 1978
Gamete Intrafallopian Transfer	GIFT	Eggs and sperm are inserted directly into the woman's fallopian tubes using a laparoscope. Embryos travel to the uterus for implantation.	United States, 1984
Zygote Intrafallopian Transfer	ZIFT	Eggs and sperm are combined in the laboratory. The resulting zygotes are then inserted into the woman's fallopian tubes and travel to the uterus for implantation.	Belgium, 1989
Preimplantation Genetic Diagnosis	PGD	Egg and sperm are united in the laboratory and the embryo is allowed to develop to 4–8 cells. One or two cells are removed and examined for harmful genes. Defective embryos are discarded; healthy ones are implanted in the woman's uterus.	United States, 1991
Immature Egg Harvest	IEH	Similar to IVF, the eggs are harvested from the ovaries while still immature, are cultured in the laboratory, fertilized, and transferred into the woman's uterus.	South Korea, 1991
Intracytoplasmic Sperm Injection	ICSI	In a laboratory setting, a single sperm cell is injected into an egg and then both are implanted in the woman's uterus.	Belgium, 1992

A Louisiana couple decided, after the death of their 3-year-old daughter from Tay-Sachs disease, not to risk having more children. They learned that they both carried one copy of the Tay-Sachs gene, which would result in a 1-in-4 chance of conceiving a child with the disease. Shortly thereafter, the couple were notified that a procedure had been developed through IVF and high-tech genetic testing (known as preimplantation genetic diagnosis [PGD]) whereby technicians can remove one or two embryonic cells from those fertilized in vitro and test for the harmful gene. This allows only healthy embryos to be transferred back to the woman's uterus. This procedure resulted in the birth of a healthy child for this couple, and one who is not a carrier of Tay-Sachs disease.

As wonderful as this may seem, concerns exist regarding what some would call the misuse of IVF. In Italy, a 62-year-old woman became pregnant using donated eggs and IVF before implantation in her uterus. She gave birth by cesarean section in 1994. A 59-

year-old woman in England delivered twins by this method. More recently, a new record was set for what is thought to be the oldest woman in the world to give birth to a healthy infant. In April 1997, it was announced that a 63-year-old woman had given birth via cesarean section on November 7, 1996. The woman, married and previously childless, is said to have told doctors she was 50 and had medical records attesting to that age. (The medical center where the IVF occurred sets an age limit of 55 on accepting patients.) A donor egg and the husband's sperm were used for the IVF (Roan, 1997).

In some countries, legislation has been passed to prevent such situations. In January 1994, the French Senate opted to prohibit the use of reproductive options in certain cases (Capron, 1994). One can readily identify some of the difficulties in starting the mothering process at age 62 or 63, not the least of which would be living long enough to see the child reach adulthood. Quality-of-life issues also may be involved. If the mother is 62 when the child is born, she will be 67 or 68 when the child starts school and 75 when the child becomes a teenager.

Other concerns focus on the fear that PGD will be used to make "perfect babies," or for sex selection, even when there is not a medical reason (such as hemophilia) for such action.

Artificial Insemination

Other discussions revolve around the topic of *artificial insemination*, which is the planting of sperm in the woman's body to facilitate conception. Although we tend to think of this as a fairly new procedure, the first time artificial insemination is said to have been used was in Philadelphia in 1884 (Fromer, 1981). There are two different kinds of artificial insemination: homologous (AIH), in which the husband's sperm is used, and heterologous (AID), in which a donor's sperm is used. Using the husband's sperm is by far the most common and creates the fewest problems legally, ethically, and morally. In some instances, the sperm from the husband and the sperm from a donor with similar physical characteristics are mixed together. As a result, if conception occurs, the couple could easily believe it was the husband's sperm that was accepted by the ovum.

Although some religious groups may have objections, few concerns arise when the husband's sperm is used. That is not true with donor sperm. If the woman is artificially inseminated with donor sperm without the knowledge and consent of her partner, the problems are multiplied. One of the major questions raised is that of adultery, which is considered a criminal act in most states. If conception occurs and the child is not biologically that of the husband, can one say that adultery has occurred? In at least one instance, the wife was found guilty of adultery after being artificially inseminated with donor sperm (Hayt, 1977). Others suggest that the child should be legally adopted by the husband, an act that, to some extent, helps to clarify issues of inheritance, child support (if the couple should later divorce), and the legal status of the child.

Single Parents

Another ethical issue has emerged as our society has granted greater acceptance to single-parent families. More single women are trying to adopt children, and some see artificial insemination as a logical solution. In some instances, these women are also lesbians. One of the couple will seek artificial insemination with a donor sperm; the child then is raised as family in the lesbian relationship. Providing a parenting option to lesbians is totally unacceptable to many people. Aside from the emotion that the issue of a lesbian relationship may introduce, there is the argument against the artificial insemination of any unmarried woman on the basis that the traditional two-parent family composed of a man and woman is in the best interest of all children.

Surrogate Mothers

Unique problems arise with surrogate mothering, a practice by which a woman agrees to bear a child conceived through artificial insemination and to relinquish the baby at birth to others for rearing. This practice has occurred with increasing frequency and in a variety of relationships. The following represents one such situation.

> A 47-year-old woman agreed to serve as gestational surrogate for her own daughter, whose uterus had been removed because of disease. The daughter's eggs were inseminated with her husband's sperm and the embryos were then implanted in the mother, who gave birth to triplets when she was 48. Thus, this woman became the gestational mother and the genetic grandmother to triplets.

As you see, these artificial means of reproduction have complicated even the language that we are accustomed to using. The term *biologic* is no longer adequate for making some critical conceptual distinctions. Macklin (1991, p. 6) states, "The techniques of egg retrieval, in vitro fertilization (IVF), and gamete intrafallopian transfer (GIFT), now make it possible for two different women to make a biological contribution to the creation of a new life." Macklin further believes that the woman who contributes her womb during gestation is also a biologic mother. We find terms such as *genetic mother* used to refer to the individual contributing the ovum, and *gestational mother* used to refer to the individual who provides the uterus in which the child develops. In some instances the surrogate mother is both.

Surrogate mothering within a family has caused fewer problems than have been seen when a stranger serves as the surrogate mother. The majority of serious conflicts have occurred in situations in which a woman has been paid to serve as a surrogate mother. A formal, contractual relationship is usually established. The couple who wish to have the child agree to pay all expenses associated with the pregnancy, and to pay the surrogate mother an agreed sum for her time and involvement. The contract must be carefully drawn up because it is illegal in all states to sell a child.

What happens if the child is born with an anomaly, as occurred with a New York couple in 1982? How are these dilemmas to be solved? What is to happen to the child? Who bears the responsibility?

> A gentleman paid a woman to be artificially inseminated with his sperm and to carry his child. When the child was born with microcephaly (an unusually small brain), the man rejected the infant, stating that he could not be the father. The surrogate mother and her husband also did not want to accept the responsibility for parenting the child.

Recently, problems associated with surrogate mothering have centered around the surrogate mother's unwillingness to give up the child after birth (Fig. 10-2).

"Baby M," as the court called her, was born to a surrogate mother after she was impregnated with the sperm of a man for whom she agreed to bear the child. This man's wife, a pediatrician, chose not to bear a child because she had multiple sclerosis. Although signed agreements existed, the surrogate mother broke the contract within days of the baby's birth and asked for custody of the child.

Such instances create great controversy, and pain for those involved. There are no easy answers.

Critical Thinking Activity

What safeguards would you recommend with regard to in vitro fertilization, artificial insemination, and surrogate mothers to ensure respect for the human condition? Be specific about how you believe these safeguards would be effective. Reflect on your proposals. Are there any you would change? Discuss your proposals with a classmate.

FIGURE 10–2   Complexities arise when surrogate mothers are unwilling to relinquish the infant after birth.

Sperm Banks

Another aspect of the artificial insemination issue is that of sperm banks. Sperm banks have been established in different parts of the United States for various reasons. Men who want to have a vasectomy may contribute to a sperm bank "just in case" they change their minds in the future. Men who will be exposed to high levels of radiation in their work, or during treatment of disease, may wish to have sperm stored because radiation may cause mutation of the genes or result in sterility. In most cases, the medical community establishes sperm banks so that sperm is available for artificial inseminations. In California, a sperm bank was started that contains only sperm of outstanding and brilliant men. The idea was to create children with this sperm who will be genetically endowed with greater intelligence and creativity. Many find this unacceptable because it brings up the issue of creating a super race. Concerns also have been raised regarding the possible number of offspring in a single community who might be genetically related without knowing it.

Are there ethical implications for the man who becomes a sperm donor and is the biologic father of a child, but assumes no ethical responsibility for who receives that sperm or for the resulting child and, in fact, has no knowledge regarding the use of his sperm? Some ask how a man can ethically father offspring and have no responsibility for their well-being.

The Right to Genetic Information

All the issues of artificial insemination using donor sperm, surrogate mothering, single parenting, and sperm banks are further complicated by a recent trend toward providing individuals with information regarding their genetic background, makeup, and history. You can readily anticipate the problems that would be created if donor sperm were used for insemination. In some instances, no record has been maintained with regard to who donated the sperm.

As society emphasizes the importance of the role of fathers and the rights of children to know their genetic heritage, will anonymous sperm donation remain an option? How many individuals would be willing to donate sperm if it were to include a detailed genetic background? What might be the ultimate legal involvement? On the other hand, what are the rights of the child to know what genetic factors he or she carries? Whose rights should take precedence? The state of Oregon has passed legislation opening birth records for adults adopted as infants to learn their backgrounds, even though anonymity of the birth mother was guaranteed at the time of the adoption. Will tracking of sperm donors also become a concern in the future?

BIOETHICAL ISSUES CONCERNING DEATH

One of the most important areas of ethical debate involves the topic of death and dying. As mentioned earlier, the advent of lifesaving procedures and mechanical devices has required redefinition of the term *death*, caused us to examine the meaning of "quality of life," and created debates about "death with dignity."

Also associated with the issue of death are several companion concerns that did not exist before the technologic advances that have occurred in the past 10 years. Some of these concerns relate to euthanasia, the right to refuse treatment, and the right to die. Other concerns relate to organs retrieved from the dying, because of the scarcity of these medical resources. Generally, the demand for donated organs far exceeds the number of organs available to meet the needs. Superimposed on all these issues is that of informed consent.

Death Defined

Until recently, the most widely accepted definition of death was from *Black's Law Dictionary*, which defines death as the irreversible cessation of the vital functions of respiration, circulation, and pulsation (Rothman & Rothman, 1977). This traditional view of death served us well until the development of ventilators, pacemakers, and other advances in medical science made it possible to sustain these functions indefinitely. We also have learned that various parts of the body die at different times. The central nervous system is one of the most vulnerable areas, and brain cells can be irreversibly damaged if deprived of oxygen, while other parts of the body will continue to function.

Newer definitions of death have been built around the concept of human potential—meaning the potential of the human body to interact with the environment and with other people, to respond to stimuli, and to communicate. When these abilities are lacking, there is said to be no potential. Because this potential is directly related to brain function, the method most often used to assess capability is electroencephalography. Brain activity, with few exceptions, is said to be nonexistent when flat electroencephalographic (EEG) tracings are obtained over a given period, often 48 hours (Rothman & Rothman, 1977). At this point the person may be considered dead, although machines may be supporting the vital functions of respiration and circulation. Many institutions now accept this definition of cerebral death and use it as a basis for turning off respirators and stopping other treatments. It is also used as a basis for determining death when there is a desire to recover organs from the patient.

Planning for End-of-Life Issues

Increasing emphasis is being placed on prior planning for end-of-life issues. Identifying futile treatments is one aspect of this process. Another important consideration relates to patient self-determination in regard to these issues. Many hope that the use of such planning will decrease the ethical dilemmas in end-of-life situations.

FUTILE TREATMENTS

Futile treatments are those that "cannot, within a reasonable possibility, cure, ameliorate, improve or restore a quality of life that would be satisfactory to the patient" (Hudson, 1994b). For example, when an individual is dying of terminal cancer, treatment for a respiratory infection may be deemed futile because it will not alter the fact that the person is dying and will not restore a satisfactory quality of life. Identifying whether further treatment is futile may be extremely difficult. However, Schneiderman and Jecker (1993) suggest that if, in the last 100 cases of the same nature, there was no change in the outcome based on the treatment, it can be considered futile. Others take a position that treatment never can be declared futile. In their thinking, the future cannot be predicted accurately, and if there cannot be absolute certainty about the outcome, then futility cannot be clearly identified.

Other problems may arise when futility is declared. Does a patient have a right to treatment even if it has been identified as futile? What about cost considerations? Should insurance companies be required to pay for treatment that has been classified as futile? What about Medicare or Medicaid? Should there be differences in decisions based on age or quality of life?

ADVANCE DIRECTIVES

When end-of-life concerns arise, the patient is often unconscious or not able to participate in decision making. This raises the question of obtaining consent. Does the responsibility for action, or the lack of action, then fall to the family, the physician, or the nurse? The law in each state specifies who may give consent when an individual is incapacitated and there is no directive as to the patient's choice for a surrogate decision maker. Would the ethical answer to this question be the same as the legal answer? Who is to decide?

In an attempt to gain greater control over the area of dying, many people are now completing a variety of documents that have been titled *advance directives*. An advance directive is a legal document that indicates the wishes of an individual in regard to end-of-life issues.

In 1990, Congress took a major step regarding this issue by passing legislation that requires all Medicare and Medicaid providers to inform patients, on admission to any agency receiving federal funds, of their right to refuse treatment. In December 1991, this federal Patient Self-Determination Act (PSDA) went into effect. The intent of this legislation was to enhance an individual's control over medical treatment decisions by promoting the use of advance directives. The PSDA requires individual institutions to inform patients of state law regarding directives, to document the existence of directives in their medical records, and to educate the community. An "interim final rule" gave considerable latitude to institutions regarding the ways that requirements could be met. Many institutions have used this as an opportunity to promote patient decision making. The entire process has not been without its problems. The time of admission to a health care facility is often filled with anxiety, making it almost impossible to consider such matters. Most patients indicate that they prefer to discuss these matters with a doctor or nurse who is involved in their care, but in some settings this task is delegated to an admissions clerk (Hudson, 1994a).

In 1991, the American Nurses Association developed *A Position Statement on Nursing and the Patient Self-Determination Act*, which was revised in 1995. They believe that nurses should play a primary role in implementation of the Act, should facilitate informed decision making for patients, and should occupy a critical role in education, research, patient care, and advocacy (ANA, 1995b).

A *living will* is a document that has been widely used as an advance directive (Fig. 10-3). In a living will, a person identifies what measures to include in care if he or she becomes terminally ill. The living will is often used to request that no extraordinary measures be implemented, although it can be used to indicate a preference that all pos-

**TO MY FAMILY, MY PHYSICIAN, MY LAWYER, MY CLERGYMAN
TO ANY MEDICAL FACILITY IN WHOSE CARE I HAPPEN TO BE
TO ANY INDIVIDUAL WHO MAY BECOME RESPONSIBLE FOR MY
HEALTH, WELFARE OR AFFAIRS**

Death is as much a reality as birth, growth, maturity and old age—it is the one certainty of life. If the time comes when I, _____
can no longer take part in decisions for my own future, let this statement stand as
an expression of my wishes, while I am still of sound mind.

If the situation should arise in which there is no reasonable expectation of my
recovery from physical or mental disability, I request that I be allowed to die
and not be kept alive by artificial means or "heroic measures". I do not fear
death itself as much as the indignities of deterioration, dependence and hopeless pain. I therefore, ask that medication be mercifully administered to me
to alleviate suffering even though this may hasten the moment of death.

This request is made after careful consideration. I hope you who care for me
will feel morally bound to follow its mandate. I recognize that this appears to
place a heavy responsibility upon you, but it is with the intention of relieving you
of such responsibility and of placing it upon myself in accordance with my
strong convictions, that this statement is made.

Signed _____

Date _____

Witness _____

Witness _____

Copies of this request have been given to _____

_____

_____

_____

FIGURE 10–3   The living will.

sible actions should be taken. Although the living will is not necessarily considered
legal consent, it does reveal the desires of the person receiving care. It may help families to make decisions more confidently.

Another approach being used with increasing frequency is the signing of a *durable
power of attorney for health care*. In this type of an agreement, an individual (referred
to as the "principal") may designate another person to have the power and authority
to make health care decisions for the principal, should the principal be unable to make
those decisions. The durable power of attorney goes into effect after the principal is no
longer capable of making decisions, but not until this point is reached. These forms can
be purchased in most office supply stores and become valid if signed before a notary
public. However, it is best to consult an attorney before entering into such an arrangement (Figure 10-4). Durable power of attorney documents may simply name the decision maker, or may contain detailed preferences of the individual.

Since 1985, New York has had a Task Force on Life and the Law, which has dealt with issues related to organ procurement and distribution, the determination of death, and surrogate motherhood. The group also has worked on the issue of appointing a surrogate to make health care decisions for an incapacitated adult patient who lacks a precise advance directive or a previously appointed health care agent.

Euthanasia

Euthanasia, meaning "good death," may be classified as either negative or positive. The word, as it is generally applied, refers to the act or method of causing death painlessly so as to end suffering.

NEGATIVE EUTHANASIA

Negative, or passive, *euthanasia* refers to a situation in which no extraordinary or heroic measures are undertaken to sustain life. The concept of negative euthanasia has resulted in what are called "no codes" (also designated as DNR—do not resuscitate) in hospital environments. In these situations, hospital personnel do not attempt to revive or bring back to life persons whose vital processes have ceased to function on their own.

It is difficult to describe what constitutes extraordinary measures, and to determine on whom they should or should not be used. Is it one thing to defibrillate a 39-year-old man who is admitted to an emergency department suffering from an acute heart attack, and quite another to defibrillate a 95-year-old man whose body is riddled with terminal cancer and whose heart has stopped? Often, people who are involved in giving medical and emergency care develop an almost automatic response to lifesaving procedures and have difficulty accepting dying as an inevitable part of the life process. It is difficult to know when it is permissible to omit certain life-supporting efforts, or which efforts should be omitted. If the 95-year-old man who is dying of terminal cancer were also to develop pneumonia, should his physician prescribe antibiotics? This brings us to the distinction between stopping a particular life-supporting treatment or machine, or withdrawing treatment, and not starting a procedure in the first place—that is, withholding treatment.

Some ethicists do not differentiate between withholding treatment in the first place and withdrawing treatment once it has been determined to be inappropriate or futile. They would see both as having the same position in terms of right and wrong. Those who support negative euthanasia support both withholding and stopping treatment. The general public often sees these as separate issues, and may support withholding treatment while not supporting the termination of treatment once it has begun. Increasingly, the legal system has supported withdrawing treatment that is determined to be futile. Even the Roman Catholic Church, which has a strong pro-life stance, has supported both the right not to institute heroic treatment and the right to withdraw it once it has begun.

POSITIVE EUTHANASIA

Positive, or active, *euthanasia* occurs in a situation in which the physician prescribes, supplies, or administers an agent that results in death. In the case (cited later in this

[PLEASE NOTE: This is a standardized legal document that may not be appropriate for a person in your particular situation. You should consult your attorney before signing this or any legal document.]

DURABLE POWER OF ATTORNEY FOR HEALTH CARE DECISIONS

I, _____ as principal, domiciled and residing in the State of Washington, hereby enter into a Durable Power of Attorney to provide informed consent for health care decisions pursuant to the laws of the State of Washington.

1. **Designation.** I designate _____ , if living, able and willing to serve, as my attorney-in-fact. If he or she is not living, able and willing to so serve, then I designate _____ , if living, able and willing to serve, as my attorney-in-fact.

2. **Powers.** The attorney-in-fact, as fiduciary, shall have all powers to provide informed consent for health care decisions on principal's behalf.

3. **Effectiveness.** This power of attorney shall become effective upon the disability or incompetence of the principal. Disability shall include the inability to make health care decisions effectively for reasons such as mental illness, mental deficiency, physical illness or disability, advanced age, chronic use of drugs, chronic intoxication, confinement, detention by a foreign power or disappearance. Disability may be evidenced by a written statement of a qualified physician regularly attending me. Incompetence may be established by a finding of a Court having jurisdiction over me.

4. **Duration.** This power of attorney shall remain in effect to the extent permitted by RCW 11.94 notwithstanding any uncertainty as to whether the principal is dead or alive.

5. **Revocation.** This power of attorney may be revoked in writing by notice mailed or delivered to my attorney-in-fact, and by recording the written instrument of revocation in the office of recorder or auditor of the county of my residence.

FIGURE 10–4   Durable power of attorney for health care. (Continued)

chapter) in which parents choose to let a newborn with Down syndrome and an intestinal blockage die, positive euthanasia would have occurred if the doctors had hastened the infant's death with medication. There may well be more instances of positive euthanasia than we know about publicly.

The issue of positive euthanasia is cloudy. On some occasions, a physician prescribes strong narcotics for a terminally ill patient and requests that the medication be given frequently enough to "keep the patient comfortable." Nurses often are reluctant to administer a medication that they realize has a potentially fatal effect when given in that dosage. In such cases, the ethical intent of the action is often considered. Medications given for the comfort of the dying patient may be ethically justifiable even if they hasten death to some extent. This is based on the ethical concept of *double effect,* in which the acceptable effect (such as pain relief) is the purpose of the medication and the secondary effect (such as depressing respiration) is not the intended effect. When nursing staff have difficulty with this issue, a patient conference with an oncology spe-

6. Termination.

   a. By Appointment of Guardian. The appointment of a guardian of the person of the principal terminates this power of attorney. The appointment of a guardian of the property only does not terminate this power of attorney.

   b. By Death of Principal. The death of the principal shall be deemed to revoke this power of attorney upon proof of death being received by the attorney-in-fact.

7. Reliance. The designated and acting attorney-in-fact and all persons dealing with the attorney-in-fact shall be entitled to rely upon this power of attorney so long as neither the attorney-in-fact nor person with whom they were dealing at the time of any act taken pursuant to this power of attorney had received actual knowledge or actual notice of the revocation or termination of the power of attorney by death or otherwise, and any action so taken, unless otherwise invalid or unenforceable, shall be binding on the heirs, devisees, legatees, or personal representatives of the principal.

8. Indemnity. The estate of the principal shall hold harmless and indemnify the attorney-in-fact from all liability for acts done in good faith and not in fraud on behalf of the principal.

9. Applicable Law. The laws of the State of Washington shall govern this power of attorney.

10. Execution. This power of attorney is signed on this _____ day of _____, 199 _____ , to become effective as provided in Paragraph 3.

Signature: _____

Print name: _____

STATE OF WASHINGTON)

) ss.

COUNTY OF KING   )

   I certify that I know or have satisfactory evidence that _____ is the person who appeared before me, and said person acknowledged that _____he signed this instrument and acknowledged it to be h_____ free and voluntary act for the uses and purposes mentioned in the instrument.

FIGURE 10–4 *(Continued)*

cialist or with a nurse skilled in the area of death and dying can help the staff to clarify values and deal with individual feelings.

Right-to-Die Issues

Right-to-die issues are gaining much more attention than in previous years. Kass (1993, p. 37) identifies four reasons for such a right to be asserted:

- Fear of prolongation of dying due to medical interventions; hence, a right to refuse treatment or hospitalization, even if death occurs as a result;
- Fear of living too long, without fatal illness to carry one off; hence, a right to assisted suicide;

- Fear of the degradations of senility and dependence; hence, a right to death with dignity;
- Fear of loss of control; hence, a right to choose the time and manner of one's death.

There has been a great deal of controversy around the issue of maintaining the lives of persons considered to be in a persistent vegetative state (PVS). Some of the issues that arise are the patient's rights, the family's wishes, and the cost to society. In most cases, the problems emerge when the life of a family member is being maintained through support measures that might be considered extraordinary.

In 1991, St. Francis-St. George Hospital in Cincinnati was sued in one of the first cases of its kind. The suit charged that the nurses should not have resuscitated an 82-year-old man when he suffered a heart attack. In so doing they disregarded the "no code" status of the patient (Hospital sued, 1991).

WITHHOLDING TREATMENT

Withholding treatment could be considered negative euthanasia. A historic case occurred in 1963.

A couple on the East Coast gave birth to a premature infant who was diagnosed as having Down syndrome, with the added complication of an intestinal blockage. The intestinal blockage could have been corrected by surgery with minimal risk; without surgery the child could not be fed and would die. The Down syndrome, however, would have resulted in some degree of permanent mental retardation. The severity of the retardation could not be determined at birth, but would range from very low mentality to borderline subnormal intelligence.

The parents, who had two normal children at home, believed that it would be unfair to those children to raise a child with Down syndrome, and refused permission for the corrective operation on the intestinal blockage. Although it was an option, the hospital staff did not seek a court order to override the decision. The staff believed it was unlikely that a court would sustain an order to operate on the child against the parents' wishes, because the child had a known mental handicap and would be a burden to the parents financially and emotionally, and perhaps a burden to society. The child was put in a side room (an interesting action) and was allowed to die, a process that took 11 days. When confronted with the possibility of giving medication to hasten the infant's death, both doctors and nurses were convinced that it was clearly illegal (Gustafson, 1973).

The situation above stimulates both ethical and legal questions. Would the approach have been the same if the infant had not been mentally retarded? Would the staff have been guilty of murder if the infant had been given medication to hasten death? If a court decision to proceed with the surgery had been requested and granted, who would have been responsible for the costs incurred? What are the rights of the child? Who advocates for those rights if the child is unable to do so?

WITHDRAWING TREATMENT

In some instances, a family has sought court orders to have extraordinary life-support measures discontinued. A landmark case is that of Karen Quinlan.

Karen Quinlan was a young woman left in a vegetative state after suffering severe brain damage from chemical abuse that involved both drugs and alcohol. She was placed on a respirator, and her physicians believed that she would live only a short time if it were to be removed. Her parents requested that the respirator be discontinued, but because she continued to manifest a minor amount of brain activity, their request was refused. After previous petitions to the Supreme Court of New Jersey had been rejected, the courts ruled on March 31, 1976, that her parents could exercise her privacy right on her behalf, and the respirator was discontinued. Much to everyone's surprise, Karen continued to live after the respirator was stopped, although she never emerged from her comatose condition; she died in 1986.

This case represents a situation in which treatment was withdrawn even though the individual was not considered immediately terminal. Such cases represent hard decisions for all involved and evoke legal, moral, and ethical questions in almost all instances. A similar case that attracted much attention was that of Nancy Cruzan.

In March 1988, Joe and Joyce Cruzan requested through the Jasper County Missouri Probate Court that they be allowed to remove the gastrostomy tube that kept their daughter Nancy alive. Nancy had been in a persistent vegetative state since an automobile accident in 1983. Although the request was granted, Missouri's attorney general appealed the decision, asking for a clear precedent from a higher court. In June 1990, the US Supreme Court effectively denied the request in asking for "clear and convincing" evidence of the patient's view. In reaching this point, a fine line was drawn between initially withholding medical treatment and later withdrawing it. In Missouri, once the family gives initial consent for treatment, they forfeit all power to undo that consent or to stop treatment. No other state has such a law (Colby, 1990). Treatment can be stopped in only two ways: if it can be demonstrated that it causes pain, or if the patient left behind clear and convincing evidence of his or her wishes prior to incompetency. The first was not an option because of Nancy Cruzan's persistent vegetative state. Therefore, her parents presented a state court with testimony from her physician and three friends that Nancy would not have wished to continue existing with irreversible brain damage. The Circuit Court judge ruled that this met the test and Nancy's feeding tube was removed on December 14, 1990. She died on December 26th.

Other cases have reached the headlines as individuals and families have striven to have more voice in determining issues related to the right to die. In all cases, much conflict exists in the arguments put forth by those supporting the right-to-die and right-to-life movements. In 1990, Congress took a major step regarding this issue by passing legislation that requires all Medicare and Medicaid providers to inform patients, on admission, of their right to refuse treatment. The matter is far from settled and is discussed in greater detail later in this chapter.

Of particular concern to nurses are their own feelings when a decision is reached to remove life-supporting measures, whether they are tube feedings or ventilators. Strong emotional attachments often form between the nurse and patient, even when the patient is in a vegetative state. Nurses who have worked to preserve the patient's dignity have great difficulty "letting go." In some instances, patients are transferred to other facilities to die in an environment where the nurses are not so emotionally involved with the patient.

POSITIONS ON WITHHOLDING AND WITHDRAWING TREATMENT

Several organizations and groups have issued guidelines for their members, and others who would find them useful, with regard to the issue of withholding or withdrawing treatment. Key to all of these guidelines is whether the patient is legally *competent* (able to make decisions for herself or himself), or *incompetent* (in need of someone else to make those decisions). Table 10-3 outlines the date, organization and major tenets of some of those positions.

ASSISTED DEATH

The activities of a retired Michigan pathologist, Jack Kevorkian, who is alleged to have assisted patients in their suicide, have received much media attention in the past few years. Although eluding criminal charges for a number of years, in March 1999, Dr. Kevorkian was convicted of second degree murder and the delivery of a controlled substance after CBS televised a video showing him administering lethal drugs. The first case in which he was charged but not convicted involved an Oregon woman with Alzheimer's disease.

In June 1997, the Supreme Court of the United States rendered a decision on physician-assisted suicide. This decision took the position that there was no constitutionally protected right to physician-assisted suicide on behalf of terminally ill patients.

In October 1997, the residents of Oregon legalized physician-assisted suicide, despite the Supreme Court decision. A study was conducted one year later of all terminally ill Oregon residents who received prescriptions for lethal medications. Of the 23 persons who received prescriptions for lethal medication, 15 died after taking the medications, 6 died from underlying illnesses, and 2 were alive as of January 1, 1999. Researchers found that the decision to request and use lethal medications was related to concern with loss of autonomy and bodily functions rather than concern with pain or financial loss. Level of education or health insurance coverage played no part in the patient's decision (Chin, et al, 1999).

The American Nurses Association has developed a position statement on assisted suicide in which they state that the nurse should not participate in assisted suicide. Such an act is viewed as a violation of the *Code for Nurses* (see Chapter 9). It is the position of the ANA that the challenge for nurses should not be in legalizing assisted suicide. Rather, the role of the nurse should be directed toward revers-

TABLE 10–3.   Positions on Withholding and Withdrawing Treatment

Date	Organization	Position
1983	President's Commission Report—*"Deciding to Forego Life-sustaining Treatment"*	Focused on the ethical, medical, and legal issues in treatment decisions. Distinguished between withholding (not starting) and withdrawing (stopping after it started) treatment without making a moral distinction between the two. Suggested that withholding may require more justification because the positive effects would not be known.
1986	American Medical Association—*"Statement on Withholding or Withdrawing Life-prolonging Medical Treatment"*	Stated that life-prolonging medical treatment and artificially or technologically maintained respiration, nutrition, and hydration, could be withheld from a patient in an irreversible coma even if death was not imminent (Fry, 1990).
1986	Office of Technology Assessment of the U.S. Congress—*"Life-sustaining Technologies and the Elderly"*	Issued the results of its study on the use of life-sustaining technologies on the elderly. Report noted that the most controversial of the technologies was that of nutritional support. Identified that the most troublesome aspect of nutritional support is whether it is intravenous feeding and hydration or a tube feeding (Fry, 1990).
1987	Hasting's Center—*"Guidelines on the Termination of Life-sustaining Treatment"*	Provided clear definitions of key terms and a general guideline for making decisions regarding treatment. Viewed nutrition and hydration as medical interventions, much as other life-sustaining measures. Placed emphasis on the patient's ability to make decisions and required case-by-case assessment (Fry, 1990).
1988	American Nurses Association—*"Guidelines on Withdrawing or Withholding Food and Fluid"*	Indicated that there were few instances under which it would be permissible for nurses to withdraw food or fluid from their patients. No distinction was made between withdrawing and withholding (ANA, 1988).
1995	American Nurses Association—*"Position Statement on Foregoing Medically Provided Nutrition and Hydration"*	Stated that the decision to withhold medically provided nutrition and hydration should be made by the patient or surrogate with the health care team. The nurse continues to provide expert and compassionate care to patients who are no longer receiving medically provided nutrition and hydration. Distinguished between medically provided nutrition and hydration and the provision of food and water (ANA, 1995a).

ing the despair and pain experienced in the last stages of life, and in fulfilling the obligation to provide competent, comprehensive, and compassionate end-of-life care (ANA, 1994).

THE RIGHT TO REFUSE TREATMENT

The right to refuse treatment is an issue closely aligned with the right to die. However, it carries special implications that require separate consideration. Although we discussed some of the parameters of this issue in the previous section on the right to die, other aspects can create even bigger problems for the nurse. The moral, if not legal, precedent for refusing treatment occurred in 1971.

Carmen Martinez was dying of hemolytic anemia, a disease that destroys the body's red blood cells. Her life could be maintained by transfusions, but her veins were such that a "cut-down" (a surgical opening made into the vein) was necessary to accomplish the transfusions. Finally, Martinez pleaded to have the cut-downs stopped and to be "tortured" no more. The physician, fearful of being charged with aiding in her suicide, asked for a court decision. The court ruled that Martinez was not competent to make such a decision and appointed her daughter as her guardian. When the daughter also asked that no more cut-downs be performed, the compassionate judge honored the daughter's request. He decided that although Martinez did not have the right to commit suicide, she did have the "right not to be tortured." She died the next day (Veatch, 1976).

People working in the health care professions often are confronted with such dilemmas. Cases such as one in which a patient refuses to have a leg amputated, even though not having the surgery undoubtedly will result in death, often will make the news. The right to refuse treatment can take on additional implications when the patient, by refusing one type of treatment, is essentially demanding alternative medical management. Our support of the right to refuse treatment is based on a basic belief in and respect for the autonomy of the patient. When the refusal of medical intervention means that the individual is no longer a patient, it is known as a *negative right simpliciter* by bioethicists. In these cases the patient's physician need only do nothing, as in cases in which the patient discharges himself or herself from the hospital. When the patient refuses treatment, but does not withdraw from the role of being the patient, the matter becomes more complex. An example would be the patient who refuses to have a gangrenous toe surgically removed and demands to have it treated otherwise. These are referred to as positive rights. In the case of a patient with a gangrenous toe, one form of treatment may be more accepted than another, but both may be successful. A case illustrating this right occurred in 1993 in Chicago, and attracted national attention.

A Pentecostal Christian mother refused to have a cesarean section when physicians recommended the procedure because her fetus was being deprived of oxygen and would die if delivered vaginally. The courts upheld the patient's right to refuse the surgery. She later gave birth to an apparently healthy boy.

When children are involved, it is even more newsworthy, and again points out that there is as yet no consensus about when minors should be allowed to refuse treatment.

In November 1994, 16-year-old Billy Best made national news when he ran away from home to avoid another 5 months of chemotherapy and radiation. Suffering from Hodgkin's disease, the high school junior was experiencing nausea, aching, and fatigue, as well as hair loss, from the treatment. He stated, ". . . I could not stand going to the hospital every week. I feel like the medicine is killing me instead of helping me." (Dorning, 1994).

Often in such cases, the parents refuse to have the treatment started, many times because of religious beliefs. The courts usually become involved in reaching a decision. A case in Illinois in 1952 is typical.

Eight-day-old Cheryl suffered from erythroblastosis fetalis (Rh incompatibility). Her parents, who were Jehovah's Witnesses, refused to authorize the administration of blood necessary to save her life. The judge in the case ruled that Cheryl was a neglected dependent and overrode the parent's refusal. In such instances, the child is usually made a temporary ward of the court and legal documents are attached to the record authorizing the needed treatment. Such court decisions usually have been based on the premise that the right to freedom of religion does not give parents the right to risk the lives of their children or to make martyrs of them (Veatch, 1976).

Sometimes, when time is not a factor, the court will recommend that treatment be delayed until the child is 15 or 16 years old and can make a decision as an older minor. Other judges will rule just the opposite, deciding that it is cruel to place the burden of the decision on this older minor.

Situations like those that have been cited are always difficult for the people involved. Because nurses have the most contact with patients, they must examine their own feelings and attitudes. Nurses must recognize that patients also have the right to attitudes and beliefs. If a nurse decides that his or her feelings are so strong that they might interfere with the ability to give compassionate care, it would be wise to ask to be assigned to other patients (Fig. 10-5).

FIGURE 10–5   People working in the health care field are frequently confronted with the dilemma of patients who may wish to refuse treatment.

ADDITIONAL BIOETHICAL CONCERNS

Most of you probably will find the area of bioethics interesting. Although many topics are central to bioethics, such as the right to die, the right to refuse treatment, and all the issues related to conception, a number of less well-defined concerns are encountered in our health care delivery system. We cannot discuss all of these without creating a separate bioethics textbook; however, several deserve some review.

Organ Transplantation

Developments in the area of *organ transplantation* have created several issues deserving consideration. *Organ transplantation* is the process by which a tissue or organ is removed and replaced by a corresponding part. Transplants can be done using tissue from one's own body (eg, skin, bone, or cartilage); this is called an autograft. Transplantation using organs from a donor's body is known as homograft or allograft; it might involve organs such as the kidney, liver, heart, cornea, or skin of another individual. Some organs (eg, the heart) must be transplanted immediately or they will die. Others, such as the kidney or skin, can be stored for short periods. The main obstacle to transplantation of organs lies in the rejection of those organs by the recipient, and has resulted in the antigenic typing of tissues and the administration of immunosuppressive drugs.

The replacement for a diseased organ typically is obtained from donors who have died, although some (eg, a kidney) can come from living individuals. This has necessitated a clearer definition of death. The supply of organs that can be used for transplantation has not been able to keep up with the demand. This is a result of the larger variety of organs that can be transplanted today. Additionally, as modern technology has been able to save more lives, organs available for transplantation have decreased.

CONCERNS ABOUT PROCUREMENT

It has been estimated that between 1990 and 1995, an annual average of 4,835 people donated organs for use after their deaths. But many more—about 48,000 individuals—remain on organ waiting lists (Cimons & Maugh, 1996). Conflicts of interest between the potential donor and the person receiving the donor organ are easy to anticipate. Certainly, no one would want to remove an organ from a donor as long as that person had any potential for recovery; on the other hand, it is imperative that donor organs be removed immediately after the death of the donor, before the organs become unusable.

Although there is lack of uniformity in the definition of death throughout the 50 states, it is generally accepted that organs can be removed from donors who have a flat electroencephalogram. This action is based on the 1975 definition of death, which states: "For all legal purposes, a human body with irreversible cessation of total brain function, according to usual and customary standards of medical practice, shall be considered dead" (Capron, 1978, p. 300).

The idea of consent again becomes important when we talk about organ transplantation. It is preferable to have the consent obtained from the donor. This has been facilitated in many states by the Uniform Anatomical Gift Act, which was drafted by a committee of the National Conference of the Commissions of Uniform State Laws in July 1968, and adopted in all American jurisdictions in 1971 (Hayt, 1977). People who are willing to donate parts of their bodies after death may indicate the desire to do so in a will or other written documents, or by carrying a donor's card. Many states now provide a space on the driver's license where individuals can authorize permission for organ donations.

The next-of-kin also must grant permission for the removal of organs after death. However, the time factor is crucial; the deaths are often accidental, and the relatives are often so emotionally distressed that the process of obtaining permission may be difficult. Most medical personnel are at least initially hesitant to request permission for donor organs at this critical time. As we have gained more experience in this process, we also have developed better ways to deal with delicate issues. It is generally recommended that two groups of personnel be involved in requesting organs. The first group (usually nurses or medical personnel) helps the family realize that death has occurred or is imminent. This allows the family to grasp the reality of the situation. The second group, often referred to as the procurement team, requests the organ donation; these are persons skilled in recognizing the stress being felt by the family and experienced in providing information that will be important to them (Fig. 10-6).

Some states have regulations that allow donation of organs from an unidentified donor. Once a diligent search has been completed for next-of-kin, organs can be recovered. A coroner's consent is required in cases of accidental death, homicide, suicide, or any questionable cause of death.

In response to the inadequate supply of organs to meet societal needs—a situation referred to as *scarce medical resources*—some states have passed legislation requiring that donor organs be requested of the family when it is apparent that the patient has no chance for survival. This brings forth other problems. Who is to be responsible for approaching the family and requesting the organs? Must it be the family's physician? Would critical time be saved if it were the emergency department nurse or hospital social worker? A growing number of hospitals are designating a nurse as transplantation coordinator to facilitate this process. An interesting and controversial case occurred in California in 1990.

An 18-year-old woman, an only child, was diagnosed as having chronic myelogenous leukemia. Although this form of leukemia responds favorably to bone marrow transplants, no compatible donor could be found after testing the girl's family and contacting the National Marrow Donor Program. In desperation, the parents decided to have another child with the hope that the new baby would have genetically matching tissue type. This required that the father have a vasectomy reversed and that the mother, age 43, go through another pregnancy that terminated in a cesarean section. The baby proved a good match and was able to provide donor tissue for her sister. The case drew considerable attention as medical ethicists voiced concern about creating one child to save another. Citing Immanuel Kant, they argued that the baby was conceived, not as

Consent for Removal of Organs from the Deceased

I, _____ , next of kin (_____)
        Name   *Relationship*

of _____
                                   Name of Donor

for humanitarian reasons hereby give consent for removal of _____

_____ from
                        Names of Organs and Tissues

_____
                                   Name of Donor

after his or her death for the purpose of transplantation, or for the retention of such
organs and tissues for any other scientific or therapeutic purposes.

I understand that some of the procedures necessary for determination of suitability for
transplantation will include testing for HBsAg (hepatitis B virus) and human immunodeficiency virus (AIDS virus antibody). I further authorize the release of medical information gathered in this process to the physicians involved in transplanting the above
stated organs and tissues.

_____
Signature

_____
Date

_____
Witness

_____
Witness

FIGURE 10–6   Organ donation consent form.

an end in itself, but for utilitarian purposes. Some medical ethicists argued in favor of the rights of the individuals involved, saying that it is not the concern of biomedical ethicists to intrude into matters affecting private citizens, especially when that intrusion approaches "intruding into a couple's bedroom." Still others say that striking cases must be brought before the public because an obligation to inform society exists.

The critical need for human organs also causes us to challenge previous decisions. A good example is that raised when considering organs removed from an anencephalic infant. An anencephalic infant is one born with only enough brain to support such vital functions as heartbeat and respiration. It has been estimated that about 60% of these infants are stillborn, and of those born alive only about 5% will live more than 3 days. Because anencephaly affects only the brain, other organs can be used for transplantation if the infant is kept alive on a respirator until an organ recipient is located. This challenges our definitions of death. How can current definitions of "brain" death be applied to a condition in which there is no brain as we normally recognize it?

Other problems also arise with regard to organ transplantations, especially because more people need organs than there are organs available. The skill of modern technology has resulted in the development and implantation of artificial organs such as the heart. Such technologic advances once were viewed as science fiction. As a result, historic cases such as the implantation of an artificial heart in Barney Clark in 1982 received a great deal of publicity. Over the years the use of artificial organs has not proven effective, and the practice of implanting artificial organs is not common today. This is not true of artificial parts, however. The use of artificial joints, heart valves, and other prostheses continues to grow.

MINORITY ATTITUDES TOWARD ORGAN DONATION

Another issue that has emerged is that of minority differences in regard to organ donation. A growing number of minorities are now on waiting lists for transplantation. The risk of end-stage renal disease for African Americans and Native Americans is three to four times higher than for the white population (Kasiske, Neylan, Riggio, et al, 1991). Minority organ donations lag behind those from the white population, with 78.5% of cadaver donations coming from whites, 11.4% from African-Americans, 8.2% from Hispanics, and 1.0% from Asians (Wheeler & Cheung, 1996). Some of this difference is attributed to the fact that minority groups have been found to lack education and information regarding organ donation.

Minority groups also have identified religious beliefs and cultural customs as forbidding organ donation, although no major Western religion prohibits organ donation. African Americans listed distrust of the medical community, fear of premature death, and racism as major barriers. Hispanics experienced language barriers and identified the importance of having the entire extended family involved in all decision making regarding donations. Puerto Ricans verbalized denial of death and fear of mutilation of the body as critical factors. Barriers to organ donation in Asian American cultures included the belief that the body should remain intact to the grave and lack of respect during the handling of the body after death. Although Native Americans are supportive of organ donations, their rate of donation is low, probably owing to lack of knowledge (Wheeler & Cheung, 1996). Although no single approach to organ donation fits all groups, efforts to decrease barriers to donation are being instituted.

Critical Thinking Activity

> Have you signed an organ donation card? If not, discuss the reasons why you have chosen not to do so. If you have, discuss the reasons why you have. Is there a possibility you will change your mind? Why or why not? What solutions can you suggest to help the nation deal with the shortage of organs needed for transplantation?

CONCERNS ABOUT XENOTRANSPLANTATION

Xenotransplantation refers to the practice of using animal organs, cells, and tissues for transplantation into human beings. It is in the stage of experimentation around the world. Xenotransplantation usually involves organs or tissues from pigs and nonhuman primates. One case receiving national publicity was that of an AIDS patient in San Francisco who received the transplant of baboon bone marrow to bolster his weakening immune system. Since 1906, some 55 animal-to-human whole organ transplants have been attempted; none was successful (Fano, et al, 1999). Cases that received particular attention were the 1984 transplant of a baboon heart into Baby Fae (who died 20 days later) and the 1992 transplant of a baboon liver into a 35-year-old man (who also died).

In addition to the obvious problems associated with immune system rejection, of particular concern to some is the possibility of transmitting serious animal viruses and other microbes, so-called zoonotic diseases, to people. Feno and associates (1999) report more than 20 known, potentially lethal viruses that can be transmitted from nonhuman primates to humans. This has prompted the use of pigs as the "donor" of choice, and has led to attempts to alter pigs genetically so that tissues would be more adaptable to transplantation. Recent concerns in England over the communicability of bovine spongiform encephelopathy through the ingestion of meat from ill animals has prompted the discussion of the potential for all animal organs to transmit diseases that would appear only years later. Even raising animals in a sterile environment has its limitations because it is now being discovered that some diseases are transmitted from mother to fetus in utero.

In September 1996, the federal government proposed strict safeguards to provide protection. The guidelines were developed by representatives from the Food and Drug Administration (FDA), the Centers for Disease Control and Prevention (CDC), and the National Institutes of Health (NIH). The guidelines urged that patients and their families be fully informed of potential risks, and further required that any planned procedure be thoroughly screened and approved by a series of local institutional review boards, and by the FDA. The recommendations also require that transplants take place at a clinical center associated with an accredited biology and microbiology laboratory.

Animal-rights activists also have expressed concern about the process. They view the transplantation experiments as costly, cruel, and hopeless.

CONCERNS ABOUT ALLOCATION

How will we determine who receives donated organs? Does "elitism" exist in their distribution—that is, does a white-collar worker have a better chance to receive an organ than a blue-collar worker? Medicaid and most insurance policies refuse to pay for the cost of many organ transplants, although Medicare usually covers the costs of corneal transplants and kidney transplants. Transplants are expensive procedures, often running into several hundreds of thousands of dollars. If money is required "up front," as it sometimes is, where can the needy person procure such funds? Other questions involve both donor and recipient. Should the donor or the donor's family be able to say who will receive the organ? How can one "get in line" for an organ, and how can that need be made known? What about selling a healthy organ, such as a kidney?

Much has been written about the problem of selecting recipients for organ transplantation when the number of applicants exceeds the number of available organs. Many criteria have been suggested, and as one might anticipate, these criteria have arguments both pro and con; the criterion requiring medical acceptability is probably the only exception. Many transplants require that compatibility exist in the tissue and blood type of donor and recipient. It would not be logical to give a much-needed organ to a person whose body would automatically reject it.

The criterion of the recipient's social worth is probably one of the hardest to defend, although it was used in the Pacific Northwest in the early 1960s to decide who should be allowed to live by kidney dialysis. Social worth, including past and future potential, was considered, and even such factors as church membership and participation in community endeavors were considered.

Some suggest a form of random selection, once the criterion of medical acceptability has been met. This could be either a natural random selection of the first come, first served variety, or an artificial selection process such as a lottery. A criticism of this method is that it removes rational decision making from the process.

We offer no suggestions to solve this problem, but merely demonstrate the difficulty it presents. Even the issue of who should serve on the decision-making committee can be touchy. The problem of personal biases is a big concern.

In an effort to gather donations and disseminate information about individuals who need various organs, an Organ Procurement Program was started in Pittsburgh, Pennsylvania. This program was established to facilitate the matching of donor with recipient and to provide a central listing agency for those in need of transplants. Today, organ procurement agencies are located in all regions of the country. These groups carry out many activities related to organ procurement, including establishing groups for individuals who have received donated organs and their families, publishing newsletters, developing educational materials, increasing public awareness of the need for organs, and serving as a clearinghouse for organ procurement and matching. They are connected through the federally funded United Network for Organ Sharing.

CONCERNS ABOUT INDIVIDUAL PROPERTY RIGHTS

Concern for an individual's property rights in regard to human tissues also has attracted attention. Developments in biotechnology allow profit-oriented companies to use human tissue to generate lucrative products such as drugs, diagnostic tests, and other medically related materials. The modern legal system has consistently held that no property rights are attached to the human body (Swain & Marusyk, 1990). In 1990, a Seattle man sued the University of California, two researchers, and two biotechnology and drug companies, because in 1976 he had sought treatment for hairy cell leukemia and subsequently had his spleen removed (which is the standard treatment). It was later discovered that the removed spleen contained unique blood cells that produced a rare blood protein, which then was used experimentally in the treatment of certain cancers and possibly AIDS. The patient was never told that his cells had great potential value, although he was brought from Seattle to Los

Angeles frequently for blood and other tests. His cells were then developed into a self-perpetuating cell line to mass produce the rare blood protein. The patient's suit claimed that the defendants wrongfully converted to their own use his personal property (ie, the blood cells) and that this was done without his consent.

Truth-Telling and Health Care Providers

The issue of "to tell" or "not to tell" may not carry the emotional and bioethical impact that one experiences with concerns such as euthanasia, but it is often encountered in the health care environment. Although informed consent has forced a more straightforward approach between physician and client, the problem of having the patient fully understand the outcome of care still exists (see Chapter 9). Sometimes the question about telling the client the expected outcome of care results from a request made by a close relative, but most of the time it results from the persistence of past medical practices.

In such instances the physician operates in a paternalistic role in relation to the client. Under this model of care, the locus of decision making is moved away from the client and resides with the physician. "Benefit and do no harm to the patient" is the dictum often cited as the ethical basis for this approach. It rationalizes that complete knowledge of his or her condition would place greater stress on the client. More recent discussions of medical ethics explore the rights of clients, particularly their right to make their own medical decisions. These discussions emphasize that in our pluralistic society, which also has fostered medical specialization to keep up with advances in knowledge and technology, physicians may be unable to perceive the "best interests" of their clients and to act accordingly.

Physicians do not agree on how much information should be provided to patients regarding their conditions. We usually experience a major controversy relating to this issue when a client has a terminal diagnosis such as cancer. Physicians may be concerned that sharing bad news will result in unhappiness, anxiety, depression, and fear, and that the client suffering from a terminal illness will "give up." Physicians who argue the other side of the issue state that there exists a common moral obligation to tell the truth. They believe that the anxiety of not knowing the accurate diagnosis is at least as great as knowing the truth, especially if the truth is shared in a humane manner. These physicians also argue that one needs to have control over one's life and, if the news is bad, to have time to get personal affairs in order. Fortunately, new regulations regarding informed consent and more aggressive treatment for all life-threatening conditions have minimized situations in which patients are not provided full knowledge of their condition.

Thus far, we have discussed situations in which information regarding a terminal illness may be shared with the client and family. At least one other circumstance that involves telling the truth is worth mentioning, although many examples could be included. One that we often see in the obstetric area of the hospital deals with sharing information with the parents of a newborn who is critically ill or who has a malformation. Sometimes physicians may want to spare the mother unpleasant news until she is stronger. This occurs frequently enough for obstetric nurses to have labeled it the *spare-the-mother syndrome*. In some instances, the physician may want to delay giving information until suspicions can be validated. If the doctor is waiting for the return of laboratory tests to confirm suspicions of genetic abnormalities, several days may be required. If good communication exists between nurse and physician, so that the nurse is well informed, the nurse can provide emotional support and meet the client's need for information.

Although to tell or not to tell (or to delay telling) is a problem that exists between client and physician, nurses often become involved. Because the nurse is in contact with the client for a more extended time, he or she may be put on the spot by the client's questions. The nurse may feel that hedging on a response compromises the ethics of nursing practice. In such instances a conference, whether formal or impromptu, that would involve the physician, nurses, and other appropriate members of the health team, may help everyone deal with the situation. The nurse who is a novice in the health care system should realize that anyone may initiate a client care conference, although appropriate channels of communication should be followed in organizing it.

The question of whether "to tell" or "not to tell" has been applied to another issue in the health care delivery system in recent years. That controversy pits the rights to privacy of the individual who is HIV positive against society's right to be protected. Dr. Cary Savitch, who has treated AIDS patients since 1981, advocates universal testing. Dr. Savich (1996, p. 140) states, "Controlling the epidemic is the only means to limit needless suffering and death. Controlling the epidemic will not come at the hands of a vaccine or miracle drug. Controlling the epidemic requires prevention. Prevention requires knowing who is communicable. Knowing who is communicable requires universal testing."

Many express concerns about privacy and confidentiality. If universal testing for AIDS is mandated, what would be next? Others argue that if health care providers exercise proper precautions, little danger exists. Still others would find the cost of universal testing too great to make it realistic. There is no agreement among health care providers, activists, civil libertarians, and all concerned citizens regarding this issue, and the controversy is certain to continue.

Ethical Concerns and Behavior Control

Before leaving this discussion of bioethical issues, we should say a few words about behavior control. Many people experience extreme discomfort when contemplating research into human behavior. Although it may be one thing to work with atoms, molecules, and genes, it seems quite another to look at the science of human behavior.

Some of the problem seems to center around the fact that people define "acceptable behavior" in different and sometimes conflicting ways. When is behavior deviant? When is the client mentally ill? An excellent example is that of homosexuality, which the American Psychiatric Association at one time listed as a mental illness. Although many people may not approve of homosexuality, they would not classify all homosexuals as being mentally ill. Increasingly, society looks on sexual orientation as a personal matter.

The world has benefited from the work of many people whose behavior might not be looked upon as normal. Van Gogh cut off his ear; Tchaikovsky had terrible periods of depression; Beethoven was known for his uncontrollable rages. Some have suggested that Florence Nightingale's flights into fantasy could better be described as neurosis. Should this behavior have been changed? If so, by what methods?

We now can change behavior by several methods. Certainly one of the most common methods in which nurses will be involved is the administration of pharmacologic agents. Tranquilizers are now one of the largest classifications of drugs in the United States. Other chemicals, such as alcohol, marijuana, cocaine, and lysergic acid diethylamide (LSD), also change behavior. Some of these are considered socially acceptable, whereas others are not. Some are socially acceptable to some people or to some cultures, yet unacceptable to other cultures.

Electroconvulsive therapy (ECT), known earlier as electric shock therapy (EST), has been used for years to treat severe depression. Although antidepressant drugs more commonly are used today, ECT is still used in many areas of the country for depression that does not respond to drugs. Opponents of this form of therapy, who see it as inhumane, are becoming an organized political force. Proponents point out that with the current safeguards, it can be an effective therapy.

Psychosurgery—for example, frontal lobotomy (portrayed in *One Flew Over the Cuckoo's Nest*)—was used in the 1930s. This is undoubtedly one of the most criticized treatment modalities because of its effect on the person. It is rarely used today, although another type of brain surgery is now being suggested for obsessive-compulsive disorder.

Psychotherapy can change other behavior. Techniques include verbal and nonverbal communication between the client and the therapist. Although psychotherapy requires considerable time, it is widely used.

When are any of these methods justified? Who makes the decision? What behavior is beyond the realm of acceptability? Who determines this? How does behavior control mesh with our beliefs about the autonomy of the individual or with concepts of self-respect and dignity? The issues of power and coercion pose a concern at this point. Problems related to involuntary commitment have moved this from the arena of ethics to that of legal determinants.

Halleck (1981, p. 268) has defined behavior control as treatment "imposed on or offered to the patient that, to a large extent, is designed to satisfy the wishes of others. Such treatment may lead to the patient's behaving in a manner which satisfies his community or his society." Halleck goes on to point out that the question of behavior control has become more critical because newer drugs and new behavior therapy (such as aversive therapy and desensitization) make it possible to change specific behavior more rapidly and effectively. Traditional psychotherapy, which works slowly, offers the patient time in which to contemplate the change and reject it if it is unacceptable.

Dworkin (1981, p. 278) has proposed a set of guidelines that preserve autonomy in behavior control, as briefly stated here. Although these guidelines are almost 20 years old, they continue to be recognized for the direction they provide.

- We should favor those methods of influencing behavior that support the self-respect and dignity of those who are being influenced.
- Methods of influence that destroy or decrease a person's ability to think rationally and in his or her own interest should not be used.

- Methods of influence that fundamentally affect the personal identity of the person should not be used.
- Methods of influence that deceive or keep relevant facts from the person should not be used.
- Modes of influence that are not physically intrusive are preferable to those that are (eg, drugs, psychosurgery, and electricity).
- A person should be able to resist the method of influence if he or she so desires, and changes of behavior that are reversible are preferable to those that are not.
- Methods that work through the cognitive and affective structure of a person are preferable to those that "short-circuit" his beliefs and desires and cause him to be passively receptive to the will of others.

 ## Critical Thinking Activity

> Review the guidelines for ethical treatment of psychiatric conditions. Which do you believe are the strongest, and why? Are there any that you question; if so, why? Are there any that you think should be added?

Rationing of Health Care

As we enter the 21st century, perhaps no issue in health care will receive more attention than the rationing of health care. Technology has allowed people to live longer. New treatment modalities have become more expensive. Dollars do not exist within our current social system to make all forms of health care available to all who wish to receive it. What should be treated and what should not? Who should receive the treatment and who should not? Should age be a factor? Mental status? Ability to contribute to society? *Rationing* is restricting the availability of some desired commodity to limited allotments. Most consider rationing to be a planned, thoughtful approach to a limited supply. Some would argue that we currently ration health care by restricting its availability to those with the financial means to pay, although none would argue that this is a carefully planned approach.

Some states have begun to address these issues. In 1989, the Oregon legislature passed several statutes that, among other things, created a process to establish health care priorities so that Medicaid and state-encouraged private coverage could provide the most cost-effective and beneficial forms of care for the largest number of persons. Implicit in this legislation was the involvement of the public in the process of building consensus on the values to be used to guide health resource allocation decisions. Oregon has continued to lead the nation in health care reform, especially at the consumer involvement level.

In Vermont, a statewide public education and discussion project was initiated to explore public attitudes and values that underlie health care and the public's priorities in the allocation of health resources. The project focused on the need for individuals to make known their preferences with regard to personal treatment.

In New Jersey, a Citizens' Committee on Biomedical Ethics has taken the position that citizens have the right and responsibility to insist that their preferences and values influence the development of health care policies and the allocation of medical resources. They have launched a community health program to clarify the ethical and social issues surrounding the provision of health care in that state.

Other states are following these examples. Citizens are being asked to make informed decisions regarding health care. As a nurse, you have a vital role to play in the sharing of information regarding the delivery of health services. It is critical for you to anticipate some of the questions you may be asked and to analyze your own values.

Critical Thinking Activity

What do you see as the major issues regarding the rationing of health care? Develop a list of the major health conditions for which you believe care should be funded. Identify those that should receive partial funding. List those that you believe should not be funded. Give a rationale for placing the various conditions on one of the three lists.

KEY CONCEPTS

- Bioethics is the study of ethical issues that result from technologic and scientific advances, especially in biology and medicine. The number of bioethical issues surrounding the delivery of health care is growing.
- The area of human genetic research has raised many ethical questions, including how this knowledge should be used, rights to privacy, and who in the health care delivery system carries the responsibility for making testing, diagnosis, and cost effective care available to patients.
- Many bioethical issues can be divided into two major categories: those related to the beginning of life and those related to the end of life.
- Family planning (and the associated concern regarding age of consent) is one issue related to the beginning of life. Personal preferences and religious beliefs are critical determinants, and nurses should be prepared to meet the needs of all clients without imposing their personal values on clients.
- Abortion, amniocentesis, chorionic villus samplying, prenatal diagnosis, genetic screening, sterilization, the concept of eugenics, in vitro fertilization, artificial insemination, surrogate mothers, single parents, sperm banks, and the right to genetic information are additional topics presenting concerns.
- Fundamental bioethical issues concerning death are the changing definition of death and the decision about when it occurs.
- End-of-life issues include identifying futile treatment and establishing patient self-determination.
- Although many courts, based on individual circumstances, have accepted negative euthanasia, positive euthanasia remains very controversial.

- Surrounding the discussion of right-to-die are many issues, including those related to withholding treatment, withdrawing treatment, assisted death, and the right to refuse treatment.
- Bioethical concerns associated with the process of organ transplantation include procurement of organs, minority attitudes, allocation of organs, individual property rights, and the appropriateness of xenotransplantations.
- Debate and controversy have long surrounded determining what degree of information should be shared with clients and their families.
- The area of behavior control is subject to bioethical review, and guidelines have been established to preserve autonomy in behavior control.
- Rationing of health care commands major attention now. Many states have begun to establish citizen committees to respond to this concern.

REFERENCES

American Nurses Association. Position Statement on Foregoing Medically Provided Nutrition and Hydration. Washington, DC: American Nurses Association, 1995a

American Nurses Association. Position Statement on Nursing and the Patient Self-Determination Act. Washington, DC: American Nurses Association, 1995b

American Nurses Association. Position Statement on Assisted Suicide. Washington, DC: American Nurses Association, 1994

American Nurses Association. Guidelines on Withdrawing or Withholding Food and Fluid. Washington, DC: American Nurses Association, 1988

Blackmun H. Majority opinion in Roe vs Wade. *In* Mappes TA, Zembaty JS: Biomedical Ethics, 2nd ed. New York: McGraw-Hill, 1981:478–482

Burley SK, Almo SC, Bonanno JB, Capel M, Chance MR, Gaasterland T, Lin D, Sali A, Studier FW, Swaminathan S. Structural genomics: Beyond the human genome project. Nat Genet 23(2):151–157, 1999

Callahan D. The goals of medicine: Setting new priorities. Hasting Cent Rep 26(6;Suppl): 518–528, 1997

Capron AM. Grandma? No, I'm the Mother! Hastings Cent Rep 24(2):24–25, 1994

Capron AM. Death, definition and determination of: Legal aspects. *In* Reich WT: Encyclopedia of Bioethics, vol 1. New York: Free Press, 1978

Chin AE, Hedberg K, Higginson GK, Fleming DW. Legalized physician-assisted suicide in Oregon—the first year's experience. N Engl J Med 340(7):577–583, 1999

Cimons M, Maugh II, TH. Rules outlined for transplants from animals. Transplant: Safeguards drafted on animal-to-human treatments. *Los Angeles Times*, September 21, 1996:A1, A15

Colby WH. Missouri stands alone. Hastings Cent Rep 20(5):5–6, 1990

Committee on Bioethics, American Academy of Pediatrics. Informed consent, parental permission, and assent in pediatric practice. Pediatrics 95(2):314–317

Dorning M. Teen-agers refusal of treatment stirs debate. *San Diego Union Tribune*, November 13, 1994:A8

Dworkin G. Autonomy and behavior control. *In* Mappes TA, Zembaty JS: Biomedical Ethics, 2nd ed. New York: McGraw-Hill, 1981:273–280

English cardinal bucks Vatican on destroying embryos. *The Herald*, August 1, 1996:7A

Fano A, Cohen MJ, Cramer M, Greek R, Kaufman SR. Of pigs, primates, and plagues: A layperson's guide to the problems with animal-to-human organ transplants. Available at *www.mrmcmed.org/pigs.html*. Accessed December 22, 1999.

Fromer MJ. Ethical Issues in Health Care. St. Louis: CV Mosby, 1981

Fry ST. New ANA guidelines on withdrawing or withholding food and fluid from patients. *In* Lindeman CA, McAthie M: Readings: Nursing Trends and Issues. Springhouse, PA: Springhouse, 1990:499–507

Grady D. How to coax new life. *Time Special Issue*, Fall 1996:37–39

Gustafson JJ. Mongolism, parental desires, and the right to life. Perspect Biomed, Summer 1973:529

Halleck SL. Legal and ethical aspects of behavior control. *In* Mappes TA, Zembaty JS: Biomedical Ethics, 2nd ed. New York: McGraw-Hill, 1981:267–273

Hayt LR. Medicolegal Aspects of Hospital Records, 2nd ed. Berwyn, IL: Physicians' Record Company, 1977:397

Hellegers AE. Bioethical debates in gynecology and obstetrics. *In* Romney SL, et al: Gynecology and Obstetrics: The Health Care of Women. New York: McGraw-Hill, 1975:36

Hospital sued for "wrongful life." Am J Nurs 91(5):111, 1991

Hudson T. Advance directives: Still problematic for providers. Hospitals and Health Networks 68(6):46, 48, 50, 1994a

Hudson T. Are futile-care policies the answer? Hospitals and Health Networks 68(4):26–32, 1994b

Human Genome Project Information. Ethical, legal, and social issues (ELSI) of the Human Genome Project. Available at *www.ornl.gov/TechResources/Human_Genome/resource/elsi.html*. Accessed December 15, 1999.

Human Genome Project Information. Frequently asked questions. Available at *www.ornl.gov/hgmis/faq/faqs1.html*. Accessed December 15, 1999.

Jonsen AR. The birth of bioethics. Hastings Cent Rep 23(6;Suppl):S1–S4, 1993

Kasiske BL, Neylan JF, Riggio RR, et al. The effect of race on access and outcome in transplantation. N Engl J Med 324:302–307, 1991

Kass LR. Is there a right to die? Hastings Cent Rep 23(1):34–43, 1993

Kelly SJ. Pediatric Emergency Nursing, 2nd ed. Norwalk, CT: Appleton & Lange, 1994

Kevles DJ. Social and ethical issues in the Human Genome Project. National Forum LXXIII(2):18–21, 1993

Macklin R. Artificial means of reproduction and our understanding of the family. Hastings Cent Rep 21(1):5–11, 1991

Mancini M. Nursing, minors, and the law. Am J Nurs 78(1):124–127, 1978

Nuland SB. An epidemic of discovery. *Time Special Issue*, Fall:8–13, 1996

O'Toole M. (Ed.) Miller-Keane Encyclopedia & Dictionary of Medicine, Nursing, & Allied Health, 5th ed. Philadelphia: WB Saunders, 1992

Pilbeam SP. Mechanical Ventilation: Physiological and Clinical Applications, 2nd ed. St. Louis: Mosby-Year Book, 1992:17

Roan S. Woman gives birth at 63: Ethical questions raised. *Los Angeles Times*, April 24, 1997:A1, A31

Roe v. Wade, 410 U.S. 113 (1973)

Rossiter BJF, Caskey CT. Medical consequences of the Human Genome Project. National Forum LXXIII(2):12–14, 1993

Rothman DA, Rothman NL. The Professional Nurse and the Law. Boston: Little, Brown, 1977

Rothstein MA. The challenge of the new genetics. National Forum 69(4):39–40, 1990

Savitch C. The Nutcracker is Already Dancing: The HIVs and the HIV-Nots. Ventura, CA: Teague House Press, 1996

Schneiderman LF, Jecker N. Futility in practice. Arch Intern Med 153:437–440, 1993

Swain MS, Marusyk RW. An alternative to property rights in human tissue. Hastings Cent Rep 20(5):12–15, 1990

Thomas CL. Taber's Cyclopedic Medical Dictionary, 17th ed. Philadelphia: FA Davis, 1993

&TOTSE. Age of consent in every state. Available at *www.totse.com/files/FA019/aoc.htm.* Accessed December 15, 1999

University of Wisconsin—Madison. Stem Cell Press Kit. Office of News and Public Affairs, November 5, 1998. Available at *www.news.wisc.edu/emediakit/release.html.* Accessed July 3, 2000.

Veatch RM. Death, Dying and the Biological Revolution. New Haven, CT: Yale University Press, 1976

Wheeler MS, Cheung A. Minority attitudes toward organ donation. Critical Care Nurse 16(1):30–34, 1996

FURTHER READING

American Nurses Association. Position Statement on Promotion of Comfort and Relief of Pain in Dying Patients. Washington DC: American Nurses Association, 1994

American Nurses Association. Position Statement on Nursing Care and Do-Not-Resuscitate Decisions. Washington DC: American Nurses Association, 1995

Arras GJ. Crazy making: Embryos and gestational mothers. Hastings Cent Rep 21(1):35–38, 1991

Arras JD. Anencephalic newborns as organ donors: A critique. JAMA 259:2284–2286, 1988

Bailey LL. Organ transplantation: A paradigm of medical progress. Hastings Cent Rep 20(1):24–28, 1990

Berrio MW, Levesque ME. Advance directives; most patients don't have one. Do yours? Am J Nurs 96(8):24–29, 1996

Callahan D. Medical futility, medical necessity: The problem without a name. Hastings Cent Rep 21(4):30–35, 1991

Chafey K. "Caring" is not enough: Ethical paradigms for community-based care. N & HC Perspective on Community 17(1):10–15, 1996

Chervenak FA, McCollough LB. Justified limits on refusing intervention. Hastings Cent Rep 21(2):12–18, 1991

Colbert T. Public input into health care policy: Controversy and contribution in California. Hastings Cent Rep 20(5):21, 1990

Cranford RE. A hostage to technology. Hastings Cent Rep 20(5):9–10, 1990

Crawford KF. How ethical dilemmas are resolved. Journal of Long-Term Care 22(3):4–9, 1994

Crawshaw R. A vision of the health decisions movement. Hastings Cent Rep 20(5):21–22, 1990

Daniels N. Duty to treat or right to refuse? Hastings Cent Rep 21(2):36–46, 1991

Downes J. Ethical issues. The ethical dilemmas of mandatory prenatal and newborn HIV testing. Nursing Connections 8(4):43–50, 1995

Dunn DG. Bioethics and Nursing. Nursing Connections 7(3):43–51, Fall 1994

Ellman IM. Can others exercise an incapacitated patient's right to die? Hastings Cent Rep 20(1):47–50, 1990

Garland MJ, Hasnain R. Health care in common: Setting priorities in Oregon. Hastings Cent Rep 20(5):16–18, 1990

Gaylin W. Fooling with mother nature. Hastings Cent Rep 20(1):17–21, 1990

Greer MB. Factors affecting opinions on life support issues in the elderly. Issues on Aging 18(2):19–23, 1995

Hill TP. Giving voice to the pragmatic majority in New Jersey. Hastings Cent Rep 20(5):20, 1990

How far should we push Mother Nature? *Newsweek* 17:54–57, January 1994

Kowalski S. Withdrawal of nutritional support: A family's choice. Gastroenterology Nursing 19(1):25–28, 1996

Lauritzen P. What price parenthood? Hastings Cent Rep 20(2):38–46, 1990

Lippman H. After Cruzan: The right to die. RN 54(1):65–68, 73, 1991

Lynn J, Glover J. Cruzan and caring for others. Hastings Cent Rep 20(5):10–11, 1990

Nurses seek a voice in right-to-die cases. Am J Nurs 91(3):26, 1991

Oregon Nurses Association. Death with Dignity Act Position Statement. Portland, Oregon: Oregon Nurses Association, 1995

Overall C. Selective termination of pregnancy and women's reproductive autonomy. Hastings Cent Rep 20(3):6–11, 1990

Pinch WJ, Dougherty CJ, McCarthy V. Ethics in nursing practice: Confidentiality for women and their children with HIV/AIDS. Medsurg Nurs 4(6):452–457, 1995

Powledge TM. Capital report—springtime for fetal tissue research? Hastings Cent Rep 21(2):5–6, 1991

Robertson JA. Cruzan: No rights violated. Hastings Cent Rep 20(5):8–9, 1990

Rothman, DJ. Strangers at the Bedside: A History of How Law and Bioethics Transformed Medical Decision Making. New York: Basic, 1991

Rousseau PC. How fluid deprivation affects the terminally ill. RN 54(1):73–74, 1991

Taylor SL. Quandary at the crossroads: Paternalism versus advocacy surrounding end-of-treatment decisions. American Journal of Hospice and Palliative Care 12(4):43–46, 1995

Weber LJ, Campbell ML. Ethics and the law. Medical futility and life-sustaining treatment decisions. J Neurosci Nurs 28(1):56–60, 1996

Wendling EM. Anencephalics as organ donors. Imprint (April/May):47–48, 1990

Wurzbach ME. The dilemma of withholding or withdrawing nutrition. Image 22(4):226–230, 1990

Zerwekh Z. Do dying patients really need IV fluids? Am J Nurs 97(3):26–31, 1997

Relevant Web Sites

Bioethics Discussion Pages *www.hsc.usc.edu/~mbernste/*

Bioethics Online Service *www.mcw.edu/bioethics/index*

Bioethics Network *www.bioethics.net*

Hastings Center *www.hastingscenter.org/*

John Hopkins University Center *www.med.jhu.edu/bioethics_institute*

Midwest Center *www.midbio.org/*

National Bioethical Advisory Commission *www.bioethics.gov/*

National Catholic Bioethics Center *www.ncbcenter.org/*

National Reference Center for Bioethics Literature *www.georgetown.edu/research/nrcbl/*

Nursing Ethics Network *www.bc.edu/nursing/ethics*

Poynter Center *www.indiana.ceu/~poynter/index.html*

University of British Columbia Center *www.ethics.ubc.ca/*

United Network for Organ Sharing Transplantation Information Site *www.unos.org/*

UNIT IV

Career Opportunities and Professional Growth

The final unit in this textbook is devoted to topics that will assist you to move into the world of employment. Information is provided about the competencies needed for the wide variety of opportunity available to nurses today. Chapter 11 also describes how to set short- and long-term goals, write resumés, and compose letters of application and letters following up on interviews.

Strategies you can use to prevent reality shock and cope with the realities of the work world (including workplace violence) are included. As you move toward employment in one of the health care environments, it is important to understand organizational structure, including the purpose of missions, organizational charts, chains of command, and approaches to governance. You can find this information in Chapter 12.

The final chapter also discusses the forms of nursing care delivery, collective bargaining in nursing, and the purpose of and what to expect in a contract. The pros and cons of having a professional nursing association serve as the bargaining agent for nurses concludes the unit.

11

Beginning Your Career as a Nurse

The art of nursing involves our ability to engage in relationship-centered care, use knowledge and wisdom with well developed cognitive skills and implement interventions safely and effectively. It is the gestalt of what we do, how we do it and why. The art of nursing cannot be formalized and regimented; like any form of art, it reflects the artist and the audience.

(Lindeman, 1999)

OBJECTIVES

After completing this chapter, you should be able to:

1. Describe a variety of employment opportunities available to nurses today and the educational requirements of each.

2. Explain the competencies needed by the new graduate as outlined by the job analysis study.

3. Analyze the eight common expectations employers have of new graduates and relate them to your own background and education.

4. Develop a list of your personal short- and long-term career goals.

5. Describe how you plan to maintain your competence in nursing.

6. Create a plan for beginning your career, including a personal resumé; sample letters of application, follow-up, and resignation; and your possible responses in an employment interview.

7. Explore strategies that you might personally use to prevent or alleviate reality shock.

8. Analyze your own values and life situation in relationship to your personal potential for burnout.

9. Discuss three areas of concern related to sex discrimination in nursing.

10. Identify hazards to the health of both yourself and others in the nursing workplace and ways that you can act to protect yourself.

When you graduate, one of your first objectives no doubt will be obtaining employment as a registered nurse. You probably look forward to practicing in the nursing role you have spent so long attaining. You may even envision the "perfect" nursing position and have thought no further ahead than this first job. For other new graduates, the desire for a job is initially general, rather than specific, in view of student loans to be repaid and the desire to move into a lifestyle different from the student one. In the past, the expectations of most new graduates were simple, but a nursing career is now much more complex. In this chapter, we try to assist you as you survey the registered nursing job market and plan for a successful approach to obtaining that important first position. We also try to provide suggestions to help you find satisfaction and growth after your initial employment.

EMPLOYMENT OPPORTUNITIES TODAY

The health care environment today is affected by all that has gone before, including the militaristic, religious, and paternalistic roots discussed in Chapter 4. Some settings still have remnants of the paternalistic attitudes that were prevalent when women were expected to accept the hospital as the family surrogate during training and employment. This attitude may coexist with one that expects today's nurse to be an independent decision maker. Emphasis is placed on the nurse's need for breadth and depth of theory to cope with the complexities of evidence-based practice for both health promotion and health restoration. At the same time, pangs of nostalgia may be expressed for the days when nurses "really knew how to work" and did not worry much about "book learning."

Unlike graduates of the hospital programs of the past, you will have spent a more limited number of hours working in the patient care setting. Although some new graduates have worked as unlicensed assistive staff or practical nurses during their education, others' contact with health care settings may have been as students rather than as employees. You may not have experienced all of the many settings in which registered nurses are employed. You may have questions regarding employer expectations and your own role as a registered nurse employee.

As the population ages and more high-intensity health care is available in hospitals, the hospital nursing job market is expected to increase by 30% by 2005 (Saver, 1999). Ambulatory care clinics in hospitals and community settings have increased employment of nurses; those in hospitals have more than doubled and those in the community increased by 137% from 1980 to 1996 (Saver, 1999). As more care is delivered outside of acute care hospitals, the percentage of nurses working outside the hospital has increased. Employment in home care is predicted to increase by 128% between 1992 and 2005 (Saver, 1999).

However, newly licensed nurses continue to be employed primarily in acute care and long-term care facilities. In its trend study, the National Council of State Boards of Nursing (NCSBN) identified changes over time in the work environments, employment characteristics, and job activities of newly licensed nurses through surveys conducted every 3 months beginning in January 1998. In January 1998, although 24% of newly licensed LPN/VNs were unemployed, only one person reported it was because of inability to find a job. By July 1999, none of the 15% who were unemployed indicated that they were unable to find a job. In both the January 1998 survey and the July 1999 survey, 55% of the newly licensed LPN/VNs were working in subacute or long-term care and 21% in acute care. In January 1998, 21% of the RNs surveyed were unemployed 4 months after licensure, with 19% indicating it was because of inability to find a job. However, by July 1999 only 10% were unemployed 4 months after licensure and only one of those individuals reported that it was because of inability to find a job. Furthermore, the survey indicated that in July 1999, 82% of the RNs were working in acute care environments, 10% were in subacute or long-term care, and 8% were in community-based care (NCSBN, 1999).

Home health care, hospice care, community mental health centers, women's health care delivery systems, maternal-infant care programs, outpatient and primary care, and long-term care facilities are hiring growing numbers of registered nurses as they care for patients with more complex needs. In Chapter 1, we discussed the many settings in which health care is delivered, and we also pointed out the nursing roles seen in those settings. The growth of autonomy for the registered nurse has been even more marked outside the hospital setting than in it. Community health nurses have always operated much more independently than hospital nurses. The focus on health care is shifting from illness to health. Because many positions in the community require a baccalaureate degree, experience, or specialized educational programs, the new graduate most often is employed in an institutional setting.

The number of positions for registered nurses in many settings other than those providing client care also has grown. Health care-oriented businesses, such as insurance companies and medical equipment supply companies, have found that it is easier to teach nurses about business than to teach business people about health care. As a result, nurses are being employed in what some individuals see as non-nursing positions. Others argue that these, too, should be considered nursing positions, because the expertise that makes the individual successful is nursing expertise.

The number of men in nursing, which remained relatively small for many years, is beginning to grow as society reassesses its attitude toward labeling jobs as women's or men's work. Only 5.4% of practicing nurses are men (HRSA, 1996). Men have been attracted by the career opportunities and improving economic picture of nursing and as of 1996 constituted 11.5% of those entering nursing programs (NLN, 2000).

The economic position of the nurse has improved for several reasons. One reason is the extension of laws governing fair labor practices to nonprofit institutions and the advent of collective bargaining. Another major factor affecting the economic position of nurses was the nursing shortage of the 1980s. The demand for nurses rose faster than the supply, and employers began increasing salaries and benefits to attract nurses. This trend was especially notable in urban communities.

In the 1990s, the pressures of a changing health care system and cost containment created still more changes for nursing. Hospital stays shortened so dramatically that hospital censuses decreased across the country. The nursing shortage appeared to end abruptly as hospitals began reassessing their needs. Some hospitals closed; many downsized. In addition, many hospitals restructured to employ more unlicensed assistive personnel. These factors contributed to layoffs of nurses from hospitals. Long-term care and home care have increased, although funding of home care remains a problem.

Now as we enter a new century, a nursing shortage is again emerging. The client of the downsized hospital is more acutely ill than before. To maintain short stays and early discharge, patient teaching and planning for discharge have assumed more importance than before. Hospitals that downsized too abruptly are finding they need to replace staff. Concerns that the nursing shortage will continue and even grow more acute are based on the convergence of several factors. The currently employed RN population is aging, with an average age in the mid 40s. The workload is high and the pace is demanding. As a consequence, older RNs often choose to work less than full time. Graduations from schools of nursing have declined somewhat. Some programs have failed to meet targets for admissions. Positions for those with baccalaureate and higher degrees and for those with specialty training, such as intensive care or operating room nursing, are growing faster than the job market in general.

All of these factors bring you, as a new graduate, into a world of uncertainty, but one also filled with opportunity and promise. Now you must determine your place in this world.

COMPETENCIES OF THE NEW GRADUATE

Recently you have heard the term *competency* used a great deal, especially as it applies to the new graduate. Competency, as used here, refers to the ability of the graduate effectively and safely to perform specified nursing skills, including the application of critical thinking skills. Some have differentiated "competency," which is an entry-level expectation, and "proficiency" which is expected of the experienced nurse (Fig. 11-1).

Competencies Identified by Nursing Organizations

The most definitive statements on the competencies needed by the newly licensed practical nurse and the registered nurse have been developed by the NCSBN, based on its job analysis studies that serve as the basis for the NCLEX-RN and NCLEX-PN licensing examinations.

FIGURE 11–1 New graduates are expected to know both their own abilities and when to seek appropriate help.

In these studies, activities reported by a stratified random sample of newly licensed, entry-level nurses were examined. Both the frequency of the nursing activities and their criticality were studied. *Criticality* refers to activities that cannot be delayed or omitted without a "substantial risk of unnecessary complications, impairment of function, or serious distress to clients" (Chornick, Yocum, & Jacobson, 1993, p 11). The most recent RN study was completed in 1999; the results of that study supported the continuation of the current test plan and passing score (NCSBN, 1999a). The most recent PN study was completed in 1997, and was the basis for the 1998 changes in the PN examination (NCSBN, 1997).

Activities expected of newly licensed registered nurses that led the list for criticality were:

- Use appropriate infection control measures
- Report significant changes in the client's condition
- Perform cardiopulmonary resuscitation
- Perform Heimlich maneuver/abdominal thrust
- Provide emergency care for a wound disruption
- Recognize the occurrence of hemorrhage
- Manage a medical emergency until a physician arrives
- Implement measures to prevent circulatory complications (eg, embolus, shock, hemorrhage)
- Respond to symptoms of fetal distress

Activities were studied further in terms of the frequency with which they were expected of newly licensed registered nurses. In all settings, nurses were expected to:

- Coordinate care through working with others on the health care team and supervising delivery of care by assistive personnel
- Preserve the quality of care through such activities as acting as an advocate for needed changes in care, documenting errors or problems, and intervening in situations involving unsafe or inadequate care
- Maintain the safety of the client as exemplified by verifying, identifying, and reporting unsafe equipment, and following infection control guidelines
- Prepare clients and families for care that is to be done, including procedures and treatments; and help them to understand expected outcomes
- Carry out procedures in a safe, effective manner

Physiologic and psychosocial integrity were supported by many individual nursing actions. Some, such as assessing vital signs, seemed almost universal. Others, such as monitoring for side effects of radiation therapy, were needed in a small minority of settings. Allowing clients to talk about their concerns and assisting them to communicate effectively were almost universal activities.

Nursing process continues to be a strong expectation for registered nurses. In the 1999 study, newly licensed RNs indicated that they spent 30% of their time on assessments, 12% on analysis, 14% on planning, 30% implementing client care, and 14% on evaluation. Seventy-eight percent stated that they were required to know nursing diagnosis and 70% used it in their current position (NCBSN, 1999).

In addition to the National Council, other organizations have explored the issue of competencies of new nursing graduates. The various educational councils of the National League for Nursing have developed statements regarding competencies of new graduates. Most recently, the NLN Council of Associate Degree Programs approved a new set of competencies of the associate degree graduate in 1999. The American Association of Colleges of Nursing developed a document titled "Essentials of Baccalaureate Education for Nursing" that includes expected competencies. Additionally, some states have developed statements of competencies for graduates of the nursing programs in those states. This often has been part of a process to improve articulation between programs at different levels.

Similarities and patterns have emerged from all of these statements. The outline of theoretical knowledge and functioning in regard to the nursing process seems to be the most consistent. The most divergent opinions seem to be in the area of specific skill or task competency (Fig. 11-2).

Employers' Expectations Regarding Competencies

Employers often ask for further clarification of competence. Have these graduates only the necessary theoretical knowledge of the skill? Have they actually performed the skill? If so, was it in a practice laboratory only, or was it in a client care situation? Does competence mean that the new graduate can function independently, or will some supervision still be needed?

FIGURE 11–2 Employers often are concerned about an applicant's specific technical skills.

Further complicating the picture is the confusion surrounding competencies of the graduates of the three types of nursing education programs preparing individuals for registered nurse licensure: the hospital-based diploma program, the associate degree program, and the baccalaureate degree program. Although statements by several organizations have distinguished among levels of functioning, many employers do not differentiate expectations. Some employers state that new graduates from different types of programs have not clearly demonstrated differences in competencies. This has created confusion in the minds of nurses, employers, and the public over the role of the registered nurse prepared in each type of educational program.

What is expected of the new graduate varies in different health care agencies and in different geographic areas. Expectations are affected by factors in the community, such as whether there are nursing programs in that community and whether new graduates come from one or from many different schools. The acuity of the client care load and the types of services offered by an agency also may affect expectations. The Joint Commission on the Accreditation of Healthcare Organizations (JCAHO) has a criterion requiring that accredited institutions monitor and assure the competence of their staff. This requires that an institution identify expected competencies for staff and then design an assessment method. As institutions move to comply with this standard, most are directing their initial efforts toward technical skills, because these are more easily identified and assessed. Other competencies will be more difficult to assess.

Based on the NCSBN job analysis studies, some general patterns of employer expectations can be seen.

1. *Possess the necessary theoretical background for safe client care and for decision making.* Many employers believe that new graduates today are very competent in this area. For instance, the new graduate should understand the signs and symptoms of an insulin reaction, recognize it when it occurs, and know what nursing actions should be taken. The new graduate must know when an emergency or complication is occurring and secure medical help for the client when that is needed.

2. *Use the nursing process in a systematic way.* This includes assessment, analysis, planning, intervention, and evaluation. New graduates should be able to develop plans of care and follow plans such as care pathways that have been developed by the agency.

3. *Recognize own abilities and limitations.* To provide safe care, the nurse must identify when a situation requires greater expertise or knowledge and when assistance is needed. Employers may be able to assist if nurses ask for help and direction, but cannot accept the risk to clients created by nurses who do not know or accept their own limitations.

4. *Use communication skills effectively with clients and coworkers.* In every setting there are clients and families who are anxious, depressed, suffering loss, or experiencing other emotional distress. The nurse is expected to respond appropriately to these individuals and to facilitate their coping and adaptation. Effective communication skills are essential to the functioning of the entire health care team. Often, the nurse is expected to help coordinate the work of others, and this cannot be done without effective communication skills.

5. *Work effectively with assistive personnel, delegating and supervising nursing care tasks in an appropriate manner.* In most settings, assistive personnel are a part of the nursing team. The registered nurse, and in some instances the practical nurse, is expected to identify what can be delegated and do so in a way that contributes to appropriate patient care outcomes.

6. *Understand the importance of accurate and complete documentation.* Employers generally recognize that the new graduate must be given time to learn the documentation system used in the facility. However, the new graduate is expected to recognize the need for recording data. It is anticipated that the nurse will keep accurate, grammatically correct, and legible records that provide the necessary legal documentation of care.

7. *Possess proficiency in the basic technical nursing skills.* This is an area in which a wide variety of expectations may be present. In most settings, proficiency in the basic skills required to support activities of daily living is expected. These skills include transferring, giving baths, and performing general hygienic measures. In some settings, nurses will be carrying out these tasks, whereas in others they will be directing or teaching others who do them, such as nursing assistants or family members. In either case, proficiency is essential to evaluating the care provided. The technical skills or tasks that are reserved for the registered nurse represent the area of widest diversity in the identification of essential

skills. The settings in which nurses practice are diverse, and therefore technical skills may be needed in one setting but not in another. Some facilities provide extensive orientation programs in which every skill is checked before the new graduate is allowed to proceed independently. Other employers expect the new graduate to perform the skill if able, and be checked off as required, or to ask for help if unable to be independent. Often employers are flexible in their expectations, so that it may be acceptable if an individual seems to have competency in a reasonable percentage of the skills required by that agency; further development of skill competency will be supported by the institution. Other employers have a list of skills in which competency is mandatory at the time of hire, although speed may not be expected. Also, there may be a difference between what the employer would wish and what the employer will accept.

In addition to these professional responsibilities as a nurse, employers also speak of their concern for worker-related competencies they want to see in all health care workers. These include:

8. *Understand and have a commitment to a work ethic.* This means that the employee will take the responsibility of the job seriously and will be on time, take only the allowed coffee and lunch breaks, and will not take "sick days" unless truly ill. It also means that the new graduate recognizes that nurses may be needed 24 hours a day, 365 days a year, and that this may require sacrifices of personal convenience, such as working evening shifts or on holidays.

9. *Function with acceptable speed.* This is another area in which expectations differ greatly. Most employers state that they expect the new graduate will be slower; however, they may vary in how much slowness is acceptable and how soon they feel that nursing actions should become more time efficient. Generally, an orientation period is planned—although, with the pressures on health care agencies, this often has been shortened considerably. An acceptable speed of function is reflected by the ability to carry out a usual registered nurse assignment within a shift. Thus, if the usual client assignment for a registered nurse is the care of six to eight moderately ill clients, the new graduate is expected to accomplish this by the end of the orientation period.

PERSONAL CAREER GOALS

In caring for clients, you are involved in the process of goal setting. Many nurses recognize the value of this in client care but never transfer the concept to their personal lives. Nursing as a profession offers many career options. Without carefully setting goals, you might drift for years.

Focusing Your Goals

You may want to focus on a broad area of clinical competency, such as pediatric nursing, or on a more restricted area, such as neonatal care. Clinical areas available for concentrated effort become more varied as health care becomes more complex. Emergency care, coronary care, neurologic and neurosurgical nursing, and specialties in the care of persons with ear, nose, and throat disorders are just a few of the clinical possibilities. Nurses specialize in aerospace nursing, enterostomal therapy, and respiratory care as well as operating room nursing and postanesthesia care. Opportunities for additional education and for practice in most clinical specialties are now available for any experienced registered nurse, regardless of the person's initial educational background.

Some specialty positions are in the primary care field, such as the woman's health care specialist, the family nurse practitioner, and the pediatric nurse practitioner. Increasing numbers of these programs require a baccalaureate degree for entry, but some admit registered nurses with experience in that specialty area.

Another approach may be to focus your goals on the setting in which care is delivered, such as acute care, long-term care, or community care. As health care needs expand, these separate realms of care delivery are all demanding more specialized knowledge. Even within the individual area of focus differences are present. For example, within the community are ambulatory care settings, public health nursing agencies, occupational health nursing departments, and day care facilities.

Yet another way of focusing your goals is according to functional categories. Although nurses are initially thought of as direct care providers, they are needed in many other positions. For example, there is need for those who would move into supervisory and administrative capacities, those who teach, and those who conduct nursing research. Nursing also lends itself to writing, to community service, and even to political involvement.

You may decide to set your goals in relation to all three foci. That is, you might identify a clinical area, a care setting, and a functional category.

Setting Your Goals

The first step in setting personal career goals is a thorough self-assessment. Determine how your abilities and competencies correspond to your own expectations, and to those of employers. Other factors to explore are your likes and dislikes and the situations or types of work you particularly enjoyed as a student. Also, it is important to recognize the area in which you were most comfortable. Were there areas in which you or your instructor felt that you were an above-average student? Consider your health and personal characteristics in relationship to types of work. Do you have physical restrictions? Do you prefer working independently or with others? How do you respond to close supervision or to relative freedom in the job setting? Do you prefer a work environment that is relatively predictable, or do you thrive in a situation that changes frequently? Do you work well with long-term goals and a few immediate reinforcements, or do you need to see results quickly? Another factor to consider is your own geographic mobility: would you be willing to move or travel as part of a job? Both your personal responsibilities and preferences operate in this arena.

As you plan ahead, you need to examine many of the options offered by nursing. What types of jobs and opportunities are open to you? What education and personal abilities are needed in these areas? Are you interested? Does the education you have meet the educational requirements? Are avenues for additional education available to you? All of these considerations are important as you plan for the future. Career goals need to be both short- and long-term. They will help you to plan your future constructively. This does not mean that goals are static. Just as client goals must be realistic, personal, and flexible, so must your own goals.

Short-term goals encompass what you want to accomplish this month and this year. What do you want to do and what do you want to be in the immediate future? For example, one recent graduate stated that her short-term goal was to have 2 years of solid experience in a busy metropolitan hospital.

Long-term goals represent where you want to be in your profession 5 to 10 years from now. The long-term goal of the graduate referred to above was to work in a small, remote community in which she would have the opportunity to function autonomously.

Although both long- and short-term goals will be revised as your life evolves, they guide you in making day-to-day decisions more effectively. In today's world of rapid health care change, you may need to keep your goals somewhat broad and flexible. Be ready to consider alternative goals and a variety of pathways to one goal. These approaches will be of value as you enter a system in transition.

Critical Thinking Activity

Write out your short- and long-term professional goals with a brief plan on how you can achieve these goals. Think critically about the obstacles you will need to overcome to reach these goals. How will you deal with the obstacles?

Maintaining and Enhancing Your Competence

Every nurse has an obligation to society to maintain competence and continue practicing high-quality, safe care. Continuing education may occur through learning on the job, reading professional publications, or attending classes. There are television courses, programmed instruction programs, and examinations related to journal articles. Any of these avenues may be appropriate, depending on the circumstances. Some nurses may want to advance through specialty or higher education. Included in your goal setting should be an approach to maintaining and enhancing your competence.

MAKING GOALS REALITY

Philosophical questions regarding goals must be resolved by practical approaches. As a new graduate, your first goal simply may be to get a job in nursing (especially if you live in an area of the country that has more limited opportunities for registered nurses).

Whatever the situation, you are more likely to realize your goals if you are prepared to present yourself in the best possible way to a prospective employer. Many of you have held different jobs in the community as students and as adults. You may be familiar with and competent in the job search process. Others have never applied for the kind of job that truly could be considered the beginning of a career. Employers and prospective employees may hold different expectations in such a situation.

Identifying Potential Employers

To begin your job search effectively, you need to identify potential employers. You might begin your review with those more familiar to you and gradually move outward in an ever-widening circle to identify others.

The clinical sites where you had experiences as a student or where you worked when a student are good places to begin. You may know these agencies, be familiar with the type of care provided, and already be oriented to many of their policies and procedures. Your prior association with these agencies may provide you with ready access to their hiring procedures. If you worked as an employee in a health care setting before graduation, you may be given preference in hiring. This is one reason for seeking health care employment during your nursing education process.

Another source of potential jobs is the classified section of the local newspaper. There you are more likely to find single jobs in small facilities as well as general recruitment announcements from larger facilities. However, just because an agency does not advertise, does not mean they will not be hiring any employees. Advertising is expensive and may result in an excess of applicants to screen. Therefore, some health care agencies do not advertise and rely on those who independently seek them out as potential employers.

Job fairs for health care employers are becoming more common. Each employer participating provides a booth or table for the various health care employers in the community to provide information on job openings in their agencies. An individual looking for employment may explore a variety of employers, learning about job openings, benefits, and opportunities in a brief time without the difficulty of searching out each employer. The employer may see many potential employees in a focused period. Thus, job fairs benefit both employers and potential employees. Job fairs may be held in the community, attracting experienced health care workers as well as students and new graduates. Some colleges arrange job fairs on campus. Nursing programs or nursing student clubs also may arrange job fairs.

The "Yellow Pages" of the telephone book may help you to locate smaller employers in your community. You could look under "nursing homes," "home care," "nursing care" and other such headings. This may help you to identify health care providers you were not aware of. Do not hesitate to call or even personally visit these settings to obtain information for a job application.

If you have the flexibility to move from your local area, you may expand your search for possible positions. The major nursing journals have sections in the back pages devoted to advertisements. Some of these advertise nursing positions. If you have a specific area in mind, you might visit your local library and consult the newspaper and the telephone directory for that area. Your nursing program may receive advertising magazines that are designed to present job opportunities for new graduates. These magazines provide a few articles about relevant job search topics, such as interviewing, as well as advertisements from health care agencies. These advertisements present information on the agency itself and how to contact them for possible application.

For those with electronic access to the World Wide Web, additional sources of potential jobs are available. Many governmental job openings also are posted online. Using your search engine, look for "employment opportunities," "jobs," or "careers." Some online service providers have additional support services for a job search that might include career guidance (for a fee), or sample documents such as resumés and cover letters.

Letter of Inquiry or Application

Writing a letter of inquiry is an excellent way to approach many prospective employers (Display 11-1). This letter is often termed a "cover letter" because it is sent with your resumé (see below). You can present yourself positively through a well-written letter. In addition, a letter may be dealt with at the recipient's convenience, whereas a telephone call may interrupt a busy schedule. There are fewer chances for misunderstanding if your request is in writing and if you receive a written reply.

Before you write your letter, you should make sure you have information about the prospective employer. What kind of facility is this? What types of clients do they serve, and what special services do they offer? It makes a poor impression to write to a prospective employer stating that your goal is to work in pediatrics when that facility does not provide any pediatric services. You might obtain this information by calling the human resources department of the facility or by contacting a public information office. In a small agency, you may simply speak with a receptionist or secretary. Be honest and straightforward in explaining that you are considering applying for employment and would like information about the agency before making that decision.

Another part of your advance planning is identifying how you will focus your letter on your special qualifications and what you want to highlight. You will want to focus on the skills or accomplishments related to the position you want. Your letter should be no more than one page in length, but should be planned to present all essential information. Introduce yourself and your purpose for writing in the first paragraph so that the reader immediately understands why you are writing. You may want briefly to state your reasons for applying for a position with this particular employer. The more specific the reasons, the better the impression you are likely to make.

Briefly highlight your qualifications for the position. This should not be a simple recitation of what is in your resumé, but should either present the information in a slightly different light or add pertinent detail that is not in the resumé. If you are responding to an advertisement, you should respond to each of the qualifications listed in the advertisement. You might include personal qualities that would make you an effective employee in the position. You should relate your skills and abilities to the needs of this particular agency. If your health care experience is limited, you should point out skills you have gained from other jobs that would be useful in nursing. These might be interpersonal skills, management skills, or adaptability.

In the final paragraph, make a summary statement indicating why you want to work for this employer and ask for an appointment for an interview. Be sure to indicate the times you can be available and how and where you can be contacted if the

Display 11-1
LETTER OF APPLICATION

Maribeth Wilson
3428 1ˢᵗ Ave. N.
Seattle, WA 98103
(206) 274-5978
e-mail: maribethw@email.com

January 30, 2001

Joyce Montgall, R.N.
Nurse Recruiter
Seattle General Medical Center
321 Heath Blvd.
Seattle, WA 98101

Dear Ms. Montgall:

Enclosed please find a copy of my resumé, along with my application to Seattle General Medical Center's New Graduate Residency Program. I will graduate from Shoreline Community College's associate degree nursing program on May 28. I expect to acquire my registered nurse license by the end of June. I am extremely interested in a medical-surgical nursing position within your upcoming residency program.

I believe that I would bring many strengths to a new graduate position. I have worked here at Seattle General as a nursing assistant for the past year, and my experience has given me an excellent foundation in understanding the philosophy and mission of the Medical Center. During this time I have been assigned to several different units, including 4 West and 4 Center, where new graduate positions are available. The nurses at Seattle General have been generous in their mentoring and have helped me to increase my understanding of the patients' conditions. They have been supportive as I developed increased problem-solving and decision-making skills.

Within my nursing student educational experience, I have had the privilege of working in a wide variety of health care institutions throughout the city. From these experiences I would bring an understanding of the community standards of care as well as a unique appreciation of the position of Seattle General in the health care community.

I hope that I will be selected for an interview and look forward to hearing from you. My phone number, email address, and home address are at the top of this letter. If I do not hear from you within the next two weeks, I will contact your office to ascertain the status of my application.

Sincerely,

Maribeth Wilson

Maribeth Wilson

employer so wishes. It is also wise to indicate that you will contact the person to whom the letter is addressed to request an appointment. This allows you to maintain some initiative in the process. Thank the person for considering your application, and close.

Another point to remember is that the letter's appearance and its content both represent you. You will be judged on spelling, grammar, clarity, and neatness in addition to content. Your letter of application should be written in standard business format on plain white or off-white business paper. Make it brief and clear. Ask a friend or family member to check your first draft if you have any questions about its correctness.

The Resumé

A resumé is a brief overview of your qualifications for a position (Display 11-2). Its purpose is to provide the employer with a way to identify quickly whether you have the basic qualifications for a position, and to present you in the most positive light to be considered for the position in which you are interested. In most instances you will want to include your resumé with your initial letter. In addition, you may leave your resumé with the employer at the end of your interview.

Critical Thinking Activity

Create an effective resumé and samples of letters to employers that present you as a positive addition to their staff.

APPEARANCE

The appearance of your resumé is important because it initially presents your image to the prospective employer. You want its appearance to reflect a competent, professional

Display 11–2
QUESTIONS TO HELP YOU PLAN A RESUMÉ

1. What educational institutions have you attended? Dates? Degrees or certificates?
2. What credentials do you have that might be useful in a nursing employment setting?
3. What jobs have you held that you want to highlight? Were any of them health care related?
4. What specific skills did you apply in your workplace that would be transferable to nursing?
5. What skills, abilities, or personal characteristics do you want to draw the employer's attention to?
6. Have you had volunteer or community experiences that demonstrate positive personal attributes?
7. Have you had any awards or recognition that identify your positive abilities or attributes?

image. It is not necessary to have a professionally produced resumé. Nursing employers, when asked, have indicated that it neither adds to nor detracts from their impression to read a resumé that has been produced by some professional printing method. The important point is that it be a somewhat formal, standard, informative document that is neat and without errors. In today's business world, a computer-produced resumé is standard (Figs. 11-3 and 11-4).

Your resumé should be on standard-sized (8.5 × 11), white or off-white, good quality paper so that it is easy to handle, file, and read. A resumé that is individually printed (or reproduced well enough so that it appears to be) usually will be more positively received than a poor-quality photocopy. If you have access to a computer and word processing, you will find it valuable to create a resumé and save it to a disk. In this way, you will be able to revise it easily, and you may even be able to tailor it to an individual job situation. In addition to the capabilities of standard word processing software, there are inexpensive software programs especially designed to facilitate the production of a well-organized and formatted resumé.

To achieve legibility, use wide margins, spacing, indentation, bullets, and numbering to separate different sections and topics. You might want to underline or bold print important items or highlight them with an asterisk or bullet to draw swift attention. When an employer is reviewing many such documents, anything that facilitates review and makes you stand out is an advantage. Ask someone to review the appearance of your resumé and identify those areas that first caught their attention. This helps you to evaluate its appearance.

CONTENT

The content of your resumé is critical. It always begins with your name, address, and telephone number (including area code). If you will be moving, indicate the date the move will be effective and provide an alternate method of contacting you after that date. A permanently settled relative or friend who would be willing to forward your mail would be appropriate. Employers are not permitted to ask about age, marital status, and dependents, and you do not need to include this information.

Objective. You should include a personal goal or objective. This may include both a short-term goal such as "employment as a registered nurse on a general medical unit" and a longer-term goal such as "with eventual move to employment in coronary care." Be sure that your goal is realistic and does not imply that you are not really interested in a beginning level position. If you state that your goal is to work in an emergency room and you do not have the experience for this kind of position, your application usually will be discarded. If you state that you want to work in maternity nursing and the only position available is in medical-surgical nursing, you may not be considered for the medical-surgical position that you would have accepted although it was not your first choice.

Credentials. You will want to include information regarding your licensure and other credentials. Indicate the date your license will be effective and whether you have a temporary permit to work as a nurse. Indicate when you expect to take your licensing examination and have a license. Your nursing license or permit number should be listed

Sarah Mitchell

5714 31st Ave. N., Seattle, WA 98117 • (206) 733-8934 • e-mail: sarahmit@email.com

Objective

An entry-level registered nurse position in an acute care hospital.

Experience

2000-present   Seattle General Medical Center   Seattle, WA

Patient Care Technician, Medical-Surgical Units

- Provide basic care and ADLs with attention to psychosocial needs for acutely ill medical-surgical patients. Assist R.N. with procedures and carry out delegated duties.
- Work collaboratively with nursing team, assuring prompt response to patient needs.
- Effectively manage time to support seven patients on evening shift.
- Document care on computerized system, maintaining accuracy and confidentiality.

1999-2000   Health Choice Urgent Care Center   Seattle, WA

Nursing Technician, Urgent Care Clinic

- Interviewed clients, took vital signs, initiated documentation, and prioritized care for urgently ill and injured adults and children.
- Under RN supervision, performed assessments, dressing changes, ECGs, nebulizer treatments, and hospital admission processes.
- Attended to psychosocial needs of family and others accompanying a sick or injured individual.

1997-1998   First United Bank   Lynnwood, WA

Bank Teller

- Maintained excellent customer service by following detailed bank policies and procedures.
- Utilized a variety of computerized systems to assure accurate and detailed documentation of all activities.
- Incorporated information from employee training classes into job skills to assure up-to-date function.

Education

1999-2001   Shoreline Community College   Seattle, WA

AAAS Nursing, to be awarded June, 2001

FIGURE 11–3   Resumé of a recent graduate: Example A.

Joseph M. Sanchez

1298 Avenida Diaz
La Quinta, CA 92252
(619) 524-4321)

OBJECTIVE: A beginning Registered Nurse position that will provide the opportunity for professional development and advancement toward critical care nursing.

SKILLS:
- Work effectively in a multicultural environment
- Communicate in a positive, supportive way with co-workers, clients, and families
- Bilingual Spanish/English
- Strong work ethic and experience in working multiple shifts/floating positions
- Excellent critical thinking and problem-solving developed in a wide variety of occupations as well as in the nursing context

EDUCATION:
College of the Desert, Palm Desert, CA
Associate in Science in Nursing, June 2001

EXPERIENCE:
Manor Care Center, Palm Desert, CA
Nursing Assistant, Certified: 1998-Present
- Maintained function and dignity of dependent elderly adults by providing direct care, strong interpersonal relationships, and effective collaboration with nursing and allied health.
- Earned promotion to position of mentor for new hires and team leader for a group of nursing assistants. Facilitated team performance to accomplish assigned responsibilities.

Northrup Corporation, Los Angeles, CA
Machinist: 1988-1997
- Performed precision skills with accuracy and attention to detail.
- Followed precise written protocols and procedures to assure quality.
- Led a team in a program of total quality management within our department.

AWARDS:
- College of the Desert Merit Scholar 2000
- Golden Acorn Award for Leadership of Parent Involvement
  Cactus Valley Elementary School PTA, LaQuinta, CA

FIGURE 11–4   Resumé of a recent graduate: Example B.

after you have it. If you do not have a license at the time you are preparing your resumé, you may choose to put information about when you expect to have your license in your letter of application.

Employment History. Work experience is of critical importance, and you should provide a meaningful employment history. If using a traditional format, for each job you held include address, dates employed, position, and duties. The prospective employer would be especially interested in a previous nursing assistant position or any other position that demonstrates your knowledge of or experience in some area of health care or the assumption of responsibility. Other positions also may be important if you are able clearly to identify skills used in those settings that are transferable to nursing.

If you have had only one or two part-time jobs during your educational program, it would be appropriate to include them in detail. However, if during your educational program you held 15 part-time jobs, it is appropriate to list significant ones that offered valuable experience. In one line write, "Various part-time jobs to finance schooling: clerk and waitress. Individual names provided on request." Include the overall dates for this period.

You may choose a more skill-focused resumé and not include details of all your previous positions. For individuals who are older and have an extensive employment history, a resumé focused on skills and types of positions rather than a chronological list of employers is often the most effective. To keep your resumé on one page, you should consider how you may most effectively present employment history. In a skill-focused resumé, you can emphasize the responsibilities you had within positions rather than each specific position. Be sure to include language proficiency if you are fluent in more than English. Computer literacy also may be a valuable skill.

Regardless of the organizational format, we suggest that you focus on accomplishments and use active verbs to describe skills. Words such as supervised, designed, managed, developed, analyzed, coordinated, documented, planned, delegated, created, completed, and operated give life to your resumé and create interest in the reader. See the accompanying display for a list of active verbs you might use (Display 11-3).

Education. Educational background should form another section and cover your nursing education and any specialized courses or postgraduate work you have done. It is appropriate to note any college-level work. Do not include high school information unless you entered your nursing program directly from high school. Then you might indicate your high school and graduation date on one line of your educational information.

In each group of information, list the most recent items first. The most common approach is to group information in the categories just mentioned. See Figures 11-3 and 11-4 for examples of this type of resumé.

If you had educational experiences in an area that especially relates to the position for which you are applying, you might individualize your resumé by briefly identifying these special experiences. For example, you might have had a senior leadership practicum on an orthopedic unit—this would be particularly relevant to an application for a nursing position in orthopedics. If you had a practicum in the facility or agency to which you are applying, indicate this in some way. Your familiarity with their poli-

Display 11–3
POWER VERBS FOR RESUMÉS

- Use of verbs without subjects is more concise and conserves space.
- Use of words such as "advanced to" rather than "promoted to," "earned" rather than "was given" indicates a person who does things rather than receives them.
- Use of "-ed" or "-ing" as verb endings can both be effective.

accompanied	displayed	installed	planned
achieved	directed	instructed	prepared
acquired	doubled	insured	presided
activated		integrated	procured
administered	earned	intensified	produced
advanced to	educated	interviewed	progressed
advised	employed	invented	promoted
analyzed	enacted		prompted
arranged	encouraged	keynoted	proposed
assembled	engineered		proved
assisted	established	led	provided
	evaluated	located	
built	executed		reconciled
	exhibited	maintained	reduced
clarified	expanded	managed	regulated
commanded	experienced	manufactured	related
composed		marketed	reorganized
conceived	facilitated	mastered	reported
concluded	formed	mediated	researched
conducted	financed	motivated	
constructed	formalized		satisfied
consulted	formulated	negotiated	secured
contrived	founded	nominated	served
controlled			serviced
converted	generated	obtained	simplified
coordinated	governed	officiated	solved
correlated	graduated	operated	sparked
corroborated		ordered	structured
created	headed	organized	succeeded
		originated	
decided	implemented	overcame	trained
delegated	improved		transferred
demonstrated	improvised	participated	transformed
designed	increased	perceived	
detailed	induced	perfected	unified
determined	influenced	performed	
developed	initiated	piloted	verified
devised	innovated	pioneered	
discovered	inspired	placed	won
			wrote

cies and procedures would be a valuable asset. If you attended any special workshops, include those in a separate section.

Additional Experience. Volunteer or community work and awards and honors form two sections when you have these experiences. You also might want to add a section for special skills such as computer familiarity or experience with special types of equipment. Choose the items you list under volunteer and community work carefully. If you are 40 years old, the fact that you were student body president in high school would probably be considered irrelevant. However, if you went from high school directly into a nursing program, this information could be important in demonstrating your leadership ability. If you are an older student, your participation in any community organizations, such as the Parent-Teacher Association, and service in any leadership roles might be significant to an employer.

In some instances, you may want to list briefly the skills or abilities gained from a particular volunteer activity. For example, if you worked as a volunteer for a Planned Parenthood clinic, you might specify that your duties included individual client counseling in relation to family planning methods. Simply stating that you were a volunteer would not communicate the level of responsibility you assumed. This is an area that you might want to individualize to target the particular skills you think are important to the position for which you are applying.

List awards, honors, and professional associations (such as NSNA) that would demonstrate your competence or leadership ability. You may omit this section if you feel that you have nothing pertinent to enter.

Personal References. References are typed on a separate page and given to the prospective employer if they are requested, or copied onto an application form. Be selective in choosing the people you list as references. Consider the people who know you and would be able to speak positively of you to a future employer, and who would have credibility with the employer.

A primary reference should be an instructor or supervisor from your basic educational program. This person would be able to affirm your ability in the nursing field. Some agencies request two instructor references, so be prepared for that. Another reference should be someone who has employed you and who can describe your work habits and effectiveness as an employee. If you have had any health care work experience, this would be the best work reference. Also look at the position in which you assumed the most responsibility. This should be reasonably recent (within the last 10 years). Again, some employers ask for two work references. You should have available as one reference someone who has known you personally for a relatively long time and who could attest to your ability to relate with others and to such attributes as personal integrity. Not all employers are interested in personal references. Some agencies indicate the type of references they want. If this is the case, supply the names of references that comply with the agency's request. Include full names with titles (if any), addresses, and telephone numbers so that the employer will be able to contact the references easily.

Seek the person's permission before giving an individual's name as a reference. When seeking permission to use someone as a work reference, you might outline what you would like the person to emphasize if contacted—for example: "If you are contacted, I would particularly like you to provide information about my work habits and effectiveness as an employee."

Employers express differences of opinion about the value of a standardized letter of reference addressed "To Whom It May Concern." Some employers may consider this a useful initial presentation of your qualifications. Other employers want the reference to address the specific position needs or the qualifications outlined on a reference form. One advantage of the general letter is that you might be able to obtain this reference from a part-time faculty member or supervisor who may no longer be employed by the institution. If you do obtain this type of letter, be sure to preserve the original carefully (perhaps in a clear, plastic sleeve) to show to a potential employer; you then would provide a good quality photocopy for the employer to place in your file. Even when an employer accepts this as an initial reference, your references will most probably be personally contacted as well.

The Interview

The interview should be a two-way conversation in which you will gain as well as give information. Think through the situation before going to the interview, and outline information that you want to obtain and questions that you want answered. It is helpful to write out your questions so that they are clearly stated, and so that you do not forget items in the tense atmosphere that often exists in an interview situation.

Time spent reflecting on your personal views in advance will be valuable for the interview. Remember that an interview is a chance to sell yourself to an employer, a chance to present yourself as a valuable addition to their nursing staff, and an opportunity to determine how you will fit into that work setting.

When planning for an employment interview, consider your appearance, your attitude and approach, and what the content of the interview will be. Your personal appearance is likely to evoke some response from the interviewer. Consider what you would like that response to be and dress appropriately. This means that what you wear when applying for one type of job might be inappropriate when applying for another type of job. For example, if you were applying for a position at a hospital, you would wear businesslike clothing, such as dress pants and shirt, or a suit or dress. Being neat and well-groomed contributes to a businesslike atmosphere. If you were applying for a position in a walk-in health care clinic that offered services to persons who are uncomfortable in a traditional environment, it might be appropriate to wear the casual clothing worn by the workers at the clinic. You need to make a conscious decision about the impression you want to create. Although some may wish that appearances had no effect on the opinions of others, remember that, in reality, appearance often does make a significant difference.

Take a copy of your resume with you to the interview. In addition, be prepared with the names, addresses, and telephone numbers of all references, and your Social Security number. If you have already received your nursing license, take that with you. Take along a black pen to fill out any forms, and a note pad with your questions listed and a place to make personal notes of important information obtained during the interview. This can increase your self-confidence if you have forms to fill out or if questions about statements on your resume arise during the interview.

Plan to arrive at an interview early. This gives you time to check your appearance and focus your thoughts. When you arrive at an interview, be sensitive to the problems and concerns of the interviewer. If it is apparent that unplanned events are demanding the interviewer's attention, state that you are aware of the difficulty and ask whether it would be more convenient if you made another appointment. Your sensitivity to the interviewer's cues are evidence of your sensitivity to clients' cues.

Your manner in the interview is also important. Although the employer expects an applicant to be nervous, he or she will be interested in whether your nervousness makes you unable to respond appropriately. Follow common rules of courtesy. Wait to be asked to sit down before you take a chair. Avoid any distracting mannerisms, such as chewing gum or fussing with your hair, face, or clothes. Be serious when appropriate, but do not forget to smile and be pleasant. The interviewer is also thinking of your impact on clients, visitors, and other staff members.

When you prepare your responses, try to anticipate possible questions from the interviewer. To do this, you must know the role of the person interviewing. In large agencies, your first interview might be with a human resources department employee, not a nursing employee; if you are successful at this stage, you might be recommended for an interview in the nursing department.

Role-playing an interview situation with a friend or relative may help you to feel more confident in your responses. Another technique is to visualize the interview situation in your mind and mentally rehearse responses to questions. Some interviewers focus on asking questions about your past experiences and your future plans. Others focus their questions on specific accomplishments and problems encountered in your past nursing experiences. Presenting hypothetical problems for you to consider, and asking you to provide appropriate nursing responses is common. See Display 11-4 for a list of questions you might reflect on as you prepare.

In most instances, be sure to answer questions that are asked rather than skirting them. However, if the interviewer asks a question that is illegal, such as a question regarding age or marital status, you might want to redirect the question to address what appears to be the concern of the interviewer. For example, in response to a question about your age you might say, "Perhaps you believe that I appear to be young and inexperienced. I want to assure you that I have demonstrated my maturity and responsibility both in my nursing education and in my position with (name of employer)." In response to a question about marital status or children, you could reply, "Perhaps you are concerned about how long I plan to stay in my first position? I want to assure you that whatever my personal situation, professionally, I am looking for a position in an organization where I can be a long-term employee and plan for advancement within the organization." Avoid simple yes or no answers, but try to describe or explain to give a more complete picture of yourself.

An interview usually covers a wide variety of subjects. The interviewer may direct the flow of topics or may encourage you to bring up the ones that concern you. Applicants who focus initial attention on the issues of wages and benefits may be viewed as more concerned about themselves than about nursing. Therefore, if you are asked to present questions, ask professional questions first. Make sure your questions are appropriate for the interviewer. In the human resources department, you might ask

Display 11–4

QUESTIONS TO HELP YOU PREPARE FOR A JOB INTERVIEW

Nursing Philosophy and Beliefs
- What is your philosophy of nursing?
- Is there a nursing theorist that you use as a basis for your nursing practice?
- What do you believe is the most central concept to support excellence in nursing?

Personal Goals and Planning
- Where do you see yourself in 1 year? 5 years? 10 years?
- Have you developed any professional goals? If so, would you share those with me?
- Why do you want to work here?
- What plans do you have for continuing education in nursing?
- What do you see as your weakest area in nursing?
- What do you see as your strengths in nursing?

Your Experiences
- What experience in your nursing education did you find the most rewarding? Why?
- What experience in your nursing education did you like the least? Why?
- In what kind of settings did you have an opportunity to work as a nursing student?
- What other job experiences have you had? What skill did you develop there that will be useful in nursing?

Problem Solving
- Identify a problem in patient care that you encountered as a student and explain how you solved that problem.
- Describe a difficult patient with whom you worked. Include why you found that patient difficult and how you managed the situation.
- Identify a situation in which you were involved in a conflict and describe how you handled that situation. If you had it to do over again, what would you do differently?
- Explain how you would use the nursing process in patient care.
- A problem may be presented to you for your solution. Plan ahead to approach it in a systematic manner.

Technical Skills
- What technical nursing skills do you feel comfortable performing?
- What skills will you require assistance with?
- What do you do when you encounter a technical skill you have not performed before?

The Employment Setting
- In what type of unit do you wish to work?
- Why do you want to work here?
- Why do you think we should hire you for this position?

about the overall mission and philosophy of the organization, its organizational structure, and how authority and accountability are determined. With a nursing interviewer, demonstrate that you are concerned about how nursing care is given and by whom, where responsibility and authority for nursing care decisions lie, the philosophy underlying care, the availability of continuing education, and where you would be expected to fit into their overall picture. However, before you leave be sure to cover such topics as hours, schedules, pay scales, and benefits.

Some interviews are conducted by a group of interviewers. This might include a person from nursing administration, a unit manager, and a staff development nurse. For an applicant to sit across the table from three to five individuals can be unnerving. You will need to look around the group, being sure to make eye contact with each individual. Make sure that you understand the role of each person present. You might actually write down individual names and roles on your notepad and then go back over your list to be sure you have them correct. This would allow you to direct a question to a specific individual or to use an individual's name when replying to a question. While replying to the person who asks the question, you might also glance at others as you make your point. Be sure that you do not ignore any individual, even if one of the interviewers does not seem to ask questions or to be as active in the process as the others. Interviews of this type are often longer than interviews with one person.

Some interviewers are less skilled than others; in these situations the questions may seem less focused and more vague. You may sometimes feel at a loss as to exactly what is being asked. Before proceeding you should seek clarification, but be careful that your manner of asking for clarification does not offend the interviewer. You might ask "Would you give me an example of the type of situation you were thinking about?" Another clarifying approach is for you to state clearly what you perceive to be the central question before continuing, "Let me clarify. You would like me to identify a situation in which I believe I responded effectively to a problem. Is that correct?" In this situation you may have to take the initiative to be sure that you have an opportunity to present your strengths and skills.

If you are unfamiliar with the interview process, you might benefit from reading books on the topic. Reading several different books will give you a variety of viewpoints and might provide you with strategies that are comfortable for you.

Follow-up Strategies

Your initial inquiry should always be followed-up. If you were granted an interview, you would follow-up with a letter as described below. If you did not obtain an interview, you should continue to contact the potential employer at intervals to learn of other job opportunities and to indicate that you are still seeking a position. When a new position opens, employers do not necessarily go back through previous employment files. They are more likely to interview a person who appears to be currently searching for a position than one who was searching several months previously.

After your interview, you should write a brief thank you letter to the person who interviewed you. If a group interviewed you, direct the letter to the person who seemed to be in charge. In that letter, thank the individual for the time and attention to your questions and concerns. Restate any agreement you feel was reached. For example, "I understand that I am to call your office next week to learn whether I have been scheduled for an interview with the maternity unit manager." Close your letter with a positive comment about the organization. Even if you are not offered a job or do not choose to work at that facility, you are leaving a positive impression. You can never tell when that will be important to you in the future (Display 11-5).

Display 11–5
INTERVIEW FOLLOW-UP LETTER

Maribeth Wilson
3428 1st Ave. N.
Seattle, WA 98103
(206) 274-5978
e-mail: maribethw@email.com

January 30, 2001

Joyce Montgall, R.N.
Nurse Recruiter
Seattle General Medical Center
321 Heath Blvd.
Seattle, WA 98101

Dear Ms. Montgall:

I want to thank you for meeting with me today to discuss your new nursing graduate residency program at Seattle General. I am particularly interested in the medical-surgical positions available on 4 West and 4 Center, although I am certainly willing to consider another unit.

My educational background, clinical experience, and commitment to excellent patient care appear to make me an ideal match with Seattle General. In addition, I feel very "at home" in the Seattle General environment, having worked there as a nursing assistant for the last year.

Again, I hope that you will consider me for one of the medical-surgical positions in the June graduate program. I am available to meet with any of the unit managers, which I understand is the next step in your hiring process. I can be contacted at the above telephone number or by e-mail. I do have an answering machine and would promptly return your call if I were not there to receive it. If I have not heard from you within two weeks, I will check with your office regarding the status of my application.

Thank you again for your time and consideration.

Sincerely,

Maribeth Wilson

Maribeth Wilson

Do not let this letter be your last contact with that potential employer. Call back as agreed. Even if you do not get a position at this time, you might ask that your application be kept on file because you are still interested in employment with that particular agency. Then continue to call back every two or three weeks to find out if any other positions are available.

Setting up your own record-keeping system often enhances managing a job search. You should have a record of when you contacted an agency, in what manner (letter or telephone call), interviews—including the interviewer's name and the content of the interview—and dates and times of any follow-up letters or calls. Have a place to record your own notes or impressions. This will enable you to keep track of details when you manage an extensive job search. By keeping this type of record you will not forget to call an agency to recheck on job availability, or mistakenly send an inquiry letter and resumé twice to the same agency.

Managing a Prolonged Job Search

In some areas of the country, new graduates may be faced with a prolonged job search because of the local employment market. Some of the concerns that arise when this happens include: "What am I doing wrong?" "Should I work in health care in another role?" "Should I accept a job that I do not feel prepared for?" "What happens if my skills get out-of-date?"

Evaluating your own job search strategies and the documents you are producing (your letters and resumé) is critical. You might ask for assistance from a career counselor, from a personnel resource, or from friends and family. You might practice your telephone skills and role-play some interview situations. You want to make sure that you are presenting your very best self to potential employers.

In regard to health care employment, you need to know what the recommendations and opinion of your Board of Nursing are regarding taking this type of position. Once you have a registered nurse license, the law usually requires that you function within the expectations of that license in regard to the public. This is true in volunteer or paid work. In many states, the Board has given the opinion that it does not matter what your job title or salary is—if you are a registered nurse, you are held to that standard of practice to assure the safety of the public. If you take a position as a nursing assistant and are a registered nurse, you could be placed in a no-win situation. The licensing board might hold you to a standard of practice that is closed to you by the employer. This might not become apparent until a problem occurred and you did not respond as a registered nurse, but rather as a nursing assistant.

You might look for a part-time position so that you can work while continuing to search for a full-time position. This would help you to keep skills you have and to grow in proficiency. The experience also will assist you in being a more effective candidate for a full-time position. Volunteer work with any number of agencies might be an avenue for you to maintain and enhance skills and provide further support for obtaining a position. This might be tailored to fit the times available to you while you maintain a non-nursing job to continue some type of income.

To maintain your knowledge and skills while involved in a prolonged job search, you should plan to attend continuing education events, read journals, and perhaps complete the examinations provided in journal articles to provide yourself with continuing education credits.

Do you need to broaden your ideas of what kind of position you will seek and accept? Have you narrowed your search too greatly? Research more extensively the positions available in your community as described above. Consider whether geographic mobility is an option for you. Based on this review, target those types of agencies where positions are more likely to arise. Focus your continuing education and volunteer efforts toward those areas most likely to yield job openings. This might make you a better candidate.

Above all, you need to maintain a positive attitude and avoid discouragement. Negative attitudes are often translated into your contacts with potential employers and do not present you as a desirable employee. You might form a support group with others who are seeking employment to maintain your perspective and give you a forum in which to discuss your feelings.

Resignation

When you decide to leave a nursing position, it is important that you provide the employer with an appropriate amount of time to seek a replacement. The more responsible your position, the more time the employer will need. For a staff nursing position, you should strive to provide a month's notice unless an urgent matter requires that less notice be given. Notice of resignation should be in a letter that is directed to the head of your department, often to the Director of Nursing. Copies should be sent to other supervisory people, such as the head nurse and the supervisor.

The letter of resignation is important in concluding your relationship with the employer on a cordial and positive basis. The feelings left behind when you resign will influence letters of recommendation and future opportunities for employment with that agency. Give a reason for your resignation and the exact date when it will be effective. If you have accrued vacation or holiday time and want to take the time off or be paid for it, clearly state that. Comment about positive factors in the employment setting and acknowledge those who have provided special support or assistance in your growth.

If you are resigning because of problems in the work setting and want to note them, do so in a clear, factual, unemotional way. Avoid attacking anyone personally and do not make broad, sweeping negative comments. Try to make the letter a clear and reasonable statement of your position as a professional (Display 11-6).

PROBLEMS EXPERIENCED BY NURSES IN THE WORKPLACE

For many of you, graduating from a nursing program and becoming a registered nurse is the realization of a long-cherished goal. You have spent years preparing for this status and now it is here! What you have viewed as an ideal state, freed from financial pressures that you felt as a student, liberated from the tyranny of the examination, may prove to be quite different from what you had expected. Let us consider some of the problems that may occur as you make this transition from student to professional.

Display 11–6

LETTER OF RESIGNATION

1546 Avenida Escuela
Palm Desert, CA 76321
February 14, 2001

Marvin Short, R.N., Unit Manager
Transitional Care Unit
Desert Hospital
509 Desert Highway
Palm Desert, CA 76320

Dear Marvin:

It is with mixed feelings that I am submitting my resignation to be effective March 23. I will be moving to Oregon and returning to school full time beginning spring quarter.

My two years here at Desert Hospital have been an excellent foundation for my future career. The nurses were supportive of me as a new graduate and have always encouraged me to think of my career as a lifetime opportunity for growth.

The last day I plan to work will be at the end of the pay period. My understanding is that my unused vacation and holiday pay will be included in my final paycheck.

Thank you again for all of your help.

Sincerely,

John Webster

John Webster, R.N.

cc: Maria Gonzales, Vice President for Patient Care Services

Moving From "Novice to Expert"

The path from novice to expert is a challenging one. Benner's (1984) work in this area has provided a basis for understanding and research into this process. She related this path to the Dreyfus Model of Skill Acquisition (Dreyfus & Dreyfus, 1980) in which the individual moves from novice, to advanced beginner, to competent, to proficient, to expert. Throughout this progression she identified exemplars of nurses performing in six different roles:

1. The helping role
2. The teaching-coaching function
3. The diagnostic and monitoring function
4. Effective management of rapidly changing situations
5. Administering and monitoring therapeutic interventions and regimens

6. Monitoring and ensuring the quality of health care practices and organizational and work-role competencies.

Through interviews with nurses, she described the depth of nursing skills and abilities found in the expert nurse. This expertise is forged over time and results from personal experience and personal knowing. One of the challenges for beginning nurses is pressure to function as an expert without this background of growth.

Reality Shock

One problem confronted by the new graduate is the seeming impossibility of delivering quality care within the constraints of the system as it exists. You may feel powerless to effect any changes and may be depressed over your lack of effectiveness in the situation.

Marlene Kramer was the first to call the feelings that result from such a situation *reality shock* (Kramer, 1979). She noted that the new graduate often experiences considerable psychological stress and that this may exacerbate the problem. The person undergoing such stress is less able to perceive the entire situation and to solve problems effectively (Fig. 11-5).

CAUSES OF REALITY SHOCK

With all of the uncertain expectations and demands, the new graduate often feels caught in the middle. As a student, you may think that you are expected to learn a tremendous amount in an alarmingly short time. The expectations may seem high and

FIGURE 11–5 Some new graduates are disillusioned by the working conditions that they find on their first job.

in some ways unrealistic. Then, as a new graduate suddenly thrust into the real world, you may feel insecure and think that your educational program did not adequately prepare you for what is expected of you. On one hand you are expected to function like a nurse who has had 10 years of experience, but on the other hand your new ideas may not be considered because you have so little experience. You may become frustrated because you do not have time to provide the same type of care you gave as a student. For example, you may not have adequate time to deal with a client's psychosocial problems or teaching needs.

As a student, you are taught that the "good nurse" never gives a medication without understanding its actions and side effects, and that evaluating the effectiveness of the drug is essential. As a staff nurse, you may find that the priority is getting the medications passed correctly and on time and that there is little or no time to look up 15 new drugs. As for evaluation, that becomes a dream. How can you evaluate the subtle effects of a medication in the 2 minutes spent passing the medication to a client you do not know? The individually and meticulously planned care that was so important to you as a student may become a luxury when you are a graduate. Often the focus is on accomplishing the required tasks in the time allotted, and it is efficiency in tasks that may earn praise from a supervisor.

Bradby (1990) suggests that reality shock is part of the passage from novice to experienced nurse. She suggests that it be treated as a normal transitional process with a focus on the growth that can occur.

EFFECTS OF REALITY SHOCK

When reality shock occurs, some nurses become disillusioned and leave nursing altogether. Others begin to "job hop" or return to school, searching for the perfect place to practice perfect nursing as it was learned. Some push themselves to the limit, trying to provide ideal care and criticizing the system. This may result in their being labeled nonconformists and troublemakers. Still others give up their values and standards for care and reject ideals as impossibly unrealistic expectations that cannot be fulfilled in the real world. These persons simply mesh with the current framework and become part of the system.

FINDING SOLUTIONS FOR REALITY SHOCK

There is an alternative to these nonproductive coping methods. It is possible to create a role for yourself that blends the ideal with the possible—one in which you do not give up ideals, but see them as goals toward which you will move, however slowly. To do this you need to be realistically prepared for the demands of the real world.

One way of meeting the challenge is to assess yourself as you approach the end of your educational program. Consider what your competencies are. Think about the areas of expectation that were discussed earlier in the chapter:

1. Theoretical knowledge for safe practice
2. Use of the nursing process
3. Self-awareness

4. Communication skill
5. Delegation
6. Documentation
7. Skill proficiency
8. Work ethic
9. Speed of functioning

Second, gain information about what the employers in your community expect from new graduates. You can do this by talking with experienced nurses, requesting interviews with nursing administrators, meeting with faculty, and contacting recent graduates who are currently employed. Try to get specific information. If you have a nursing student organization, setting up a forum for speakers from various agencies might be one avenue to gaining this insight.

After you have gathered this information, try to correlate it with a realistic appraisal of your own ability to function in accordance with an employer's expectations. If you identify any shortcomings, the time to try to remedy them is before graduation. If you identify a lack in certain technical skills, you might register for extra time in the nursing practice laboratory to increase your proficiency. You could even time yourself and work to increase speed as well as skill. You might consult with your clinical instructor to arrange for experiences that would help you gain increased competence. If you recognize that you consistently have difficulty functioning within a time frame, you might obtain employment in a hospital or other health care facility while still in school; this will give you more experience in organizing work within the time limits that the employer sees as reasonable.

As you plan for your first job, you can examine the psychological challenges to be met. Understanding that you are not alone in your feelings of frustration is often helpful. It may be useful to form a support group of other new graduates who meet regularly to discuss problems and concerns and seek solutions jointly. You can also gain valuable reinforcement from other nurses in your work setting. Many have dealt successfully with the problems you face and are able to provide support and help. This "mentor" relationship is an important one and needs to be cultivated.

When confronted with areas of practice that you would like to see changed, weigh the importance of an issue. Use your energies wisely. The "politics of the possible" is important to you. Learn how the system in which you are employed functions and how to use that system for effective change. You, as a person, are important to nursing, so it is important that you neither burn yourself out nor abandon the quest for higher-quality nursing care; you should be able to continue to work toward improving nursing and bringing it closer to its ideals.

Some hospitals attempt to help new graduates deal with reality shock by making orientation programs more comprehensive and by providing an experienced nurse to work as a preceptor to the new graduate. Nurse internships or residencies in some settings have been created to provide a planned and organized transition time during which the new graduate participates in a formal program, including classes, seminars, and rotations to various units of the hospital. Unfortunately, restructuring in many health care agencies has greatly limited orientation time and decreased the support available to the new graduate. The new graduate is required to be more self-directed in identifying needs and the ways that those might be met within the constraints of the system.

Some hospitals provide an opportunity for nursing students to work during the summer before the last year of their basic program to become familiar with the hospital and the nursing role. In this type of program the nursing student may be employed as a nursing assistant, but participate in a planned program that introduces the role of the registered nurse. In other instances, nursing students work as nursing assistants and the orientation to the nursing role in the agency depends upon the initiative the individual takes. You may wish to inquire whether hospitals in your area have developed any of these or other programs to assist you when you are a new graduate.

 Critical Thinking Activity

> With a group of nursing students, develop personal strategies for managing reality shock. Discuss your rationale for any strategy you propose.

Burnout

Burnout is a form of chronic stress related to one's job. This problem arises after you have been in practice for a period of time. It can be identified by feelings of hopelessness and powerlessness, and accompanied by a decreased ability to function both on the job and in personal life. Burnout primarily occurs in nurses who work in particularly stressful areas of nursing, such as critical care, oncology, or burn units. It also occurs in other areas when staffing is inadequate or interpersonal relationships are strained. The downsizing of nursing staff and the rapid changes in the health care environment have contributed to burnout in some settings.

SYMPTOMS OF BURNOUT

Symptoms of burnout include both physical changes and psychological distress. Exhaustion and fatigue, frequent colds, headaches, backaches, and insomnia all may occur. There may be changes in disposition, such as being quick to anger or exhibiting all feelings excessively. Individuals experience a decreased ability to solve problems and make decisions as burnout progresses. This frequently results in an unwillingness to face change and a tendency to block new ideas. There may be feelings of guilt, anger, and depression because one cannot meet the expectations for doing a "perfect job."

In response to these feelings, some nurses quit their jobs and move on to other settings that may not even be in nursing. Others remain in their jobs, but develop a personal shell that tends to separate them from real contact with clients and coworkers; they may become cynical about the possibility of anyone doing a good job and may function at a minimal level. A few become more and more unable to function and find themselves in jeopardy of losing their positions.

CAUSES OF BURNOUT

Many causes of burnout have been discussed in the literature. Prominent among them is the conflict between ideals and reality. Just as this is a problem for the new graduate, it is also a problem for the experienced nurse. In trying to achieve the ideal, the nurse drives harder and harder and becomes critical of the environment and of himself or herself. Nurses see themselves as being responsible for all things to all people and often take on more and more responsibility, thus increasing their own stress level.

Another cause of burnout is the high level of stress that results from practicing nursing in areas that have high mortality rates. Continually investing oneself in clients who die can take a tremendous toll on personal resources. In addition, the demand is constant for optimal functioning.

Inadequately staffed institutions may also place great stress on nurses. The clients are in need of care, the nurse has the skills to provide the care, and yet the clients do not receive good care. The nurse typically tries to accomplish more, staying overtime, skipping breaks and lunch, and running throughout the shift. Despite this effort, there is little job satisfaction because the things that are left undone or that are not done well seem to be more apparent than all the good that is accomplished.

PREVENTING BURNOUT

Mounting a stress-reduction effort involving the nursing staff, supervisory personnel, the hospital administration, and other health care workers can best prevent burnout. The most important objective seems to be bringing burnout into the open and acknowledging the existence of the problems. This alone helps the individual nurse move away from the feelings of separation and alienation that often accompany burnout. Whatever the problems, they seem less frightening if they are defined as "normal" and if the individual nurse does not see himself or herself as the only person not performing as the "perfect nurse."

A second step is to provide for group discussions during which nurses can share feelings and specific concerns in an accepting atmosphere. This sharing may lead to concrete plans to reduce the stress created by the setting. For example, if one source of stress is conflicting orders between two sets of physicians involved in care, a plan might be developed whereby the nurses no longer take responsibility for the conflict, but refer the problem to some authority within the medical hierarchy. This type of resolution is possible only when the whole health care team is addressing the problem of burnout. However, it also requires that nurses give up trying to control "everything."

Giving nurses more control over their own practice often decreases stress. Assuming more control is limited by the constraints of the setting, but it may involve flexible scheduling, volunteering for specific assignments, and participating in committees that determine policies and procedures.

As an individual nurse, you also can take actions to prevent burnout. These are the same general actions that are designed to control stress in any aspect of life. Paying attention to your own physical health is an important preventive measure; this includes maintaining a balanced program of rest, nutrition, and exercise. Another important point is not to subject yourself to excessive changes over short periods of time, because changes increase stress. You may decide, for example, not to move at the same time you change to a different shift. A period of "wind down" or "decompression" after work helps you to avoid carrying the stress of the workplace into your private life; this period may involve physical exercise, reading, meditation, or any different activity. The activity you choose should not create more demands and increase stress. An important resource is someone who is willing to listen while you ventilate your feelings and talk about your problems. Sometimes this is a family member or personal friend, but it may be more appropriate for this to be a coworker or counselor.

Rotating out of a high-stress area, such as a burn unit or pediatric oncology, before you become "burned out" may allow you to rebuild resources and return to the job with enthusiasm. This can be done only if there is no stigma or blame attached to the need to rotate and if other nurses are available for replacement. In client care areas that are known to be stressful, it is helpful to have a counselor available for nurses. Consulting with this counselor should be viewed by the staff as a positive step and not as an admission of some lack or fault. The counselor needs to be someone who understands the setting and who has the skills to assist people in coping with stress.

Another strategy is to focus on those positive aspects of nursing that drew you to it initially. Much is being written about cognitively reframing situations and settings to focus on those parts that are positive and affirming. The art of nursing reflects that positive view of nursing. Lindeman (1999) suggests that the art of nursing is composed of three central aspects. The first, informed caring, refers to behaviors that make a difference for patients; attending to what patients say, analyzing and synthesizing information; and acting as an advocate for patient and family. The second aspect is thoughtful doing. She characterizes nursing practice as a "continuous, interactive, unbroken spectrum of thought and action" (p. 3). The third aspect is lifelong learning. Lifelong learning is an essential foundation for the informed caring and thoughtful doing that are the first two components. Looking at the art of nursing and focusing your energy and attention on this may help you surmount the everyday pressures you encounter.

Burnout is a serious concern in the nursing profession, but there are strategies for managing it. If you are in a high-stress situation, you need to plan for prevention before you become burned out.

Critical Thinking Activity

> Compare burnout with the stress response you have studied in relation to client care. Compare the strategies that you have taught clients with those suggested for preventing burnout.

DISCRIMINATION IN NURSING

Discrimination relates to treating others differently based on stereotypes about groups of people. Two major areas in which discrimination may occur are those of racial or ethnic background and the area of gender or sex. Three major areas in which there is concern about sex discrimination in nursing are the issues of comparable worth, discrimination against men in nursing, and sexual harassment.

Racial/Ethnic Discrimination

While nursing reflects the society in which it operates, there are indications that nurses have moved into greater acceptance of all individuals in advance of some other portions of society. Nursing united the American Association of Colored Graduate nurses with the American Nurses Association before the general civil rights movement in the United States. There have always been prominent nurses of color. The immediate past president of the American Nurses Association, Beverly Malone, and the past president of the National League for Nursing, Rhetaugh Dumas, are both African American women who have been leaders for all of nursing. However, the number of minorities in nursing does not reflect the number of minorities in the general population. According to the Health Resources and Services Administration, only 10% of nurses come from racial/ethnic minority backgrounds (HRSA, 1996). This contrasts with a general population that has 17% racial/ethnic minorities (U.S. Census Bureau, 1999). This difference may stem from many different causes but is of concern because a workforce that reflects the population is more likely to meet the health care needs of that population in a culturally sensitive manner. Some of the root causes of the lower participation of minorities in nursing have to do with access to education, support for high career goals, economic status, the image of nursing, institutionalized racism, and other general societal problems.

Nurses are challenged to examine this situation and be a part of the solution. All of us need to recognize and welcome diversity in the nursing profession. We need to acknowledge that a diversity of views and life experiences will enrich nursing as a profession and support excellence in patient care. When we see discrimination occurring, whether in education or in the workplace, we need to speak up as agents for change. The National Student Nurses' Association (NSNA) has supported a program called Breakthrough to Nursing, in which nursing students mentor minority individuals in nursing education. These and similar efforts help nursing to move forward as a profession that welcomes and provides opportunities for all.

Comparable Worth

Nursing has been, and still is, a profession dominated by women. Laws exist in many states that prohibit explicit sex discrimination in salary for a given job. For example, if a health care provider hires both men and women as registered nurses, they must be compensated on the same basis. This principle has been expanded to encompass jobs that involve essentially the same work, although the titles may differ. The janitor and the maid may have different titles, but if they have essentially the same tasks, then they must be paid on the same basis. In one case, nurse practitioners (who were primarily women) in an agency argued that they should receive the same compensation as the physician's assistants (who were primarily men) because they performed basically the same tasks. These nurses saw the difference in the salaries as a form of sex discrimination.

The next step that many women would like to see accepted is the principle of compensation based on comparable worth. Jobs may be studied and assigned points or rank based on educational requirements, skills required, level of responsibility, and authority. Those with the same points or rank are considered to be of comparable worth although the actual substance of the work may differ. Alaska has a law barring discrimination in pay for work of comparable character.

Many women believe that different jobs of comparable worth are not compensated equally because of sex discrimination. Many jobs that are found to score high in education requirements, skill, and responsibility, and yet have low salaries, are jobs that historically have been held by women, such as nursing. For example, physicians' assistants are primarily men and nurse practitioners are primarily women. The average salaries for physicians' assistants have tended to be higher than the average salaries for nurse practitioners in many areas. Where different job descriptions exist for these two groups, equity would need to be based on determining comparable worth. Groups of women have brought suit against employers, charging sex discrimination based on failure to provide equal pay for jobs of comparable worth.

Currently, the political climate does not support positive responses to claims of discrimination based on comparable worth; the argument against this premise is that jobs requiring comparable education and skills commonly have different wages based on market forces. When these jobs are held primarily by men or primarily by women, this does not constitute discrimination but simply reflects the realities of the marketplace. This will continue to be an issue in the field of nursing.

Discrimination Against Men

Men in nursing also have expressed concern about sex discrimination. Their concern is not monetary, but is related to being allowed to practice in all areas of nursing and being accepted within the profession. Anti-male sexism in the United States was discussed by Kus (1985), who pointed out that society stereotypes men just as feminists have criticized that it stereotypes women. He made a strong case for the importance of nurses examining the stereotypes they hold about men. Stereotypes narrow our thinking and interfere with people being able to develop to their fullest potential. It is appropriate for women in nursing to examine their own behavior and identify whether they have been guilty of perpetuating outmoded stereotypes of the nurse and supporting a type of discrimination toward men that they would fight to eliminate for women.

In some facilities or areas, men are not allowed to care for women clients, or if they are allowed to care for women, restrictions are placed on them in terms of obtaining consent for care from each client. Those who support the limitations on the practice of men in nursing state that it is a matter of providing for the modesty and privacy of female clients. This position was upheld by a court decision in favor of a hospital that refused to assign a man to a nursing position in labor and delivery (Arkansas judge, 1981). The argument was made that the client did not have free choice of a nurse but rather was assigned a nurse for care, and therefore the restrictions were appropriate.

In an article in *The American Nurse*, Ketter (1994) presented the situations of men who have felt discrimination in the workplace based on their gender. One of these men has filed three complaints with Equal Employment Opportunities Commission (EEOC) regarding discrimination in employment in obstetric/gynecologic settings in the 3 years he has been in nursing. His case is expected to end up in federal court.

Those who oppose limitations on the practice of men in nursing state that, as a professional, a nurse (whether a man or woman) should always consider the privacy and modesty of a client of either gender. This can be done without excluding anyone from providing care in any area. By careful assessment, the nurse can determine the true needs of the client and plan for appropriate avenues to deliver that care. Furthermore, the point has been made that men as physicians have not been excluded from any branch of medicine and this has not created problems. The client does not always choose physicians, either. House staff are assigned, referrals are made to specialty physicians, and many group plans designate a physician to provide care. Female nurses care for male clients in all situations. This has been accepted because women are seen in a nurturing, mothering role that the public associates with nursing.

The American Assembly for Men in Nursing (see Appendix B) provides a forum for the concerns of men in nursing and those who are concerned about the problems of sex discrimination. This organization seeks to educate people and opposes any limitations on opportunities available to men.

Critical Thinking Activity

Review the advertisements for nursing positions in three current journals and analyze them for gender bias.

Sexual Harassment

Sexual harassment has been identified as behavior of a sexual nature that creates a work environment that is perceived as hostile and unduly stressful. Sexual harassment may take the form of comments about an individual's body, persistent unwanted attempts to initiate a personal relationship, the ongoing use of suggestive or obscene language, unwanted touching, or direct sexual advances. Both men and women may be the objects of sexual harassment. Issues of sexual harassment have been in the news in many ways in the last few years. Sexual harassment is a concern in nursing. Because nurses are involved with personal care of individuals of the opposite sex, there is sometimes the unspoken assumption that they will not be offended by sexual comments, jokes, or innuendo.

Harassers in the health care workplace may be clients, coworkers, or physicians. According to Kaye (1996) and Williams (1995), most harassers in the health care workplace are physicians; this follows the general data showing that sexual harassment is a demonstration of personal power over others. Historically, physicians have had the most power in health care environments. Temper tantrums, verbal abuse, and inappropriate sexual remarks often were tolerated from physicians because other health professionals knew that they did not have the power to change these behaviors. While recognizing the problem, it is important not to stereotype physicians, because the majority of physicians are professional and appropriate in their relationships.

Individuals should take steps to stop sexual harassment by giving clear, direct verbal messages indicating that the behavior in question is unwanted, unpleasant, and must stop. Sometimes this action alone stops inappropriate behavior. If clear, direct messages are not successful, the individual then should report the matter in writing to an immediate supervisor. Any individual who believes that he or she has been the victim of sexual harassment would be wise to keep records of the behavior and of all attempts to stop the behavior in question. If you belong to a collective bargaining group, that group can serve as a resource to assist you if you believe you are the victim of sexual harassment.

Employers are legally and ethically responsible for having clear policies that prohibit sexual harassment, and for providing an appropriate work environment. These policies should be publicized so that everyone is aware of them. The courts support the responsibility of the employer to maintain a work environment free of sexual harassment (Neuhs, 1994; Wolfe, 1996).

Critical Thinking Activity

Formulate an appropriate response to experiencing sexual harassment in the workplace. Include specific statements you would use and each step you would take if the harassment continued.

WORKPLACE SAFETY AND HEALTH FOR NURSES

Nurses have expressed concern regarding safety in the working environment for many years. Employees have a right to expect their employers to provide the safest working environment possible. Some hospitals employ an occupational health nurse to examine the working environment, and use employment practices to promote health and safety on the job. Nurses themselves, however, often have been lax in recognizing on-the-job hazards and acting for self-protection; this can be likened to the response of those who continue to smoke despite their knowledge of the health hazards of smoking, or those who fail to wear seatbelts even though statistics show fewer fatalities in automobile accidents when seatbelts are worn. Some people continue to do those things that they know are detrimental to their health and well-being. Unfortunately, nurses are no exception (Fig. 11-6).

The Bureau of Labor Statistics tracks and reports data related to occupational hazards. Reports have identified that hospitals have an incidence of work-related illness or injury of 11.8 per 100 full-time workers. Nursing homes are even more hazardous, with an incidence of 17.3 per 100 workers. Nurse aides were even more at risk than registered nurses (RNs Facing, 1995). Personal awareness is the first step in attempting to control this growing problem.

FIGURE 11–6 Needle-stick injuries are a major concern in all health care environments.

Infection as an Occupational Hazard

Transmission of infection is a major concern when caring for infected clients. The presence of resistant organisms causes extra concern and makes treatment difficult. All hospitals have an infection control officer, usually a registered nurse, who has the expertise to guide the staff in planning appropriate infection control procedures. Staff in other settings may not have access to such an expert.

The hidden danger for nurses lies in those clients who have not been diagnosed as having an infection and for whom specific infection control measures have therefore not been prescribed. Universal precautions have been mandated by the Occupational Safety and Health Administration (OSHA) for use with all clients in all settings (that is, universally) to protect staff from blood-borne pathogens. These precautions prevent the spread of HIV, hepatitis B, and other such blood-borne pathogens. Nurses who have frequent contact with blood and blood products, and those engaged in intravenous therapy, have a special risk for exposure to hepatitis B. Although a vaccine exists to protect against this disease, the vaccine itself is not without side effects; therefore, a discussion with a physician regarding risks versus benefits for you as an individual is appropriate before undertaking immunization. OSHA has developed standards that require employers to pay for hepatitis B immunization for those employees with significant exposure to blood and body fluids that can transmit blood-borne organisms.

AIDS has created a reevaluation of all approaches to infection control and of health care workers' obligations to provide care for those with communicable diseases. AIDS remains a serious concern for all health care workers. One of the first employer actions toward preventing AIDS and other blood-borne diseases was the provision of "sharps" containers wherever needles were used. Another important employer responsibility is the provision of a supply of gloves and protective eyewear for employee use. OSHA mandates these measures as part of universal precautions. However, not all cases of transmission of blood-borne pathogens can be prevented by universal precautions. Needle-stick injuries—especially those with large-bore needles (eg, bone marrow aspiration needles)—continue to be the most frequent transmission source. Wearing gloves does not prevent these injuries.

More attention is now being given to designing needles and other sharp devices in new ways that provide greater protection. For example, a needle with a protective plastic housing is available for injections. These needles are unlikely to injure an individual even if they are not handled properly. Needleless intravenous connections are also available. Syringes are available that have a protective cover into which the needle retracts immediately after use. These safer devices are more expensive; therefore, some employers have been reluctant to make the change, because they are not required to do so. Nurses have a legitimate interest in requesting that hospitals provide safer equipment. To participate knowledgeably in decisions regarding needle systems and devices, nurses need to seek information about what devices are available. Nurses have lobbied both in states and nationally for legislation requiring safe needle devices. In 1999, legislation setting up this requirement was introduced into the US Congress (Willard, 1999). Although it did not pass then, it will be introduced again. Several states have introduced needle safety legislation; it has been passed in California.

Blood-borne pathogens are not the only pathogens of concern in the health care environment. The new Standard Precautions recommended by the Centers for Disease Control and Prevention (CDC, 1996), often referred to as Body Substance Precautions, are used in many places—but they are not required by OSHA. These precautions protect clients and staff from infections that might be transmitted by any body substance. When these new Standard Precautions were being formulated, OSHA indicated that regulations would likely be changed from the current requirement for Universal Precautions to a requirement for the more extensive Standard Precautions. Because of the antiregulatory stance of the Congress through 1999, OSHA did not proceed with formulating new requirements for employers. This may occur in the future.

The incidence of tuberculosis is again on the rise, with drug-resistant strains of the organism appearing. Although rooms with special ventilation and special masks that are impervious to the tuberculosis organism are available, individuals with the disease may be in contact with health care providers long before they are clearly diagnosed. Should nurses in high-risk areas, such as the emergency room, wear special masks during all client contact, or is this unrealistic? These are important questions to consider.

Although the details of infection control are beyond the scope of this text, we remind you that you hold the key to protecting yourself in many ways. Health care workers often become lax in their attention to the use of gloves or eye protection because these measures are inconvenient. It is your responsibility to use the very best techniques for self-protection. Nurses must assume responsibility for their own protection by conscientiously carrying out appropriate measures at all times. Employers must be held accountable for providing the supplies and environment to make this possible.

Hazardous Chemical Agents

Anesthetic gases can increase the risk of fetal malformation and spontaneous abortion in pregnant women who are exposed to them on a regular basis. Standards exist for waste-gas retrieval systems and the allowable level of these gases in the air. Nurses working in operating rooms should seek information on the subject and expect hospitals to provide a safe work environment.

Chemotherapeutic agents used in the treatment of cancer are extremely toxic, and nurses who work in settings where such agents are prepared and administered should seek additional education regarding their administration, not only in relation to the client's safety but also in relation to personal safety. The employer is responsible for providing the equipment needed to maintain safety when handling these agents. In many settings, protocols now require the routine use of personal protective equipment when handling chemotherapeutic agents.

Contact with many medications, especially antibiotics, during preparation and administration may cause the nurse to develop sensitivity. This can create transitory problems (eg, a hand rash), and may be a threat if treatment for a serious infection is compromised later. Other medications are absorbed through the skin and may produce an undesirable effect. Nurses must take personal responsibility for their own safety in regard to these agents. Nurses who understand these hazards handle all drugs with discretion and are careful not to expose themselves to these agents.

Cleaning agents and disinfectants used in the hospital also may be hazardous if used improperly. Employers are now required by OSHA to maintain a list of all chemicals used in the work environment, along with information on their possible effects, and the appropriate treatment if individuals are accidentally exposed to them. If you work with these agents, you should seek out this information, found in the Material Safety Data Sheets (MSDS), and be sure that you handle chemicals correctly.

Back Injuries

Because nursing includes providing direct care to incapacitated individuals, back injuries are a common occupational hazard. Back injuries in general are a serious concern because they interfere with the working life of people in their most productive years. Nursing assistants in long-term care facilities have the highest incidence of back injuries. As staff numbers are reduced, remaining staff often feel pressure to move and lift people and equipment without essential assistance. Back injuries then increase (RNs facing, 1995).

Some institutions provide instruction in lifting, transfer, posture, body mechanics, and other back-saving strategies to help prevent injury. Mechanical lifting devices provide a means of moving clients without danger to staff. More types of lifting devices are now available, and more employers are open to purchasing equipment to prevent these costly injuries. You need to be aware of the potential for back injury and examine your own work habits. Some nurses feel that they must accomplish certain tasks even if the necessary assistance is not available, and therefore carry out actions of danger to themselves. Nurses must learn to be assertive in regard to their own safety.

Violence in the Workplace

Most nursing students think of hospitals as places where victims of violence are helped. Rarely do they think of themselves as potential victims of violence in their own workplace. According to OSHA, two thirds of nonfatal workplace assaults happen in health and social services facilities. The majority of these are assaults by clients on nursing staff, and more occur in psychiatric mental health settings than in other settings. Assaults on staff by visitors and outsiders also occur; most of these take place in emergency rooms. In addition to assaults, 18 RNs and 88 other health care workers died in workplace homicides between 1980 and 1990 (Violence is still, 1996). Although statistics for the 1990s are not yet available, many health care workers do not believe that it has diminished. However, the general statistics for violent crime show a decrease nationally, and there is hope that this will be reflected in decreased violent incidents in health care workplaces.

OSHA has issued guidelines for use by facilities trying to establish a safer workplace. These are not enforceable rules, but may represent what is termed the "General Duty" clause in the OSHA Act. The guidelines call for clear programs designed to protect workers. These programs would include an assessment and analysis of the workplace for hazards and a plan for prevention of problems. One form of prevention is to train employees in the management of hostile and violent behavior. Ways of identifying hostile and assaultive clients should be developed so that staff can be warned to take extra personal safety precautions. Other important environmental safeguards include the use of such devices as metal detectors, panic buttons, and bulletproof glass where appropriate. Adequate staff to manage potentially violent behavior is of particular concern in psychiatric/mental health settings. The addition of security personnel is important in some environments. There should be an attitude throughout the institution of zero tolerance for abusive or assaultive behavior.

In addition to preventing and managing problem situations, there should be clear guidelines for reporting both verbal and physical abuse and following through on all complaints. Health care institutions should work with law enforcement professionals when abusive or assaultive behavior occurs to assure that legal procedures are carried out correctly.

Those who report incidents should receive support and assistance and be assured that there will be no reprisals or blaming. Some nurses have been reluctant to report verbal and physical abuse or assault because of personal and institutional beliefs that health care staff should be able to handle these behaviors independently. Another common belief in health care environments is that all behavior has meaning for the individual and that staff should accept inappropriate behaviors on the part of clients. Social constraints and adverse consequences related to inappropriate behavior are a valuable ally in redirecting the behaviors of those who are cognitively impaired, mentally ill, or developmentally delayed. Nurses need support from their work environments in accessing these avenues to protect themselves.

Critical Thinking Activity

Research the occupational health program offered by a local employer of nurses. Evaluate that program in relation to health hazards in the workplace of which you are aware.

Workers' Compensation

If you believe that you have a work-related injury or illness, you must follow the policies and procedures prescribed by your facility or by state regulation. This includes reporting the injury as soon as possible after it happens. In most institutions this is done on an incident or quality assurance report. A common error is to delay reporting in the belief that you should report something only if you know it will be serious or require medical care. By the time you know this, it may be much more difficult to prove that the problem was work related.

Employers may seek to have workers' compensation claims disallowed to limit their financial liability. Because back injuries are the most common work-related injuries, and often have no clear objective evidence of damage even when pain is present, stigma frequently is attached to those who have back injuries. HIV and hepatitis B are transmitted through needle-stick injuries, but they are also transmitted through other unsafe behaviors. These factors may underlie attempts by an employer to disallow claims for care and time lost from work due to these work-related illnesses or injuries. Prompt, thorough reporting is essential to future claims.

You also should have any injury assessed by an appropriate health care provider. If your agency has an occupational health nurse, you may be required to be seen there for initial screening. One concern is whether you may receive care from the provider of your choice or whether you must receive care from a designated provider. This varies based on the regulations governing work-related injury and illness in your state. You should ask this question of your employer and then research it through your state workers' compensation office. If the laws allow the employer or a state agency to designate the provider and you go to another of your choice, you may not be reimbursed for expenses incurred.

Compensation for time off work is another concern when a work-related problem occurs; you usually are required to use your sick leave, but additional time may be available through the workers' compensation program. In general, these programs do not match your working salary, so your income will be lessened. This is one reason why many individuals choose to have private disability insurance that provides replacement income when they cannot work because of illness or disability.

The Americans With Disabilities Act requires that employers seek ways to provide reasonable accommodation for individuals with disability so that they can continue to work. This might include transferring an individual to a different position or modifying the work environment to provide a setting in which the individual can function. Employers have been known to refuse to make accommodations and to try to terminate an individual who has an ongoing disability. Those with work-related illness and disability do have legal rights within the system. Sometimes it requires considerable effort to sustain those rights.

KEY CONCEPTS

- Throughout the history of nursing, employment patterns have changed, moving from a focus on the home and the community in the first part of this century to a focus on acute care institutions.
- In today's health care world, the percentage of nurses employed in hospital inpatient settings is diminishing as more outpatient, home care, long-term care, and community settings are established for the delivery of care.
- Competencies needed by the newly licensed registered nurse can be categorized by criticality and by frequency.
- Employers have expectations in eight basic areas: theoretical knowledge for safe practice and decision making; ability to use the nursing process; self-awareness; communication skills; understanding the importance of documentation; commitment to a work ethic; proficiency in specified technical skills; and speed of functioning.
- Developing a successful career pathway involves setting personal short- and long-term goals and developing a plan for maintaining and enhancing your own competence.
- To obtain a nursing position, you will need to identify potential employers, develop a professional resumé, write appropriate letters to employers, and interview effectively.
- Reality shock occurs when an idealistic new graduate enters the real world of practice and has difficulty with the expectations and demands found there. You can prepare for this transition by attending to your own expectations and developing personal strategies for coping.
- Burnout is a stress response experienced by nurses and others who work in occupations that make many emotional demands. Burnout may be alleviated by planned actions, but it may be necessary to change job settings when stress accumulates.
- Nurses may see discrimination in the workplace manifested as racial/ethnic discrimination, wage discrimination against women, job opportunity discrimination against men, and sexual harassment in the workplace.
- Occupational safety and health are special concerns for nurses because of the infectious nature of the illnesses with which they come in contact, the toxicity of some chemicals in the nursing environment, and the potential for back injury and violence.
- Nurses who experience a work-related injury must carefully follow all relevant rules and regulations for reporting the injury, completing appropriate forms, and seeking care to assure that they receive assistance for any medical care and lost wages.

REFERENCES

An HIV-infected RN finds a cause: Universal use of safer needles. Am J Nurs 96(4):69–70, 1996

Arkansas judge rules male nurse out of labor/delivery. Am J Nurs 81(7):1253, 1981

Benner P. From Novice to Expert. Menlo Park, CA: Addison-Wesley, 1984

Bradby M. Status passage into nursing: Another view of the process of socialization into nursing. J Adv Nurs 15(10):1220–1225, 1990

Chornick N, Yocom CJ, Jacobson J. 1992–1993 Job Analysis Study of Newly Licensed, Entry-Level Registered Nurses. Chicago: National Council of State Boards of Nursing, 1993

Dreyfus SE, Dreyfus HL. A five-stage model of the mental activities involved in directed skill acquisition. Unpublished report supported by the Air Force Office of Scientific Research (AFSC), USAF (Contract F49620-79-C-0063), University of California at Berkeley, 1980 (as reported in Benner P, From Novice to Expert, Menlo Park, CA: 1984)

Health Resources and Services Administration (HRSA)-Bureau of Health Professions. Notes from the National Sample Survey of Registered Nurses, March 1996. Available at *www.hrsa.dhhs.gov/bhpr/dn/sample.htm.* Accessed July 15, 2000

Injured on the job? Nursing 24(6):28, 1994

Kaye J. Sexual harassment and hostile environments in the perioperative area. AORN J 63(2):443–446, 448–449, 1996

Kaye J, Donald CG, Merker S. Sexual harassment of critical care nurses: A costly workplace issue. Am J Crit Care 3(6):409–415, 1994

Ketter J. Sex discrimination targets men in some hospitals. Am Nurse 26(4):3, 24, 1994

Kramer M. Reality Shock. St. Louis: CV Mosby, 1979

Kus RJ. Stages of coming out: An ethnographic approach. West J Nurs Res 7(2):177–194, 1985

Lindeman C. The Art of Nursing. Creative Nursing 5(3):3–4, 1999

National League for Nursing. Educational Outcomes of Associate Degree Nursing Programs: Roles and Competencies. Publication No. 23-2348. New York: National League for Nursing, 1991

National Council of State Boards of Nursing. National Council Completes 1997 Job Analysis of Newly Licensed Practical/Vocational Nurses. Issues 18(4), 1997. Available at *www.ncsbn.org/files/publications/issues/vol184/lpnjob184.asp.* Accessed January 21, 2000

National Council of State Boards of Nursing. Current NCLEX-RN Test Plan Under Review. Issues 20(4), 1999. Available at *www.ncsbn.org/files/publications/issues/vol204/test-plan204.asp.* Accessed January 21, 2000

National Council of State Boards of Nursing. Employment and Work Environment Trends in Newly Licensed Nurses: Findings from the January 1998 Survey. Available at *www.ncsbn.org/research/studies/qja9801.asp.* Accessed January 21, 2000

National Council of State Boards of Nursing. Employment and Work Environment Trends in Newly Licensed Nurses: Findings from the July 1999 Survey. Available at *www.ncsbn.org/research/studies/employment9907.asp.* Accessed January 21, 2000

Neuhs HP. Sexual harassment: A concern for nursing administrators. J Nurs Admin 24(5):47–52, 1994

RNs facing new danger at work. Am J Nurs 95(10):78, 81, 1995

Saver C. Nursing in the new millenium. Imprint (January):32, 1999. Available at *www.nsna.org/pubs/imprint/janfeb99/nursing.html.* Accessed January 10, 2000

U.S. Census Bureau. Statistical Abstract of the United States, National Data Book, 1999

Williams M. The prevalence and impact of violence and sexual harassment of registered nurses in the workplace. Chart 92(4):5–6, 1995

Wolfe S. Legally speaking: If you're sexually harassed. RN 59(2):61–64, 1996

FURTHER READING

Alward R, Monk T. The Nurse's Shift Work Handbook. Washington, DC: American Nurses Publishing Co., 1993

Brady B. How I was sexually harassed. Nursing 24(5):52–56, 1994

Busy nurses need stressbusters. Am Nurse 26(2):5–6, 1994

Butts BJ, Witmer DM. New graduates: What does my manager expect? Nurs Management 23(8):46–48, 1992

Career Guide. Nursing2000, monthly feature

Career Planning Guide. New York: National Student Nurses Association, annual publication

Carroll PL. Reducing the risk of needlestick injury associated with implanted ports. Home Healthcare Nurse 16(4):225–234, 1998

Coleman S, Hansen S. Reducing work-related back injuries. Nurs Management 25(11):58, 60–61, 1994

Foley ME. Change signals need for career security versus job security. Am Nurse 26(2):1, 3, 1994

Fulmer H, Cashman S, Bushnell K. Community-oriented primary care: A model for the future. Am Nurse 26(2):19, 1994

Job Focus. American Journal of Nursing, monthly feature

Johnson C. Coping with compassion fatigue. Nursing 22(4):116, 118–119, 120, 1992

Kairns DM. Protect yourself: Set boundaries. RN 55(3):19–22, 1992

Ketter J. Nurses, HIV exposure and the burden of proof. Am Nurse 26(5):14, 21, 1994

Ketter J. Retraining programs benefit staff nurses. Am Nurse 26(4):1, 3, 1994

Leiter, MP. The correspondence of patient satisfaction and nurse burnout. Soc Sci Med 47(10):1611–1618, 1998.

Libbus MK, Bowman KG. Sexual harassment of female registered nurses in hospitals. J Nurs Admin 24(6):26–31, 1994

Lovejoy RL. When are you entitled to worker's compensation? RN 53(3):81–83, 1990

Miya PA. Ethical dilemmas: Touchy subject . . . sexual harassment. Am J Nurs 94(9):56, 1994

Owen BD. Preventing back injuries. Am J Nurs 99(5):76, 1999

RN Nursing Opportunities. RN Magazine, annual publication

Schuldenfrei P. No heavy lifting: Making safety work. Am J Nurs 98(9):46, 1998

Sullivan P. Stress and burnout in psychiatric nursing. Nurs Standards 8(2):36–39, 1993

Survival Skills in the Workplace: What Every Nurse Should Know. Washington, DC: American Nurses Publishing Co., 1990

Tammelleo AD. Hurt at work? Who dictates where you get care? RN 57(12):64, 1994

Travel nursing: Get up and go! Nursing93 23(12):60–62, 1993

Willard J. Sharps injury prevention. Nursing99 29(9):69–70, 1999

Workplace safety. Am J Nurs 98(9):58, 1998

Relevant web sites

Advanced Resource Solutions, Inc. *www.arsjobs.com/*

American Nurses Association *www.nursingworld.org*

American Nurses Association Online Classified
www.nursingworld.org/market/classifi/classifi.htm

Lippincott Williams & Wilkins Career Center Online *www.nursingcenter.com/career*

Nursing Jobs.com *www.nursing-jobs.com*

Nurse Jobz *www.nursejobz.com/*

Nurse Options USA *www.nursingjobs.org*
  www.nurseoptions.com
Occupational Safety and Health Administration *www.osha.gov*
RN magazine *www.rnweb.com/career.html*
RN Wanted.com *www.rnwanted.com*
Springhouse Corporation Online *www.springnet.com/career.htm*
  www.nursingmanagement.com/careers9800.htm

12

Preparing for Workplace Participation

We are born in
organizations, educated by
organizations, and most of
us spend much of our
lives working for
organizations.

(Etzioni, 1964)

OBJECTIVES

After completing this chapter, you should be able to:

1. Discuss the purpose of mission statements.

2. Analyze the relationships among organizational charts, chains of command, and channels of communication within the structure of organizations.

3. Delineate the characteristics of shared governance, analyzing the advantages of a shared governance approach.

4. Describe various patterns of nursing care delivery, identifying the major characteristics of each.

5. Discuss the history of collective bargaining as it applies to nursing.

6. Analyze the processes through which resolution is achieved in collective bargaining issues.

7. Identify at least four professional concerns that should be addressed in a contract for nurses.

8. Discuss the concerns nurses have regarding membership in a collective bargaining group and the reasons for each of these concerns.

9. Outline the advantages and disadvantages of having the state nurses' association serve as a bargaining agent for nurses.

10. Compare and contrast the characteristics of a grievance and a complaint.

KEY TERMS

Accountability

Agency shop

Authority

Authoritative mandate

Bargain in good faith

Binding arbitration

Broad span of control

Bureaucratic

Case method

Chain of command

Channels of communication

Clinical ladder

Collective action division

Collective bargaining

Common interest bargaining

Concession bargaining

Contract

Cross-training

Deadlock

Division of labor

Final offer

Flat organization

Functional method

Government seizure

Grievance process

Injunction

Impasse

Job description

Informational picketing

Lock out

Mediation

Mission statement

Narrow span of control

National Labor Relations Act

National Labor Relations
  Board

Negotiate–negotiation

Organization

Organizational chart

Organizational hierarchy

Path of authority and
  accountability

Policy

Professional collectivism

Protocol

Ratify

Reinstatement privilege

Role transition

Shared governance

Span of control

Standards of care

Statements of philosophy

Structure of an organization

Tall organization

Team nursing

Total patient care

Unfair labor practice

Unions

Union busting

Organizations surround us. Wherever you look you will find organizations. And, like most other new nursing graduates, when you complete your studies you probably will seek employment in an organization—a health care organization. This may be in an acute care hospital, a long-term care facility, an intermediate care facility, or a variety of other organizations that offer challenging opportunities. Accepting employment in a health care organization requires that you adapt to the policies and procedures established by that organization. You will go through what we refer to as *role transition*, the process of assuming and developing a new role. This process occurs most comfortably when you have a basic understanding of the organization, how it operates and functions, and how you can participate effectively in the activities of that workplace. It is also helpful to be able to anticipate some of the frustrations you may encounter.

This chapter presents content that we believe can assist you in your transition from student to employee. We begin with a brief discussion of the structure of organizations and some of the most common conditions of employment, and then present the most common avenues through which employees participate in workplace decisions. Because we can only touch on these topics, students are encouraged to gain greater depth in this area by reading books devoted to this topic.

UNDERSTANDING ORGANIZATIONS

An *organization* may be defined as a formally constituted group of people, with identified tasks, who work together to achieve a specific purpose defined by the organization. All organizations have structure and purpose. Organizations that have the delivery of health care as their primary objective usually are considered *bureaucratic* organizations, which means that they operate and are administered through a number of departments and subdivisions, with designated individuals responsible for carrying out various functions.

The Mission Statement and the Philosophy

All organizations have a purpose, or a reason for existing. This purpose typically is expressed in the form of a *mission statement*, which outlines what the organization plans to accomplish. Sometimes mission statements incorporate *statements of philosophy* (beliefs), purpose, and goals or objectives into a single statement; other times the philosophy, purposes, and goals are addressed in addition to the mission statement. These statements serve as a benchmark against which an organization's performance can be evaluated. A large research hospital might incorporate into their mission statement an obligation to research, teaching, and the care of clients with complex problems. A smaller community hospital may reflect a goal of meeting the health care needs of citizens of the community in their mission statement. The hospital's ability to meet these goals then would be reviewed as part of the overall evaluation of the organization.

Critical Thinking Activity

Based on your perception of the needs of the community in which you live, write a mission statement for a hospital that would serve the needs of the area. How did you arrive at the decision to offer the services you outlined? What facts support this decision?

Organizational Structure

To survive, any organization must make enough money to meet expenses and to improve and develop; some also seek to provide a profit return to investors. This is as true in health care as it is in Wall Street businesses. A central goal of most organizations is to seek an organizational structure that is efficient while providing maximum effectiveness. As the values and priorities of our society change, and as new technology becomes available, health care organizations also must make adaptations. Thus, today we encounter a health care system experiencing tremendous transformation (see Chapters 1 and 2).

In organizational theory, the concept of management is associated with structure. The *structure* of an organization may be defined as "the sum total of the ways its labor is divided into distinct tasks and then coordination is achieved among these tasks" (Huber, 1996, p. 226). In other words, the structure of an organization refers to the way it is "put together" to accomplish its goals. Breaking work into pieces or tasks, which are assigned to various individuals or groups, is known as *division of labor*. Size, age, services, technical components, and environment influence the structure of an organization.

Types of Structure

The power to make decisions is a key factor in the structure and function of any organization. With regard to the decision-making process, organizations may be described as having a centralized (or tall) or a decentralized (or flat) structure. An organization is depicted as *centralized* when the authority to make decisions is vested in a few individuals (Fig. 12-1). Conversely, when the decision making involves a number of indi-

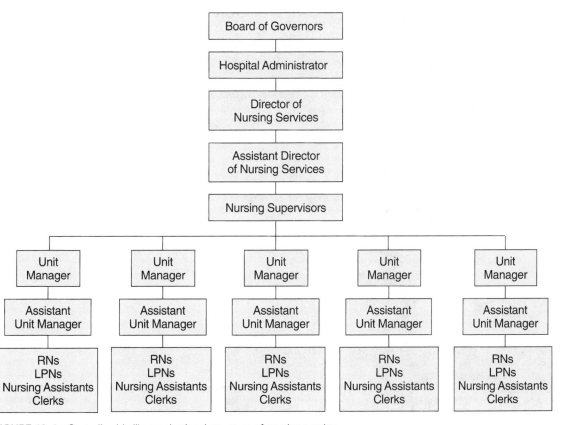

FIGURE 12-1 Centralized (tall) organizational structure of nursing service.

viduals, and filters down to the individual employee, the organization is said to operate in a *decentralized* fashion. Later in this chapter we discuss the concept of shared governance, which embraces a decentralized structure and function (Fig. 12-2).

Another organizational structure may be either flat or tall—the matrix structure. The unique characteristic of the *matrix structure* is that a second structure overlies the first, creating two directions for lines of authority, accountability, and communication. The relationship that exists among individuals is outside the regular chain of command. We typically see the matrix structure in very large, multifaceted organizations. Individuals with special expertise or authority in an area serve as resource persons for several departments, all of which can benefit from the knowledge. For example, in Figure 12-3, three different types of expertise (financial services, planning and marketing, and quality assurance) are demonstrated to cross all aspects of this large hospital corporation, which includes acute care, long-term care, and home care. Another example of a matrix-type relationship could be illustrated by a nurse with expertise in gerontologic nursing who provides assistance, advice, and information to employees in each branch of this hospital organization. This individual would have authority, responsibility, and accountability in each of the health care settings.

AUTHORITY, RESPONSIBILITY, AND ACCOUNTABILITY

Authority, responsibility, and accountability are three terms often used when discussing the ways that groups or organizations operate. *Authority* refers to the official power an individual has to approve an action, to command an action, or to see that a decision is enforced. It is based on one's position in the hierarchy of the organization. For

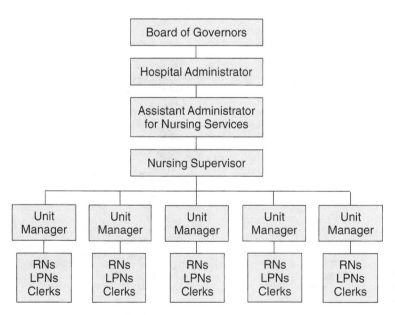

FIGURE 12-2 Decentralized (flat) organizational structure of nursing service.

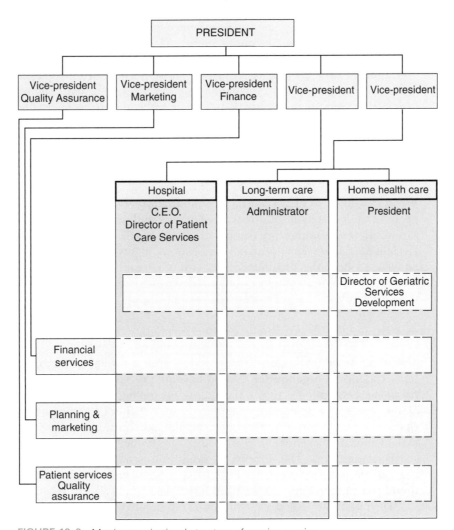

FIGURE 12–3   Matrix organizational structure of nursing service.

example, the team leader has the authority to determine which team members will provide care to which patients. The team leader also might assign a nursing assistant to
work with you.

   Accountability refers to the process of answering or being responsible for what
occurs, and carries legal implications for task performance. Accountability flows
upward in the organizational hierarchy and can be interpreted to mean "the buck stops
here." For example, if you delegate to the nursing assistant the responsibility for checking the vital signs of your four patients, you are still accountable for that activity. You
need to be sure that the vital signs are taken, that they are accurate, and that they are
reported and documented. Accountability cannot be delegated; you must answer for
the care you give and for the care you ask others to complete. This has become a very

sensitive issue for nurses as more unlicensed assistive personnel are hired to replace licensed staff in an effort to contain costs.

Responsibility refers to the distribution and acceptance of a task or job, or the obligation to take on and accomplish an assignment. For example, the team leader assigns you to the care of four patients and you agree to that assignment; therefore, their care is your responsibility. You have an obligation to secure the desired outcome with regard to that care.

ORGANIZATIONAL RELATIONSHIPS

When looking at an organization, it is important that you identify relationships among people and departments and realize where the authority is placed within that organization. All organizations are composed of individuals who are relating to one another. Explaining relationships within organizations in several different ways helps us to understand how the organization functions. Organizational charts, chains of command, channels of communication, job descriptions, and policies and procedures provide different views of organizational relationships.

The Organizational Chart

The structure of any large group comprises both a formal and an informal organization. The formal organization can be seen on an *organizational chart*. The organizational chart is a graphic, pictorial means of portraying roles and patterns of interaction among parts of a system. It identifies formal chains of command, communication channels, and the authority for decision making. In most groups, we also find an informal organization, sometimes called the "grapevine," which represents informal or social relationships. The informal organization is not depicted on an organizational chart or formally acknowledged in any specific manner, but it can often have a profound effect on how an organization functions.

The organizational chart typically is represented by boxes stacked in a pyramid-shaped chart. The greatest authority exists at the top of the chart (often a single box), and authority declines as you move toward the base (many boxes). Persons occupying jobs at the top of the organizational chart are considered administrators, executives, or "the management," and individuals with jobs closer to the base are considered employees or staff. Located between these two levels is an area known as "middle management," comprising those who coordinate and control activities of specified groups of workers.

The organizational chart may take one of several forms, reflecting the type of administration operating within that organization. One term used to describe these forms is *span of control*, which refers to the number of employees supervised by a manager. A *narrow span of control* exists when a manager has responsibility for only three to five subordinates. If, however, the organization operates with a *broad span of control*, it places authority and responsibility for decision making in the hands of fewer individuals, with each manager supervising a large number of employees. The larger the number of individuals to be supervised, the more difficult it is to control each worker through direct observation. If two organizations of equal size were to exist—one with a narrow span of control and the other with a broad span of control—the organization choosing to implement a narrow span of control would have more managers.

The Chain of Command

All organizations have a *chain of command*. The chain of command represents the *path of authority and accountability* from individuals at the top of the organization to those at the base of the organization. It is often referred to as the *organizational hierarchy*. Thus, in hospitals we typically find that the nursing administrator gives directions to and evaluates the performance of the assistant administrator, who in turn gives directions to and evaluates the performance of the nursing unit manager, and so forth. When we look at this process from the base of the organization to the top, we often use the language "reports to"—which indicates that the unit manager is accountable to the assistant administrator, and the assistant administrator is accountable to the nursing administrator. Similarly, we find the registered nurse giving direction to and overseeing the activities of the practical (vocational) nurse and the nursing assistant. The length of the chain of command varies depending on the size of the organization.

Almost without exception, the salaries commanded by persons at the top of the organizational hierarchy are greater than those of persons close to the base. Accordingly, the experience, educational requirements, hours worked, and responsibilities are greater for persons with positions near the top of the organizational chart.

Channels of Communication

Channels of communication are, as the name implies, the patterns through which messages are delivered within an organization. The channels of communication usually reflect the chain of command. Thus, the nurse manager communicates concerns and information to the assistant administrator, who may have the authority and responsibility to deal with the problem, or who relays the concern to the nursing administrator. The nursing assistant reports her concerns to the staff nurse, who may have the authority to deal with the issue, or who reports it to the head nurse or manager. For a nurse manager to report a concern directly to the administrator is referred to as "looping" the system; it is generally considered improper and inappropriate to skip or bypass any level in the communication system. For example, if a staff nurse disagrees with a pharmacy technician who delivers medications to the unit, and takes this problem directly to the supervisor without first discussing it with the unit manager, this is considered "looping" the system. You readily can see how this would put the unit manager at a distinct disadvantage, should the supervisor ask about the incident.

Channels of communication run up and down the organizational chart, moving from one level of responsibility and authority to the next.

Job Descriptions

Job descriptions form another important aspect of any organization. *Job descriptions* are written statements, usually found in policy manuals, that stipulate the duties and functions of the various jobs within the organization, and the scope of authority, responsibility, and accountability involved in each position. Job descriptions should explain the role of each individual working for the company or organization, from the chief executive officer to the janitor.

Sometimes job descriptions are very specific; other times they are more broadly stated. If broadly stated, policy and procedure manuals may help to specify a task or responsibility. Job descriptions provide the foundation for performance standards for each position, and should provide the basis for evaluation. Job descriptions also may include competencies expected of employees, and can provide the basis for Competency-Based Orientation (CBO)—a program used especially for new graduates and for cross-training. *Cross-training* involves teaching one member of the health care team to perform functions usually associated with another position. For example, a respiratory therapist might learn to perform basic patient care skills and, when not needed for respiratory therapy treatments, be available to answer lights and respond to patient needs. Cross-training is viewed by some administrators as a method by which costs can be reduced through the efficiency of having an individual able to do more than one set of tasks within the organization. The effectiveness of cross-training between different disciplines has not been well documented. However, cross-training of nurses between differing specialties has become common, and many nurses welcome the employment flexibility this provides.

Job descriptions also may be in the form of *clinical ladders*. A clinical ladder differentiates and defines the skills and performance expected of nurses in terms of advancing levels. Typically, three or four levels of performance are defined, with each higher level having greater responsibility and authority than the previous one. A new graduate usually enters the system as a Clinical Nurse One (or similar title), moves to Clinical Nurse Two, and then to Clinical Nurse Three as that individual becomes more proficient. Salary increases typically accompany movement from one level to another. Sometimes additional formal education or continuing education is required for advancement. Through this process the nurse is supported and encouraged to develop greater clinical expertise. The clinical ladder also serves as a mechanism for recognizing and rewarding nurses who wish to remain in direct care positions rather than seek administrative positions.

Policies, Procedures, and Standards of Care

A *policy* may be defined as a designated plan or course of action to be taken in a specific situation. In organizations, the governing board holds the responsibility and authority for assuring that appropriate policies are adopted. The governing board usually delegates the development of policies to the chief administrative officer. The administrator usually delegates the responsibility for development of policies for a specific department to individuals or groups in the department that will be most affected by the policy. Once their work is completed, the policy is returned to the governing board for review, possible revision, and adoption. The management within the organization is responsible for assuring that the policies are followed and that more specific policies are developed if necessary.

Written copies of all policies usually are placed in a policy manual that is available in each department, or a current copy may be available online in the institution's computer network. Online policy manuals assure that all departments are referring to the most current policy and that the information is always available. Depending on the area in which you are employed, you will find varying needs for referring to the policy manual in your role as a new employee. As you might anticipate, the need for special policies related to occurrences in an emergency department, delivery room, or a critical care unit is greater than in a general medical or surgical unit in a hospital. When you are confronted with a new nonclinical problem to solve and you are unsure of what action to take, always check your policy manual to see if it offers guidance.

Special unit policies are sometimes termed *protocols*. For example, the protocol for dealing with a patient seen in the emergency department suffering from a dog bite determines which local authorities should be notified, who is responsible for seeing that they are notified, and perhaps general management of the wound.

Procedure manuals also are found in each unit or department. *Procedure manuals* spell out how a particular nursing activity is to be completed, often describing it in a number of steps. For example, you may find a procedure for changing the dressing on a central intravenous line, for administering chemotherapy agents, and for doing many other procedures, such as catheterizations.

Institutions are giving nurses more responsibility for effecting and developing institutional policies and procedures, and serving as representatives to various committees that monitor, review, and update policies and procedures. As hospitals move to broader spans of control and to greater involvement of all employees in decision making, grassroots participation in policy formation is becoming more common. The nature of a policy and the breadth of its scope will determine whether it needs further review within the organization.

Standards of care are authoritative statements that describe a common or acceptable level of client care or performance that have some similarity to policies and procedures. Thus, standards of care define professional practice. The American Nurses Association (1991) has formulated general standards and guidelines for nursing practice. They apply across the nation and are broad and general in nature. They are now in their second edition, and 24 areas of specialty practice have been added. Similarly, state practice acts contain language describing the standard of practice that applies to all nurses licensed in that state. Each agency also may develop standards of care for patients with selected health care problems. These more detailed and specific standards may take the form of standard nursing care plans. Some standards are being incorporated into documents termed *care pathways* or *critical pathways*. These identify both outcomes and care activities that are expected to be appropriate for each 24-hour period of hospitalization. These specific standards of care become the basis for evaluation of care and for quality improvement within the organization.

SHARED GOVERNANCE

Few industries have felt the impact of technology as much as health care. Ranging from new systems of information and communication to different administrative structures, to changing approaches to systems of evaluation, the health care delivery system has seen a radical acceleration in all forms of technology. In the realm of administrative structure, one of the more important changes has been the recent move to a pattern of shared governance within health care agencies.

Shared governance is a professional practice model in which the nursing staff and the nursing management are both involved in decision making, as opposed to the administrative decision area being controlled by management. It originated during the mid-1980s and gained status and recognition as an alternative to bureaucratic management during the 1990s. This structure allows nursing staff to make major decisions within the organization and attempts to get the decision-making process as close to where the action is occurring as possible. Often this pattern of organization is paired with the concept of total quality improvement (TQI), which has as its hallmark emphasis on the customer. Alexander, Bourgeois, and Goodman (1994, p. 283) state "TQI and shared governance (1) empower all employees, (2) encourage decision making at the appropriate level within the organization, (3) promote teamwork with consensus and shared responsibility, (4) encourage and recognize employee contributions, and (5) provide opportunities for personal growth."

There is no single model for shared governance. The shared governance format may take several approaches, including a councilar model in which committees and councils have defined authority and functions, a congressional model that involves an elected representative system, or an administrative model consisting of committees or forums in which people communicate and share ideas (Porter-O'Grady, 1987). The committees or councils result in staff actively participating in management, and, as a consequence, gaining autonomy, control over the work environment, and greater job satisfaction. Often, councils report to a nursing executive board that serves as a coordinating and approval body. Within this framework, the nurse is held to greater accountability within the context of peer-defined and peer-operated parameters (Porter-O'Grady, 1990). The traditional role of the supervisor as one who hires, evaluates, promotes, and fires becomes a thing of the past. This change has been a major impediment to the success of shared governance. Many managers find their new and changing role difficult to accept.

The shared governance model has become widespread in hospitals. Its implementation requires that staff nurses participate in professional development sessions that increase nurses' understanding of the decision-making process, team building, group dynamics, leadership, and budgeting (Jacoby & Terpstra, 1990).

The continuance of shared governance models in today's health care system has been questioned by many. The reengineering and restructuring of the health care delivery system, which has resulted in multihospital systems, consolidations, mergers, and the use of nurses as primary care providers and case managers, also may result in the demise of shared governance, or in its assuming a different format. The time involved in shared governance is costly to an organization, and the cost-effectiveness of shared governance in terms of patient outcomes is being questioned. Today's health care system is experiencing much change.

Critical Thinking Activity

> Interview some nurses who are working in a shared governance environment. Identify what they find satisfying about shared governance. How would they like to see it changed? If shared governance is not used in your area, interview nurses about the concept of shared governance and how they believe it would improve patient care.

PATTERNS OF NURSING CARE DELIVERY

The nursing department of any health care institution carries major responsibility for the quality of nursing care delivered. Throughout the years, the structure of the delivery of care has taken many different formats. The astute student will note that the particular pattern of care that was in vogue has changed about every 20 years. Among the factors influencing the delivery pattern selected in each era were the types of patients served, the type of care provided, the cost of the care, and the number and education of potential employees. Perhaps a wider variety of patterns of care is being used today than at any other time in nursing's history. In the following section we describe the typical implementation of several patterns of care delivery. However, it is important to remember that you might find a particular pattern of care practiced a little differently in different settings.

The Case Method

The *case method* was the first system used for the delivery of nursing care in the United States (around the beginning of the 20th century) and should not be confused with the term "case management" used today (discussed later). With the case method, the nurse worked with one patient (or case) only, and was expected to meet all of that patient's needs. The nurse often lived in the patient's home, and was expected to assume other household duties, such as cooking for the patient and family, and light housekeeping when not busy with the patient. Nurses worked long hours and were poorly paid. Advancing technology and increasing costs made this type of care delivery impractical, but vestiges of its structure can be seen in today's home health nursing. However, the role of the registered nurse in home health care is typically one of assessment, planning, skilled intervention, supervision of care provided by a home health aide, and evaluation of the client's progress.

The Functional Method

The *functional method* of care delivery emerged during the Great Depression of the 1930s. This method allowed for the care of greater numbers of patients in hospitals and for use of advancing technology. At this time, the industrial model of narrowly defined and frequently repeated tasks was revolutionizing manufacturing. The idea that this would transfer into all types of work environments was widely accepted. Typically, the head nurse assigned nursing tasks to the various persons employed on the unit, according to the level of skills required for performance. One nurse might take all temperatures, another would do all dressings, while yet another administered all medications, charted them, and provided a list of replacement needs to the head nurse. Assignments varied depending on the size of the unit, the number of personnel available, and the skill level of the personnel. The head nurse gave a report to the next shift. Although economical and efficient, this system of care delivery had the disadvantage of fragmenting care—no single individual was responsible for the planning of the care. Patients were confused about who was caring for them, and communication among caregivers was lacking. Individual nurse-patient relationships were limited. Nursing care came to be viewed as a list of procedures and tasks. This pattern of care still may be used in long-term care facilities or sub-acute units, largely because of the educational preparation of the care providers. Some nurses are concerned that the economic push in today's health care institutions may see many hospitals returning to functional approaches to care.

Team Nursing

The concept of *team nursing* was introduced in the early 1950s, with a promise that it would result in more patient-centered care. This approach to care was based on the premise that each unit would have at least two teams composed of variously educated care providers. For example, a team might be composed of two nurse aides, an orderly, a licensed practical (vocational) nurse, and a registered nurse. A more experienced registered nurse would be the "team leader." Team members worked together, each performing those tasks for which they were best prepared. The team leader made assignments, had overall responsibility for the care of patients on her unit, might give all medications, and gave a report to the team that followed on the next shift. An important part of this form of nursing was the "team conference," at which members of the team met to communicate about the needs of their patients and to plan for care. Without the conference and the communication, team nursing might be little different from functional nursing. Today, as we see more health care facilities decreasing the number of registered nurses and adding more unlicensed assistive personnel, team nursing may again become a prevalent method of care delivery (Fig. 12-4).

Total Patient Care

During the late 1970s and early 1980s, many hospitals returned to a *total patient care* type of assignment, in which a registered nurse or licensed practical (vocational) nurse is assigned for all care needs. A nurse is assigned to the care of a group of four to six patients, depending on how acutely ill each patient is, and depending on patient needs. This returns a greater sense of control to nurses, gives them a greater sense of autonomy, and fosters a greater sense of involvement in the whole spectrum of care and in patient outcomes. This type of care focuses on the total person (from which its name is derived) rather than on a collection of tasks or procedures.

FIGURE 12–4 Team conference, planning, and communication are critical elements of team nursing.

Primary Care Nursing

In a pattern of *primary care*, which came into popular application in the 1980s, one nurse is assigned the responsibility for the care of each patient from the time the patient is admitted to the hospital until that patient's discharge. The primary nurse is responsible for initiating and updating the nursing care plan, patient teaching, and discharge planning. An associate nurse works with this same patient on other shifts and on the primary nurse's day off, carrying out the plan of care developed by the primary nurse. Obvious benefits of this method include the continuity of care for the patient and job satisfaction for the nurses because they have more autonomy and control. Whether this method is more expensive has been the subject of debate. Health care administrators argue that the salary costs for RNs make this a more costly approach to care. Some data would indicate that decreased complication rates, shorter length of stays, and decreased readmission rates for patients, plus the employment of fewer assistive personnel who have greater turnover rates, offset the additional direct care costs. The ANA has urged research to explore this concern.

Under this system every nurse is a primary nurse for a few patients and an associate nurse for others. Sometimes the nurse functioning in an associate role has difficulty following the plan of the primary nurse, or may disagree with the established plan of care. The patient's condition also may change rapidly, requiring the plan to be changed without consulting the primary nurse. Another concern is the level of expertise and commitment required of all nurses, and the fact that nurses who work autonomously with patients soon forget how to delegate responsibilities.

Case Management

Case management is a process of monitoring an individual patient's health care for the purpose of maximizing positive outcomes and containing costs. A key to case management is the identification of a critical pathway for care and treatment that includes specific timelines and protocols. The case manager typically follows the patient from the diagnostic phase through hospitalization, rehabilitation, and back to home care, ensuring that plans are made in advance and that the patient receives care that will achieve the most positive outcomes. The case manager may not provide direct care, but is responsible for managing the patient's interaction with the entire health care system (Fig. 12-5).

Registered nurses are the health care professionals who most often act as case managers. In some settings social workers also act as case managers. Case managers may be employed by third-party payers (such as insurance companies) or by health care agencies (such as hospitals or long-term care facilities). Case managers employed by a par-

FIGURE 12–5 The case manager may follow the patient from the diagnostic phase through hospitalization, rehabilitation, and back to home care.

ticular institution also might be involved in wellness programs such as blood pressure management, stress management, smoking cessation programs, and exercise classes.

Some objections to this form of care delivery come from physicians, who see the role of the case manager as an infringement on their historic rights of autonomy in decision making. Providers may also believe that the case manager is more concerned with cost factors than with what is best for the individual, arguing that quality is sacrificed to cost containment.

Critical Thinking Activity

Compare the various patterns of nursing care delivery with the pattern being used in a facility where you currently receive clinical experience. Analyze the pattern in current use and evaluate whether another pattern of care delivery would be more or less effective. Provide a rationale for your answer.

DELEGATION

Delegation occurs when you authorize a competent person to act for you or in your stead. In so doing, you authorize another person to carry out the action, but you retain the accountability for the activities performed. The appropriate and effective assignment of work to others is a part of all organizations and work groups. Those individuals who are most able to delegate tend to be the most successful. Those lacking skills in delegation will not be able to complete their duties, tasks, or responsibilities and will find that they are stressed and exhausted by having more to do than can easily be accomplished by one person.

The delegation of responsibilities to others has become a major concern in nursing within recent years. As hospitals strive toward restructuring and cost containment, more categories of caregivers who have minimal nursing education and experience have been hired to assist in the provision of nursing care, and are viewed as nurse extenders. In most instances this has resulted in fewer registered nurses working on a unit. These unlicensed assistive personnel have a variety of titles, and in all instances have less formal education than the registered nurse; in some instances it may be minimal.

National Council of State Boards of Nursing Guidelines to Delegation

In response to this situation, in 1995, the National Council of State Boards of Nursing, Inc. (NCSBN) developed conceptual and historic papers on delegation that defined terms, provided general guidelines to be followed, and outlined actions to be taken. Among these were the five rights of delegation. They are as follows:

1. Right task
2. Right circumstance

3. Right person
4. Right direction/communication
5. Right supervision/evaluation

As a beginning staff nurse, you may have had little experience in delegating tasks to others. However, this skill, like many others, can be learned. It requires critical thinking and analysis on your part. You must know the level of competence of each of your team members, including each individual's strengths and weaknesses; the requirements of the tasks you plan to delegate (that is, the degree of complexity they involve); and the amount of time available to supervise the tasks. You should be knowledgeable about the nurse practice act of the state and any practice limitations that might exist. Specifically, you need to know the scope of practice defined for each individual to whom you plan to delegate responsibilities. You also must possess good communication skills, which are critical to communicating assignments, setting down your expectations, and providing ongoing follow-up and evaluation.

Assigning the Right Task to the Right Person

It is important that you assign the right task to the right person. This is where your knowledge of your workers, their scope of practice, and the job descriptions of the institution are critical. It helps you know how closely you must supervise an individual. Generally speaking, the tasks that have the highest level of predictive outcome (those that are routine and standard) are the best ones to delegate to others. For example, if you delegate to a nursing assistant the responsibility for getting a patient into a wheelchair, you can anticipate that the assistant will be able to carry out this task. However, you would not want to delegate a task requiring a high level of nursing judgment and evaluation, such as assessing the condition of a patient. You also want to consider the potential for harm and how difficult a task is to perform. Remember, in all instances you remain accountable for the care you have delegated and must answer for anything that is not done or is not completed correctly.

Communicating Your Expectations Clearly

Once you have decided which tasks can be delegated to which team members, it is important that you give clear and complete directions to those responsible for completing the assignments (Fig. 12-6). After giving instructions, ask questions that will provide an indication of whether your directions have been clearly understood. Asking a team member to repeat your instructions to you is one approach that can be used; it is particularly effective if working with individuals who have English as a second language.

Providing Team Members With Authority to Act

It is also necessary to provide to your team members the authority to complete the assigned work once it has been delegated. When you first learn to delegate, there may be a tendency to want to do everything yourself, or to "hold on" to all responsibilities.

FIGURE 12–6 Good communication skills are critical to communicating assignments, setting down expectations, and providing ongoing follow-up and evaluation.

This response may be due to a lack of confidence in the abilities of others, concern that to be done correctly something must be done by yourself, or even concern that someone else may do it better. However, constraints on your own time are such that many tasks must be delegated, and you need to accomplish some of your responsibilities by using the skills of others.

Monitoring Progress and Outcomes

In all instances you need to monitor the outcomes of the care that has been delegated. You also want to provide your team members with feedback regarding their performance, emphasizing the things done well and offering constructive assistance to those who have not met reasonable expectations.

Nurses, as a group, have been concerned about the use of nurse extenders because of the effect on patient care and the legal responsibility that nurses must assume for tasks performed by others. Many state boards also have expressed concern about the safety of the public (which is their primary responsibility) and are issuing statements regarding the use of unlicensed assistive personnel. Be certain that you know whether such a statement is in effect in your state and, if so, the nature of the content and guidelines.

Critical Thinking Activity

As a new graduate, you must delegate some aspects of care of patients assigned to you to a nursing assistant. What factors should you consider when delegating? What is your responsibility once the care is delegated?

COLLECTIVE BARGAINING

Collective bargaining is a process that allows employees who are members of the union to participate in management decisions with regard to terms of employment, salaries, benefits, working conditions, and similar issues. Because of nursing's long history as a profession of dedication, altruism, and service, initially collective bargaining was a controversial issue within nursing. Some saw this process as detracting from the professional role of the nurse.

Today, however, nurses are vitally concerned about contracts, services, third-party payers, comparable worth, patients' rights, shared governance, staffing ratios, and a host of issues that can be discussed at the bargaining table. Nurses believe that people who choose nursing as a career should have the opportunity to have some voice in patient care assignments, length of the work day and week, fringe benefits, and wages, without losing face with the public at large, members of the medical profession, or other colleagues. This thinking was succinctly outlined in a statement by Janet Muff (1988, p. 245):

We are not in this business out of charity, as altruists and nightingalists would have us believe. We are here to make money, to use our minds and our skills, to provide services to patients on our own terms. We need no longer apologize and feel guilty.

History of Collective Bargaining

As early as the 1850s, Horace Greeley, a reformer, publisher, and politician, was generating interest in and giving impetus to collective bargaining issues in his editorial columns in the *New York Tribune*. During the early part of the 20th century, efforts by workers to organize were met with opposition from employers, governmental officials, and some members of the public. After the Great Depression that immobilized the United States in the late 1920s and early 1930s, several laws were enacted to help improve workers' conditions. Franklin D. Roosevelt was elected president in 1932, and his New Deal administration saw the passage of the National Industrial Recovery Act. One result of this act was the creation of the National Recovery Administration, whose purpose was to administer codes of fair practice within given industries. The nation was called on to accept an interim blanket code that established a 35- to 40-hour work week for workers, minimum pay of 30 to 40 cents an hour, and prohibition of child labor—all issues that had long been advocated by nurses.

PASSAGE OF THE NATIONAL LABOR RELATIONS ACT

On July 5, 1935, the National Labor Relations Act (NLRA) became the national labor policy of the United States. Also known as the Wagner Act, for Senator Robert F. Wagner (who introduced the legislation), the NLRA gave workers federal protection in their efforts to form unions and organize for better working conditions. It listed as unfair practice any actions on the part of employers that would interfere with this process. Senator Wagner wanted management and labor to resolve their mutual problems through a system of self-government. This act also created the National Labor Relations Board (NLRB), a quasi-judicial body that was to ensure proper enforcement of the conditions of the legislation.

The NLRB has the responsibility for administering the NLRA. In addition, it has two primary functions: to conduct secret-ballot elections that will determine that the majority of employees of a unit desire the representation of a given union in collective bargaining procedures, and to prevent and rectify unfair labor practices committed by employers or unions. It also has the responsibility for determining into which bargaining units, of the eight established for health care workers in acute care facilities, various employees will be assigned. This is important to nurses because it enables them to have a separate unit and, therefore, to deal with issues important to their role in health care delivery. Of interest is recent discussion regarding the unit to which nursing practitioners and advance practice nurses should be assigned (O'Meara & O'Meara, 1995).

The original NLRA used the term labor organization, which was defined in language that could be interpreted to exclude nursing and several other professions, such as teaching and medicine, that were organized through professional organizations. These early labor unions often were viewed negatively by the public—an image that was reinforced in movies, in newspapers, and on radio. Often portrayed as rowdy, aggressive, and hostile, unions did not seem to fit well in nursing.

In 1947, the original NLRA was amended through the Taft-Hartley Act (also known as the Labor Management Relations Act). Because of heavy lobbying by hospital management, the act was written in such a way as to specifically exclude nonprofit hospitals from the legal obligation of bargaining with their employees. Although the administrations of some hospitals chose to negotiate salaries and working conditions with their employees, many did not, and no legal action could be taken to force the process.

ACTIVITY OF THE AMERICAN NURSES ASSOCIATION

By 1931, the American Nurses Association (ANA) was publicly recognizing its obligation with regard to the general welfare of its members, and developed within its organization a legislative policy addressing this concern. Some suggest that this effort was spurred by the fact that other groups, particularly the Service Employees International Union (SEIU), an affiliate of the American Federation of Labor/Congress of Industrial Organizations (AFL/CIO), were actively working to organize health care workers. Other factors also were important. Before 1930, most nurses were employed in public health, visiting nurse, or private duty positions. Students, aides, and orderlies, under the direction of a head nurse, delivered much of the care in hospitals. As more care was delivered in the hospital setting, the number of nurses employed by these facilities grew. The existing working conditions affected more people.

In 1945, a committee was appointed by the ANA to study employment conditions. This study culminated in the creation of an ANA Economic Security Program in 1946. This action was followed by the enactment of a resolution that would encourage state nurses' associations to act as exclusive bargaining agents for their respective memberships in the important areas of economic security and collective bargaining. Also in 1946, the SEIU formed its first RN Guild in New York City.

The concept of professional collectivism, which emphasizes that good care depends on satisfactory working conditions and satisfaction with nursing itself, began to take shape. However, concern for the image of the nurse and nursing prompted a no-strike policy to be adopted officially by the ANA in 1950, and it remained in effect until it was rescinded in 1968.

By 1947, with the impetus provided by the Economic Security Program of ANA, collective bargaining between nurses and hospital administrations had been implemented in several states, and negotiated contracts were in effect. Many hospital employers were voluntarily developing contracts with employees and were showing genuine concern about working conditions. Some states were mandating that state hospitals negotiate with all employees, but there was no federal requirement for this process.

Federal legislation passed in 1962 enabled employees of federal health care institutions to participate in collective bargaining. In 1967, investor-owned hospitals and nursing homes also were included, and the ANA was identified as the bargaining agent for the nurses of the Veterans Administration hospitals. Legislation passed in 1970 saw the inclusion of nonprofit nursing homes in the collective bargaining process. Concurrently, SEIU and other labor-related organizations were also bargaining for nurses.

THE TAFT-HARTLEY LAW AMENDED

Finally, on August 25, 1974, Public Law 93-360 was put into effect; it amended the Taft-Hartley Act to provide economic security programs for those employed in nonprofit hospitals, and brought health care facilities and their employees under the jurisdiction of the NLRB. Nonprofit hospitals were legally required to bargain with nurses for better wages, hours, staffing conditions, patient-nurse ratios, and a voice in hospital governance. To ensure that the public would be protected from strikes or work stoppage, several amendments were attached to the NLRA passed in 1974, including the requirement of longer notification periods and provisions mandating participation in mediation.

Understanding the Basic Language

Intelligent bargaining begins with an awareness of the process itself. Collective indicates that employees act together. Bargaining involves a formal negotiation process. *Collective bargaining* consists of a set of procedures by which employee representatives and employer representatives negotiate to obtain a signed agreement (contract) that spells out wages, hours, and conditions of employment that are acceptable to both. A key word in this definition is *negotiate*.

BARGAINING AND NEGOTIATING

To negotiate means to bargain or confer with another party or parties to reach an agreement. *Bargaining* implies a discussion of the terms of the agreement and suggests that there will be give and take—that neither party will obtain all items asked for in the contract. Ideally, negotiations would proceed in a somewhat philosophical vein, moving toward reasonable compromises that would allow each side to achieve many of the conditions it requested, but this does not always occur.

Common interest bargaining refers to a process in which the employer and employee representatives begin by identifying those areas in which they agree and those goals or values held by both parties. Based on shared values and goals, the two parties then begin to work out their differences in regard to specific policies and conditions. Although relatively new as an approach to collective bargaining, common interest bargaining is gaining attention as a less adversarial process that may preserve effective working relationships and lessen feelings of alienation between supervisory personnel and employees involved in the union.

UNIONS AND COLLECTIVE ACTION

Collective bargaining allows employees working together as an organized unit to negotiate. A *union* is a legally authorized organized group of employees that negotiates and enforces labor agreements. Its major concern is improvement in the wages, hours, and working conditions of its members. Collective bargaining units tend to become organized when a group of persons in an institution identifies common problems and concerns and becomes interested in forming a unit (Flanagan, 1992). When a branch or part of a professional association assumes this responsibility, as often occurs in nursing, the negotiating group may be known as a *collective action division*. The activity of the group may be referred to as *professional collectivism*, which supports the premise that the quality of patient care is directly tied to working conditions and that collective action is a professional responsibility. Nursing collective bargaining units point out that while shared governance provides input from nurses, that can be unilaterally changed. A contract can provide a legal commitment to including the voice of nursing in decisions. A professional organization must work under the same legal constraints as a union. It provides legal counsel and representatives to assist with negotiations, may lobby on behalf of issues, or may participate in other activities that would further the economic welfare of nurses. It oversees the development of the contract.

THE CONTRACT

The conclusion of the bargaining process should result in a signed contract that converts to writing the agreements that have been reached. A *contract* is "an agreement between two or more people to do something, especially one formally set forth in writing and enforceable by law" (Neufeldt, 1996; Webster's, p. 302). This signed contract is enforceable under law and cannot be changed by either party acting unilaterally.

The contract may be the most important product of the collective bargaining process because it converts to an agreement all issues that have been discussed. It provides the foundation for further activities. In most instances a contract need not be in writing, but it is much easier to implement when written and signed by all involved. The contract remains in effect until breached or terminated. Most negotiated contracts define the period of time—usually 2 or 3 years—during which the established conditions are effective.

Before being put into effect, a contract must be *ratified*. This means that the members of the bargaining group must accept the terms of the contract. This is usually done by a vote of the membership.

RULES GOVERNING LABOR RELATIONS

When two parties agree to begin the negotiation process, it is understood that both will *bargain in good faith*. Bargaining in good faith is a poorly understood concept, but generally it means that the parties will meet at regular times to discuss (with the intent to resolve) any differences over wages, hours, and other employment conditions. Failure to carry out these activities could lead to an unfair labor practice.

An *unfair labor practice* is any action that interferes with the rights of employees or employers as described in the amended NLRA. It is not possible to discuss all of these in detail; however, some examples follow. An employer must not interfere with the employee's right to form a union or other organized bargaining group, join the group, or participate in the group's activities. The employer may not attempt to control a group, once organized, or to discriminate against its members in regard to hiring or tenure. Most important, the employer must bargain collectively and in good faith with representatives of the employees.

Likewise, labor organizations have constraints placed on their activities. They, too, must bargain in good faith. They must not restrain or coerce employees in selecting a bargaining group to bargain collectively. They may not pressure an employer to discriminate against employees who do not belong to the labor organization.

One of the issues frequently brought up in negotiations that usually results in a dispute is that of *agency shop*. When an agency shop clause is in effect, all employees are required to pay dues for membership. The obvious advantage of this requirement, from the workers' point of view, is encouraging membership in the union. The union is required to represent all employees, both members and nonmembers. Negotiating a contract, monitoring compliance with its provisions, and facilitating the grievance process may be costly. The union, therefore, desires to have a greater percentage of paying members to support these activities. There are several variations in provisions related to agency shop. If, because of religious or philosophical beliefs, employees are unwilling to pay dues to the bargaining group, provisions may be made to pay the same sum to a nonprofit group, such as a church or foundation. In some instances, those who are already members of the union are required to remain members for the life of the contract, although no one is required to become a member. In some states, laws referred to as "right to work laws" forbid the establishment of an agency shop.

Settling Labor Disputes

When labor disputes arise, several actions can be taken to help resolve the differences. Initially, of course, the parties continue to negotiate, and may agree to extend the negotiation period if progress in settling differences is being made.

When the two parties doing the negotiating cannot come to agreement on an issue, they are considered to be *at impasse*, or are *deadlocked* on the issue.

MEDIATION AND ARBITRATION

Perhaps the most commonly used method of seeking agreement between parties is through *mediation* and *arbitration*. A *mediator* is a third person who may join the bargainers in early sessions to assist the parties in reconciling differences and arriving at a peaceful agreement. Mediation involves finding compromises, and the mediator assists with this. He or she must gain the respect of both parties and must remain neutral to the issues presented.

An *arbitrator* is technically defined as a person chosen by agreement of both parties to decide a dispute between them. The primary difference between a mediator and an arbitrator is that the mediator assists the parties in reaching their own decision, whereas the arbitrator has the authority to actually make the decision for the parties if necessary. However, the terms mediator and arbitrator and mediation and arbitration often are used interchangeably; in fact, a mediator may also serve as an arbitrator (Fig. 12-7).

FIGURE 12–7 The arbitrator's decision may not really please either side.

Arbitration may take several forms. It may be mediation-arbitration, in which a third person joins the parties in the negotiation process before any serious disputes arise. This person's role is to act as a mediator who attempts to keep the parties talking, suggests compromises, and helps establish priorities. If an agreement is not reached by a specified date, or if it appears that the issue is deadlocked with neither party willing to compromise, the mediator then assumes the role of an arbitrator and makes a decision based on the information gained in the role of mediator.

Another form of arbitration is called *binding arbitration*. This means that both parties are obligated to abide by the decision of the arbitrator. Some people see this as the least desirable alternative in settling disputes because it may result in a decision that is not satisfactory to either side, but one by which both must abide. It has been suggested, in instances in which binding arbitration is used, that the parties spell out exactly which of the issues are to be decided by the arbitrator. Binding arbitration has the advantage of resolving deadlocked issues without a strike. It also encourages both parties, knowing that the arbitrator's decision may not please either side, to reach a compromise on their own.

The *final offer* approach is a type of binding arbitration. Employer and employee bargaining representatives reach agreement on as many issues as possible. The deadlocked issues and a final position from each side are then presented to the arbitrator, who is obligated to select only the most reasonable package. The arbitrator may not develop a third alternative, which would "split the difference." The final offer approach encourages both sides to come up with a fairly realistic package and serves to close the gap on issues as each side seeks to maintain some control over the outcome of the deliberations.

One criticism of any type of arbitration is the expense involved. Arbitrators must be paid for their services. Arbitration is also criticized because it undermines voluntary collective bargaining and allows parties to avoid unpleasant confrontation with their own difficulties by shifting that responsibility to a public authority. However, it is useful in preventing the disruption of services.

Arbitration may be requested from the American Arbitration Association or from available state, public, and private mediation and conciliation services. The American Arbitration Association is a nonprofit, nonpartisan organization that, for a nominal fee, can provide a list of qualified arbitrators. Most states have available groups, such as the Public Employees Relations Commission, that also can provide a list of mediators and arbitrators.

STRIKES AND LOCKOUTS

When the negotiation process breaks down, lockouts and strikes are likely to occur. A *lockout* occurs when an employer closes a place of business to force employees to agree to the terms offered by the employer. One readily can see how undesirable this would be in the health care system, but it has occurred in some instances.

A *strike* occurs when workers refuse to continue to work until certain demands are met, thus imposing economic hardship and pressure on the employer. When the negotiation process breaks down, employees may use the strike to emphasize their position. Workers may be striving to improve their own working conditions, salaries, and benefits. The most recent strikes by nurses, however, have been over issues related to patient care rather than those related to the economic status of the nurses. Striking places a serious economic hardship on employees and therefore is not undertaken lightly. Sometimes a strike is used to gain public attention to the labor dispute and to create public pressure for a settlement. This is only successful if the public agrees with the position of the striking workers.

At one time, nurse's strikes were viewed by some as unprofessional and detrimental to the health of the community. When strikes occurred they drew major media attention. Today that thinking has largely changed, and less attention is drawn to the strikes other than in nursing publications.

Strikes in nursing are undertaken only with advance notice, to enable patients to be transferred to another facility. Typically, arrangements are made with another hospital to admit patients during the strike and all elective procedures are canceled. The striking nurses may also agree to provide staffing to critical care, labor and delivery, and emergency departments of the facility in which the strike is occurring. Often the notification that nurses intend to strike on a certain date is sufficient incentive to move negotiations to the point of settlement, as occurred in Hawaii at the end of 1999.

REINSTATEMENT PRIVILEGE

A *reinstatement privilege* is a guarantee offered to striking employees that they will be rehired after the strike, provided that they have not engaged in any unfair labor practices during the strike, and provided that the strike itself is lawful. The hospital may replace a striking nurse during the strike. If strikers agree unconditionally to return to work, the employer is not required to rehire a striking nurse at that time. However, recall lists are developed, and if the nurse cannot find regular and equivalent employment, he or she is privileged to recall and preference on jobs before new employees may be given employment.

Nurses may lose their reinstatement privileges because of misconduct during a lawful strike. For example, strikers may not physically block other nurses and personnel from entering or leaving a struck hospital. Strikers may not threaten nonstriking employees and may not attack management representatives. These types of activities usually do not occur in strikes conducted by nurses, but are not outside the realm of possibility.

OTHER METHODS OF INFLUENCING SETTLEMENT

There are a wide variety of methods by which solutions can be reached in the negotiating process. The following discussion addresses the more formal and far-reaching of these activities.

One method of reaching solution is to employ an *authoritative mandate*, in which a peaceful settlement is encouraged by a president, secretary of labor, or other high-ranking or influential person. This is usually employed when the situation becomes critical and when continuance of a strike would cause problems for a great number of people.

Another technique is *informational picketing*, which involves employees carrying informational signs outside of the institution. Informational picketing is not designed to stop work, but rather to inform the public of the concerns under dispute. This tactic is designed to create public pressure on behalf of the union and the employees, and is seen frequently. Other methods of obtaining community support also may be employed. These include newspaper editorials, letters to the editor, and even paid advertisements. Rallies and marches may be used to draw public attention to the issues.

In some instances, an *injunction* may be requested. This results in a court order that requires the party or parties involved to take a specific action or, more commonly, to refrain from taking a specific action. Employers may use this measure to forestall or end a strike. Unions may use this measure to stop a lock-out.

In still other instances, an institution or company may be subjected to *government seizure and operation*. Government employees are then used to run the plant, firm, or industry in question. This is seldom seen in the health care industry, for obvious reasons. However, this option was used in Montana in 1991, when state employees decided to strike. The National Guard was called in to replace striking state patrolmen.

What to Look for in a Contract

The negotiation process should ultimately conclude in the development of a written contract that is signed by both bargaining groups and management representatives. The contract establishes guidelines for working conditions such as overtime, floating, work schedules, job security, and retention and recruitment of staff (Boisvert, 1991). It usually spells out certain other privileges to be provided to employees, such as in-service education, leaves, health and safety provisions, committee participation, and tuition reimbursement (Flanagan, 1992). The contract also may provide guidelines for the grievance process.

A contract must meet certain specified criteria to be legally binding. It must result from mutually agreed-on items arrived at through a "meeting of minds." Something of value must be given for a reciprocal promise, that is, professional duties for an agreed-on sum. Contracts can be enforceable whether written or oral, but it is easier to work with those that are written (Rothman & Rothman, 1977).

Although each agreement will differ, most contracts have a fairly general format that includes:

- A preamble stating the objectives of each party
- A statement recognizing the official bargaining groups
- A section dealing with financial remuneration, including wages and salaries, overtime rates, holiday pay, and shift differentials
- A section dealing with nonfinancial rewards, that is, fringe benefits such as retirement programs, types of insurance available, free parking, and other services provided by the employer
- A section dealing with seniority in respect to promotions, transfers, work schedules, and layoffs
- A section establishing guidelines for disciplinary problems
- A section describing grievance procedures
- A section that may explicitly state codes of conduct or professional standards

Several other areas that are negotiable are important and should be incorporated into a contract for nurses. These may be included in the section dealing with professional standards or nursing care. The following are generally accepted as items that should be considered in a contract involving professional nurses.

First, the contract should provide for shared governance—that is, professional policy decisions should be developed by professional staff and administration who work jointly on the policy. This often takes the form of a nursing practice council or a professional performance committee. The committees should be identified, duties described, and benefits and rights clarified.

Second, the contract should provide for individual professional accountability. It establishes the guidelines for such issues as floating, overtime, and scheduling. It should include areas related to evaluation, such as peer evaluation of a practitioner's competence. It also should assure job security, stipulate retention and recruitment efforts, and deal with issues of promotion or dismissal.

Third, the contract should define the collective professional role. This spells out the responsibility of registered nurses as professional practitioners and describes their part in the planning of patient care. The purpose of this is to strengthen nurses' influence on the quality of care. It should discourage the encroachment of non-nursing staff into nursing practice and might include guidelines for staffing ratios.

Other items that should be included in contracts relate to health and safety provisions, in-service education or continuing education, tuition reimbursement, and leaves of absence. All of these affect the quality of the work experience (Fig. 12-8).

It is important that, as a new graduate, you know whether there is a contract in effect in the institution in which you seek employment or in the community in which you plan to work. You should also be knowledgeable about the terms of the existing contract so that you might best fulfill your obligations, and recognize and benefit from the provisions to which you are entitled. The organization to which you are applying for employment can provide you with a copy of the current contract. The state nurses' associations can be contacted for information regarding the organization that represents nurses in a particular hospital or facility. They can also provide a copy of any contracts that have been negotiated for which they represented the nurses.

The Grievance Process

Effective contracts include, in addition to wages, hours, working conditions, and other items, a section that spells out the grievance procedure. A *grievance* is a circumstance or action believed to be unjust and in violation of a contract (or of policies if a contract is not in place). The *grievance process* represents an established and orderly method to be used in the adjustment of grievances between parties. In this sense, it represents a problem-solving mechanism.

The steps to be used in mediating grievances are usually included in the collective bargaining contract. Some organizations that lack formal collective bargaining agreements have developed internal policies that outline grievance procedures. Perhaps you are aware of grievance processes from your students' handbook, where the processes in place in an educational program are shared with students.

FIGURE 12–8   As a new graduate, you may find yourself poorly prepared to make decisions that are involved in bargaining issues.

Grievances are usually related to interpretations of a contract. They generally occur as a result of a misunderstanding or difference of opinion about the contract or its language, or as a result of direct violations of the contract. Although either the management or an employee can file grievances, in most instances it is an employee who instigates the case.

The grievance process spells out in writing in the contract a series of steps to be taken to resolve the area of dissension. Initially the employee and the immediate supervisor attempt to resolve the disagreement through an informal talk. If no resolution occurs, the discussion moves to the steps of the grievance process, involving others within the organization. The steps include providing notifications and responses in writing, adhering to strict time lines for action, and eventually involving people at higher levels within the organization (eg, representatives from the bargaining unit, a grievance chairman, the personnel director, and administrative representatives). Perhaps the services of an arbitrator will be needed toward the end of the dispute. Failure of either side to comply with the time lines that are in effect regarding their own actions or responses ends the process. If an arbitrator is involved, that person's decision is usually binding (Fig. 12-9).

It is important to differentiate between complaints and grievances. Employees may have complaints that are not violations of the contract. For example, Nurse No. 1 may object that she was required to float from the postpartum unit to the nursery; she had

FIGURE 12–9 It is important to discriminate between complaints and grievances.

been oriented to the nursery but preferred to work in the postpartum unit. Nurse No. 2 was required to float from a medical unit to a surgical unit to which she had not been oriented. If the contract in this hospital stipulates that no one would be floated to a unit to which he or she had not been oriented, Nurse No. 1 had a complaint, whereas Nurse No. 2 had a grievance.

The absence of grievances may not be the best indicator of the health of an organization. It is entirely possible that problems are not being addressed. On the other hand, a high number of grievances may indicate problems within the organization. These problems also may relate to the language of the contract or the education of the employee regarding the conditions of the contract. Another barometer of the health of an organization is the level at which the grievances are resolved. It is most desirable to settle most grievances at the informal level, without the involvement of an arbitrator.

The grievance procedure may sound like many steps that take a great deal of time, and indeed this is true. Although most grievances are settled short of arbitration, they are still time and energy consuming. Grievances can best be avoided if everyone has a good understanding of the terms of the contract and if sound personnel policies are developed and applied consistently and equitably. Open discussions between the employees and management to review mutual concerns and share information help reduce the number of grievances. Mutual respect is a critical element in any organization.

Critical Thinking Activity

What are the reasons that grievance processes need to be spelled out in a contract? How would you determine whether an issue is a grievance or a complaint?

Issues Related to Collective Bargaining and Nursing

Four major issues of collective bargaining affect the nursing profession. The first of these relates to the fact that some nurses see collective bargaining as unprofessional. The second is the issue of which bargaining group will represent nursing when nurses participate in collective bargaining. The third issue is an individual one and relates to the question of whether to join a union when one exists; the fourth deals with the role of the supervisor.

These issues may take on greater or lesser importance depending on the area of country involved, the length of time the nurses in that area have been participating in collective bargaining, and the group chosen to represent the nurses at the bargaining table. As a staff nurse you may, at some time, have to make a decision regarding whether to strike. In making this decision, you want to be well grounded in the issues at hand, and the arrangements that have been made for continuing to provide services in emergency situations and in special hospital areas such as labor and delivery.

COLLECTIVE ACTION AND PROFESSIONALISM

The strain that exists between professionalism and collective action has probably received more space in recent nursing literature than any other issue related to collective bargaining. The argument against unionism has its roots in the history of nursing itself. Nursing was perceived by many, including nurses, as a selfless, all-serving, altruistic calling. The act of caring for others, even if that meant subordinating the individual to the goals of that care, was to be compensation enough for the services rendered. The strong religious influence that pervaded the early development of nursing added to this concept of the profession. Early leaders in nursing espoused this dedication to its arts. In 1893, Lavinia Dock stated:

Absolute and unquestioning obedience must be the foundation of the nurse's work, and to this end complete subordination of the individual to the work as a whole is as necessary for her as for the soldier. (Cited in Bullough & Bullough, 1966)

Another factor that has hampered the strong development of unionization in nursing is the fact that nursing is primarily a woman's profession. Although more men now enter nursing, only about 5.4% of the registered nurses in the United States are male.

Early social beliefs that a woman's role should be submissive, supportive, and obedient were extremely compatible with the expectations that our society placed on nurses. The paternalism that has existed in the health care delivery system has also made the process of collective bargaining for nurses a slow one (see Chapters 4 and 5). The combination of the role of women and the role of the nurse under earlier paternalistic practices had the nurse caring for the "hospital family," looking out for the needs of all (from patient to physician) and being responsible for keeping everyone happy (Ashley, 1976). The tendency to see the physician as the father figure in the health care system, the nurse as the corresponding mother figure, and the patients as the children has done little to promote the autonomy of nursing as a profession. A quote by Campbell (1980, p. 1286) demonstrates the use of the family concept in health care: "If we are to keep unions out of the profession we, as nurses, must make every effort to build loyalty and a family feeling among our fellow nurses."

Despite nursing's history of ambivalence toward union negotiations, today we see nurses involved in collective bargaining in greater numbers than ever before. Several factors are responsible for this change. Wilson and colleagues (1990) have identified these as: the focus on the continued high cost of health care and the need to examine this rise; the scrutiny that has been placed on employee's salaries as part of this process; the fact that nurses constitute the largest number of employees in hospitals (nearly half); and changes in the NLRA allowing nurses to bargain collectively. Various sources differ with regard to whether unionization of hospital employees results in higher hospital costs.

In the early years of collective bargaining by nurses, there was some reticence to use the term "unionism." Much of the nursing literature surrounding the issue used appropriate and less emotionally charged synonyms. Today the term "unionism" is used with increasing frequency, reflecting a change in sentiment supporting the belief that nurses should be involved in collective bargaining, and also reflecting the general acceptance of the process by the public at large.

Many have come to believe that the collective action of nurses provides one of the best avenues for achieving professional goals and exercising control over nursing practice. As nurses are called on to assume greater responsibility for complicated decisions, collective bargaining through a professional organization may provide the means to implement the concept of collective professional responsibility.

Certainly the way that collective bargaining is perceived by the nurse, and by the public that is served, is determined by the manner in which the bargaining is conducted. Nurses as a group need to develop the skills necessary to communicate to the public the importance of their role in health care delivery. They must be able to handle conflicts and work toward resolution while maintaining integrity and dignity. Nurses need to become enlightened and informed, and they need more than a superficial understanding of the process of collective bargaining.

Nurses may benefit from broadening their perceptions. This applies to many issues in nursing practice—particularly bioethical issues—in addition to collective bargaining (see Chapter 10). Many nurses dichotomize issues into categories such as good/bad, right/wrong, best/worst. Nurses need to work toward understanding and accommodating different points of view and acknowledging that areas of compromise do exist.

Of perhaps greater concern to many nurses is the issue of whether nurses should participate in strike activities if negotiations break down. Many nurses believe that the withholding of services from patients is unprofessional, and therefore, personally unacceptable. Others view the strike as a final method for bringing attention to the needs of the nurse as a citizen. Fortunately, as bargaining groups representing nurses become more knowledgeable and skilled in the process, strikes occur less frequently. Disagreements at the bargaining table are more commonly resolved through mediation and arbitration, much to the relief of many professionals.

Critical Thinking Activity

Do you support the concept of nurses becoming members of a union? If so, should all employees of an organization be required to pay membership fees? Analyze your response to this question and provide the rationale to support your views.

REPRESENTATION FOR NURSES

Of far greater controversy than whether nurses should unionize is the issue of which organization should represent nurses at the bargaining table. This is determined by elections that are supervised by the NLRB. To become the certified collective bargaining representative of a group of employees, the organization in question must receive 50% of the votes cast, plus one.

When nurses first began to organize, the ANA, through the state nurses' associations, was the bargaining representative. This group still represents more nurses than all other organizations combined. In 1991, across the country, state associations represented more than 139,000 registered nurses through more than 840 bargain units (Fuller-Jonap, 1994). However, there has been a strong movement on the part of other organizations to vie for the representative position. It has been estimated that more than 30 labor organizations represent health care workers (Miller, 1980). The ANA has been representing nurses since 1946. The National Union of Hospital and Health Care Employees (representing nurses since 1977) and the SEIU have voted to unite, creating something of a "super union" for health care workers. The Federation of Nurses and Health Professionals began organizing nurses in 1978. Other groups representing nurses in various parts of the country include the United Food and Commercial Workers, the Teamsters Union, and the American Federation of Teachers.

Nurses face a difficult decision when trying to decide which group can represent them best. In recent years, this decision has occupied perhaps more time and effort on the part of nurses than has the actual bargaining. Those who have strong allegiance to the ANA contend that only registered nurses should bargain for registered nurses. One of the reasons given for this position is that in collective bargaining, nurses face different issues than other workers. In addition to concerns about salary, benefits, working conditions, and the like, nurses also want to negotiate questions pertaining to staffing, patient care concerns, and participation on joint hospital committees. Many believe that only nurses can effectively negotiate such items. These people contend that hospital administrations, fearing the power of labor unions, will bargain more constructively and positively with nurses themselves. They also believe that the ANA will be a stronger, more united organization if it serves as both the professional association and the bargaining agent.

Others believe that nurses compromise their collective bargaining powers when the recognized union is a group other than the state nurses' association. They think that when nurses do not bargain for themselves, the "organization shrivels and their influence on health care weakens" (Mallison, 1985, p. 943).

Some parts of the country are experiencing a trend toward having an organization other than the professional nurses' association represent nurses. Chief among the arguments for bargaining conducted by another group is the issue of supervisor membership in the professional association (discussed later in this chapter). Proponents of this position also would contend that it is not realistic for one group (ie, the ANA) to work with the professionalism aspect of nursing as well as with the issues of wages, benefits, and working conditions.

Some would argue for two organizations—one to represent issues related to professionalism, and another to negotiate salaries. If nurses choose to have one group involved in professional concerns (eg, codes of ethics, standards of care, and updating skills required in the practice of the profession) and a second group representing them at the bargaining table, there are some obvious drawbacks. First and foremost is the matter of cost, because both organizations would be collecting dues. Many consider the cost of belonging to the ANA and to the state association to be very high, with dues of approximately $350.00 per year. Additional, equally expensive, membership dues in another organization might be prohibitive. Second, many believe that the union would become the dominant force between the two groups, because money and working environment issues both speak strongly.

There are no easy answers to this question, and it will certainly be one of the biggest issues facing nurses in the future.

 ## Critical Thinking Activity

> If the collective bargaining agent in the hospital in which you worked was other than the state nurses' association, would you belong to both organizations? What factors would you use to support your decision? Why are these factors important to you?

TO JOIN OR NOT TO JOIN

Once an individual nurse has gained an understanding of collective bargaining and has developed a personal philosophy about the professional role of the nurse, he or she is ready to make a decision regarding membership in the bargaining unit.

In working with students who are soon to embark on professional careers, we find that it is easier for them to decide whether to bargain collectively than it is to decide to part with the money that is required for membership. Many nurses want better working conditions and higher salaries, but are all too willing to let someone else fund these endeavors and work to achieve them.

It is in response to these concerns that many "agency shop" clauses have been added to contracts. Those who are members and are active in the negotiation process believe it is inappropriate for some to benefit from the labors of the bargaining process without having contributed, at least financially, to the effort. The presence of agency shop clauses may serve as either an asset or a deterrent to recruitment, depending on the applicant's viewpoint.

THE SUPERVISOR AND COLLECTIVE BARGAINING

In 1994, a nursing home argued before the Supreme Court that the licensed practical nurses in its employ were supervisors (because of their role in directing nursing assistants in patient care) and, therefore, were not protected by the National Labor Relations Act. The Supreme Court, in a 5 to 4 decision, ruled in favor of the nursing home. Nursing organizations engaged in collective bargaining have expressed serious concern regarding the implications of this ruling for all nurses. Labor groups expect to lobby for legislation that would alter this interpretation of the NLRB ("Striking at Bargaining," 1994).

This issue was again addressed in February 1996, when the National Labor Relations Board ended nearly 2 years of deliberation by ruling that charge nurses at Alaska's Providence Medical Center could not be called "supervisors" simply because the role requires some direction of other workers. The Board stated that the essence of the nurse's role was "judgment," and went on to explain that authority that arises from professional knowledge is distinct from the authority of a front-line manager (NLRB to the Supreme Court, 1996).

Changing Trends With Regard to Collective Bargaining

At one time economic concerns and working conditions may have been the principal motivators for collective action. However, by the mid-1980s subtle, and at times not so subtle, changes were occurring throughout the United States with regard to collective bargaining, unionism, and labor-management relations. Some working in the area of contract management reported a shift from the adversarial relationship that historically had existed between the employee and the employer (which focused on salaries, work hours, and the like) to one that placed greater emphasis on the quality of work life.

The focus of collective bargaining issues also changed during the 1990s. Originally focusing on wages and benefits, today the major concern of nurses is often staffing patterns, involvement in decisions affecting patient care, cross-training, the use of unlicensed assistive personnel, and workplace safety. This shift in emphasis reflects the general acceptance of the process of collective bargaining by nurses and the fact that significant headway has been made through this process with regard to basic issues. This change of thinking is borne out by the recent vote of the House of Delegates of the American Medical Association to develop an affiliated national labor organization, under the National Labor Relations Act, which would support the development and operation of local negotiating units to represent employed physicians. Self-employed physicians are currently barred from joining collective bargaining units by antitrust laws (Docs vote, 1999).

CONCESSION BARGAINING

Concession bargaining is a process in which there is an explicit exchange of reduced labor costs for improvements in job security. This has been occurring with increasing frequency. An example would be a shift in emphasis from one that asks for increases in salary to one that focuses on eliminating the practice of calling nurses and telling them not to report for work because the census has dropped (on such days, the nurses do not receive salary). These changes have been seen in industry more than in nursing, although the strike of 6,000 Minnesota nurses in 1984 was triggered by hospital practices related to the layoff of staff and the involuntary reduction of hours (6,000 Minnesota RNs, 1984).

"UNION BUSTING"

A trend seen in health care institutions during the 1980s, and persisting in some areas today, is an effort toward "union busting." Although technically illegal when referring to methods used to get rid of an existing union, the term *union busting* has been expanded to include a wide range of legal activities that slow down collective bargaining. Pressured by rapidly escalating health care costs, and influenced by the changing attitudes toward work, hospital administrators have hired consultants and law firms to assist and advise in discouraging and impeding organizational activities. This is also a counteraction to the courting by unions of the expanding groups of previously unorganized professionals, such as physicians and nurses. Antiunion organizing campaigns usually are aimed at strategies that will delay and thus drag down the momentum of organizing efforts. This could include challenging union membership, attempting to decertify elections, and failing to bargain in good faith—thus drawing out the negotiating process (Ballman, 1985).

ISSUES OF DISCRIMINATION

As nurses have become more comfortable and knowledgeable about the bargaining process, their energies have been directed toward many issues. These include such concerns as pay equity, discrimination against female employees, comparable worth, and the rights of employees to know the hazards within a work environment (see Chapter 11). In some instances, discriminatory practices against male nurses also have been an issue.

CHANGES IN THE NUMBER OF BARGAINING UNITS

Within hospitals are many different positions and job titles ranging from professional staff through office staff to those responsible for hospital maintenance. In nursing alone, there are groups of registered nurses, licensed practical nurses, and nursing assistants. As these groups have been granted authority to organize into bargaining units, concern has been expressed about the number of unions with which any hospital administration must bargain at any given time. Some fairly elaborate estimates have been made regarding the amount of time demanded by the collective bargaining process.

When the NLRA was first passed in 1974, the NLRB specified that seven employee bargaining units would exist within the health care industry (Wilson, Hamilton, & Murphy, 1990, p. 37). The seven groups were registered nurses, physicians, other professional employees, technical employees, business office or clerical employees, and skilled maintenance employees.

In 1984, the NLRB determined that bargaining units would be decided on a case-by-case basis. This resulted in the number of bargaining units being reduced to three: all professionals, all nonprofessionals, and guards.

In 1989, the NLRB proposed a new rule that resulted in the establishment of eight collective bargaining units. At this time it was also determined that the rule would apply to all hospitals of all sizes. In response, the American Hospital Association (AHA) sought and obtained a permanent injunction against the rule. Subsequently, "all-RN" units were legally approved. As might be expected, the AHA and the ANA occupied opposite points of view with regard to this issue.

The latest activity regarding this issue occurred in April 1991. The US Supreme Court upheld the NLRB in its authority to define bargaining units for health care workers in acute care hospitals, and allowed for all-RN bargaining units (Supreme Court, 1991).

CURRENT ACTIVITY OF THE ANA IN COLLECTIVE BARGAINING

In 1991, the ANA embarked on a Workplace Advocacy Initiative. The focus of this initiative was to improve the work environment and ensure that nurses are involved in decisions affecting the quality of their work environments. Ideally this would assure that patients would receive the best possible nursing care.

Other aspects of the ANA Workplace Advocacy Initiative included providing data about salaries and related economic and employment issues; providing information related to health, safety, and other workplace concerns; developing systems of analysis of compensation packages; consultation; and supporting networks for sharing information and providing mutual support.

In 1999 the ANA House of Delegates reorganized ANA's approach to collective action for nurses (Actions, 1999). The delegates approved the development of an autonomous arm of ANA titled United American Nurses. This organization will coordinate efforts between state nurses associations that are engaged in collective bargaining and act on the behalf of all nurses in relationship to workplace issues.

The Impact of Shared Governance on Collective Bargaining

The greater involvement of staff nurses in health care agency decision making may have a significant impact on the collective bargaining process. Many of the issues that historically were resolved at the bargaining table, such as the use of agency nurses, work load, and policies regarding floating from one unit to another, are now resolved at the committee or council level. Each nurse has greater accountability for participation in decision making outside of the bargaining process and for implementing decisions that have been made. With mechanisms for change built into the operational pattern of the health care agency, nurses may find less to negotiate at the bargaining table and, in reality, the processes may provide some duplication of one another.

KEY CONCEPTS

- One of the critical elements of any organization is its mission statements. Mission statements explicitly outline the purpose of the organization and may also contain the philosophy and goals of the group.
- Organizations may be structured a number of different ways. Some are tall and centralized, whereas others are flat and decentralized.
- All organizations have chains of command, channels of communication, and spans of control that describe lines of authority and accountability. These can be depicted in organizational charts that represent the formal organization. An informal organization also exists within organizations.
- Organizations have developed job descriptions that outline the responsibilities of all employees, and policies and protocols to guide the activities of the employees.
- Many hospitals are now using a shared governance process, a form of practice model that involves shared decision making by nursing staff and management. It results in a decentralized organization and often results in greater job satisfaction for nurses.
- Many patterns of nursing care delivery have existed over the years. These include the case method, the functional method, team nursing, total patient care, primary nursing, and case management.
- Since 1974, it has been possible for nurses to bargain collectively for salaries, working conditions, and fringe benefits. This process also allows for their participation in committees focused on improving patient care and patient care standards.
- The collective bargaining process culminates in a contract that places in writing the decisions reached at the bargaining table. As a new graduate, you should know whether the health care agency at which you are seeking employment has a contract in effect.
- A contract usually includes a section that spells out the process to be used in a grievance. Should a grievance arise, it is essential that all steps be followed as outlined in the contract. Nurses need to be able to distinguish between issues that are grievances and those that are simply complaints.
- One of the issues surrounding nurses and collective bargaining is related to which group should do the bargaining for nurses. Many believe this process is best conducted by a professional nursing organization; others believe they are served best by an organization that has collective bargaining as its major focus.
- Trends with regard to the collective bargaining process include concession bargaining, "union busting," issues of discrimination, and changes in the number of bargaining units.

REFERENCES

Alexander MK, Bourgeois A, Goodman LR. Total quality improvement: Bridging the gap between education and service. *In* Strickland OL, Fishman DJ: Nursing Issues in the 1990s. Albany, NY: Delmar Publishers, 1994:280–289

Ashley JA. Hospitals, Paternalism and the Role of the Nurse. New York: Teachers' College Press, 1976

Ballman CS. Union busters. Am J Nurs 85(9):963–966, 1985

Boisvert SC. Collective bargaining: Another view. Maine Nurse 78(4):5, 1991

Bullough V, Bullough B. Issues in Nursing: Readings Selected From Books and Periodicals to Form a Basis for Discussion of Problems in Nursing Today. New York: Springer-Verlag, 1966:96

Campbell GJ. *In* Opinions: Is bargaining unprofessional for nurses? AORN J 31(6):1289, 1980

Docs vote for unionization. Available at *www.nursingworld.org/tan/julaug99/inbrief.htm*. Accessed January 8, 2000

Etzioni A. Modern Organizations. Englewood Cliffs, NJ: Prentice-Hall, 1964:1

Flanagan L. How collective bargaining benefits nurses. Directions: American Nurse Supplement. October:8–9, 22, 1992

Fuller-Jonap F. Collective bargaining in nursing: Benefits, issues, and problems. *In* Strickland OL, Fishman DJ: Nursing Issues in the 1990s. Albany, NY: Delmar Publishers, 1994:33–45

Huber D. Leadership and Nursing Management. Philadelphia: WB Saunders, 1996

Jacoby J, Terpstra M. Collaborative governance: Model for professional autonomy. Nurs Management 21(2):423–444, 1990

Mallison MB. Weathering the economic climate. Am J Nurs 85(9):943, 1985

Miller RU. Collective bargaining: A nursing dilemma. AORN J 31(6):1197, 1980

Muff J. Altruism, socialism and nightingalism: The compassion traps. *In* Muff J: Women's Issues in Nursing: Socialization, Sexism, and Stereotyping. Prospect Heights, IL: Waveland Press, 1988:234–247

NLRB to the Supreme Court: Labor law protects nurses. Am J Nurs 96(4):67, 72, 1996

Neufeldt V. (Ed.). Webster's New World Dictionary, 3rd ed. New York: Macmillan, 1996

O'Meara SM, O'Meara DP. NLRB to issue landmark decision on nurse practitioners. Nurse Practitioner 20(12):14, 16, 24, 1995

Porter-O'Grady T. Nursing governance in a transitional era. *In* Chaska NL: The Nursing Profession: Turning Points. St. Louis: CV Mosby, 1990:432–439

Porter-O'Grady T. Shared governance and new organizational models. Nursing Economics 5(6):281–286

Rothman DA, Rothman NL. The Professional Nurse and the Law. Boston: Little Brown, 1977

6,000 Minnesota RNs strike back at layoff trend. Am J Nurs 84(7):941, 948, 1984

Striking at bargaining rights, court says RNs are supervisors. Am J Nurs 94(7):67, 70–71, 1994

Supreme Court okays all-RN unit. Am Nurse (June):1, 1991

Wilson CN, Hamilton CL, Murphy E. Union dynamics in nursing. J Nurs Admin 20(2):35–39, 1990

FURTHER READING

Actions of the 1999 ANA House of Delegates. Online at *www.nursingworld.org/about/summary/99hodact.htm*. Accessed January 11, 2000

Beletz E, Meng MT. The grievance process. Am J Nurs 77(2):256–260, 1977

Castrey BG, Castrey RT. Mediation: What it is, what it does. J Nurs Admin 10(9):18–21, 1980

Eldridge I, Levi J. Collective bargaining as a power resource for professional goals. Nurs Admin Q (Winter):29–40, 1982

Flanagan L. All-RN rule to have major impact. Am Nurse (March):26, 1982

Gross JA. Conflicting statutory purposes: Another look at fifty years of NLRB law making. Indust Labor Rel Rev 39(10):7–18, 1985

Hudacek SS. Collective bargaining—not a dinosaur of the past. Adv Clin Care 5(1):27–28, 1990

Ketter J. Staff nurses celebrate 20 years of NLRB protection. Am Nurse 26(6):3, 9, 1994

McCarty P. ANA launches workplace initiative—SNAs get grants for RN advocacy, new organizing. Am Nurse 22(April):7, 1991

Pettengill MM. Collective bargaining: Impact on nursing. *In* Chaska NL: The Nursing Profession: Turning Points. St. Louis: CV Mosby, 1990:454–463

Pettengill MM. Multilateral collective bargaining and the health care industry: Implications for nursing. J Prof Nurs 1(5):275–282, 1985

Scott K. SNA representation means increased job satisfaction. Am Nurse 25(January):24, 1993

Smith GR. Unionization for nurses: An issue for the 1980s. J Prof Nurs 1(4):192–201, 1985

Stickler KB. Union organizing will be divisive and costly. Hospitals 64(13):68–70, 1990

Targeting charge nurses, hospitals move to prove RN "supervisors." Am J Nurs 94(9):75, 1994

Relevant web sites

Nurses' Call *www.nurses-call.org/*
Nurses' Station *www.hci.net/~nursecline/*
Nurseweek *www-nurseweek.webnexus.com*
NursingNet *www.nursingnet.org/*

APPENDIX

A

Nursing Licensing Authorities (Boards of Nursing) United States and U.S. Territories

Note: For specific information regarding licensure requirements, regulations, and fees, contact the specific state licensing authority. Current addresses, telephone numbers, and directors also can be obtained on the Internet through the National Council of State Boards of Nursing at *www.ncsbn.org*

ALABAMA
Alabama Board of Nursing
RSA Plaza, Ste 250
770 Washington Avenue
Montgomery, AL 36130-3900
Phone: (334) 242-4060
FAX: (334) 242-4360
Contact Person: N. Genell Lee, MSN,
    JD, RN, Executive Officer
Web Site: *www.abn.state.al.us*

ALASKA
Alaska Board of Nursing
Dept. of Comm. & Econ. Development
Div. of Occupational Licensing
3601 C Street, Suite 722
Anchorage, AK 99503
Phone: (907) 269-8161
FAX: (907) 269-8196
Contact Person: Dorothy Fulton, MA,
    RN, Executive Director
Web Site:
    www.dced.state.ak.us/occ/pnur.htm

AMERICAN SAMOA
American Samoa Health Services
Regulatory Board

LBJ Tropical Medical Center
Pago Pago, AS 96799
Phone: (684) 633-1222
FAX: (684) 633-1869
Contact Person: Etenauga Lutu, RN,
    Executive Secretary

ARIZONA
Arizona State Board of Nursing
1651 E. Morten Avenue, Suite 150
Phoenix, AZ 85020
Phone: (602) 331-8111
FAX: (602) 906-9365
Contact Person: Joey Ridenour, MN,
    RN, Executive Director
Web Site: *www.azboardofnursing.org*

ARKANSAS
Arkansas State Board of Nursing
University Tower Building
1123 S. University, Suite 800
Little Rock, AR 72204
Phone: (501) 686-2700
FAX: (501) 686-2714
Contact Person: Faith Fields, MSN,
    RN, Executive Director
Web Site: *www.state.ar.us/nurse*

CALIFORNIA

California Board of Registered Nursing
400 R St., Ste. 4030
Sacramento, CA 95814-6239
Phone: (916) 322-3350
FAX: (916) 327-4402
Contact Person: Ruth Ann Terry, MPH,
    RN, Executive Officer
Web Site: *www.rn.ca.gov*

California Board of Vocational Nursing
    and Psychiatric Technicians
2535 Capitol Oaks Drive, Ste. 205
Sacramento CA 95833
Phone: (916) 263-7800
FAX: (916) 263-7859
Contact Person: Teresa Bello-Jones,
    MS, JD, RN, Executive Officer
Web Site: *www.bvnpt.ca.gov*

COLORADO

Colorado Board of Nursing
1560 Broadway, Suite 880
Denver, CO 80202
Phone: (303) 894-2430
FAX: (303) 894-2821
Contact Person: Patricia Uris, PhD,
    RN, Program Administrator
Web Site: *www.dora.state.co.us/nursing*

CONNECTICUT

Connecticut Board of Examiners for
    Nursing
Division of Health Systems Regulation
410 Capitol Avenue, MS 12HSR
P.O. Box 340308
Hartford, CT 06134-0328
Phone: (860) 509-7624
FAX: (860) 509-7553
Contact Person: Dorothy Pacyna, MS,
    RN, Supervisor of Nursing
    Consultants
Web Site: *www.state.ct.us/dph*

DELAWARE

Delaware Board of Nursing

861 Silver Lake Blvd.
Cannon Building, Suite 203
Dover, DE 19904
Phone: (302) 739-4522
FAX: (302) 739-2711
Contact Person: Iva Boardman, MSN,
    RN, Executive Director

DISTRICT OF COLUMBIA

District of Columbia Board of Nursing
Department of Health
825 N. Capitol St., N.E., 2nd Fl.
Room 2224
Washington, DC 20002
Phone: (202) 442-4778
FAX: (202) 442-9431
Contact Person: Denise Pope, MSN,
    RN, Acting Executive Officer

FLORIDA

Florida Board of Nursing
4080 Woodcock Drive, Suite 202
Jacksonville, FL 32207
Phone: (904) 858-6940
FAX: (904) 858-6964
Contact Person: Ruth R. Stiehl, PhD,
    MN, MA, BS, RN, Executive
    Director
Web Site: *www/doh.state.fl.us/mqa/
    nursing/rnhome.htm*

GEORGIA

Georgia Board of Nursing
237 Coliseum Drive
Macon, GA 31217-3858
Phone: (912) 207-1640
FAX: (912) 207-1660
Contact Person: Shirley Camp, BSN,
    JD, RN, Executive Director
Web Site: *www.sos.state.ga.us/ebd-rn*

Georgia State Board of Licensed
    Practical Nurses
237 Coliseum Drive
Macon, GA 31217-1640
Phone: (912) 207-1633

FAX: (912) 207-1633
Contact Person: Jacqueline Hightower, JD, Executive Director
Web Site: *www.sos.state.ga.us/ebd-lpn*

GUAM
Guam Board of Nurse Examiners
P.O. Box 2816
1304 East Sunset Boulevard
Barrgada, GU 96913
Phone: (671) 475-0251
FAX: (671) 477-4733
Contact Person: Margarita Bautista-Gay, RN, BSN, MN, Chairperson and Acting Executive Director

HAWAII
Hawaii Board of Nursing
Professional and Vocational Licensing Division
P.O. Box 3469
Honolulu, HI 96801
Phone: (808) 586-3000
FAX: (808) 586-2689
Contact Person: Kathleen Yokouchi, Executive Officer

IDAHO
Idaho Board of Nursing
280 N. 8th Street, Suite 210
P.O. Box 83720
Boise, ID 83720
Phone: (208) 334-3110
FAX: (208) 334-3262
Contact Person: Sandra Evans, MA, Ed., RN, Executive Director
Web Site: *www.state.id.us/ibn/ibnhome.htm*

ILLINOIS
Illinois Department of Professional Regulation
James R. Thompson Center
100 West Randolph, Suite 9-300
Chicago, IL 60601

Phone: (312) 814-2715
FAX: (312) 814-3145
Contact Person: Jacqueline Waggoner, MSN, RN, Nursing Act Coordinator
Web Site: *www.dpr.state.il.us/*

INDIANA
Indiana State Board of Nursing
Health Professions Bureau
402 W. Washington St., Room W041
Indianapolis, IN 46204
Phone: (317) 232-2960
FAX: (317) 233-4236
Contact Person: Laura Langford, RN, Executive Director
Web Site: *www.ai.org/hpb*

IOWA
Iowa Board of Nursing
RiverPoint Business Park
400 S.W. 8th Street
Suite B
Des Moines, IA 50309-4685
Phone: (515) 281-3255
FAX: (515) 281-4825
Contact Person: Lorinda Inman, MSN, RN, Executive Director
Web Site: *www.state.ia.us/government/nursing/*

KANSAS
Kansas State Board of Nursing
Landon State Office Building
900 S.W. Jackson, Suite 551-S
Topeka, KS 66612
Phone: (785) 296-4929
FAX: (785) 296-3929
Contact Person: Mary Blubaugh, MSN, RN, Executive Administrator
Web Site: *www.ksbn.org*

KENTUCKY
Kentucky Board of Nursing
312 Whittington Parkway, Ste. 300
Louisville, KY 40222

Phone: (502) 329-7000
FAX: (502) 329-7011
Contact Person: Sharon Weisenbeck,
    MS, RN, Executive Director
Web Site: *www.kbn.state.ky.us*

LOUISIANA

Louisiana State Board of Nursing
3510 N. Causeway Blvd., Ste. 501
Metairie, LA 70002
Phone: (504) 838-5332
FAX: (504) 838-5349
Contact Person: Barbara Morvant,
    MN, RN, Executive Director
Web Site: *www.lsbn.state.la.us*

Louisiana State Board of Practical
    Nurse Examiners
3421 N. Causeway Blvd., Ste. 203
Metairie, LA 70002
Phone: (504) 838-5791
FAX: (504) 838-5279
Contact Person: Claire Glaviano, BSN,
    MN, RN, Executive Director

MAINE

Maine State Board of Nursing
158 State House Station
Augusta, ME 04333
Phone: (207) 287-1133
FAX: (207) 287-1149
Contact Person: Myra Broadway, JD,
    MS, RN, Executive Director
Web Site: *www.state.me.us/nursingbd*

MARYLAND

Maryland Board of Nursing
4140 Patterson Avenue
Baltimore, MD 21215
Phone: (410) 585-1900
FAX: (410) 358-3530
Contact Person: Donna Dorsey, MS,
    RN, Executive Director
Web Site: *dhmh1d.dhmh.state.md.us/
    mbn*

MASSACHUSETTS

Massachusetts Board of Registration in
    Nursing
Commonwealth of Massachusetts
239 Causeway Street
Boston, MA 02114
Phone: (617) 727-9961
FAX: (617) 727-1630
Contact Person: Theresa Bonanno,
    MSN, RN, Executive Director
Web Site: *www.state.ma.us/reg/
    boards/rn*

MICHIGAN

Michigan CIS/Office of Health Services
Ottawa Towers North
611 W. Ottawa, 4th Floor
Lansing, MI 48933
Phone: (517) 373-9102
FAX: (517) 373-2179
Contact Person: Cathy Seyka, Licensure
    Manager
Web Site: *www.cis.state.mi.us/bhser/
    genover.htm*

MINNESOTA

Minnesota Board of Nursing
2829 University Avenue SE
Suite 500
Minneapolis, MN 55414
Phone: (612) 617-2270
FAX: (612) 617-2190
Contact Person: Shirley Brekken, MS,
    RN, Executive Director
Web Site: *www.nursingboard.state.
    mn.us/*

MISSISSIPPI

Mississippi Board of Nursing
1935 Lakeland Drive, Suite B
Jackson, MS 39216
Phone: (601) 987-4188
FAX: (601) 364-2352
Contact Person: Marcia Rachel, PhD,
    RN, Executive Director

MISSOURI
Missouri State Board of Nursing
3605 Missouri Blvd.
P.O. Box 656
Jefferson City, MO 65102-0656
Phone: (573) 751-0681
FAX: (573) 751-0075
Contact Person: Calvina Thomas, PhD,
   RN, Executive Director
Web Site: *www.ecodev.state.mo.us/*
   pr/nursing

MONTANA
Montana State Board of Nursing
Arcade Building, Suite 4C
111 North Jackson
Helena, MT 59620-0513
Phone: (406) 444-2071
FAX: (406) 444-7759
Contact Person: Jill Caldwell, MSN,
   RN, Acting Executive Director
Web Site: *www.com.state.mt.us/*
   License/POL/index.htm

NEBRASKA
Nebraska Health and Human Services
   System
Dept. of Regulation and Licensure
Nursing Section
301 Centennial Mall South
P.O. Box 94986
Lincoln, NE 68509-4986
Phone: (402) 471-4376
FAX: (402) 471-3577
Contact Person: Charlene Kelly, PhD,
   RN, Executive Director
Web Site: *www.hhs.state.ne.us/crl/*
   nns.htm

NEVADA
Nevada State Board of Nursing
1755 East Plumb Lane
Suite 260
Reno, NV 89502
Phone: (775) 688-2620

FAX: (775) 688-2628
Contact Person: Kathy Apple, MS, RN,
   Executive Director
Web Site: *www.nursingboard.state.*
   nv.us/

NEW HAMPSHIRE
New Hampshire Board of Nursing
78 Regional Drive, Bldg. B
P.O. Box 3898
Concord, NH 03302
Phone: (603) 271-2323
FAX: (603) 271-6605
Contact Person: Doris Nuttelman, EdD,
   RN, Executive Director
Web Site: *www.state.nh.us/nursing/*

NEW JERSEY
New Jersey Board of Nursing
124 Halsey Street, 6th Floor
P.O. Box 45010
Newark, NJ 07101
Phone: (973) 504-6586
FAX: (973) 648-3481
Contact Person: Patricia Lynch
   Polansky, MS, RN, Executive
   Director
Web Site: *www.state.nj.us/lps/ca/*
   medical.htm

NEW MEXICO
New Mexico Board of Nursing
4206 Louisiana Boulevard, NE
Suite A
Albuquerque, NM 87109
Phone: (505) 841-8340
FAX: (505) 841-8347
Contact Person: Debra Brady, PhD,
   RN, Executive Director
Web Site: *www.state.nm.us/clients/*
   nursing

NEW YORK
New York State Board of Nursing
State Education Department

Cultural Education Center
Room 3023
Albany, NY 12230
Phone: (518) 474-3845
FAX: (518) 474-3706
Contact Person: Milene Sower, PhD,
   RN, Executive Secretary
Web Site: *www.nysed.gov/prof/ nurse.htm*

NORTHERN MARIANA ISLANDS
Commonwealth Board of Nurse
   Examiners
Public Health Center
P.O. Box 1458
Saipan, MP 96950
Phone: (670) 234-8950
FAX: (670) 234-8930
Contact Person: Elizabeth Torres-
   Untalan, RN, Chairperson

NORTH CAROLINA
North Carolina Board of Nursing
3724 National Drive
Raleigh, NC 27602
Phone: (919) 782-3211
FAX: (919) 782-9461
Contact Person: Polly Johnson, MSN,
   RN, Executive Director
Web Site: *www.ncbon.com*

NORTH DAKOTA
North Dakota Board of Nursing
919 South 7th Street, Suite 504
Bismarck, ND 58504
Phone: (701) 328-9777
FAX: (701) 328-9785
Contact Person: Constance Kalanek,
   PhD, RN, Executive Director
Web Site: *www.ndbon.org*

OHIO
Ohio Board of Nursing
17 South High Street, Suite 400
Columbus, OH 43215-3413
Phone: (614) 466-3947
FAX: (614) 466-0388

Contact Person: Dorothy Fiorino, MS,
   RN, Executive Director
Web Site: *www.state.oh.us/nur*

OKLAHOMA
Oklahoma Board of Nursing
2915 N. Classen Blvd., Suite 524
Oklahoma City, OK 73106
Phone: (405) 962-1800
FAX: (405) 962-1821
Contact Person: Kimberly Glazier,
   MEd, RN, Executive Director

OREGON
Oregon State Board of Nursing
800 NE Oregon Street, Box 25
Suite 465
Portland, OR 97232
Phone: (503) 731-4745
FAX: (503) 731-4755
Contact Person: Joan Bouchard, MN,
   RN, Executive Director
Web Site: *www.osbn.state.or.us*

PENNSYLVANIA
Pennsylvania State Board of Nursing
124 Pine Street
P.O. Box 2649
Harrisburg, PA 17101
Phone: (717) 783-7142
FAX: (717) 783-0822
Contact Person: Miriam Limo, MS,
   MSN, RN, Executive Secretary
Web Site: *www.dos.state.pa.us/bpoa/
   nurbd/mainpage.htm*

PUERTO RICO
Commonwealth of Puerto Rico
Board of Nurse Examiners
800 Roberto H. Todd Avenue
Room 202, Stop 18
Santurce, PR 00908
Phone: (787) 725-8161
FAX: (787) 725-7903
Contact Person: Beverly Davila
   Morales, Executive Director

RHODE ISLAND
Rhode Island Board of Nurse
   Registration and Nursing Education
105 Cannon Health Building
Three Capitol Hill, Room 104
Providence, RI 02908
Phone: (401) 222-5700
FAX: (401) 222-3352
Contact Person: Charles Alexandre,
   MSN, RN, Executive Officer

SOUTH CAROLINA
South Carolina State Board of Nursing
110 Centerview Drive
Suite 202
Columbia, SC 29210
Phone: (803) 896-4550
FAX: (803) 896-4525
Contact Person: Debbie Herman, MS,
   RN, Executive Officer
Web Site: *www.llr.state.sc.us/bon.htm*

SOUTH DAKOTA
South Dakota Board of Nursing
4300 South Louise Ave., Suite C-1
Sioux Falls, SD 57106-3124
Phone: (605) 362-2760
FAX: (605) 362-2768
Contact Person: Diana Vander Woude,
   MS, RN, Executive Secretary
Web Site: *www.state.sd.us/dcr/nursing/*

TENNESSEE
Tennessee State Board of Nursing
426 Fifth Avenue North
1st Floor—Cordell Hull Building
Nashville, TN 37247
Phone: (615) 532-5166
FAX: (615) 741-7899
Contact Person: Elizabeth Lund, MSN,
   RN, Executive Director
Web Site: *www.170.142.76.180/bmf-
   bin/BMFproflist.pl*

TEXAS
Texas Board of Nurse Examiners

333 Guadalupe St., Suite 3-460
Austin, TX 78701
Phone: (512) 305-7400
FAX: (512) 305-7401
Contact Person: Katherine Thomas,
   MN, RN, Executive Director
Web Site: *www.bne.state.tx.us/*

Texas Board of Vocational Nurse
   Examiners
William P. Hobby Bldg., Tower 3
333 Guadalupe St., Suite 3-400
Austin, TX 78701
Phone: (512) 305-8100
FAX: (512) 305-8101
Contact Person: Mary Strange, RN,
   Executive Director
Web Site: *www.link.tsl.state.tx.us/
   tx/bvne/*

UTAH
Utah State Board of Nursing
Heber M. Wells Bldg., 4th Floor
160 East 300 South
Salt Lake City, UT 84111
Phone: (801) 530-6628
FAX: (801) 530-6511
Contact Person: Laura Poe, MS, RN,
   Executive Administrator
Web Site: *www.commerce.state.ut.us/*

VERMONT
Vermont State Board of Nursing
109 State Street
Montpelier, VT 05609-1106
Phone: (802) 828-2396
FAX: (802) 828-2484
Contact Person: Anita Ristau, MS, RN,
   Executive Director
Web Site: *www.vtprofessionals.org/
   nurses/*

VIRGIN ISLANDS
Virgin Islands Board of Nurse
   Licensure
Veterans Drive Station

St. Thomas, VI 00803
Phone: (340) 776-7397
FAX: (340) 777-4003
Contact Person: Winifred Garfield,
CRNA, RN, Executive Secretary

VIRGINIA
Virginia Board of Nursing
6606 W. Broad Street, 4th Floor
Richmond, VA 23230
Phone: (804) 662-9909
FAX: (804) 662-9512
Contact Person: Nancy Durrett, MSN,
RN, Executive Director
Web Site: *www.dhp.state.va.us/*

WASHINGTON
Washington State Nursing Care Quality
Assurance Commission
Department of Health
1300 Quince Street SE
Olympia, WA 98504-7864
Phone: (360) 236-4740
FAX: (360) 236-4738
Contact Person: Paula Meyer, MSN,
RN, Executive Director
Web Site: *www.doh.wa.gov/nursing*

WEST VIRGINIA
West Virginia Board of Examiners for
Registered Professional Nurses
101 Dee Drive
Charleston, WV 25311
Phone: (304) 558-3596
FAX: (304) 558-3666

Contact Person: Laura Rhodes, MSN,
RN, Executive Director
Web Site: *www.state.wv.us/nurses/rn/*
West Virginia State Board of Examiners
for Licensed Practical Nurses
101 Dee Drive
Charleston, WV 25311
Phone: (304) 558-3572
FAX: (304) 558-4367
Contact Person: Nancy Wilson, RN,
Executive Secretary
Web Site: *www./pnboard.state.wv.us/*

WISCONSIN
Wisconsin Department of Regulation
and Licensing
1400 E. Washington Avenue
P.O. Box 8935
Madison, WI 53708
Phone: (608) 266-2112
FAX: (608) 267-0644
Contact Person: Kimberly Nania,
Director, Bureau of Health Service
Professions
Web Site: *www.state.wi.us*

WYOMING
Wyoming State Board of Nursing
2020 Carey Avenue, Suite 110
Cheyenne, WY 82002
Phone: (307) 777-7601
FAX: (307) 777-3519
Contact Person: Cheryl Lynn Koski,
MS, RN, CS, Executive Director
Web Site: *http://nursing.state.wy.us/*

APPENDIX

B Nursing-Related Organizations

Overall Professional Organizations

American Nurses Association (ANA)
600 Maryland Ave. SW
Suite 100 West
Washington, DC 20024-2571
Phone: (800) 274-4ANA or (202) 554-4444
FAX: (202) 554-2262
E-mail: See Web site under "Contact Us" for various departments
Web Site: *http://www.ana.org*
Publications: *American Journal of Nursing, The American Nurse, Online Journal of Issues in Nursing*

International Council of Nurses (ICN)
3, Place Jean Marteau
1201 Geneva 20, Switzerland
Phone: 41-22-908-01-00
FAX: 41-22-908-01-01
E-mail: *webmaster@icn.ch*
Web Site: *http://www.icn.ch*
Publication: *International Nursing Review*

National Association for Practical Nurse Education and Service
1400 Spring Street, Suite 310
Silver Spring, Maryland 20910
Phone: (301) 588-2491
Publications: *Journal of Practical Nursing, NAPNES Forum*
E-mail:*napnes@aol.com*

National Council of State Boards of Nursing (NCSBN)
676 N. St. Clair, Suite 550
Chicago, IL 60611-2921
Phone: (312) 787-6555
E-mail: See "How to Contact Us" on the Web site for various departments
Web Site: *http://www.ncsbn.org*
Publication: *Issues* (see Web site for others)

National Federation of Licensed Practical Nurses, Inc.
1418 Aversboro Rd.
Garner, NC 27529
Phone: (919) 779-0046
FAX: (919) 779-5642
E-mail: *cbarbour@ntwrks.com*
Web Site: *http://www.nflpn.com*

National Federation of Specialty Nursing Organizations (NFSNO)
875 Kings Highway
West Deptford, NJ 08096
Phone: (609) 256-2333
FAX: (609) 589-7463
E-mail: *nfsno@mail.ajj.com*
Web Site: *www.nfsno.org*

National League for Nursing (NLN)
61 Broadway
New York, NY 10006
Phone: 1 (800) 669-1656 or (212) 363-5555

FAX: (212) 812-0390
E-mail: *nlnweb@nln.org*
Web Site: *http://www.nln.org*
Publication: *Nursing and Health Care Perspectives*

National Student Nurse Association (NSNA)
55 West 57th Street, Suite 1327
New York, NY 10019
Phone: (212) 581-2211
FAX: (212) 581-2368
E-mail: *nsna@nsna.org*
Web Site: *http:www.nsna.org*
Publications: *Imprint, NSNA News*

Organizations Related to Scholarship and Leadership in Nursing

Alpha Tau Delta
150 Cruickshank Drive
Folson, CA 95630
Phone: (916) 984-9150
Publications: *Captions of Alpha Tau Delta* (biennial), *President's Letter*

American Academy of Nursing (AAN)
c/o American Nurses Association
600 Maryland Ave., SW
Suite 100 West
Washington, DC 20024-2571
Phone: (800) 274-4ANA
Web Site: *http://www.ana.org/aan/index.htm*
Publication: *Nursing Outlook* (bimonthly)

Sigma Theta Tau International
550 West North Street
Indianapolis, IN 46202-3163
Phone: (888) 634-7575 or (317) 634-8171
FAX: (317) 634-8188
Web Site: *http://www.nursingsociety.org*

Publications: *Journal of Nursing Scholarship, Reflections on Nursing Leadership*

Groups Related to Ethnic/Racial Origin

American Indian Nurses Association (AINA)
PO Box 1588
Norman, OK 73071
Publication: *Newsletter of the AINA* (bimonthly)

Association of Black Nursing Faculty, Inc. (ABNF)
1708 N. Roxboro Rd.
Durham, NC 27701

National Association of Hispanic Nurses
1501 Sixteenth St., NW
Washington, DC 20036
Phone: (202) 387-2477
FAX: (202) 483-7183
E-mail: *info@nahnhq.org*
Web Site: *http://www.nahnhq.org*
Publication: *Newsletter* (quarterly)

National Black Nurses Association, Inc.
8630 Fenton Stree, Suite 330
Silver Spring, MD 20910-3803
Phone: (301) 589-3200
FAX: (301) 589-3223
Web Site: *http:www.nbna.org*
Publications: *Journal of National Black Nurses' Association* (twice yearly), *NBNA Newsletter* (4 times/year)

Phillipine Nurses Association of America, Inc.
Check Web site for address of regional office
E-mail: *LCOMPAS@Pna-America.org*
Web Site: *http://www.pna-america.org*
Publication: *The Philippine American Nurse* (published twice a year)

Educationally Oriented Associations

American Association of Colleges of
   Nursing (AACN)
One Dupont Circle, NW
Suite 530
Washington, DC 20036-1110
Phone: (202) 463-6930
FAX: (202) 785-8320
E-mail: *webmaster@aacn.nhe.edu*
Web Site: *http://www.aacn.nche.edu*
Publications: *Journal of Professional
   Nursing* (bimonthly), *Syllabus—The
   Newsletter of the American
   Association of Colleges of Nursing*
   (bimonthly)

Commission on Graduates of Foreign
   Nursing Schools (CGFNS)
3600 Market St., Suite 400
Philadelphia, PA 19104-2651
Phone: (215) 222-8454
FAX: (215) 662-0425
Web Site: *http://www.cgfns.org*

Council on Collegiate Education for
   Nursing for the Southern Regional
   Education Board (SREB)
1340 Spring Street, NW
Atlanta, GA 30309
Phone: (404) 875-9211
FAX: (404) 872-1477
E-mail: *eula.aiken@sreb.org*
Web Site: *http://www.sreb.org/
   Programs/nursing/nursing.html*

Mid-Atlantic Regional Nursing
   Association (MARNA)
350 Hudson Street
New York, NY 10014
Publication: *Marnagram* (quarterly)

Midwest Alliance in Nursing, Inc.
   (MAIN)
2511 East 46th Street, Suite E-3
Indianapolis, IN 46205

Publication: *MAINlines* (bimonthly
   newsletter)

National Organization for Associate
   Degree Nursing (NOADN)
11250 Roger Bacon Drive, Suite 8
Reston, VA 20190
Phone: (703) 437-4377
FAX: (703) 435-4390
E-mail: *noadn@noadn.org*
Web Site: *http://www.noadn.org*

North American Nursing Diagnosis
   Association (NANDA)
1211 Locust St.
Philadelphia, PA 19107
Phone: (215) 545-8105
FAX: (215) 545-8107
E-mail: *infor@nanda.org*
Web Site: *http.//www.nanda.org*
Publication: *Nursing Diagnoses*

New England Organization for Nursing
   (NEON)
Hewitt Hall, University of New
   Hampshire
Durham, NH 03824

Western Institute of Nursing (WIN)
PO Drawer P
Boulder, CO 80302

Occupational or Specialty-Related Organizations

Academy of Medical Surgical Nurses
East Holly Ave., Box 56
Pitman, NJ 08071
Phone: (609) 256-2323
FAX: (609) 589-7463
E-mail: *amsn@mail.ajj.com*
Web Site: *http:www.medsurgnurse.org*
Publication: *Certification Review
   Course Manual*

Aerospace Nursing Association (ANRA)
North Carolina Central University

Dept. of Nursing, PO Box 3369
Chapel Hill, NC 27514
Phone: (919) 560-6431
FAX: (919) 560-5343
E-mail: *yspencer@wpo.nccu.edu*

Air and Surface Transport Nurses
    Association (formerly National Flight
    Nurses)
915 Lee Street
Des Plaines, IL 60016-6569
Phone: (847) 460-1170
FAX: (847) 460-4001
Web Site: *http://www.astna.org*
Publications: *The Air Medical Journal*
    (4 times/year), *Air Med* (6 times/
    year), *Across the Board* (newsletter)

Alliance for Psychosocial Nursing
6900 Grove Rd.
Thorofare, New Jersey 08094
Phone: (856) 848-1000
Web Site: *http://www.psychnurse.org*
Publication: *Journal of Psychosocial
    Nursing and Mental Health Service*

American Academy of Ambulatory
    Care Nurses
East Holly Avenue
Box 56
Pitman, NJ 08071
Phone: (609) 256-2350
FAX: (609) 589-7463
E-mail: *aaacn@mail.ajj.com*
Web Site: *http://aaacn.Inurse.com*

American Academy of Nurse
    Practitioners (AANP)
Capital Station
PO Box 12846
Austin, TX 78711
Phone: (512) 442-4262
FAX: (512) 442-6469
E-mail: *admin@aanp.org*
Web Site: *http://www.aanp.org*

Publication: *Journal of the American
    Academy of Nurse Practitioners*

American Assisted Living Nurses
    Association
846 Williamston Street, Suite 205
Vista, CA 92084
Phone: (760) 806-5361
FAX: (760) 806-5342
E-mail: *advhs@aol.com*
Web Site: *http://www.aalna.org*

American Association for the History
    of Nursing, Inc.
PO Box 175
Lanoka Harbor, NJ 08734
Phone: (609) 693-7250
FAX: (609) 693-1037
E-mail: *AAHN@aahn.org*
Web Site: *http://www.aahn.org/*
Publication: *The Bulletin* (4 times/year)

American Association of Critical-Care
    Nurses (AACN)
101 Columbia
Aliso Viejo, CA 92656-1491
Phone: (800) 899-2226 or (949) 362-
    2000
FAX: (949) 362-2020
E-mail: *info@aacn.org*
Web Site: *http://www.aacn.org*
Publications: *AACN News, Critical
    Care Nurse, American Journal of
    Critical Care, AACN Clinical Issues:
    Advanced Practice in Acute &
    Critical Care*

American Association of Diabetes
    Educators
600 N. Michigan Ave.
Suite 1400
Chicago, IL 60661
E-mail: *mhorn@aadenet.org*
Web Site: *http://www.aadenet.org*
Publication: *The Diabetes Educator*

American Association of Legal Nurse
  Consultants
4700 West Lake Ave.
Glenview, IL 60025
Phone: Toll free (877) 402-2562
FAX: (877) 375-6313
E-mail: *info@aalnc.org*
Web Site: *http://www.aalnc.org*
Publication: *The Journal of Legal Nurse
  Consulting* (published quarterly)

The American Association of Managed
  Care Nurses
PO Box 4975
Glen Allen, Virginia 23058-4975
Phone: (804) 747-9698
FAX: (804) 747-5316
Web Site: *http://www.aamcn.org*
Publication: *The Journal of Managed
  Care Medicine*

American Association of Neuroscience
  Nurses (AANN)
224 Des Plaines, No. 601
Chicago, IL 60661
Phone: (312) 993-0043
FAX: (312) 993-0362
E-mail: *assnneuro@aol.com*
Web Site: *http://www.aann.org*
Publications: *Journal of Neuroscience
  Nursing, Synapse* (newsletter),
  *Clinical Guidelines Series, Core
  Curriculum for Neuroscience
  Nursing*

American Association of Nurse
  Anesthetists (AANA)
222 South Prospect Avenue
Park Ridge, IL 60068-4001
Phone: (847) 692-7050
FAX: (847) 692-6968
E-mail: *info@aana.com*
Web Site: *http://www.aana.com*
Publications: *AANA Journal*
  (bimonthly), *AANA NewsBulletin*

American Association of Nurse
  Attorneys (AANAT)
7794 Grow Drive
Pensacola, FL 32514-7072
Phone: (850) 474-3646
FAX: (850) 484-8762
E-mail: *TAANA@puetzamc.com*
Web Site: *http://www.taana.org*

American Association of Occupational
  Health Nurses (AAOHN)
2920 Brandywine Road
Atlanta, GA 30341
Phone: (770) 455-7757
FAX: (770) 455-7271
Web Site: *http://www.aaohn.org*
Publication: *AAOHN Journal*

American Association of Office Nurses
109 Kinderkamack Rd.
Montvale, NJ 07645
Phone: (201) 391-2600
Web Site: *http://www.aaon.org*

American Association of Spinal Cord
  Injury Nurses (AASCIN)
75-20 Astoria Blvd.
Jackson Heights, NY 11370-1178
Phone: (718) 803-3782
FAX: (718) 803-0414
E-mail: *info@epva.org*
Web Site: *http://www.aascin.org*
Publication: *SCI Nursing* (quarterly
  journal; also educational and practice
  guidelines

American Burn Association
Burn Treatment Center
Crozier-Chester Medical Center
15th and Upland Avenue
Chester, PA 19013
Web Site: *www.ameriburn.org*

American College of Nurse Midwives
  (ACNM)
818 Connecticut Avenue NW

Suite 900
Washington, DC 20006
Phone: (202) 728-9860
FAX: (202) 728-9897
Web Site: *http://www/midwife.org*
Publications: *Journal of Nurse
Midwifery, Quickening* (newsletter)

American College of Nurse
Practitioners
503 Capitol Court NE, Suite 300
Washington, DC 20002
Phone: (202) 546-4825
FAX: (202) 546-4797
E-mail: *acnp@nurse.org*
Web Site: *http://www.nurse.org/acnp*

American Forensic Nurses
255 N. El Cielo, Suite 195
Palm Springs, CA 92262
Web Site: *http://www.amrn.com*

American Holistic Nurses
Association
PO Box 2130
Flagstaff, AZ 86003-2130
Phone: (800) 278-AHNA
Web Site: *http://www.ahna.org*
Publications: *Journal of Holistic
Nursing* (annual), *Beginnings*
(newsletter)

American Nephrology Nurses
Association (AANA)
North Woodbury Road, Box 56
East Holly Avenue
Pitman, NJ 08071
Phone: (609) 256-2320
FAX: (609) 589-7463
E-mail: *anna@mail.com*
Web Site: *http://anna.inurse.com*
Publications: *Nephrology Nursing
Journal, Contemporary Nephrology
Nursing*, and various practice
guidelines

American Nursing Informatics
Association (ANIA)
PMB 105
10808 Foothill Blvd., Suite 160
Rancho Cucamonga, CA 91730
E-mail: *mbrs@ania.org*
Web Site: *http://www.ania.org*

American Nurses in Business
Association (ANBA)
Maryland Avenue
Suite 100 West
Washington, DC 20024-2571

American Organization of Nurse
Executives (AONE)
325 Seventh St. NW
Suite 700
Washington, DC 20036
Phone: (202) 626-2240
FAX: (202) 626-2345
Web Site: *http://www.aone.org*

American Psychiatric Nurses
Association (APNA)
1200 Nineteenth St. NW
Suite 300
Washington, DC 20036
Phone: (202) 857-1133
FAX: (202) 223-4579
E-mail: *apna@dc.sba.com*
Web Site: *http://www.apna.org*
Publications: *Journal of the American
Psychiatric Nurses Association,
APNA Newsletter*

American Public Health Association
(APHA)
Public Health Nursing Section
800 I Street
Washington, DC 20001-3710
Phone: (202) 777-APHA
E-mail: *comments@apha.org*
Web Site: *http://www.apha.org/* link to
sections

Publications: *American Journal of Public Health, The Nation's Health*

American Radiological Nurses Association (ARNA)
2021 Spring Rd, Suite 600
Oakbrook, IL 60521
Phone: (630) 571-9072
FAX: (630) 571-7837
E-mail: *arna@rsna.org*
Web Site: *http://www.arna.net*
Publication: *ARNA Images* (4 times/year)

American School Health Association (ASHA)
7263 State Route 43
PO Box 708
Kent, OH 44240
Phone: (216) 678-1601
FAX: (216) 678-4526
Web Site: *http://www.asha.web.org*

American Society for Long-Term Care Nurses
660 Lonely Cottage Drive
Upper Black Eddy, PA 18972-9313
Publication: *ASLTCN Journal* (bimonthly)

American Society for Parenteral and Enteral Nutrition–Nurses' Committee
8630 Fenton Street, Suite 412
Silver Springs, MD 20910-3803
Phone: (301) 587-6315
FAX: (301) 587-2365
E-mail: *aspen@nutr.org*
Web Site: *http://www.clinnutr.org*

American Society of Ophthalmic Registered Nurses, Inc., (ASORN)
PO Box 193030
San Francisco, CA 94119
Phone: (415) 561-8513
FAX: (415) 561-8575

E-mail: *asorn@aao.org*
Web Site: *webeye.ophth.uiowa.edu/asorn/*
Publication: *Insight* (newsletter)

American Society of Pain Management Nurses
7794 Grow Drive
Pensacola, FL 32514-7072
Phone: (850) 473-0233
FAX: (850) 484-8762
E-mail: *ASPMN@puetzamc.com*
Web Site: *www.aspmn.org*
Publication: *ASPMN Pathways* (quarterly newsletter)

American Society of PeriAnesthesia Nurses (ASPAN)
6900 Grove Rd.
Thorofare, NJ 08086
Phone: (609) 845-5557
FAX: (609) 848-1881
E-mail: *aspan@slackinc.com*
Web Site: *https://www.aspan.org*
Publications: *The Journal of PeriAnesthesia Nursing* (bimonthly), *Breathline* (newsletter)

American Society of Plastic and Reconstructive Surgical Nurses
East Holly Avenue, Box 56
Pitman, NJ 08071-0056
Phone: (609) 256-2340
FAX: (609) 589-7463
E-mail: *asprsn@mail.ajj.com*
Web Site: *http://asprsn.org*
Publications: *Plastic Surgical Nursing* (available on-line), *ASPRS News* (available on-line)

American Urological Association Allied
11512 Allecingie Parkway, Suite C
Richmond, VA 23235
Publications: *AUAA Journal* (quarterly), *Urogram* (newsletter)

Association of Child and Adolescent
 Psychiatric Nursing
1211 Locust Street
Philadelphia, PA 19107
Phone: (800) 826-2950 or (215) 545-
 2843
FAX: (215) 545-8107
Web Site: *http://www.acapn.org*
Publications: *Journal of Child and
 Adolescent Psychiatric Nursing,
 ACAPN Newsletter*

Association for Practitioners in
 Infection Control and Epidemiology,
 Inc.
1275 K Street, NW, Suite 1000
Washington, DC 20005-4006
Phone: (202) 789-1890
FAX: (202) 789-1899
E-mail: *APICinfo@apic.org*
Web Site: *http://www.apic.org*
Publications: *American Journal of
 Infection Control (AJIC)*, plus many
 texts, standards, and guidelines.

Association of Nurses in AIDS Care
 (ANAC)
11250 Roger Bacon Drive, Suite 8
Reston, VA 20190
Phone: (202) 462-1038
E-mail: *AIDSNURSES@aol.com*
Web Site: *http://www.anacnet.org*
Publications: *JANAC: the Journal of
 the Association of Nurses in AIDS
 Care, ANACdotes* (quarterly
 newsletter)

Association of Nurses in Substance
 Abuse
120 Wilton Road
London, SW1V 1JZ
Phone: 171 630 0346 or 171 233 8322
 (24 hrs)
FAX: 171 233 7779
E-mail: *profbriefings@msn.com*

Web Site: *http://www.profbriefings.co.
 uk/assoc/ansa.htm*

Association of Pediatric Oncology
 Nurses (APON)
4700 West Lake Avenue
Glen View, IL 60025-1485
Phone: (708) 966-3723
FAX: (708) 375-4777
Web Site: *www.apon.org*
Publication: *APON Newsletter*

Association of periOperative Registered
 Nurses (AORN)
2170 S. Parker Road, Suite 300
Denver, CO 80231-5711
Phone: (800) 755-2676 or (303) 755-
 6300
FAX: (303) 752-3212
Web Site: *http://www.aorn.org*
Publication: *AORN Journal*

Association of Rehabilitation
 Nurses
4700 West Lake Rd.
Glenview, IL 60025-1485
Phone: (800) 229-7530 or (847) 375-
 4710
FAX: (847) 375-4777
E-mail: *info@rehabnurse.org*
Web Site: *http://www.rehabnurse.org*
Publications: *Rehabilitation Nursing*
 (bimonthly journal), *ARN Network*
 (newsletter)

Association of Women's Health,
 Obstetric, and Neonatal Nurses
 (AWHONN) (formerly NAACOG)
2000 L Street, NW
Suite 740
Washington, DC 20036
Phone: (202) 261-2400
FAX: (202) 728-0575
E-mail: *kathied@awhonn.org*
Web Site: *http://www.awhonn.org*

Publications: *Journal of Obstetric, Gynecologic, and Neonatal Nursing (JOGNN) (bimonthly), AWHONN Lifelines*

Baromedical Nurses Association (BNA)
PO Box 24113
Halethorpe, MD 21227
Phone: (410) 789-5690
FAX: (410) 328-3758
E-mail: *norvellh@worldnet.att.net*
Web Site: *http://www.hyperbaricnurses.org*

Department of School Nurses of the
    National Education Association
    (NEA)
1201 Sixteenth Street, NW
Washington, DC 20036
Publication: *The School Nurse*

Dermatology Nurses' Association
East Holly Avenue, Box 56
Pitman, NJ 08071-0056
Phone: (609) 256-2330
FAX: (609) 582-1915
Web Site: *http://dna.inurse.com*
Publication: *DNA Focus* (bimonthly
    newsletter)

Developmental Disabilities Nurses'
    Association
Willow Creek Circle, Suite 515
Eugene, OR 97402
Phone: (800) 888-6733
FAX: (541) 485-7372
Web Site: *http://www.ddna.org*
Publication: *DDNA Network*
    (quarterly newsletter)

Emergency Nurses Association (ENA)
216 Higgins Rd.
Park Ridge, IL 60068
Phone: (847) 698-9400
FAX: (847) 698-9406

Web Site: *http://www.ena.org*
Publications: *Journal of Emergency
    Nursing International, Journal of
    Trauma Nursing*

Home Health Care Nurses Association
228 7th Street, SE
Washington, DC 20003
Phone: (800) 558-HHNA
FAX: (202) 547-3540
E-mail: *HHNA@puetzamc.com*

Hospice and Palliative Nurses
    Association
5512 N. Umberland St.
Pittsburgh, PA 15217-1131
Phone: (412) 687-3231
FAX: (412) 687-9095
Web Site: *http://www.hpna.org*

International Association for
    Enterostomal Therapy, Inc.
    (IAET)
2081 Business Center Drive, Suite 290
Irvine, CA 92715
Publication: *Journal of Enterostomal
    Therapy*

International Society of Nurses in
    Genetics, Inc.
7 Haskins Road
Hanover, NH 03755
Phone: (603) 643-5706
FAX: (603) 643-3169
E-mail: *erawn@valley.net*
Web Site: *http://147.134.136.150/*

International Transplant
    Nurses Society
1739 E. Carson St., Box #351
Pittsburgh, PA 15203-1700
Phone: (412) 488-0240
FAX: (412) 431-5911
E-mail: *itns@msn.com*
Web Site: *www.itns.org*

Publication: *Progress in Transplantation: A Journal for Procurement and Clinical Professionals*

Intravenous Nurses' Society, Inc.
Fresh Pond Square
10 Fawcett Street
Cambridge, MA 02138
Phone: (617) 441-3008
FAX: (617) 441-3009
Web Site: *http://www.ins1.org*
Publication: *Journal of Intravenous Nursing* (bimonthly)

Midwest Alliance for Nursing Informatics
PO Box 48
Mount Prospect, IL 60056-0048
E-mail: *InternetChair@maninet.org*
Web Site: *http://www.maninet.org*
Publication: *MANI Newsletter* (online)

National Alliance of Nurse Practitioners
325 Pennsylvania Ave., SE
Washington, DC 20003-1100

National Association of Clinical Nurse Specialists
4700 W. Lake Avenue
Glenview, IL 60025
Phone: (847) 375-4740
FAX: (847) 375-4777
E-mail: *info@nacns.org*
Web Site: *http://www.nacns.org*
Publications: *CNS: The Journal for Advanced Practice Nursing, NACNS News*

National Association of Directors of Nursing Administration in Long Term Care (NADONA/LTC)
10999 Reed Hartman Hwy., Suite 229
Cincinnati, OH 45242
Phone: (513) 791-3679

FAX: (513) 791-3699
E-mail: *gary@nadona.org*
Web Site: *http://www.nadona.org*

National Association for Health Care Recruitment
PO Box 5769
Akron, OH 44372
Publication: *Recruitment Directions* (10 times/year)

National Association of Neonatal Nurses
701 Lee Street, Suite 450
Des Plaines, IL 60016
Phone: (847) 299-NANN (6266) or (800) 451-3795
FAX: (847) 297-6768
E-mail: *info@nann.org*
Web Site: *http://www.nann.org*
Publications: *NANN Central Lines* (quarterly journal), *The NANN Pages* (newsletter)

National Association of Nurse Practitioners in Reproductive Health (NANPRH)
2401 Pennsylvania Avenue, NW
Washington, DC 20037
Phone: (202) 466-4825
FAX: (202) 466-3826

National Association of Orthopedic Nurses
East Holly Avenue, Box 56
Pitman, NJ 08071
Phone: (609) 256-2310
FAX: (609) 589-7463
E-mail: *naon@mail.ajj.com*
Web Site: *http://naon.inurse.com*
Publication: *Orthopaedic Nursing J*

National Association of Pediatric Nurse Associates and Practitioners (NAPNAP)
1101 Kings Highway North, Suite 206

Cherry Hill, NJ 08034-1912
Phone: Toll free: (877) 662-7627 or
  (856) 667-1173
FAX: (856) 667-7187
Web Site: *http://www.napnap.org*
Publications: *The Journal of Pediatric
  Health Care, The Pediatric Nurse
  Practitioner* (newsletter)

National Association of Physicians
  Nurses
900 South Washington St.
Suite G-13
Falls Church, VA 22046
Phone: (703) 237-8616
FAX: (703) 533-1153

National Association of School Nurses
Eastern Office
PO Box 1300
Scarborough, ME 04074-1300
Phone: (207) 883-2117
FAX: (207) 883-2683
Web Site: *http://www.nasn.org*
Western Office
111 Cantril Street
Castle Rock, CO 80104
Phone: (303) 663-2329
FAX: (303) 663-0403
Publication: *School Nurse Journal NAS
  Newsletter* (quarterly)

National Consortium of Chemical
  Dependency Nurses (NCCDN)
1720 Willow Creek Circle, Suite 510
Eugene, OR 97402
Phone: (800) 876-2236
FAX: (541) 485-7372

National Gerontological Nurses
  Association
7794 Grow Drive
Pensacola, FL 32514-7072
Phone: (850) 473-1174
FAX: (850) 484-8762
E-mail: *NGNA@puetzamc.com*

National HIV Nurses Association—UK
c/o The Foundation for Nursing Studies
32 Buckingham Palace Rd.
London SW/WORE
E-mail: *admin@fons.org*
Web Site: *http://www.fons.org/
  home.htm*
Publication: *AIDS Treatment Update*
  (published annually)

National Nurses in Business
  Association (NNBA)
56 McArthur Avenue
Staten Island, NY 10312
Phone: (800) 331-6534
FAX: (718) 317-0858
Web Site:
  *http://www.greatnurses.com/NNBA.
  html*
Publication: *Revolution: the Journal of
  Nurse Empowerment*

National Nurses Society on
  Addictions
4101 Lake Boone Trail, Suite 201
Raleigh, NC 27607
Phone: (919) 783-5871
FAX: (919) 787-4916
Web Site: *http://www.nnsa.org*
Publications: *Journal of Addictions
  Nursing, NNSA Today* (newsletter)

Nursing Ethics Network
c/o Boston College School of
  Nursing
Cushing Hall
140 Commonwealth Avenue
Chestnut Hill, MA 02467
E-mail: *riley@emmanuel.edu* (Chair)
Web Site: *http://www.bc.edu/bc_org/
  avp/son/nen/nen.html*

National Nursing Staff Development
  Organization
7794 Grow Drive
Pensacola, FL 32514

Phone: (850) 474-0995
FAX: (850) 484-8762
E-mail: *NNSDO@puetzamc.com*
Web Site: *http://www.nnsdo.org*
Publication: *Journal of Nursing Staff Development*

Navy Nurse Corps Association
Check Web site for Regional
   addresses
Web Site: *http://www.nnca.org*
Publication: *NNCA Newsletter*

Nurse Healers Professional Associates,
   Inc.
PO Box 444
Allison Park, PA 15101-0444
Phone: (412) 355-8476
Web Site: *http://www.therapeutic-touch.org*

Nurses Organization of Veteran's
   Affairs
1726 M Street NW
Suite 1101
Washington, DC 20034
Phone: (202) 296-0888
FAX: (202) 833-1577
E-mail: *nova@vanurse.org*

Oncology Nursing Society
501 Holiday Drive
Pittsburgh, PA 15220
Phone: (412) 921-7373
FAX: (412) 921-6565
E-mail: *customer.service@ons.org*
Web Site: *http://www.ons.org*
Publication: *Oncology Nursing*

Pediatric Endocrinology Nursing
   Society
PO Box 2933
Gaithersburg, MD 20886-2933
E-mail: *webmaster@PENS.org*
Web Site: *http://www.pens.org*
Publication: *PENs Newsletter*

Respiratory Nursing Society
7794 Grow Drive
Pensacola, FL 32514-7072
Phone: (850) 474-8869
FAX: (850) 484-8762
E-mail: *RNS@puetzamc.com*

Society for Vascular Nursing (SVN)
7794 Grow Drive
Pensacola, FL 32514-7072
Phone: (850) 474-6963
FAX: (850) 484-8762
E-mail: *SVN@puetzamc.com*
Publication: *SVN Journal* (quarterly)

Society of Gastroenterology Nurses and
   Associates, Inc.
401 N. Michigan Ave.
Chicago, IL 60611
Phone: (800) 245-7462
FAX: (312) 321-5194
E-mail: *sgna@sba.com*
Web Site: *http://www.sgna.org*
Publication: *Gastroenterology Nursing*
   (bimonthly)

Society of Gynecologic Nurse
   Oncologists
14628 Stonegate Drive
Lockport, IL 60441
Phone: (708) 301-7868

Society of Otorhinolaryngology and
   Head-Neck Nurses, Inc.
116 Canal St., Suite A
New Smyrna Beach, FL 32168
Phone: (904) 428-1695
FAX: (904) 423-7566
E-mail: *sohnnet@aol.com*
Web Site: *http://www.sohnnurse.com*
Publication: *ORL—Head and Neck
   Nursing* (quarterly), *Update*
   (monthly newsletter)

Society of Pediatric Nurses
2170 South Parker Road, Suite 350

Denver, CO 80231-5711
Phone: (800) 723-2902
FAX: (303) 750-3212
Web Site: *http://www.pednurse.org*
Publication: *Journal of the Society of Pediatric Nurses*

Society of Trauma Nurses
PMB 193 2743 S. Veterans Parkway
Springfield, IL 62704-6536
Phone: (217) 787-3281
FAX: (217) 787-3285
E-mail: *stnexecdir@aol.com*
Web Site: *http://www.traumaNurseSoc. org*
Publication: *Journal of Trauma Nursing*

Transcultural Nursing Society
College of Nursing
Madonna University
36600 Schoolcraft Rd.
Livonia, MI 48150
Phone: (888) 432-5470
FAX: (734) 432-5463
E-mail: *barnes@smtp.munet.edu*
Web Site: *http://www.tcns.org*
Publication: Biannual newsletter

World Federation of Neuroscience Nurses
PO Box 3703
Parramotta, NSW
2150 Australia

Wound Ostomy and Continence Nurses (WOCN)
2755 Bristol Street, Suite 110
Costa Mesa, CA 92626
Phone: (714) 476-0268
FAX: (714) 545-3643
Web Site: *http://www.wocn.org*

Miscellaneous Nursing Organizations

American Assembly for Men in Nursing

c/o NYSNA
11 Cornell Road
Latham, NY 12110
Phone: (518) 782-9400 x 346
FAX: (518) 782-9530
E-mail: *aamn@nysna.org*
Web Site: *http://www.freeyellow.com/ aamn*

The Florence Project
Check Web site for regional contact
Web Site: *http://www.florenceproject. org*

National Nurses for Life
1998 Menold
Allison Park, PA 15104

Nurse Advocate: Nurses and Workplace Violence
Web Site: *http://www.nurseadvocate.org*
E-mail: *carriejl@home.com* (an international e-mail list about nurse-experienced workplace violence)

Nurses Christian Fellowship
6400 Schroeder Road
PO Box 7895
Madison, WI 53707
Phone: (608) 274-4823 x 402
E-mail: *ncf@ivcf.org*
Web Site: *http://www.gospelcom.net/ iv/ncf*
Publication: *Journal of Christian Nursing* (quarterly)

Nurses Educational Funds
555 West 57th Street
New York, NY 10019
Publication: Semiannual newsletter

Nurses' House, Inc.
350 Hudson Street
New York, NY 10014

C

Commonly Used Acronyms

AACN	American Association of Colleges of Nursing
AACN	American Association of Critical–Care Nurses
AAN	American Academy of Nursing
ABNS	American Board of Nursing Specialties
AD	Associate degree
ADN	Associate degree nursing
AHA	American Hospital Association
AHCPR	Agency for Health Care Policy and Research (now the AHRQ)
AHRQ	Agency for Healthcare Research and Quality (formerly the Agency for Health Care Policy and Research—AHCPR)
AMA	American Medical Association
ANA	American Nurses Association
ANA–PAC	American Nurses Association Political Action Committee
ANCC	American Nurses Credentialing Center
ANF	American Nurses Foundation
APIC	Association for Professionals in Infection Control
APN	Advanced practice nurse
BSN	Bachelor of science in nursing
CADP	Council of Associate Degree Programs of the NLN
CAT	Computer adaptive testing
CBHDP	Council of Baccalaureate and Higher Degree Programs of the NLN
CCNE	Commission on Collegiate Nursing Education (related to American Association of Colleges of Nursing)
CDC	Centers for Disease Control and Prevention
CDPN	Council of Diploma Programs in Nursing of the NLN
CE	Continuing education
CEU	Continuing education unit
CHAP	Community Health Accreditation Program
CINAHL	Cumulative Index to Nursing and Allied Health Literature
CNA	Canadian Nurses Association
CNPE	Congress on Nursing Practice and Economics of the ANA
CNS	Clinical nurse specialist

CPNP	Council of Practical Nursing Programs of the NLN
CQI	Continuous quality improvement
DHHS	Department of Health and Human Services
DOE	Department of Education
DRG	Diagnosis-related group
FAQs	Frequently asked questions
FDA	Food and Drug Administration
HCFA	Health Care Financing Administration
HGP	Human Genome Project
HHS	Health and Human Services
HMO	Health maintenance organization
ICN	International Council of Nurses
IOM	Institute of Medicine
JCAHO	Joint Commission on Accreditation of Healthcare Organizations
MSN	Master's of science in nursing
NANDA	North American Nursing Diagnosis Association
NAPNES	National Association for Practical Nurse Education and Service
NCLEX–PN	National Council Licensing Examination for Practical Nursing
NCLEX–RN	National Council Licensing Examination for Registered Nursing
NCSBN	National Council of State Boards of Nursing
NFLPN	National Federation of Licensed Practical Nurses
NFSNO	National Federation for Specialty Nursing Organizations
NIC	Nursing Interventions Classifications
NIH	National Institutes of Health
NINR	National Institute of Nursing Research
NIOSH	National Institute of Occupational Safety and Health
NLM	National Library of Medicine
NLN	National League for Nursing
NLNAC	National League for Nursing Accrediting Commission (related to the National League for Nursing)
NLRA	National Labor Relations Act
NLRB	National Labor Relations Board
NOADN	National Organization for Associate Degree Nursing
NOC	Nursing Outcomes Classification
NP	Nurse practitioner
NSNA	National Student Nurse Association
NSNCO	National Specialty Nursing Certifying Organization
OASIS	Outcomes and Assessment Information Set
OBRA	Omnibus Budget Reconciliation Act
OSHA	Occupational Health and Safety Administration
PA	Physician's assistant
PN	Practical Nurse
PPOs	Preferred provider organizations
PPS	Prospective payment system
QA	Quality assurance
QAI	Quality assessment and improvement

RUGs	Resource utilization groups
SBNs	State Boards of Nursing
TQM	Total quality management
UAP	Unlicensed assistive personnel
VN	Vocational nurse
WHO	World Health Organization
WWW	World Wide Web

INDEX

I

Page references with "t" denote tables, "d" denotes displays, and "f" denote figures

A

abbreviations, 553–554
Abdellah, Faye, 167t
abortion
  age of viability and, 404
  bioethical issues regarding, 402–404
  elective, 402
  legal aspects of, 403
  spontaneous, 402
  therapeutic, 402
academic degree, 255
access, to health care
  economic, 66–67
  geographic, 67–68
  sociocultural, 68
accountability, 495–496, 517
accreditation
  body of knowledge to support, 172
  definition of, 256
  of education programs, 32
  of health care institutions and agencies, 69–71
  National League for Nursing, 110–111
  national programs, 257
  specialized, 256–257
acronyms, 553–554
acuity measures, 64–65
acupuncture, 39–40
acute care
  acuity measures for, 64–65
  definition of, 7
  facilities that provide, 5
  hospital services, 10d
advance directives, 321–322, 415–417
advanced practice nurses
  definition of, 268
  licensure requirements, 268–269

agency shop, 512, 523–524
age of consent, 400–401
AIDS, 482
Alcott, Louisa May, 142t
allied health care workers
  accreditation organizations, 27d
  administrative, 28
  description of, 26
  dietary services, 29
  diversity of, 26–27
  education requirements, 22t, 26
  electrocardiographic technician, 28
  medical laboratory technician, 28
  medical technologist, 28
  occupational therapist, 30
  pharmacists, 29
  physical therapist, 29–30
  prosthetic and assistive device makers, 28–29
  radiology technician, 28
  respiratory therapists, 29
Alpha Tau Delta, 115, 540
alternative care
  acupuncture, 39–40
  Asian medicine, 39–40
  bioelectromagnetic therapies, 35–36
  biofeedback, 38–39
  considerations in choosing, 42
  description of, 34–35
  dietary changes, 36
  folk medicine, 40
  herbal medicines, 36–37
  homeopathy, 40
  indigenous systems, 40
  manual healing, 37–38
  mind-body therapies, 38–39
  naturopathy, 41
  pharmacologic and biologic, 39

liability (*continued*)
  individual, 310–311, 311d
  institutional, 310
licensed practical nurses
  certification of, 290
  description of, 209
  nursing organizations, 112–113
licensed vocational nurse, 209
licensing authorities, 531–538
licensing examination
  administering of, 274–275
  administration of, 270–271
  computerized adaptive testing, 275–276
  content of, 271–274
  description of, 270
  future trends in, 278
  history of, 270
  NCLEX-PN. *See* NCLEX-PN
  NCLEX-RN. *See* NCLEX-RN
  preparation for, 274–275
  scoring of, 277
licensure
  of advanced practice nurses, 268–269
  definition of, 257
  by endorsement, 278–279
  by examination. *See* Licensing examination
  fees, 266
  for foreign nursing school graduates, 283–284
  international, 284–285
  interstate endorsement, 235
  laws. *See* Licensure laws
  limiting of, 282
  mandatory, 257, 260–262
  multistate. *See* Multistate licensure
  organizations that provide, 531–538
  permissive, 257, 259–260
  qualifications for, 264–265
  reciprocity in, 278
  renewals, 266
  requirements for, 257
  revocation of, 282
  rules and regulations, 262–263
  state board test for, 230, 257
  state organizations that provide, 531–538
  sunset laws, 283
  suspension of, 385
licensure laws
  applicant qualifications, 264–265
  content of, 263
  continuing education requirements, 266
  definitions, 263–264
  disciplinary actions, 266–267
  exceptions, 268
  fees, 266
  grandfathering, 265
  nursing education programs, 266

purpose of, 263
renewal requirements, 266
titling, 265
violations of, 267
limiting of license, 282
Livermore, Mary, 142t
living will, 415–416, 416d
lobbying
  American Nurses Association, 89
  limitations, 94
  political action committees, 90–91
lockout, 514
long-term care
  acuity measures, 64–65
  assisted-living facilities, 5, 15–16
  description of, 5, 13
  hospital, 10d, 11
  nursing homes. *See* Nursing homes
  quality indicators, 73
  rehabilitation centers, 16–17
  retirement communities, 16

M

male nurses
  discrimination against, 478–479
  employment opportunities for, 444–445
malpractice
  case study examples of, 308–309
  contributing factors, 330–331
  definition of, 306
  elements of, 307d
  prevention of, 332–334
managed care
  definition of, 62
  health maintenance organizations. *See* Health maintenance organizations
  "prudent consumer" standard of, 63
  structure of, 62–63
mandatory licensure, 257, 260–262
manual healing, 37–38
master's program, 216–218, 225
mature minor, 323, 401
medex. *See* Physician's assistant
mediation
  of grievance, 517
  of labor dispute, 513
Medicaid
  certification, 70
  cost-containment initiatives, 54, 66
  fraud, 66
  funding of, 53
  history of, 53, 159
  nursing effects, 53–54
  nursing home reimbursements, 14
Medi-Cal, 14